Asthma and Allergy in Pregnancy and Early Infancy

ALLERGIC DISEASE AND THERAPY

Series Editor

DAVID G. TINKELMAN

Medical College of Georgia
Augusta, Georgia, and
Atlanta Allergy Clinic
Atlanta, Georgia

1. Histamine and H_2 Antagonists in Inflammation and Immunodeficiency, *edited by Ross E. Rocklin*
2. Asthma as an Inflammatory Disease, *edited by Paul M. O'Byrne*
3. Childhood Rhinitis and Sinusitis: Pathophysiology and Treatment, *edited by Charles K. Naspitz and David G. Tinkelman*
4. Allergen Immunotherapy, *edited by Richard F. Lockey and Samuel C. Bukantz*
5. Clinical Management of Urticaria and Anaphylaxis, *edited by Alan L. Schocket*
6. Childhood Asthma: Pathophysiology and Treatment. Second Edition, Revised and Expanded, *edited by David G. Tinkelman and Charles K. Naspitz*
7. Asthma and Allergy in Pregnancy and Early Infancy, *edited by Michael Schatz and Robert S. Zeiger*

Additional Volumes in Preparation

Asthma and Allergy in Pregnancy and Early Infancy

edited by
Michael Schatz
Robert S. Zeiger

Kaiser-Permanente Medical Center and University of California, San Diego, School of Medicine, San Diego, California

Marcel Dekker, Inc. New York • Basel • Hong Kong

Library of Congress Cataloging-in-Publication Data

Asthma and allergy in pregnancy and early infancy / edited by Michael Schatz, Robert S. Zeiger.

p. cm. — (Allergic disease and therapy ; 7)

Includes bibliographical references and index.

ISBN 0-8247-8795-1 (alk. paper)

1. Allergy in pregnancy. 2. Asthma in pregnancy. 3. Allergy in infants. I. Schatz, Michael, M.D. II. Zeiger, Robert S., M.D. III. Series: Allergic disease and therapy ; v. 7.

[DNLM : 1. Asthma—in infancy & childhood. 2. Asthma—in pregnancy. 3. Hypersensitivity—in infancy & childhood. 4. Hypersensitivity—in pregnancy. W1 AL538 v.7]

RG580.A47A87 1993
616.2′38—dc20
DNLM/DLC
for Library of Congress 92-48684
CIP

This book is printed on acid-free paper.

Marcel Dekker, Inc.
270 Madison Avenue, New York, New York 10016

Current printing (last digit):
10 9 8 7 6 5 4 3 2 1

PRINTED IN THE UNITED STATES OF AMERICA

To our teachers and patients, who have taught us what we know, and to our families, who have been so supportive in our endeavor to implement that knowledge.

Series Introduction

Allergic disease and its therapy has long been a topic of discussion. The development of theories on the cause of allergic symptoms has consumed volumes of medical literature dealing with virtually all organ systems. From these postulations have come practical approaches to the diagnosis and management of allergic disorders. Despite the continuum of medical "breakthroughs," the answers to many of the questions relating to allergy remain unknown.

In this series, Allergic Disease and Therapy, the authors will attempt to concisely put forth reviews of past approaches as well as the most up-to-date information relating to a variety of different allergic states. Basic scientists, clinical researchers, and experts will combine their efforts to establish rational approaches to the diagnosis and management of the complex allergic problems of today. This will be a multidisciplinary approach by individuals spanning the globe in an effort to cover these topics from many different perspectives. From the genetics laboratories where complex questions concerning the role of certain gene pools in the development of immunologic competence are being studied to the research facilities of pharmaceutical companies where new therapeutic products are being tested, this series will address many unanswered questions in the rapidly growing field of allergy and immunology. The goal of the series is to provide the practitioner with the background knowledge and tools with which to approach the allergic problems that are so common in today's society.

David G. Tinkelman

Preface

Pregnancy and early motherhood represent a very special time in a woman's life. Although it is often a time of much joy and fulfillment, it often entails formidable challenges as well. For the allergic or asthmatic pregnant woman, this period may provide many additional difficulties: a variety of uncomfortable symptoms during pregnancy, which may range from mild to life-threatening and which may require medication; concerns about the effect of the illness or the medicine on the baby; concerns about the baby's development of allergies or asthma; and then the care of a baby who may have inherited allergies or asthma. This book is devoted to that special period in the allergic or asthmatic woman's life. Its main purpose is to improve her medical care as well as that of her allergic or asthmatic infant.

The first four chapters of the book concentrate on the relevant physiology of normal pregnancy, including hormonal changes, pulmonary physiology, immunological changes, and determinants of fetal oxygenation. Chapters 5–9 explore general therapeutic principles such as avoidance measures, immunotherapy, psychological care, and pharmacological management, including gestational safety data on specific allergy and asthma medications and medicolegal considerations. Chapters 10–13 detail the interrelationships between asthma and pregnancy and provides medical and obstetric management guidelines from several perspectives. Chapters 14–17 describe in detail the relationships to pregnancy and gestational management of other allergic or related conditions including rhinitis, sinusitis, anaphylaxis, cutaneous diseases, and adverse drug reactions. Chapters 18–23 cover allergy and asthma in infancy. It reviews genetic and environmental factors in the development of allergy, the natural history of allergy and asthma during childhood, and prospects for prevention of allergy in infancy. It also describes the diagnosis and management of food hypersensitivity, atopic dermatitis, and wheezing in infants. Finally, the Appendix presents the recently published (1992) guidelines for the management of gestational asthma formulated by the National Asthma Education Program Working Group on Asthma and Pregnancy.

The term "allergy" is classically defined as a reaction mediated by IgE antibody against a specific antigen, in which mediators (such as histamine) are released from basophils and mast cells, and in which the effects of these mediators on blood vessels, smooth muscle, and inflammatory cells cause the clinical reaction. Indeed, this book describes many clinical illnesses that may be mediated by this mechanism, including allergic asthma, allergic rhinitis, urticaria/angioedema, anaphylaxis, and probably some aspects of atopic dermatitis. However, clinical asthma, rhinitis, urticaria/angioedema, eczema, and even anaphylaxis may all occur through non-IgE-mediated mechanisms as well. In addition, certain of the illnesses discussed in this book appear to be due to other immunological mechanisms, such as herpes gestationis and some types of food and drug reactions.

A great deal of our interest in editing this book stems from our research on the subjects of asthma during pregnancy and the prevention of allergy in infancy. We acknowledge the supports of grants number AI20426, AI22639, and N0 1-HV-92832 from the Allergy and Asthma Branch of the National Institute of Allergy and Infectious Diseases and the support of Kaiser Foundation Hospital Research Foundation in performing these studies. In addition, we would like to thank Asthma and Pregnancy Research Coordinator Kathy Harden for her editorial assistance with this book, Pat Stanwood and Laurie Zeiger for secretarial assistance, and the Kaiser Foundation Hospital medical library staff for assistance with the references.

It is often said that the future of any society depends on its children. We hope that the information presented in this book will be used to improve the health of our children, both directly through the prevention and appropriate treatment of allergies and asthma in infancy and indirectly through promoting healthier pregnancies in women with allergies and asthma.

Michael Schatz
Robert S. Zeiger

Contributors

Richard S. Abrams, M.D. Staff Physician, Rose Medical Center, and Associate Clinical Professor, Departments of Medicine and Obstetrics/Gynecology, University of Colorado School of Medicine, Denver, Colorado

Joseph Alcalay, M.D. Department of Dermatology, Beilinson Medical Center, Sackler School of Medicine, Tel-Aviv University, Tel-Aviv, Israel

Sami L. Bahna, M.D., Dr.P.H. Professor, Department of Pediatrics, University of South Florida, and Co-Director, Allergy-Immunology Training Program, All Children's Hospital, St. Petersburg, Florida

Bengt Björkstén, M.D., Ph.D. Professor, Department of Pediatrics, Faculty of Health Sciences, University Hospital, Linköping, Sweden

S. Allan Bock, M.D. Department of Pediatrics, National Jewish Center for Immunology and Respiratory Medicine, and University of Colorado Health Sciences Center, Denver, Colorado

Walter A. Brown, M.D. Professor, Psychiatry and Human Behavior, Department of Psychiatry, Brown University School of Medicine, Providence, Rhode Island

David B. Brushwood, R.Ph., Esq. Professor, Department of Pharmacy Health Care Administration, College of Pharmacy, University of Florida, Gainesville, Florida

Valerian A. Catanzarite, M.D., Ph.D. Associate Director, Maternal-Fetal Medicine, Sharp Memorial Hospital Women's Center, San Diego, California

Larry Cousins, M.D. Director, Maternal-Fetal Medicine, Sharp Perinatal Center, Sharp Memorial Hospital, San Diego, California

Frederick H. Fern, R.Ph., Esq. Partner and Attorney, Lester Schwab Katz & Dwyer, New York, New York

Gillian M. P. Galbraith, M.D. Associate Professor, Department of Microbiology and Immunology, Medical University of South Carolina, Charleston, South Carolina

Robert Michael Galbraith, M.D. Professor and Chairman, Department of Microbiology and Immunology, Medical University of South Carolina, Charleston, South Carolina

Joan C. Gluck, M.D. Allergy Associates, Miami, Florida

Paul A. Gluck, M.D. Associate Clinical Professor, Department of Obstetrics and Gynecology, University of Miami School of Medicine, Miami, Florida

Paul A. Greenberger, M.D. Professor, Division of Allergy-Immunology, Department of Medicine, Northwestern University Medical School, Chicago, Illinois

Gunnar Hattevig, M.D. Department of Pediatrics, Kärnsjukhuset, Skövde, Sweden

Gary A. Incaudo, M.D. Associate Clinical Professor, Department of Internal Medicine, University of California, Davis, School of Medicine, Davis, California

Alan F. Isles, M.D. Pediatric Respiratory Physician, Royal Children's Hospital, Brisbane, Australia

Elizabeth F. Juniper, M.C.S.P., M.Sc. Assistant Professor, Department of Clinical Epidemiology and Biostatistics, McMaster University, Hamilton, Ontario, Canada

Janet Kershaw-McLennan, M.D. Private practice and Department of Medicine, Cedars-Sinai Medical Center, Los Angeles, California

N-I M Kjellman, M.D., Ph.D. Associate Professor, Department of Pediatrics, University Hospital, Linköping, Sweden

Armand Lione, Ph.D. Associated Pharmacologists and Toxicologists, Washington, D.C.

Eric Macy, M.D. Staff Allergist, Department of Allergy, Kaiser-Permanente Medical Center, and Clinical Instructor, Department of Medicine, University of California, San Diego, School of Medicine, San Diego, California

Joseph F. Mortola, M.D. Associate Professor, Obstetrics and Gynecology, Departments of Obstetrics, Gynecology, and Reproductive Biology, Harvard Medical School, Boston, Massachusetts

Michael T. Newhouse, M.D., M.Sc., FRCPC, FACP, FCCP Clinical Professor, Department of Medicine, McMaster University, Hamilton, Ontario, Canada

Christopher J. L. Newth, MB, FRCP(C) Head, Division of Pediatric Intensive Care, Children's Hospital of Los Angeles, and Professor, Department of Pediatrics, University of Southern California School of Medicine, Los Angeles, California

Lennart Nilsson, M.D. Department of Pediatrics, University Hospital, Linköping, Sweden

Roy Patterson, M.D. Professor, Department of Medicine, and Chief, Division of Allergy-Immunology, Department of Medicine, Northwestern University Medical School, Chicago, Illinois

Steven Rubinstein, M.D. Assistant Clinical Professor, Division of Allergy/Immunology, Department of Medicine, Stanford University Medical Center, Stanford, California

Hugh A. Sampson, M.D. Professor, Department of Pediatrics, and Director of Pediatric Clinical Research Center, Johns Hopkins University School of Medicine, Baltimore, Maryland

Michael Schatz, M.D. Staff Allergist, Department of Allergy, Kaiser-Permanente Medical Center, and Associate Clinical Professor, Department of Medicine, University of California, San Diego, School of Medicine, San Diego, California

Anthony R. Scialli Associate Professor, Department of Obstetrics and Gynecology, Georgetown University Medical Center, and Director, Reproductive Toxicology Center, Columbia Hospital for Women Medical Center, Washington, D.C.

Sheldon L. Spector, M.D. Clinical Professor, Department of Medicine, and Director, Allergy Research Foundation, University of California, Los Angeles, California

Brita Stenius-Aarniala, M.D., FCCP Associate Professor, Department of Pulmonary Medicine, University Central Hospital, Helsinki, Finland

Andrea B. Stone, M.D. Assistant Professor, Department of Psychiatry, University of Massachusetts Medical School, Worcester, Massachusetts

Stephen I. Wasserman, M.D. Helen M. Ranney Professor and Chairman, Department of Medicine, University of California, San Diego, San Diego, California

Robert S. Zeiger, M.D., Ph.D. Chief, Department of Allergy, Kaiser-Permanente Medical Center and Clinical Professor, Department of Pediatrics, University of California, San Diego, School of Medicine, San Diego, California

Contents

1

Hormonal Changes During Normal Pregnancy and Their Consequences

Joseph F. Mortola

Harvard Medical School, Boston, Massachusetts

The unique endocrine milieu of pregnancy is the result of the introduction of hormonal products of the fetal–placental unit into the prior homeostatic balance of the mother. During pregnancy, a production rate of both steroid and peptide hormones is achieved that is unparalleled in any other physiological state. The ability of the mother to tolerate these changes is largely dependent on the development of buffering systems and antihormones. Although these buffering systems usually prevent the development of pathological sequellae that may otherwise result from the hormonal excess, an increase in hormone action prevails that induces the physiological adaptation to pregnancy.

PROGESTERONE

Progesterone exists as the hormone most clearly associated with maternal adaptation to pregnancy. It is essential for the maturation of the uterine endometrium into a tissue capable of accepting implantation. Initially, progesterone is produced by the corpus luteum until its involution, which usually occurs at the end of the normal menstrual cycle. After the tenth week of pregnancy, the placenta produces almost all of the body's progesterone. In early pregnancy, however, the corpus luteum's capacity to produce both estrogen and progesterone is extended by the stimulatory action of placentally derived human chorionic gonadotropin (hCG). This hormone can be detected in the maternal circulation within 1 day of implantation. It is almost entirely unique to pregnancy (with the exception of a small production by the pituitary in the nonpregnant state), and its detection serves as the basis for modern pregnancy tests (1). In the corpus luteum, progesterone synthesis proceeds through a series of sequential steps from cholesterol (2). The synthesis of progesterone in addition to estrogen distinguishes the corpus luteum from the preovulatory follicle from which it arises, in which estrogen predominates as the end product of the steroidogenic pathway.

The shift from estrogen production in the follicular (preovulatory) phase to production of both estrogen and progesterone in the luteal (postovulatory) phase is crucial to maintenance of the normal menstrual cycle. These events serve to trigger ovulation and to prepare the endometrium for implantation of the dividing fertilized egg at the blastocyst stage, approximately 7 days later. Adequate endometrial maturation is dependent on the addition of progesterone to an estrogen-primed endometrium. As a result of progesterone, the glandular component of the endometrium undergoes marked secretory changes, and the structural matrix undergoes a characteristic edematous change (3). Progesterone administration without prior estrogen influence produces quite a different effect, with widely spaced glands lined by atrophic cuboidal epithelium (4). Progesterone, therefore, has effects that are dependent on the previous estrogen priming of the uterus. With prolonged progesterone exposure accompanied by sufficient estrogen, such as is seen in pregnancy, the uterine endometrium undergoes even more marked changes, termed *decidualization*. In this process, stromal cells adopt a distinct polyhedral shape, with clearly delineated borders that are believed to be the result of glycoprotein deposition in the cell membrane (5). Within the glandular epithelial cells the nuclei become hyperchromatic. These nuclei are polyploid and are surrounded by expanded cytoplasm, a series of changes thought to reflect hypersecretory activity. The development of such large hypersecretory cells is referred to as the *Arias–Stella reaction*, and is considered a characteristic histological marker for pregnancy (6). The actions of progesterone on the uterus, which both prepare the endometrium for implantation and maintain the pregnancy once implantation has occurred, may be the result not only of progesterone itself, but a metabolite, 20α-hydroxypregn-4-ene-3-one, synthesized within the endometrium (7).

Although the most widely recognized effects of progesterone and its metabolites are on endometrial tissue, progesterone is assumed to be largely responsible for many of the marked systemic physiological changes that accompany pregnancy. Progesterone levels increase at least tenfold between the 6th and 36th week of pregnancy (Figure 1). Progesterone or its metabolites have been shown to decrease vascular responsiveness to angiotensin II through a prostaglandin-mediated mechanism (9) and may thereby contribute to the decreased peripheral vascular resistance seen in pregnancy (10). The decreased total pulmonary vascular resistance of pregnancy has long been postulated to be the result of progesterone action as well (11). Among the most important adaptive changes in pregnancy is the increased maternal oxygen uptake that results from increased minute ventilation. This increased ventilatory effort results from a marked increase in tidal volume without necessitating a change in the respiratory rate (see Chapter 3).

The increased respiratory effort appears to be a progesterone-mediated event through central nervous system actions of the hormone. In 1975, Sutton et al. were able to demonstrate an increased respiratory drive when nonpregnant obese patients who hypoventilate were given medroxyprogesterone acetate (12).

In addition to changes in the vascular and pulmonary systems, pregnancy is characterized by a decreased gastrointestinal transit time. This includes both slower gastric emptying and prolonged intestinal transit. These alterations have been hypothesized, but not proved, to be the result of progesterone action. The urinary tract in pregnancy is also characterized by marked changes in architecture. Both hydronephrosis and hydroureter are widely reported. Typically, the hydronephrosis and hydroureter are more marked on the right side (13), suggesting that mechanical compression by the dextrorotated uterus may be a factor. There is, however, evidence that hormonal influences also play a part. Pregnant monkeys with the fetus removed, but the placenta allowed to remain intact, continued to be hydronephrotic (14). Such a result would not be expected if the effect were estrogen dominated, since most of the precursor for placental estrogen production is of fetal origin. This evidence suggests, therefore, that this may also be a progesterone-induced change.

ESTROGEN

The second major class of steroid hormone produced during pregnancy is estrogen. Pregnancy is characterized by a marked increase in both of the estrogens produced in the nonpregnant state, estradiol and estrone (15), as well as the appearance of abundant quantities of a third estrogen, estriol (16), which is produced in only trace amounts in the nonpregnant state (Figure 2). (A fourth estrogen, estetrol, is also produced in

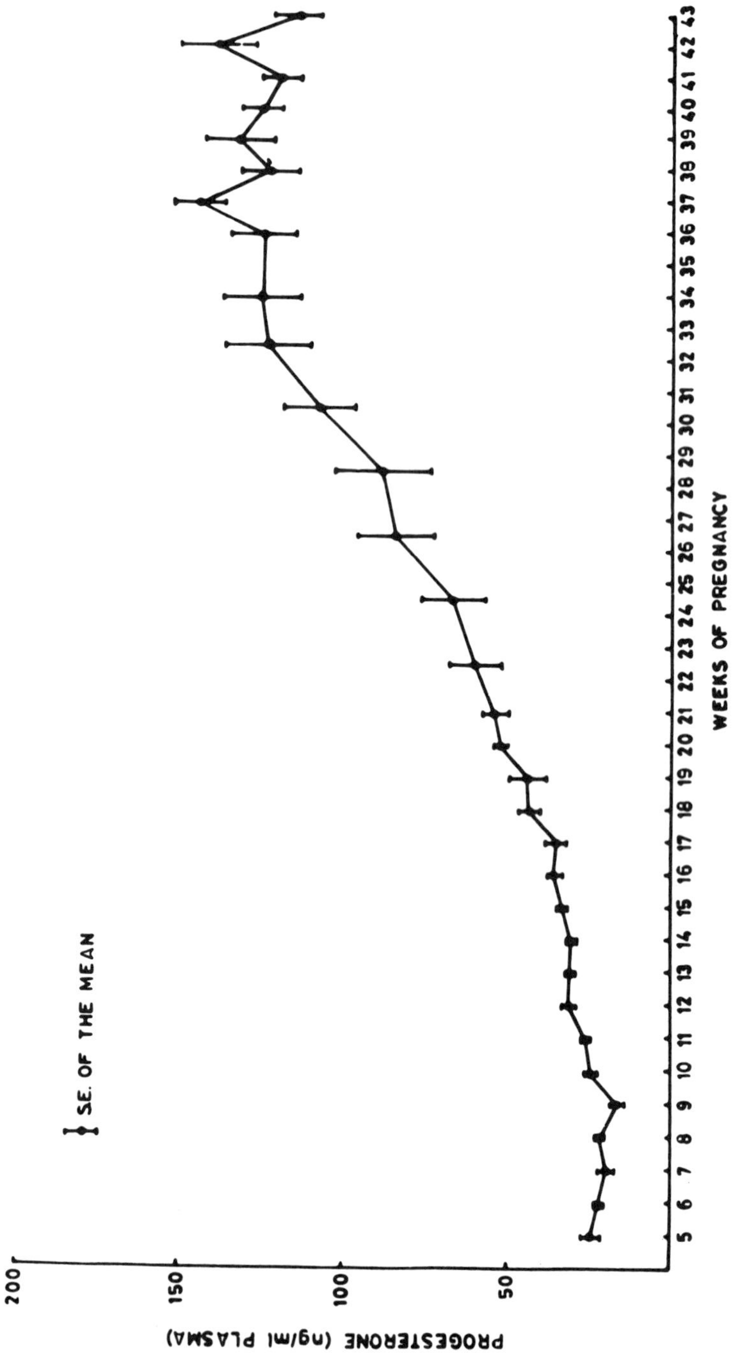

Figure 1 Plasma progesterone levels during normal pregnancy. (From Ref. 8.)

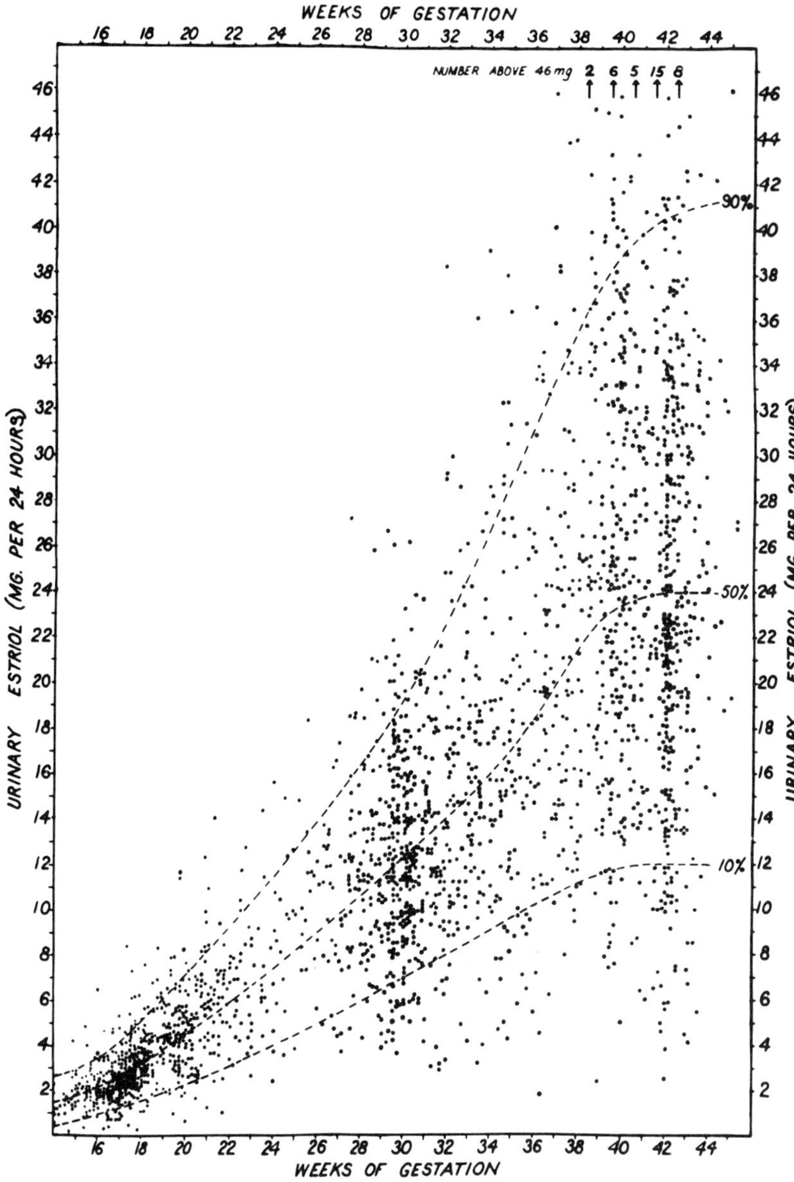

Figure 2 Urinary estriol values from 14 to 44 weeks of pregnancy demonstrating 10th, 15th, and 90th percentiles. (From Ref. 17.)

pregnancy, although its quantity is negligible and its only interest is that it is entirely unique to pregnancy with no measurable amounts found in the serum of nonpregnant women.)

The biosynthesis of estrogen is quite different from that of progesterone. Although the placenta is capable of producing large amounts of progesterone from a low-density lipoprotein (LDL) precursor of maternal origin, a placental 17α-hydroxylase/17,20-desmolase block renders the production of C_{19} steroids (androgen) and C_{18} steroids (estrogens) directly from the HDL precursor impossible in the placenta. As a result, the placenta is almost entirely dependent on the provision of C_{19} steroids for estrogen production. Studies of total estrogen levels in the circulation of women with anencephalic fetuses (which are incapable of adrenal steroid synthesis) reveal that these levels are very low. These studies support the concept that the largest production of estrogen is from fetal adrenal precursors (18). The fetal adrenal glands secrete more than 200 mg of the C_{19} compound dehydroepiandrosterone sulfate (DHEA-S) daily, which corresponds to a tenfold increase over that of maternal production (19). Extensive sulfatase activity in the placenta liberates DHEA from DHEA-S for subsequent conversion by 3β-ol-hydroxysteroid dehydrogenase/Δ^4,Δ^5-isomerase to androstenedione. Androstenedione is then rapidly converted to either estrone by aromatase or to estradiol by a two-step process (first to the more potent androgen testosterone and later to estradiol). Accordingly, the large contribution of DHEA by the fetal adrenal gland has an essential role in the production of both estrone and estradiol in pregnancy. However, direct utilization of DHEA to form these estrogens from the placenta is a relatively minor pathway for this compound to follow. Only 50% of maternal circulating estrone and estradiol at term are estimated to be derived from fetal DHEA, with maternal DHEA providing the precursor for the remaining 50%. The fate of most fetal DHEA is to undergo 16-hydroxylation in the fetal liver and, to a smaller extent, the fetal adrenal gland itself (20). This leads to the products formed from 16α-OH-DHEA, which is converted by the placenta to a series of 16α-hydroxylated variants of the same steroids along the pathway of estradiol production, including 16α-hydroxyandrostenedione, and ending in the production of estriol. At term, more than 90% of estriol is derived from fetal adrenal precursors. Suppression of maternal and fetal adrenal activity by pharmacologic doses of either dexamethasone or prednisone (10–20 mg/day) decreases estrone, estradiol, and estriol. The greater suppression of estrone and estradiol than of estriol suggests that this is primarily an effect on maternal adrenal function (21).

It has been estimated that the potency of estriol is 1/10 the potency of estrone and 1/100 the potency of estradiol, the most potent mammalian estrogen in most biological systems. Estriol has a high affinity for the estrogen receptor, but has an inordinately high dissociation constant as well. Thus, it has a poor ability to form a stable hormone–receptor complex necessary for biological action (22). It has been postulated that estriol may, in many cases, act as more of an antiestrogen than an estrogen, offering some protection against the effects of the extraordinary hyperestrogenic state of pregnancy. Such estrogenic effects include thromboembolic phenomena and perhaps an increased tendency for breast cancer. It has been shown, for instance, that an early age of first pregnancy is protective against breast cancer, perhaps because of a shortening of the time of unopposed estrogen influence (23). In addition to the potential antiestrogenic effects afforded by estriol, as a result of its ability to compete for the estrogen receptor without initiating biological action in most systems, estrogens are able to induce synthesis of sex hormone-binding globulin (SHBG) (24), which then serves to bind estrogen itself as well as androgens. Despite the availability of these buffering mechanisms to protect against massive hyperestrogenism, pregnancy must be viewed as a hyperestrogenic state. In fact, it appears that hyperestrogenism is carefully maintained by the fetal–placental unit. All steroid hormones are inhibitory of the 3β-ol-dehydrogenase enzyme; however, estrogen appears to be the most potent here (25). Thus, the block in conversion of fetal adrenal precursors to glucocorticoids, mineralocorticoids, and potent sex steroid products may be the result of the high estrogen environment. This high estrogen environment then produces an abundance of Δ^5-androgens (DHEA and DHEA-S), which the placenta can rapidly and efficiently convert to more estrogen. It has been demonstrated that the hypertrophy of the fetal zone of the adrenal gland is not the result of peptide hormones (26). This zone, which is the production site of DHEA and DHEA-S and which regresses rapidly after birth, may, therefore, primarily reflect estrogenic influence.

In addition to the actions of estrogen during pregnancy directed at producing more estrogen, there are clear effects of the estrogenic state on the mother. One mechanism by which this occurs relates to the ability of the otherwise weak estrogen estriol to have potent effects on uterine circulation. This has led to speculation that the prime function of estriol may be to provide increased uteroplacental blood flow necessary for oxygenation and nutritional needs of the fetus. The effects of estrogen on the uterine vascular bed have been shown to be mediated through prostaglandin mechanisms (27). The increased uterine blood flow is only one of a myriad of cardiovascular effects exerted by estrogen, primarily though prostaglandin-mediated mechanisms. Greiss and Anderson have shown that estrogen administration to mammals produces a decrease in vascular resistance (28). Among the most notable increases in blood flow seen in pregnancy, which reflect selective dilation of vascular beds, is a 30–80% increase in renal blood flow (29–31) and an increase in skin perfusion (32). The latter results in an increase in skin temperature and claminess of the extremities. Vascular spiders and palmer erythema are additional manifestations of increased cutaneous flow. Nasal congestion, which is one of the most persistently bothersome complaints of pregnancy, is also believed to result from increased vascular flow to the nasal mucosa (33). Other mucous membranes, notably the gums, undergo hyperemic changes as well, leading to increased tendency to bleed during minor trauma. Occasionally, a highly vascular lesion of the mouth may develop, called the pregnancy epulis. This regresses spontaneously after delivery.

In addition to vasodilatation and development of a low-resistance uteroplacental vascular bed, pregnancy is marked by dramatic increases in circulating blood volume. Although wide variations have been reported, review of the literature indicates that the best estimate is that a 50% increase in blood volume occurs, compared with that of the nonpregnant state (34). The increase in blood volume is most pronounced in the first half of pregnancy (35). From experimental evidence using estrogen treatment in a variety of nonpregnancy-related conditions, it appears that estrogen may be the key mediator of the hypervolemia (Figure 3) (36–38). Several investigators have demonstrated that renin is stimulated by estrogen (39,40). The estrogen-induced increase in renin initiates a cascade of events in which angiotensin II levels increase, aldosterone increases and, as a result, sodium and water absorption is increased, with the net effect of increasing blood volume substantially. Of interest is the well-described resistance of the vasculature of pregnant women to constriction with increased angiotensin II levels (41). This decreased sensitivity can be reversed by administration of indomethacin or aspirin (42), suggesting a prostaglandin-mediated mechanism. Vasodilatation in pregnancy appears to be estrogen-mediated, either by a direct influence of estrogen on vascular prostaglandin synthesis or through increased prostaglandin synthesis mediated by angiotensin II, which is itself increased by increased estrogen (see Figure 3).

The increase in the plasma compartment during pregnancy exceeds that of the increase in erythrocyte production, leading to the

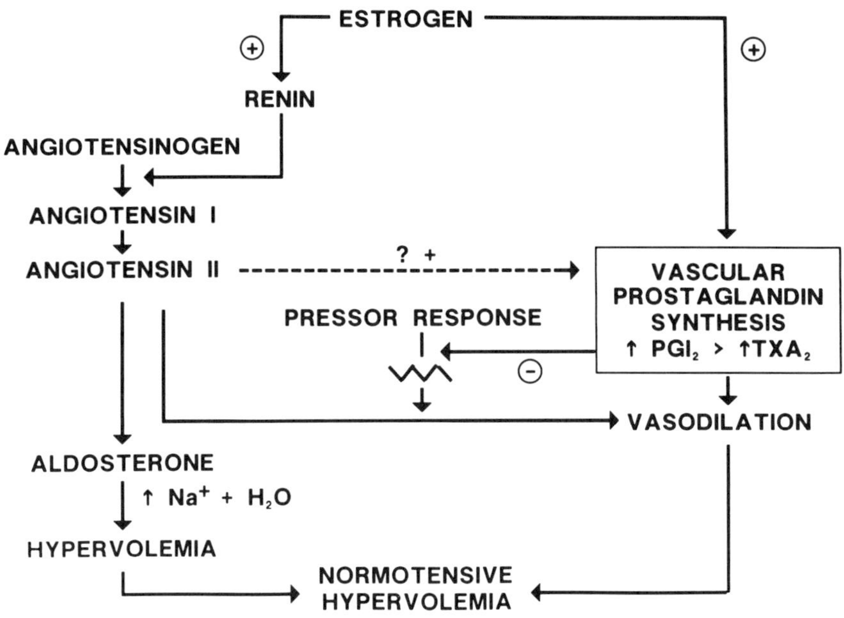

Figure 3 Diagramatic representation of the effects of estrogen on the renin-angiotensin system and vascular prostaglandin synthesis.

"physiologic anemia of pregnancy." Nonetheless, a 33% increase in red cell mass has been observed (43). The possibility that this may be due to placental lactogen-induced increases in erythropoietin has been suggested by animal studies (4,5). Leukocytosis in pregnancy has also been seen (46), although the range is highly variable, (5000–12,000/mm^3).

The expanded circulatory volume resulting from both increased plasma and erythrocytes results in the typical changes seen during examination of the pregnant patient (47). These include exaggerated splitting of the first heart sound, a third heart sound, and a systolic murmur in 90% of patients. Soft diastolic murmurs are heard in 19% of patients and a continuous murmur, believed to result from increased breast vasculature, in 10%.

The well-known hypercoagulability of pregnant women is also believed to be the result of estrogen action. During pregnancy clotting factors, particularly those that are vitamin K-dependent (II, VII, IX, X), are increased. Similar effects are seen when estrogens are administered in oral contraceptive pills (48). The hypercoagulability is furthered by an estrogen-mediated decrease in antithromboplastin III, which is also seen in women taking estrogen-containing oral contraceptives (49,50). As a result of these changes in the clotting cascade, coupled with a decreased venous return from the stasis produced by a growing uterus, pulmonary embolic phenomena have been noted to be more common during pregnancy.

PROSTAGLANDINS

During pregnancy, circulating levels of prostaglandin (PG)E_2 and PGF_2 are unchanged until just before the onset of labor. However, with the onset of labor, a dramatic rise in both of these prostaglandins occurs (51). Extensive evidence suggests that these prostaglandin changes are essential for the onset of normal labor (52). Both the fetal membranes (amnion and chorion) and uterine decidua have been demonstrated to produce PGE_1 and PGF_2 from arachidonic acid (53–55). It has been suggested that the initiation of labor is the result of decreasing progesterone concentration (56). This fall in progesterone may result in the disappearance from the amniotic epithelium of a specific prostaglandin synthetase inhibitor (57). Earlier in pregnancy, although no clear changes in circulating prostaglandins occur, PGE_2 and PGF_2 concentrations in the local area of the uterus are undoubtedly increased. Local effects of increased prostaglandin synthesis outside of the reproductive system have been postulated based on evidence that estrogen directly influences prostaglandin synthesis (58,59). Pregnancy-induced hypertension (PIH) is a common and potentially life-threatening complication of pregnancy. The aforementioned resistance of pregnant women to the pressor effects of angiotensin II, which appears to be prostaglandin-mediated, is lost in those women destined to develop PIH, a finding that may occur as early as 10–14 weeks (60). The predominant current hypothesis for the development of PIH is a decreased prostacyclin (PGI_2)/thromboxane (TXA_2) ratio (see Figure 3). Prostacyclin is a potent vasodilator, and TXA_2 is a platelet-derived vasoconstrictor. Both PGI_2 and TXA_2 levels are increased in normal pregnancy, although the increase in PGI_2 exceeds that of TXA_2 (61). Several studies have shown a decrease in PGI_2 in PIH, compared with that in a normal pregnancy (62,63). As with the loss of resistance to the pressor effects of angiotensin II, the decreased PGI_2 levels precede the development of the clinical manifestations of PIH (64). Low-dose aspirin treatment has prevented PIH in high-risk individuals (65,66). When used at low doses, aspirin will decrease TXA_2 selectively, whereas at higher doses, inhibition of the true prostaglandins (such as PGI_2) occurs as well (67,68). Thus, use of aspirin in treating PIH should be limited to low-dose regimens.

CORTISOL AND DEOXYCORTICOSTERONE

In addition to sex steroids, pregnancy is also characterized by marked increases in serum cortisol. In 1979, Judziewitsch reported that 9 AM cortisol values increased from a nonpregnant range of 4–21 mg/dL to 25–46 mg/dL in the last trimester (69). Despite the increased levels, the circadian rhythm of cortisol is maintained (70). Although cortisol-binding globulin (CBG) levels triple during pregnancy, an increase in free cortisol has also been reported (71). The increase in cortisol is accompanied by, and perhaps driven by, an increase in corticotropin (adrenocorticotropic hormone; ACTH) as well. The magnitude of the increase in cortisol would clearly be sufficient to produce pathological manifestations, were it not for the increase in CBG induced by the hyperestrogenism. Thus, a clear buffering mechanism is involved in pregnancy that produces only a moderate increase in free cortisol. Nonetheless, the hypercortisolism is at least one mechanism whereby insulin resistance is induced by pregnancy (72), the others being the result of peptide hormones, to be discussed later. The effects of the hypercortisolism on immunological function in pregnancy may also be profound. As early as 1938, Hench observed a decrease in symptoms in 43 patients with rheumatoid arthritis and used the hypercortisolism of pregnancy as a rationale for treating nonpregnant patients with cortisone (73). More recently, however, Unger et al. reported an inverse correlation between pregnancy-associated α_2-globulin levels and symptoms in rheumatoid arthritis patients (74), suggesting that other factors may be of greater significance when remission is observed.

Although normal during most of gestation, a dramatic increase in deoxycorticosterone (DOC) levels is found in late gestation. The possibilities include that this arises directly from the fetus or from the conversion of progesterone derived from the placenta (75). In favor of fetal production is the finding that dexamethasone, which suppresses maternal ACTH levels, does not reduce DOC levels. The significance of the higher levels of DOC in late gestation is poorly understood. Deoxycorticosterone, as well as progesterone and aldosterone, competitively binds to the corticosteroid receptor, albeit with a lower affinity than glucocorticoids and, therefore, may serve as important additional buffers of the hypercortisolemia of pregnancy (76–78).

HUMAN CHORIONIC GONADOTROPIN

Without question, many of the changes characteristic of pregnancy result from the occurrence of increased levels of steroid hormones. Production of several of these steroid hormones, however, is regulated by protein hormones, of which the placenta is an abundant source. These hormones, when produced by the placenta, impinge on the steroidogenic capacity of the maternal–fetal–placental unit.

Certainly the most prominent peptide hormone of pregnancy is human chorionic gonadotropin (hCG), which is produced by the developing embryo, even before implantation. Its presence in the maternal circulation is detectable as early as 24 hours after implantation. It is structurally homologous and has physiological function similar to luteinizing hormone (LH). Its first action in early pregnancy is to maintain the corpus luteum, which it does more effectively than LH itself, probably because its increased carbohydrate content markedly prolongs its half-life in the circulation. Serum hCG values in the first trimester of pregnancy rise rapidly from nearly undetectable levels to values exceeding 100,000 IU/L. Subsequent to the first trimester, hCG levels decline markedly compared with their first-trimester peak, although they remain several thousand-fold higher than in the nonpregnant state (Figure 4).

In addition to functioning as a gonadotropin in maintenance of the corpus luteum, Jaffe and colleagues (80) have demonstrated that hCG may regulate DHEA production by the fetal zone of the fetal adrenal gland during early gestation, implicating a dual role for the hormone as a corticotropin as well as a gonadotropin. Moreover, hCG also pos-

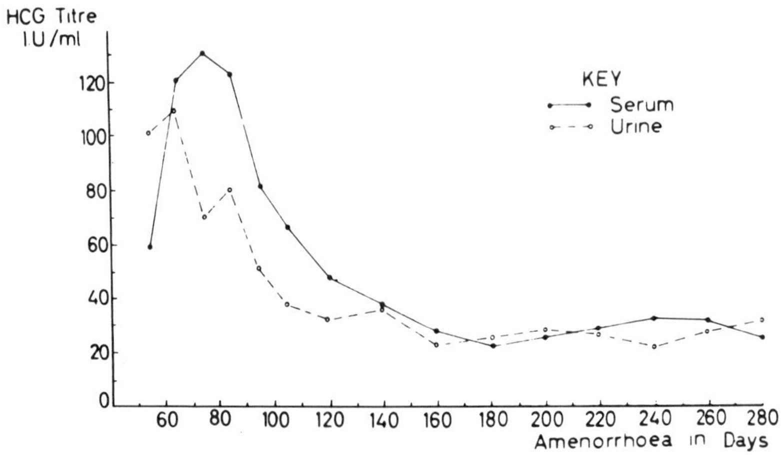

Figure 4 Mean levels of serum and urine human chorionic gonadatropin (hCG) in 600 normally pregnant women. (From Ref. 79.)

sesses thyrotropin activity. This is likely to be one mechanism for the increased thyroxine (T_4) levels seen in pregnancy (81). Of particular interest has been the suggestion that, similar to progesterone (82), hCG may have immunosuppressive effects in addition to its endocrine actions (83). Teasdale et al. (84) have shown that hCG inhibits blast cell transformation induced by either phytohemagglutinin or mixed lymphocyte reactions.

HUMAN CHORIONIC SOMATOMAMMOTROPIN

The placental analogue of growth hormone (GH) is human chorionic somatomammotropin (hCS), better known as human placental lactogen (hPL) because of its lactogenic properties in animals (85). The levels of this hormone are shown in Figure 5. Circulating concentrations of hCS are directly proportional to placental weight (86) and, therefore, maternal serum levels rise steadily until the 36th week of gestation. Dubbed the growth hormone (GH) of pregnancy, hCS possess somatotrophic effects similar to GH in most animal models, although its biological activity is only 3% or less than that of GH. Interestingly, all placental tropic hormones that ultimately result in steroid production are to some degree compensated by binding protein increases. Since GH results in no steroidal hormone production, it becomes the exception to the rule. It is elegant that the one hormone showing large increases in pregnancy, without a significant mechanism for buffering its ultimate biological action, is produced in a less potent form, sparing pregnant women from acromegaly. In fact, a normal pregnancy has been reported in the absence of hCS (87). That it does not appear to be essential in a patient with good nutritional health should not be construed to indicate that hCS does not have significant biological effects during normal pregnancy. By the last 4 weeks of pregnancy, mean hCS levels reach 5.4 mg/mL, at least a thousandfold higher than GH levels. In addition to production of hCS, the placenta also produces insulin-like growth factor I (IGF-I), providing possible increased potential for hCS action. The extent to which this IGF is buffered by changes in IGF-binding protein changes is unknown (88,89).

Largely because of the actions of hCS, pregnancy has been described by Felig as a "state of accelerated starvation" (90). The growth hormone-like effects of hCS confer an insulin-resistant state on pregnancy that is augmented by the anti-insulin actions of estrogen and of cortisol. Placental levels of hCS are regulated by circulating glucose

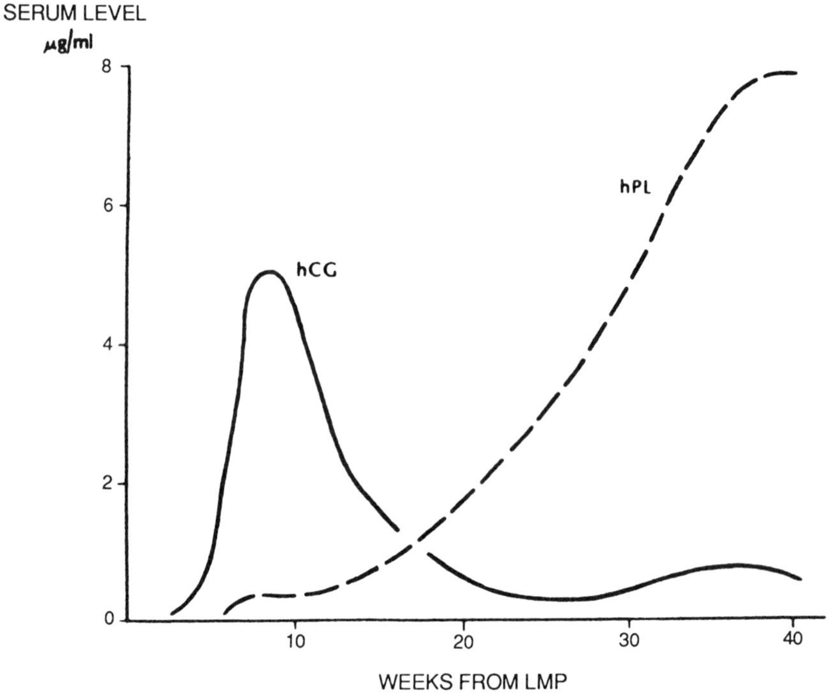

Figure 5 Concentrations of human chorionic somatomammotropin (here called HPL) during normal pregnancy. (From Ref. 43.)

levels, analogous to the control of pituitary growth hormone. Therefore, in hypoglycemic conditions there is an accelerated release of free fatty acids (accelerated starvation) caused by increased hCS levels. In the fed state, when glucose levels increase, the anti-insulin action of hCS serves to maintain higher serum glucose levels. Consequently, more glucose is available for transport to the fetus. As a further result of the anti-insulin effects of hCS, pregnancy is characterized by an increase of free fatty acids, in excess of the increased total lipids, with no change in the percentage of esterified cholesterol (91).

In pregnancy, therefore, during periods of fasting, there is more ketonuria than in the nonpregnant state. Because of the anti-insulin effect of hCS (and cortisol), pregnant patients are also prone to develop gestational diabetes. As expected, in women who develop this condition, infection is more common and more difficult to treat than in nondiabetic pregnancies.

OTHER PEPTIDE HORMONES

In addition to hCG and hCS, the placenta secretes human chorionic thyrotropin (hCT). Yen has postulated that the placenta acts as an endocrine brain, capable of producing the same hypothalamic hormones that influence the adult hypothalamic–hypophyseal axis. The entire proopiomelanocortin (POM-C) family of peptides has also been identified in the placenta. Moreover, the placenta has the capability of producing hypothalamic-releasing factors, including corticotropin-releasing hormone (CRH), thyrotropin-releasing hormone (TRH), gonadotropin-releasing hormone (GnRH), and somatostatin. The role of these hormones in autoregulation of placental hormone production is poorly understood. However, there is evidence, at least for CRH, that steroids regulate expression of the placental gene (92).

The mechanisms of buffering the increased gestational cortisol levels through the induction of CBG by estrogen have been previously addressed. To an even greater degree, there is a compensating mechanism for the increase in thyroid hormone production that results from hCG and human chorionic thyrotropin (hCT). Although total T_4 levels are increased in pregnancy, a marked increase in thyroid-binding globulin (TBG) is stimulated by estrogen, such that free T_4 and free triiodothyronine (T_3) levels are normal. The increase in TBG is apparent by the marked decrease in T_3 resin uptake (T_3RU) seen in pregnancy, since T_3RU serves as an indirect measure of TBG.

PROLACTIN

The influence of pregnancy on a prolactin (PRL), a hormone closely related to hCS and GH, is rather unique. Estrogen increases pituitary production of prolactin. In the pregnant state, prolactin levels reach at least four times the nonpregnant value as a result of hyperestrogenism. This increase is accompanied by a doubling in size of the pituitary gland because of lactotroph hypertrophy. Unlike most hormones of pregnancy, PRL is produced primarily by the fetal membranes, rather than the placenta itself. It has been demonstrated to play an osmoregulatory role in amniotic fluid, reminiscent of its primary role in lower vertebrates. However, most prolactin released into the maternal circulation is of maternal pituitary origin. Again, a buffering mechanism is present. Estrogen, which hypertrophies the lactrotroph in preparation for its formidable postpartum task of producing adequate prolactin to stimulate milk production, simultaneously inhibits prolactin action in the breast. It is only after the clearance of estrogen from the circulation, which results from placental expulsion at delivery, that the effects of hyperprolactmenia are manifest in milk production.

CALCITROPIC HORMONES

The need for calcium represents one of the most dramatic requirements of the growing fetus. During pregnancy 30 g are deposited into the fetus for incorporation into bone. It is expected, then, that specific mechanisms must exist for this transfer. One such mechanism is altered vitamin D metabolism in pregnancy. As in the nonpregnant state, the conversion of vitamin D_3 to 25-hydroxyvitamin D_3 takes place in the maternal liver. It is the 1-hydroxylation step, however, that is the rate-limiting step in production of the active metabolite 1,25-dihydrocholecalciferol (1,25$(OH)_2D_3$). In pregnancy, 1α-hydroxylase is present in the placenta and endometrial decidua, as well in the proximal convoluted tubules of the kidney, where it is found in both the pregnant and nonpregnant state. The increased hydroxylation sites as well as the increased availability of the precursor 25-OHD_3 explain the increased levels of vitamin D_3 during pregnancy (93). The twofold rise in circulating levels of vitamin D_3 might be sufficient for the development of toxic manifestations, except that a concomitant twofold increase in the buffering hormone, vitamin D_3-binding protein (DBP), is also observed. The effect of the increased vitamin D_3 is primarily to enhance intestinal calcium absorption. Parathormone (PTH) levels have also been reported to be somewhat elevated in pregnancy. The PTH is secreted in response to decreased levels of ionized calcium in the extracellular fluid. The minimal (if any) increase in PTH during pregnancy reflects the careful homeostasis of calcium metabolism. Calcium is obtained from maternal serum for fetal use by an active ATP-dependent calcium pump within the placenta (94). However, the maternal hypocalcemia that may result from such shunting appears to be offset by the increased rate of calcium absorption. Consequently, only a minimal PTH response is noted. This minimal increase in PTH has earned pregnancy the reputation of physiological hyperparathyroidism. Hypercalcemia, on the other hand, which may result from increased absorption as a result of increased 1,25-vitamin D_3 is compensated for by increased calcitonin. Calcitonin levels have been reported to be increased in pregnancy (95). This may serve as a protective mechanism against the hypercalcemia that would result from both increased absorption and increased bone resorption caused by increased PTH levels.

SUMMARY

From an endocrinological perspective, then, pregnancy appears to be a state of tremendous hormonal excess, providing optimal reserves for the maternal adaptations designed to protect the requirements of the developing fetus. This excess, however, is compensated by a variety of buffering systems, such as estriol and SHBG for estrogen, TBG for thyroid, and CBG for cortisol. Nonetheless, the hormonal milieu of the pregnant woman is usually such that the slight excesses in active hormones that persist over the attempts to buffer them produce profound effects in the mother. This system of "checked excess" provides for both physiological adaptation in normal circumstances and a reserve for periods of physiological stress. It is clear that many of these hormones exert their influence through second messengers, even the steroids (i.e., prostaglandins). Of particular interest to the field of allergy are the effects of these hormones on prostaglandin synthesis and the immunosuppressive actions of progesterone, cortisol, and perhaps the most crucial regulator of the endocrine events of pregnancy, hCG itself.

REFERENCES

1. Catt KJ, Dufau ML, Vaitukaitis JL. Appearance of hCG in pregnancy following the initiation of implantation of the blastocyst. J Clin Endocrinol Metab 1975; 40:537–540.
2. Hellig HD, Gattereau D, Lefevre Y, Bolte E. Steroid production from plasma cholesterol: I. Conversion of plasma cholesterol to placental progesterone in humans. J Clin Endocrinol Metab 1970; 30:624–631.
3. Noyes RW, Hertig AT, Rock J. Dating the endometrial biopsy. Fertil Steril 1950; 1:3–25.
4. Roberts DK, Horbelt DV, Powell LC. The ultrastructural response of human endometrium to medroxyprogesterone acetate. Am J Obstet Gynecol 1975; 123:811–881.
5. Wynn RM. Electron microscopy of the developing decidua. Fertil Steril 1965; 16:16–26.
6. Arias-Stella J. Atypical endometrial changes associated with presence of chorionic tissue. Arch Pathol 1968; 58:112–128.
7. Collins JA, Jerkes DM. Progesterone metabolism by proliferative and secretory human endometrium. Am J Obstet Gynecol 1974; 118:179–185.
8. Johansson ENB. Acta Endocrinol (Copenh) 1979; 61:607.
9. Gant NF, Worley RJ, Everett RB, MacDonald PC. Control of vascular responsiveness during human pregnancy. Kidney Int 1980; 18:253–258.

10. Metcalfe J, Ueland K. Maternal cardiovascular adjustments to pregnancy. Prog Cardiovasc Dis 1974; 16:363–374.
11. Gee JBL, Packer BS, Millen JE, Robin ED. Pulmonary mechanics during pregnancy. J Clin Invest 1967; 46:945–952.
12. Sutton FD, Zwillich CW, Creagh E, Pierson DJ, Weil JV. Progesterone for the outpatient treatment of pickwickian syndrome. Ann Intern Med 1975; 83:476–479.
13. Shulman A, Herlinger H. Urinary tract dilation in pregnancy. Br J Radiol 1975; 48:638–645.
14. Van Wegenen G, Jenkins RH. An experimental examination of factors causing ureteral dilation of pregnancy. J Urol 1939; 42:1010–1020.
15. Buster JE, Abraham GE. The applications of steroid hormone radioimmunoassays to clinical obstetrics. Obstet Gynecol 1975; 46:489–499.
16. Goebelsmann U, Chen LC, Saga M, Nakamura RM, Jaffe RB. Plasma concentration and binding protein of oestriol and its conjugates in pregnancy. Acta Endrocrinol (Copenh) 1973; 74:592–604.
17. Beischer, et al. Am J Obstet Gynecol 1969; 103:483.
18. Siiteri PK, MacDonald PC. Placental estrogen biosynthesis during human pregnancy. J Clin Endocrinol Metab 1966; 26:751–761.
19. Madden JD, Gant NF, MacDonald PC. Study of the kinetics of conversion of maternal plasma dehydroisoandrosterone sulfate to 16α-hydroxydehydroisoandrosterone sulfate, estradiol and estriol. Am J Obstet Gynecol 1978; 132:392–395.
20. Perez-Palacios G, Perez AE, Jaffe RB. Conversion of pregnenolone 7O-^{3}H-sulfate to other Δ^5-Δ^4-3β-ol-hydroxysteroid sulfates by the human fetal adrenal in vitro. J Clin Endocrinol Metab 1968; 28:19–25.
21. Challis J, Patrick J, Richardson B, Tevaarwerk G. Loss of diurnal rhythm in plasma estrone, estradiol and estriol in women treated with glucocorticoids at 34 to 35 weeks' gestation. Am J Obstet Gynecol 1981; 139:338–343.
22. Clark JH, Paszko Z, Peck EJ Jr. Nuclear binding and retention of the receptor estrogen complex: relationship of the agonistic and antagonistic properties of estriol. Endocrinology 1977; 100:91–96.
23. Korenman SG. Estrogen window hypothesis of the etiology of breast cancer. Lancet 1980; 1:700–701.
24. Anderson DC. Sex hormone binding globulin. Clin Endocrinol (Oxf) 1974; 3:69–96.
25. Byrne GC, Perry YS, Winter JSD. Steroid inhibitory effects upon human adrenal 3β-hydroxysteroid dehydrogenase activity. J Clin Endocrinol Metab 1986; 62:413–418.
26. Fujieda K, Faiman C, Feyes FI, Winter JSD. The control of steroidogenesis by human fetal adrenal cells in tissue culture: III. The effects of various hormonal peptides. J Clin Endocrinol Metab 1981; 53:690–693.
27. Resnik R, Brink GW. Modulating effects of prostaglandins on the uterine vascular bed. Gynecol Invest 1977; 8:10.

28. Greiss FC, Anderson SG. Effect of ovarian hormones on the uterine vascular bed. Am J Obstet Gynecol 1970; 107:829–836.
29. Nunlap W. Serial changes in renal hemodynamics during normal human pregnancy. Br J Obstet Gynaecol 1981; 88:1–9.
30. Little B. Water and electrolyte balance during pregnancy. Anaethesiology 1965; 26:400–408.
31. Chesley LC. Renal function changes in normal pregnancy. Clin Obstet Gynecol 1960; 3:349–363.
32. Katz M, Sokal MM. Skin perfusion in pregnancy. Am J Obstet Gynecol 1980; 137:30–33.
33. Fabricant ND. Sexual functions and the nose. Am J Med Sci 1960; 239:498–502.
34. Pritchard JA, Rowland RC. Blood volume changes in pregnancy and the puerperium. III. Whole body and large vessel hematocrits in pregnant and nonpregnant women. Am J Obstet Gynecol 1964; 88:391–395.
35. Lund CJ, Donovan JC. Blood volume during pregnancy. Am J Obstet Gynecol 1967; 98:393–403.
36. Longo LD. Maternal blood volume and cardiac output during pregnancy: a hypothesis of endocrinologic control. Am J Physiol 1983; 245:R720–R729.
37. Friedlander M, Laskey N, Silbert T. Effect of estrogenic substance on blood volume. Endocrinology 1936; 20:329–332.
38. Tapia HR, Johnson CE, Strong CG. Effects of oral contraceptive therapy on the renin–angiotensin system in normotensive and hypertensive women. J Obstet Gynecol 1973; 41:643–649.
39. Crane MG, Heitsch J, Harris JJ, Johns VJ Jr. Effect of ethinyl estradiol (Estinyl) on plasma renin activity. J Clin Endocrinol Metab 1966; 26:1403–1406.
40. Hsueh WA, Luetscher JA, Carlson EJ, Grislis G, Fraze E, McHargue A. Changes in active and inactive renin throughout pregnancy. J Clin Endocrinol Metab 1982; 54:1010–1016.
41. Abdul-Karim R, Assali NS. Pressor response to angiotonin in pregnant and nonpregnant women. Am J Obstet Gynecol 1961; 82:246–251.
42. Everett RB, Worley RJ, MacDonald PC, Gant NF. Effect of prostaglandin synthetase inhibitors on pressor response to antiotensin II in human pregnancy. J Clin Endocrinol Metab 1978; 46:1007–1010.
43. Pritchard JA, Adams RH. Erythrocyte production and destruction during pregnancy. Am J Obstet Gynecol 1960; 79:750–757.
44. Cotes PM, Canning CE, Lind T. Changes in serum immunoreactive erythropoietin during the menstrual cycle and normal pregnancy. Br J Obstet Gynecol 1983; 90:304–311.
45. Jepson JH, Friesen HG. The mechanism of action of human placental lactogen on erythropoiesis. Br J Haematol 1968; 15:465–471.
46. Efrati P, Presentey B, Margalith M, Rozenszajn L. Leukocytes of normal pregnant women. Obstet Gynecol 1964; 23:429–432.

47. Cutforth R, MacDonald CB. Heart sounds and murmurs in pregnancy. Am Heart J 1966; 71:741–747.
48. Ambrus CM, Niswander KR, Courey NG, Mink IB. Effect of contraceptive drugs on the blood coagulation system. Hematol Rev 1970; 2:163–168.
49. Zuck TF, Bergin JJ, Raymond JM, Dwyre WR. Implications of depressed antithrombin-III activity associated with oral contraceptives. Surg Gynecol Obstet 1971; 133:609–612.
50. Ambrus JL, Ambrus CM, Lillie MA, Browne BJ, Hanson FW, Niswander K, Witul M, Jung OS, Bartfay-Szabo A. Effects of various estrogen treatment schedules on antithrombin-III levels. Res Commun Chem Pathol Pharmacol 1976; 14:543–549.
51. Davidson BJ, Murray RD, Challis JRG, Valenzuela GJ. Estrogen, progesterone, prolactin, prostaglandin E_2, prostaglandin F_2, 13,14-dihydro-15-ketoprostaglandin $F_2\alpha$, and 6-keto-prostaglandin $F_1\alpha$ gradients across the uterus in labor and not in labor. Am J Obstet Gynecol 1987; 157:54–59.
52. Nelson GH, Fadel HE. Prostaglandins and parturition. Semin Reprod Endocrinol 1985; 3:231–237.
53. Gustavii B. Release of lysosomal acid phosphatase into the cytoplasm of decidual cells before the onset of labor in humans. Br J Obstet Gynaecol 1975; 82:177–182.
54. Schwartz BE, Schultz FM, MacDonald PC, Johnston JM. Initiation of human parturition: III. Fetal membrane content of prostaglandin E_2 and $F_2\alpha$ precursor. Obstet Gynecol 1975; 46:564–570.
55. Curbelo V, Bejar R, Benirschke K, Gluck L. Premature labor: 1. Prostaglandin precursors in human placental membranes. Obstet Gynecol 1981; 57:473–478.
56. Khan-Dawood FS. In vitro conversion of pregnenolone to progesterone in human term placenta and fetal membranes before and after the onset of labor. Am J Obstet Gynecol 1987; 157:1333–1337.
57. Mortimer G, Hunter IC, Stimson WH, Govan ADT. A role for amniotic epithelium in the control of human parturition. Lancet 1985; 1:1074–1076.
58. Auletta FJ, Agins H, Scommegna A. Prostaglandin F_2 mediation of the inhibitory effect of estrogen on the corpus luteum of the rhesus monkey. Endocrinology 1978; 103:1183–1189.
59. Auletta FJ, Caldwell BV, Speroff L. Estrogen induced luteolysis in the rhesus monkey: reversal with indomethacin. Prostaglandins 1976; 11:745–752.
60. Gant NF, Daley GL, Chand S, Whalley PF, MacDonald PC. A study of angiotensin II pressor response throughout primagravid pregnancy. J Clin Invest 1973; 52:2682–2689.
61. Fitzgerald DJ, Mayo G, Catella F, Entman SS, Fitzgerald GA. Increased thromboxone biosynthesis in normal pregnancy is mainly derived from platelets. Am J Obstet Gynecol 1987; 157:325–331.

62. Ylikorkala O, Pekonen F, Viinikka L. Renal prostacyclin and thromboxane in normotensive and preeclamptic pregnant women and their infants. J Clin Endocrinol Metab 1987; 63:1307–1312.
63. Goodman RP, Killam AP, Brash AR, Branch RA. Prostacyclin production during normal pregnancy and pregnancy complicated by hypertension. Am J Obstet Gynecol 1982; 142:817–822.
64. Fitzgerald DJ, Entman SS, Mulloy K, FitzGerarld GA. Decreased prostacyclin biosynthesis preceding the clinical manifestations of pregnancy-induced hypertension. Circulation 1987; 75:956–963.
65. Beaufils M, Donsimoni R, Uzan S, Colau JC. Prevention of pre-eclampsia by early antiplatelet therapy. Lancet 1985; 2:240–243.
66. Wallenberg HCS, Dekker GA, Makovitz JW, Rotmans P. Low dose aspirin prevents pregnancy-induced hypertension and preeclampsia in angiotensin-sensitive primigravidal. Lancet 1986; 1:1–6.
67. Masotti G, Poggesi L, Galanti G, Abbate R, Neri Serneri GG. Differential inhibition of prostaglandin production and platelet aggregation by aspirin. Lancet 1979; 2:1213–1216.
68. Ritter JM, Farquhar C, Rodin A, Thom MH. Low dose aspirin treatment in late pregnancy differentially inhibits cyclo-oxygenase in maternal platelets. Prostaglandins 1987; 34:717–721.
69. Judzewitsch R. Thyroid and adrenal function. In: Shearman RP, ed. Reproductive physiology. 2nd ed. Oxford: Blackwell Scientific, 1979.
70. Carr BR, Parker CRP Jr, Madden JD. Maternal plasma adrenocorticotropin and cortisol relationships throughout human pregnancy. Am J Obstet Gynecol 1981; 139:416–422.
71. Nolten WE, Rueckert PA. Elevated free cortisol index in pregnancy: possible regulatory mechanisms. Am J Obstet Gynecol 1981; 139:492–498.
72. Fain JN. Inhibition of glucose transport in fat cells and activation of lipolysis by glucocorticoids. In: Glucocorticoid hormone action. Baxter JD, Rousseau GG, eds. New York: Springer-Verlag, 1979; 547–560.
73. Hench PG. Ameliorating effect of pregnancy on chronic atrophic (infectious rheumatoid) arthritis, fibrositis and intermittent hydrarthrosis. Proc Mayo Clin 1938; 13:161–168.
74. Unger A, Kay A, Griffin AJ, Panayi GS. Disease activity and pregnancy associated α_2-glycoprotein in rheumatoid arthritis. Br Med J 1983; 286:750–752.
75. Winkel CA, Parker CR Jr, Milewich L, Simpson ER, Gant NF, MacDonald PC. The conversion of plasma progesterone to deoxycorticosterone (DOC) in men, nonpregnant and pregnant women and adrenalectomized subjects: evidence for steroid 21-hydroxylase activity in non-adrenal tissues. J Clin Invest 1980; 66:803–812.
76. Munch A, Brinck-Johnsen T. Specific and nonspecific physiochemical interactions of glucocorticoids and related steroids with rat thymus cells in vitro. J Biol Chem 1968; 10:5556–5565.

77. Bell PA. Agonists, antagonists and models for glucorticoid-receptor interactions. Biochem Soc Trans 1977; 5:639–642.
78. Rousseau GG, Baxter JD, Tomkins GM. Glucocorticoid receptors: relations between steroid binding and biological effects. J Mol Biol 1972; 67:99–115.
79. Teoh.J Obstet Gynaecol Br Commonw 1967; 74:77.
80. Seron-Ferre M, Lawrence CC, Jaffe RB. Role of hCG in the regulation of the fetal zone of the human fetal adrenal gland. J Clin Endocrinol Metab 1978; 46:834–837.
81. Nisula BC, Ketlslegers JM. Thyroid stimulating activity and chorionic gonadotropin. J Clin Invest 1974; 54:494–499.
82. Siiteri PK, Febres LE, Clemens LE, Chang RJ, Gondus B, Stites D. Progesterone and the maintenance of pregnancy: is progesterone nature's immunosuppressant? Ann NY Acad Sci 1977; 286:384–397.
83. Carr MC, Stites DP, Fudenberg HH. Cellular aspects of human fetal maternal relationship. II. In vitro response of gravida lymphocytes to phytohemagglutinin. Cell Immunol 1973; 8:448–454.
84. Teasdale FE, Adcock EW III, August CS, Cox S, Battaglia FC, Naughton MA. Human chorionic gonadotropin: inhibitory effect on mixed lymphocyte cultures. Gynecol Invest 1973; 4:263–269.
85. Josimovich JB, MacLaren JA. Presence in human placenta and term serum of highly lactogenic substance immunologically related to pituitary growth hormone. Endocrinology 1962; 71:209–220.
86. Selenkow HA, Saxena BM, Dana CL, Emerson K Jr. Measurements and pathologic significance of human placental lactogen. In: Peck A, Fenzi C, eds. The foeto-placental unit. Amsterdam: Excerpta Medica, 1964.
87. Nielsen PV, Pederson H, Karpmann E. Absence of human placental lactogen in an otherwise uneventful pregnancy. Am J Obstet Gynecol 1979; 135:322–326.
88. Kaistinen R, Kalkkinen N, Huhtala M-L, Seppala M, Bohn H, Rutanen E-M. Placental protein 12 is a decidual protein that binds somatomedin and has an identical N-terminal amino acid sequence with somatomedin binding protein from human amniotic fluid. Endocrinology 1986; 118:1375–1378.
89. Baxter RC, Martin JL, Wood MH. Two immunoreactive binding proteins for insulin-like growth factors in human amniotic fluid: relationship to fetal maturity. J Clin Endocrinol Metab 1987; 65:423–431.
90. Felig P, Lynch V. Starvation in human pregnancy: hypoglycemia, hypoinsulinemia and hyperketonemia. Science 1970; 170:990–992.
91. Hollingsworth DR. Alterations of maternal metabolism in normal and diabetic pregnancies in insulin-dependent, non insulin dependent and gestational diabetes. Am J Obstet Gynecol 1983; 146:417–429.
92. Robinson BG, Emanuel RL, Frim RM, Majzoub JA. Glucocorticoid stimulates expression of corticotropin releasing hormone gene in human placenta. Proc Natl Acad Sci 1988; 85:5244–5248.

93. Weisman Y, Harrell A, Edelstein S. 1α-25-dihydroxyvitamin D_3 and 24,25-dihydroxyvitamin D_3 in vitro synthesis by human decidua and placenta. Nature 1979; 281:317–319.
94. Fleishman AR. Fetal parathyroid gland and calcium homeostasis. Clin Obstet Gynecol 1980; 25:791–802.
95. Pitkin RM, Reynold WA, Williams GA, Hargis GK. Calcium metabolism in normal pregnancy: a longitudinal study. Am J Obstet Gynecol 1979; 133:781–790.

2

Fetal Oxygenation and Acid–Base Balance as It Relates to the Pregnancy Complicated by Asthma or Anaphylaxis

Larry Cousins and Valerian A. Catanzarite

Sharp Memorial Hospital, San Diego, California

Asthma, the most common, chronic respiratory disease seen in pregnant women, affects between 1:80 and 1:200 gravidas (1,2). This overall rate, combined with the 0.2–0.5% prevalence of life-threatening asthma or status asthmaticus in pregnancy (1,3) emphasizes the frequency of risk to which the asthmatic gravida and her fetus may be exposed.

The objectives of this chapter are to review the general issues related to fetal oxygenation, including determinants of uteroplacental–fetal oxygenation and blood flow considerations; to review the impact of alterations in fetal acid–base status on perinatal outcome and methods of assessing fetal well-being; and to recommend an approach to fetal evaluation in pregnancies complicated by asthma or anaphylaxis.

This chapter will not deal in detail with issues addressed elsewhere in the book that may indirectly influence fetal oxygenation: for example, hormonally induced alterations in respiratory center function, carbon dioxide sensitivity, or bronchodilator muscular tone; changes in ventilatory mechanics as a result of the enlarging, gravid uterus or alterations in large or small airway function; the natural history of asthma in pregnancy; or the medical management of asthma in pregnancy.

RESPIRATORY GAS EXCHANGE

Respiratory Gas Transport Between the Atmosphere and the Fetus

Introduction

The transport of oxygen from the atmosphere to fetal tissues and, conversely, of carbon dioxide from the fetus to the atmosphere, represent a series of steps occurring within the maternal–fetal diad (Figure 1). If one assumes normal respiratory muscle function, airway dimensions, and ventilatory control mechanisms, there is a volume exchange between the atmosphere and the alveoli that results in alveolar oxygen (Po_2) and carbon dioxide pressures (Pco_2) being maintained within certain limits. The diffusional transfer of oxygen and carbon dioxide across the maternal alveolar membrane is influenced by the Po_2 and Pco_2 gradients between the alveolar lumen and capillaries. Oxygen transport is further influenced by the rate of chemical reaction between oxygen and hemoglobin.

The transport of oxygen from the lungs to the placenta or of carbon dioxide from the placenta to the lungs is controlled, in part, by the blood flow between these organs. Most of the oxygen transported is in the bound state, and oxygen content is determined by Po_2, hemoglobin concentration, and the affinity of hemoglobin for oxygen. At physiological arterial and venous Po_2 (45–105 mmHg), hemoglobin saturations are greater than 75% and, accordingly, the quantity of oxygen per milliliter of blood is roughly equal to the product of oxygen saturation and hemoglobin concentration (4). In contrast with oxygen, carbon dioxide is carried primarily as bicarbonate, with smaller (but significant) amounts carried as dissolved CO_2 and in carbamino compounds.

The rate of transfer of oxygen and carbon dioxide across the placental membrane is again primarily determined by the pressure gradients for these two gases between the villus capillary (fetal compartment) and intervillous space (maternal compartment). The movement of oxygen from the placenta to fetal tissues or carbon dioxide from fetal tissues to the placenta is dependent on blood flow—in a volume sense—and an intact microcirculation. Furthermore, the quantity of oxygen transported from the placenta to fetal tissues is influenced by the hemoglobin concentration and the fetal hemoglobin affinity for oxygen. The oxygen crossing the placental membrane is equivalent to the sum of the oxygen exiting the placenta through the umbilical venules and the placental utilization of oxygen.

The constant uptake of oxygen and production of carbon dioxide within fetal tissue creates relatively low oxygen and high carbon diox-

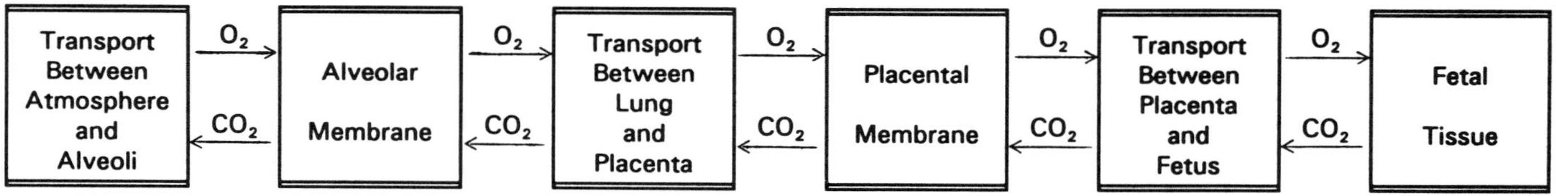

Figure 1 Transport of oxygen (O_2) and carbon dioxide (CO_2) between the atmosphere and fetal tissue. (Revised from Ref. 13.)

ide pressures in and around cells. In the intact organism these oxygen and carbon dioxide pressure gradients from blood to tissues explain the undirectional flow of oxygen to and carbon dioxide from tissues.

To better understand the processes suggested by Figure 1, we should consider how pregnancy or asthma may influence each step.

Minute Ventilation

The most consistently demonstrated, physiologic respiratory change during pregnancy is an increase in resting ventilation (5) (see also Chapter 3), Prowse and Gaensler reported a 48% increase in minute ventilation (6). Other investigators have reported a similar pattern (reviewed in 5). The currently accepted explanation for the hyperventilation of pregnancy is respiratory center stimulation by increasing concentrations of progesterone (5).

Diffusing Capacity of the Lung

During early pregnancy the diffusing capacity of the lung is felt to be generally unchanged or increased over nonpregnant values in the same patient. The diffusing capacity then frequently decreases to a plateau during the latter half of pregnancy, at a level that is equivalent to or slightly less than nonpregnant levels (5). The relative roles of alterations in pulmonary capillary blood volume, membrane diffusing capacity, and changes in maternal hemoglobin concentration on diffusing capacity remain to be clarified.

Oxygen Consumption

Oxygen consumption increases in pregnancy (6–9). The increase in uteroplacental–fetal tissue mass and increased physiological work (cardiac, respiratory, or other) would demand such an increase in oxygen consumption in the normal gravida. Interestingly, it appears there is a difference in the relative increase in oxygen consumption and minute ventilation. As noted earlier, minute ventilation increases approximately 50% in pregnancy over nonpregnant control levels (6). Furthermore, the increase in minute ventilation peaks well before the increase in oxygen consumption. The same investigators reported a 21% increase in oxygen consumption. Knuttgen and Emerson (7) and Pernoll and associates (8,9) reported a 50% increase in minute ventilation during exercise and a 30–35% increase in oxygen consumption in late pregnancy compared with postpartum measurements.

Oxygen Uptake and Ventilation in Labor

Oxygen uptake and minute ventilation are increased in women in labor compared with nonlaboring gravidas (10). Minute ventilation increases from 12 (±0.7) L/min in early labor to 23 (±0.2)L/min by the end of second-stage labor (Table 1). A similar, nonlinear increase in oxygen uptake occurs with progression of labor (see Table 1). Oxygen uptake is greater during contractions than between contractions. Dependent on the duration and strength of a contraction, mean oxygen uptake increases more than twofold from 281 (±30)mL/min between contractions to 703(±32)mL/min during contractions (10).

Arterial Blood Gases and Acid–Base Status

The increase in minute ventilation in pregnancy has been associated with a decrease in alveolar P_{CO_2} (P_{ACO_2}) and arterial P_{CO_2} (Pa_{CO_2}) to the range of 27–32 mmHg (11,12; see also Chapter 3). The increase in minute ventilation in pregnancy and the resultant relative hypocarbia produce a rise in maternal blood pH. This respiratory alkalosis-induced rise in pH is blunted by increased renal excretion of bicarbonate. The net effects of the respiratory alkalosis and increased renal bicarbonate excretion are a pH in the range of 7.40–7.45 (11,12), a serum bicarbonate decrease to 18–21 mEq/L, and a base deficit of approximately 3–4 mEq/L (11,12). In a normally ventilating gravida, exercise (11) and uterine contractions (10,11) increase minute ventilation and produce a further decrease in Pa_{CO_2}.

The Placenta as a Concurrent Exchange Mechanism

To better understand respiratory gas exchange between the maternal and fetal compartments requires an understanding of the exchange mechanism in the human (hemochorial) placenta. The placenta may be thought of as a membrane that separates maternal uterine blood flow

Table 1 Mean (±SEM) Oxygen Uptake and Minute Ventilation in the First and Second Stage of Labor

	Oxygen uptake ($mL\ min^{-1}\ m^{-2}$)	Minute ventilation ($L\ min^{-1}$)
1st stage of labor		
1 cm dilation	145 ± 18	12 ± 0.7
5 cm	204 ± 23	20 ± 0.3
8 cm	225 ± 19	21 ± 0.2
10 cm	259 ± 27	22 ± 0.2
2nd stage of labor		
Pelvic floor	266 ± 23	23 ± 0.2

Source: Ref. 10.

and umbilical blood flow. Maternal perfusion of the placenta is by the uterine arteries, which divide into progressively smaller vessels, ultimately ending in the spiral arterioles. These arterial microvessels perfuse the intervillous space and thereby bathe fetal villi. Maternal blood exits the intervillous space by uterine venules that join to form ever-larger venous structures, ultimately exiting the uterus through the uterine veins (primarily) or the venous collaterals through the ovary, bladder, and vagina. Relatively deoxygenated and hypercarbic fetal blood enters the placenta from the umbilical arteries, courses through the villus capillaries, and returns to the fetus through the umbilical vein as oxygenated and eucarbic blood.

How are these maternal and fetal microcirculations arranged? Possibilities include countercurrent and concurrent models of placental perfusion. In a countercurrent placenta the Po_2 of umbilical venous blood tends to equilibrate with the Po_2 of maternal arterial blood. As a consequence, in this model umbilical venous Po_2 can be higher than uterine venous Po_2. There is no persuasive morphological evidence of a circulatory arrangement within the human placenta whereby fetal venous blood equilibrates its Po_2 with the Po_2 of maternal arterial blood (13). The limited data from humans (10) and more extensive data in the rhesus monkey (14) have demonstrated that umbilical venous Po_2 may approximate, but does not exceed, uterine *venous* Po_2. These clinical and experimental data are most consistent with a concurrent model of placental perfusion. A concurrent mechanism, or venous equilibration model (13), suggests that umbilical venous Po_2 cannot exceed uterine venous Po_2. Umbilical venous Po_2 can equilibrate with uterine venous Po_2 only if there is no limitation of diffusing capacity across the trophoblastic membrane. The concurrent placental perfusion or venous equilibration model emphasizes the importance of the uterine venous site as the reference point for understanding umbilical venous blood gas changes.

The surprisingly low Po_2 in the oxygenated umbilical venous blood of 30–37 mmHg contrasts with the normal maternal arterial Po_2 of 100 mmHg. The fetus tolerates this relatively low Po_2 environment by several mechanisms. These include increased oxygen-carrying capacity, differences between adult and fetal oxygen–hemoglobin dissociation curves, high fetal cardiac output, and a unique distribution of fetal cardiac output. Fetal hemoglobin concentrations are significantly higher than adult blood, 15–18 g/L versus 12–13 g/L. The oxygen–hemoglobin dissociation curve of fetal blood lies to the left of the maternal curve, resulting in relatively high oxygen saturation of umbilical venous blood, despite the low Po_2. This characteristic of the fetal oxygen–hemoglobin dissociation curve also allows significant desaturation of fetal hemoglobin at the Po_2 levels found in fetal tissues. Lastly, the maximally oxygenated fetal umbilical venous blood is preferentially shunted through the foramen ovale to vital organs, such as the brain and heart. The less well-oxygenated blood is distributed to lungs, gut, and other vascular beds less vital in fetal life.

Factors Determining Uterine Venous Oxygen Pressure

Given that the human placenta functions as a concurrent exchanger of Po_2 respiratory gases, uterine venous Po_2 levels best reflect the Po_2 in fetal oxygenated (umbilical venous) blood. Therefore, it is important to be aware of factors influencing uterine venous Po_2 levels. The primary determinants of uterine venous Po_2 are the oxyhemoglobin dissociation curve of maternal blood and oxygen saturation in uterine venous blood (Table 2).

The oxyhemoglobin dissociation curve of maternal blood is influenced by the type of hemoglobin (hemoglobin A, F, S, or other), temperature, 2,3-diphosphoglycerate (DPG) levels, and pH. Changes in pH shift the oxyhemoglobin dissociation curve (Figure 2), so that at any given O_2 saturation, the Po_2 is inversely related to pH (i.e., a decrease in pH is associated with an increase in Po_2 and vice versa). Oxygen saturation of uterine venous blood is determined by arterial O_2 saturation, uteroplacental blood flow, oxygen-carrying capacity of maternal blood, and uteroplacental and fetal oxygen consumption.

Therapeutically, the clinician has little influence over the factors influencing the oxyhemoglobin dissociation curve (see Table 2). In contrast, the clinician may influence the factors determining oxygenation in uterine venous blood. Maternal position may influence arterial oxy-

Table 2 Determinants of Uterine Venous Po_2

Oxyhemoglobin dissociation curve
Hemoglobin type: A, S, F, other
Temperature
2,3-diphosphoglycerate (DPG)
pH
O_2 saturation of uterine venous blood
Arterial O_2 saturation
Uteroplacental blood flow
O_2-carrying capacity
Uteroplacental–fetal O_2 consumption

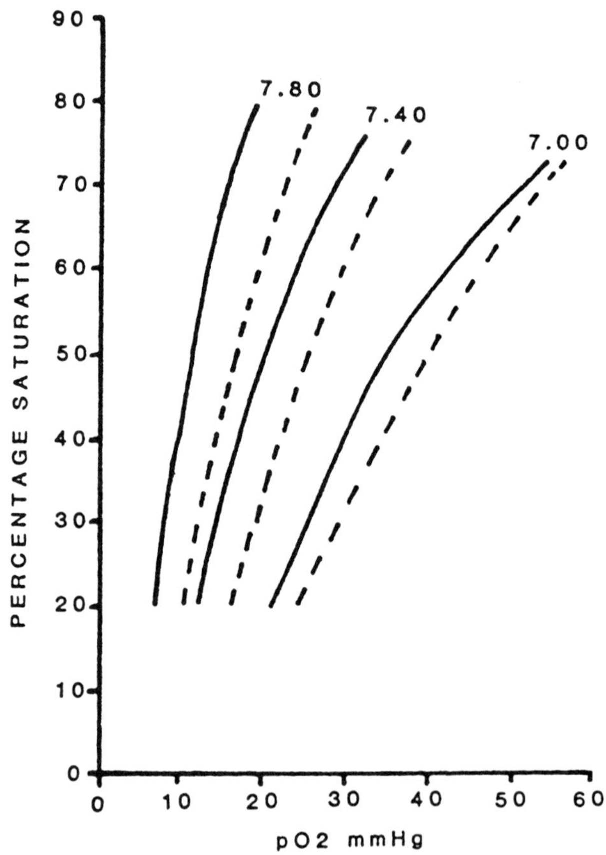

Figure 2 Oxygen dissociation curves of fetal (——) and maternal (---) human blood prepared at pHs 7.00–7.80 and 38°C. (Revised from Hellegers and Schruefer. Am J Obstet Gynecol 1961.)

gen tensions. Awe and associates (15), studying 23 nonsmoking, medically uncomplicated gravidas within 6 weeks before delivery, demonstrated that only 1 subject when tested in the sitting position had a Po_2 less than 90 mmHg. Among these late pregnant women tested after 15 minutes in the supine position, 26% had a Po_2 less than 90 mmHg (15). The frequency (26%) of modest hypoxemia found in normal, late pregnant, supine gravidas appears to be prevented by a 15° left uterine displacement (12). These investigators studying 20 nonsmoking, medically normal women at 38 weeks gestation in the supine position with 15° left uterine tilt found the arterial Po_2 to be 101.8 $\pm$1.0 mmHg (mean ±SE). This value is remarkably similar to the mean (±SD) of 101.2(±7.0) mmHg of the late pregnant gravidas sampled by Awe et al. in the sitting position (15).

Maternal oxygen therapy can remarkably alter maternal arterial oxygenation. The oxygen therapy-induced rise in maternal arterial Po_2 is accompanied by a small increase in fetal umbilical artery Po_2 levels (10). It is important not to conclude from the surprisingly small umbilical artery Po_2 changes with oxygen therapy that maternal oxygen therapy does not benefit the oxygenation status of the fetus. The venous equilibration model of placental exchange and the characteristics of maternal and fetal oxyhemoglobin dissociation curves explain why the changes in fetal arterial Po_2 with maternal oxygen therapy is numerically small (13). In a gravida with a normal Po_2, if oxygen therapy increases her arterial oxygen content 1 mM and there is no appreciable change in uterine blood flow or uterine oxygen consumption, the 1 mM increase in maternal arterial oxygen content would result in approximately a 0.7 mM increase in fetal oxygen content (Figure 3). Interestingly, and relevant to the pregnant asthmatic patient, maternal oxygen therapy of a gravida who is hypoxic could conceivably result in a greater

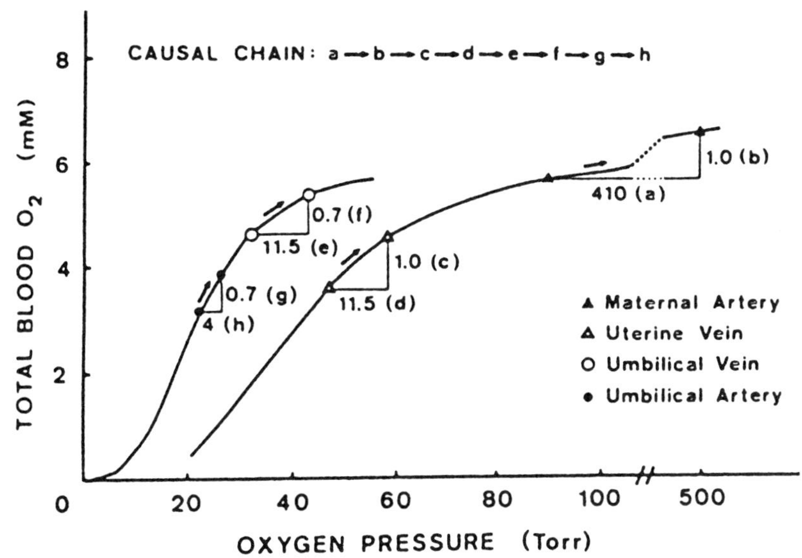

Figure 3 Example of the relationship between oxygen content and Po_2 in maternal and fetal blood before and after maternal inhalation of 100% oxygen. (From Ref. 13.)

increase in fetal oxygen content than maternal oxygen content (Figure 4). Thus, it can be seen that maternal oxygen therapy has the potential to significantly increase fetal oxygen content and, therefore, be especially beneficial in the circumstance in which fetal hypoxia is a direct consequence of maternal hypoxia.

Uteroplacental blood flow is influenced by the degree of hydration, cardiac output, and maternal position. Uteroplacental blood flow can be optimized by normalizing hydration and avoiding circumstances that compromise cardiac output. An enlarging uterus increases the gravida's predisposition to supine hypotension. This is secondary to venocaval obstruction, venous pooling in the pelvis and lower extremities, decreased cardiac return, and reduced cardiac output. This sequence of events is especially likely in the third trimester. A reduction in cardiac output in the supine position has been convincingly demonstrated (16), and such impairment could account for significant reductions in arterial Po_2 (17).

Steps taken during the antepartum period to ensure a normal maternal hemoglobin will optimize the woman's oxygen-carrying capacity. Maternal anemia (hemoglobin values lower than 10 g/L) should be evaluated and treated.

Fetal hyperglycemia stimulates endogenous insulin secretion and, subsequently, increased oxygen consumption. It then follows that iatro-

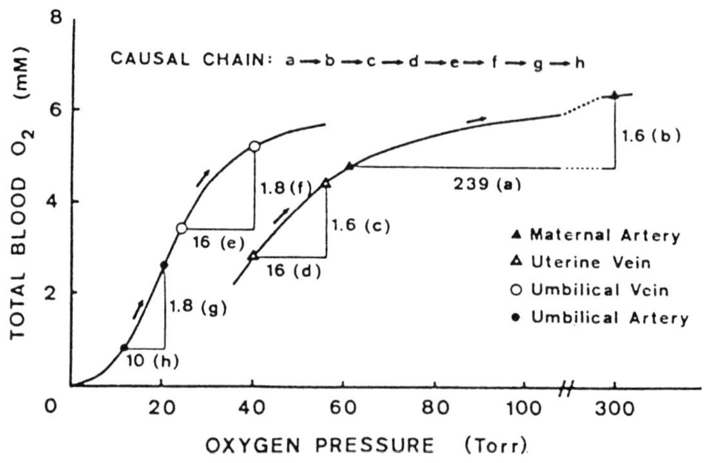

Figure 4 Example of the pronounced effect of oxygen therapy on fetal oxygen content in a case of fetal hypoxia secondary to maternal hypoxia. (From Ref. 13.)

genic hyperglycemia secondary to bolus infusions of dextrose may increase fetal oxygen consumption. Hyperglycemia, whether spontaneous, as in diabetes, or iatrogenic, should be avoided because it may precipitate fetal hypoxia and acidosis (18).

In summary, maternal venous PO_2 is optimal when the gravida is ventilating normally, afebrile, has a normal hemoglobin level, is normotensive, is euglycemic, and is sitting or supine with a 15° left uterine displacement. In situations complicated by maternal hypoxia, maternal oxygen therapy should improve uterine venous PO_2 and, therefore, umbilical venous PO_2.

UTEROPLACENTAL–FETAL OXYGEN UTILIZATION

Measurement

Oxygen uptake across a vascular bed can be calculated by simultaneously measuring arterial–venous oxygen content differences and blood flow. Application of this rationale, the Fick principle, to the uteroplacental–fetal mass indicates that measurements of uterine arterial–venous oxygen content differences will allow calculation of the combined oxygen utilization of the uterus, placenta, and fetus. The Fick principle, when applied to the umbilical circulation, allows calculation of fetal oxygen uptake. Simultaneous application of these measurements to both the uterine and umbilical circulations allows calculation of oxygen uptake of the uterus, placenta, and fetus combined, and the fetus alone. The difference between these two measurements would be the oxygen uptake of the uterus and placenta. In the late pregnant, continuously catheterized sheep model, oxygen uptake of the uterus, placenta, and fetus was 9.6 mL $min^{-1}kg^{-1}$ (13). Fetal oxygen uptake was 6.6 mL $min^{-1}kg^{-1}$ (13). Consequently, uteroplacental oxygen uptake was 3.0 mL $min^{-1}kg^{-1}$. Similarly precise measurements in humans are not available. As pointed out by Meschia (13), extrapolation from nonhuman data should be made cautiously. Among species, differences in body composition (e.g., brain mass and adipose tissue), body temperatures, and growth rates would suggest that fetal oxygen uptakes could be remarkably different. Other information, however, indicates that oxygen uptake rates in humans could approximate other species. Despite between-species differences in growth, body size, and composition, different species appear to have comparable fetal oxygen uptakes per kilogram of body weight. It is currently possible to obtain maternal arterial and uterine venous and umbilical arterial and venous samples at the time of cesarean section. Confirmation of human fetal oxygen uptake measurements awaits the availability of a practical method for obtaining simultaneous uterine and umbilical blood flow determinations.

Increased Rate of Fetal Metabolism and Placental Reserve

Increased fetal oxygen utilization has been produced in experimental animal models using fetal infusions of norepinephrine and triiodothyronine (19). In the continuously catheterized fetal lamb model, infusions of norepinephrine and triiodothyronine resulted in increased fetal oxygen consumption, without any demonstrable change in placental diffusing capacity or fetal venous and arterial blood gas measurements. The authors concluded that increases in fetal oxygen consumption in the range of 25–30% did not exceed the capacity of the placenta to provide increased oxygen for fetal requirements.

UTEROPLACENTAL AND FETAL BLOOD FLOW

Uterine Blood Flow

The importance of maintaining an adequate and uninterrupted uterine blood flow is emphasized by calculations that suggest that, if uterine blood flow ceases, there is only a 2-min fetal reserve of oxygen (20). The normal 30–50% increase in cardiac output with progression of pregnancy in large part provides for the increase in uterine blood flow that is necessary to nourish and "ventilate" the growing fetal–placental mass. Pathological conditions, such as chronic hypertension, preeclampsia, and other conditions (long-standing diabetes, systemic lupus erythematosus, other collagen vascular disorders), known to affect large and small arterial vessels may reduce placental perfusion as a result of the vascular changes.

Exaggerated maternal hyperventilation may have a deleterious effect on fetal oxygenation through several mechanisms. One mechanism involves a reduction in uterine blood flow associated with the mechanical effects of hyperventilation. Because hyperventilation, as well as hypocarbia, may influence uterine blood flow, it has been difficult to sort out the relative contribution of these alterations to fetal acid–base changes. Levinson and associates (14) constructed an experimental protocol in which they were able to control both P_{CO_2} levels and respiratory rate in chronically catheterized sheep. In hyperventilating pregnant ewes, they demonstrated a reduction in uterine blood flow that was maintained even when maternal P_{CO_2} levels were kept in a eucarbic range. Uterine blood flow returned to normal only when hyperventilation ceased. Although this study seems to have effectively ruled out a direct effect of hypocarbia in reducing uterine blood flow, the precise mechanisms by which hyperventilation reduced uterine blood flow remains to be clarified. Possible mechanisms include a compensatory response to decreased cardiac output that results from the following:

1. A decreased cardiac return secondary to hyperventilation.
2. The decreased venous return associated with hyperventilation may decrease distention of the right and left atria and pulmonary vascular bed. These changes stimulate a sympathetic response that may decrease uterine blood flow (see later section on catecholamine-induced decrease in uterine blood flow.)

Other mechanisms linking maternal hyperventilation with reductions in fetal oxygenation include

1. A left shift in the oxyhemoglobin dissociation curve, resulting in increased affinity of maternal hemoglobin for oxygen and, therefore, decreased transfer of oxygen from the maternal to the fetal compartment (see Figure 2).
2. Maternal alkalosis may increase intraplacental shunting, resulting in a mismatching of maternal and fetal circulations (21).
3. To whatever extent hyperventilation results in a decrease in cardiac output, there is the potential for a disproportionate reduction in blood flow to the uterine vascular tree.

Uterine blood flow is sensitive to adrenergic stimulation. The first systematic examination of the effect of catecholamines on uterine blood flow was by Robson and Schild (22). They found that uterine arteries of pregnant or spayed cats constricted in response to epinephrine. Subsequently, studies in dogs (23), sheep (24), and rhesus monkeys (25) reported reductions in uterine blood flow with varying maternal infusion regimens of catecholamines. Rosenfeld et al. (24) found that epinephrine infusions into gravid sheep produced 39% reduction in total uterine blood flow. The infusion rates used during the blood flow experiments did not produce a change in maternal blood pressure. The demonstrated reduction in total uterine blood flow was explained by reductions in myometrial, cotyledonary, and endometrial flow. Adamson and associates (25) found, in rhesus monkeys, that epinephrine and norepinephrine infusions to the mother sufficient to raise blood pressure were also associated with increased uterine contractions and decreased uterine blood flow. They concluded that the fetal hypoxia, hypercarbia, and acidosis resulting from catecholamine infusions placed the fetus in double jeopardy of hypoxia and acidosis by directly decreasing uterine blood flow and by increasing uterine activity, which will further decrease placental perfusion. An awareness of these adrenergic-induced changes in uterine blood flow is especially relevant to the asthmatic patient who may be exposed to epinephrine or other catecholamines in the course of her medical treatment.

Umbilical Fetal Circulation

Chronic hypoxia may increase erythropoietin levels and, consequently, red blood cell production. A significant increase in hematocrit may be associated with increased viscosity and a compromise in small-vessel perfusion. Umbilical compression is another potential source of reduced fetal perfusion. Umbilical cord compression can occur persistently with fetal entanglement in its umbilical cord (e.g., nuchal cord), with a true knot in the cord, and with oligohydramnios. Whether umbilical compression occurs suddenly or over time, it may result in a reduction in umbilical circulation and consequent impairment of respiratory gas exchange across the placental membrane, hypercarbia, and hypoxia.

RELATION OF ALTERATIONS OF MATERNAL OXYGENATION ON FETAL OXYGENATION AND ACID–BASE STATUS

The most common cause of maternal hypoxemia in patients with asthma is pulmonary ventilation–perfusion imbalance (26). The absolute or relative hypoxemia that results from the admixture of pulmonary venous effluent from normally ventilated and poorly ventilated areas of lung parenchyma thereby compromises available oxygen perfusing the placenta. Wulf et al. (10) found that a reduction in maternal P_{O_2} from 92 to 65 mmHg resulted in a reduction in umbilical venous P_{O_2} from 32 to 26 mmHg. Changes of this degree result in a significant reduction in fetal oxygen content. Even during a mild asthmatic attack, the alterations that occur (decreased P_{O_2}, decreased P_{CO_2}, increased pH, increased respiratory rate), each individually predispose to impaired fetal oxygenation. The mild hypoxemia was addressed in the foregoing. The maternal hyperventilation and decrease in P_{CO_2} are associated with a decrease in fetal P_{O_2} levels (10). The rise in maternal pH results in a shift of the oxyhemoglobin dissociation curve to the left and, consequently, to a reduction in the availability of oxygen to the fetus (see Figure 2). As the severity of an asthmatic attack evolves from mild to moderate (lower Po_2, normal pH, and normal Pco_2) to severe (even lower Po_2, low pH, and hypercarbia), the increased risk to the mother is proportional to the worsening fetal state (27). If maternal arterial Po_2 falls below 60 mmHg, the fetus is at an especially high risk (3).

EFFECT OF ANAPHYLAXIS ON THE FETUS

Anaphylaxis is problematic in any situation, but especially so during pregnancy (see also Chapter 15). This is because both anaphylaxis as well as its treatment have significant implications for the fetus. The clinical features of anaphylaxis that may occur individually or in combination include upper airway obstruction, lower airway (bronchial) constriction, hypotension, and myocardial dysfunction. The maternal and fetal implications of hypoxia, hypercarbia, and hyperventilation, secondary to upper and lower airway obstruction, no doubt explain in part the high mortality rate associated with anaphylactic reactions (28). Maternal hypotension, with or without myocardial dysfunction (e.g., arrhythmias, ischemia), will result in a reduction in uterine perfusion. This reduction may be disproportionately large, given that the uterine vasculature is not a protected vascular bed, such as the cerebral or cardiac vasculature.

Epinephrine continues to be the drug of choice for the treatment of anaphylaxis (28). It has retained this position in the treatment armamentarium for anaphylaxis because of its ability to counteract vasodilation, bronchial constriction, and other adverse effects of anaphylactic mediators on target tissues, and to inhibit the further release of mediators from mast cells and basophils (28). Treatment of the gravid woman experiencing an anaphylactic reaction is complicated by her pregnancy. Reduction in uterine perfusion that may result from anaphylaxis-induced hypotension may be exaggerated by the profound α-adrenergic effects of epinephrine. Epinephrine-induced uterine vasoconstriction produces decreased uterine perfusion (24,25). Thus, the fetal risk inherent with maternal anaphylaxis may be compounded by α-adrenergic effects of epinephrine on uterine perfusion. This concern led Entman and Moise (29) to suggest that ephedrine, a noncatecholamine adrenergic drug, may be preferable for provision of cardiovascular support in allergic reactions in pregnant women. Ephedrine supports blood pressure by a β-agonist effect of increasing cardiac output. Ephedrine doses of 25–50 mg by intravenous push can be useful in supporting maternal systemic blood pressure without compromising uterine blood flow. Higher doses are associated with an α-adrenergic effect (30).

FETAL ASSESSMENT

Fetal compromise occurs uncommonly in mild or in well-controlled asthma, but acute and chronic fetal effects may result from severe or poorly controlled asthma. Acute exacerbations of asthma that result in impaired maternal oxygenation may directly impair that of the fetus. If this reaches a critical threshold, fetal distress or death may result. In patients with chronically impaired oxygenation, placental oxygen transfer may be sufficiently restricted to interfere with fetal growth, resulting in long-term effects on the fetus; for example, growth impairment (intrauterine growth retardation; IUGR), which predisposes to fetal distress, fetal death in utero, and neonatal morbidity.

In this section, modalities available for fetal assessment are detailed. In the next, their integration into the obstetrical management of the pregnant asthmatic is described.

Gestational Age

Accurate pregnancy dating is a cornerstone of optimal obstetric care. Dating is essential to evaluate fetal growth, to anticipate fetal maturity, and to time obstetrical interventions.

By convention, obstetricians calculate gestational age from the last menstrual period, presuming a regular, 28-day menstrual cycle. In this situation, conception occurs at 2 weeks after the first day of the last menstrual period (also 2 weeks before the missed menstrual period). Full-term gestation is considered to be 40 weeks from the last menstrual period. If the cycle length is shorter or longer than 28 days, the estimated date of confinement can be calculated by adding 38 weeks to the ovulation or conception date, if this is known, since ovulation and conception regularly occur 2 weeks before the missed menstrual period. Alternatively, the estimated date of confinement can be calculated by adding 36 weeks to the date of the first missed menstrual period (31).

In the past, the menstrual history and physical examination findings from the first trimester of pregnancy were used in pregnancy dating. However, many women either do not have regular menstrual cycles or do not record them. In particular, women with chronic disease states are prone to menstrual irregularities, which invalidate the use of menstrual dating in gestational age assessment.

Fortunately, ultrasound has become a simple, reliable, and accurate means of dating pregnancy. If fetal measurements from an ultrasound examination fit with the gestational age of 7–13 weeks, the error is ±7 days; if measurements fit with 13–22 weeks, the error is ±10 days (32). Because biological variation in fetal growth increases with increasing gestational age, particularly during the latter half of gestation, the accuracy of sonography for pregnancy dating decreases as the pregnancy advances. Between 22- and 28-weeks gestation, the accuracy of sonography is ±2 weeks, and beyond 28 weeks, sonographic measurements are less reliable as a predictor of gestational age (±21 days).

Fetal Growth

Once the gestational age is established, uterine and sonographic measurements are used for fetal growth assessment.

In asthma, IUGR may occur secondary to diminished uteroplacental transfer of oxygen to the fetus. The mechanism is as follows: When the intrauterine environment is suboptimal, the fetal response is to redistribute blood flow to vital organs (i.e., heart, brain, and adrenal glands) (33). The skin, muscles, and viscera are relatively hypoperfused. Although this adaptation is useful in protecting the fetus from sudden changes, continued stress of this nature results in an *asymmetric growth retardation* pattern, in which head growth, and to a lesser extent, linear growth of the fetus are relatively spared, whereas abdominal girth, skin thickness, and muscle mass are diminished (34).

Intrauterine growth retardation represents a significant risk factor for in utero fetal death, fetal distress during labor, and neonatal morbidity (35). Thus, it is considered to be an indication for intensive fetal surveillance, and it may be an indication for delivery (see later under Obstetric Management).

For the low-risk pregnant patient, screening for fetal growth retardation is by serial measurements of the uterine fundal height. Between 20- and 35-weeks gestation, the distance from the symphysis to the top of the fundus, measured in centimeters, matches gestational age within about 2 weeks. If a significant discrepancy between fundal height and gestational age occurs, the more sensitive and specific sonographic assessment is used to assess for fetal growth problems. For the high-risk patient, sonography is used as the screening and confirmatory tool.

Typically, during sonography, the placental location, fetal presentation and position, amniotic fluid volume, and biometry of the fetus are evaluated. Measurements include the biparietal diameter, head circumference, abdominal circumference, and femur length. These individual measurements may be plotted against gestational age to infer patterns of growth disturbance. For example, in asymmetric intrauterine growth retardation, the biparietal diameter and head circumference may fall in the 40th percentile range for gestational age, the femur length at the 20th or 30th percentile, and the abdominal circumference less than the 3rd percentile. Ratios between head and abdominal measurements, and also between femur and abdominal measurements have also been useful in the diagnosis of IUGR (36). Estimation of fetal weight is available through a number of formulas involving combinations of biometric parameters (e.g., biparietal diameter and abdominal circumference, head circumference and abdominal circumference, femur length and abdominal circumference) (37). The use of an estimated fetal weight of less than 10th percentile for dates as the diagnostic criterion for IUGR has sensitivity and specificity in the 80–90% range. These levels are comparable with the sensitivity and specificity measurements for any other tested means of detecting IUGR. Fetal weight estimation is the standard in the assessment of fetal growth (38).

In addition to overall estimation of fetal weight, ultrasound and Doppler ultrasound provide the means for inferential assessment of the perfusion of at-risk fetal organ systems. The best-validated tool for such is assessment of amniotic fluid volume. Amniotic fluid is produced continuously during pregnancy by efflux of fluid from the fetal trachea and, quantitively more important, production of urine. Reduction of renal blood flow, as may occur with redistribution of blood flow in IUGR, results in diminished fetal urine production and, thereby, decreases amniotic fluid volume. The "four-quadrant technique" for assessing amniotic fluid volume during pregnancy has been reproducible and reliable as a screening tool for impaired amniotic fluid production (39). The deepest vertical fluid pocket in each of the four quadrants of the uterus is measured, and these four measurements are summed to form the *amniotic fluid index* (AFI). An AFI of less than 6 cm is abnormal at any time during the third trimester. Decreased amniotic fluid volume, as assessed by this technique, has been predictive of adverse fetal outcomes, including fetal distress in labor and adverse neonatal outcomes. Decreased amniotic fluid volume occurs commonly in patients with IUGR; however, even in the absence of IUGR, a diminished AFI is a presumptive indicator of chronic uteroplacental insufficiency.

Measurements of blood flow to various fetal organs are now available. Pulse-wave and continuous-wave Doppler techniques have been used to measure systolic and diastolic flow in the intracranial circulation, descending aorta, ductus arteriosus, umbilical cord, and other vascular structures of the fetus. Of these measurements, umbilical flow velocity wave forms have been best studied in relation to pregnancy surveillance. It is clear that elevated placental vascular resistance may reduce diastolic umbilical flow and result in an increased ratio of systolic to diastolic blood flow (S/D ratio) in the umbilical artery. A significantly elevated S/D ratio is suggestive of fetal compromise, even in the absence of IUGR or oligohydramnios. Elevated S/D ratios are considered to be an indicator for intensive fetal surveillance. If diastolic flow ceases, or is reversed, the fetus is at high risk for in utero death, and delivery is often indicated (40).

Relation of Fetal Maturity to Survival

Obstetrical intervention in complicated pregnancies is determined by balancing risks to the fetus from remaining in utero against those of extrauterine life, and balancing these against risks to the mother from intervention. Before about 25 weeks gestation, neonatal survival ex utero is very poor and, thus, if fetal jeopardy is implied, interventions, if any, must be directed toward improving the intrauterine environment. However, the rate of fetal survival at 25 weeks is about 10%, advancing to 60% at 26 weeks gestation, 80% at 28 weeks gestation, and over 90% at 30 weeks gestation (41). In the context of neonatal morbidity and the high rate of abnormal neurological outcomes in very low birth weight babies, obstetric intervention is generally reserved for pregnancies beyond 26 weeks gestation.

The threshold for delivery of the fetus, rather than continued in utero management, steadily declines as gestation advances. Fetal survival and long-term outcome relate well to three factors: fetal weight, condition at delivery, and lung maturity. For the fetus delivered in good condition, with mature lungs, and a weight in excess of 1.8–2 kg, neonatal mortality is virtually nil, and significant morbidity is uncommon.

Fetal weight estimation, as mentioned earlier, is performed by sonographic measurements and application of any of a number of weight-estimation formulas. Lung maturity can be assessed only invasively by amniocentesis. Several biochemical assessments of lung maturity have been developed, but the standard is determination of the lecithin/sphingomyelin (L/S) ratio within amniotic fluid and of the presence or absence of phosphatidylglycerol (42). Amniocentesis is performed by directing a needle, under ultrasound guidance, into the amniotic cavity. In experienced hands, amniocentesis carries minimal risk to the pregnancy.

A mature lung profile—an L/S ratio higher than 2.0 and the presence of phosphatidylglycerol—predicts that the fetus will not have respiratory distress syndrome. If the L/S ratio is higher than 2.0 in the absence of phosphatidylglycerol, as long as the patient is not diabetic, the prediction is that the baby will have at worst moderate respiratory disease and that at most short-term ventilator therapy will be required.

Fetal Health

One major goal of fetal surveillance is to prevent stillbirth and fetal distress near the time of delivery.

The simplest test of fetal health has been known since ancient times. This is the presence of an actively moving fetus. Both maternal observations and sonographic studies of the fetus confirm that a sleep–wake or activity–inactivity cycle develops in utero as early as 20-weeks gestation. Normally, a fetus will not be inactive for more than 30–45 min at a time. During the third trimester, when intervention for fetal jeopardy would be undertaken, mothers easily perceive fetal movement, and this can be used as a screening test for fetal health. One simple screening tool is to ask patients to count kicks for 1 hr daily; if ten kicks or discrete movements are not felt during the hour of monitoring, the patient is asked to report for more careful evaluation (43).

For high-risk patients, or for the patient with an inability to perceive fetal movement, fetal heart rate monitoring is used as a sensitive means of assessment of fetal health in utero. Fetal heart rate accelerations occur regularly in response to fetal movement beyond 28-weeks gestation and are often seen as early as 26-weeks gestation. Empirically, accelerations of the fetal heart rate of 15 beats per minute or more (which typically occur during fetal movements) are associated with fetal health in utero. In fact, the presence of such accelerations (*reactive nonstress test*) is associated with a very low rate of fetal death in utero within 3–4 days of testing, as long as the clinical situation is stable and the fetal heart rate tracing is otherwise normal (44).

Although a reactive nonstress test is an excellent predictor of fetal health, the fetus who does not show acceleration is not necessarily compromised. Nonreactive tracings may occur in pregnancies of fewer than 32 weeks, in the fetus with central nervous system anomalies, when the mother has taken sedative–hypnotic drugs or alcohol, or rarely, when a prolonged "sleep" state of the fetus is present. There are two alternative means of accessing fetal health in utero in this situation.

The first is the biophysical profile (BPP). The biophysical profile consists of a nonstress test, followed by sonographic observation of the fetus for up to 30 min.

The biophysical profile test is scored as follows (45):

Amniotic fluid volume: Normal if a pocket at least 2 × 2 cm is present
Fetal tone: Normal if at least one episode of limb or trunk extension followed by return to flexion is seen
Limb movement: Normal if at least three discrete movements are seen

Breathing: Normal if at least one episode of breathing lasting at least 30 sec is seen

Nonstress test: Normal if a reactive fetal heart rate pattern is seen

Each normal observation is scored 2 points, and the sum is added to form the BPP score (range: 0–10). A BPP score of 8 or 10 is highly reassuring for fetal well-being, and the risk of fetal demise within 3–4 days of testing is extremely low. A score of 4–6 is intermediate, and a score of zero or 2 is indicative of fetal compromise and, usually, delivery is recommended. As with the nonstress test, the BPP is not robust to effects of alcohol or sedative drugs on the mother; fetal tone, limb movements, and breathing movements are absent when such drugs are present.

A third test of fetal health is the contraction stress test (46). Here, the fetal heart rate is continuously monitored while mild uterine contractions are induced, either my means of maternal nipple stimulation or oxytocin infusion. If there are no "late decelerations" of the fetal heart rate following uterine contractions, with a contraction frequency of at least three per 10 min, the contraction stress test is read as "negative," and the chance of fetal death in utero within the next week is extremely low. A tracing showing persistent late decelerations is usually considered an indication for delivery; for tracings showing intermittent late decelerations (late deceleration accompanying less than half of contractions), management is individualized.

Oxygenation

Fetal oxygenation and acid–base status cannot be directly monitored on a continuous basis in utero. The fetal circulation is intermittently accessible to percutaneous umbilical blood sampling (PUBS). Under ultrasound guidance, a needle may be introduced into the fetal umbilical cord and a blood sample directly obtained for assessment of acid–base status and oxygenation (47). However, this procedure may be technically difficult (or impossible), depending on fetal and placental position and maternal size. Also, PUBS carries a risk of 2–5% for fetal distress in most series. Because it gives only a single assessment of fetal oxygenation, its use for this purpose is quite limited.

When the intrauterine environment is unstable (i.e., when maternal oxygenation is unstable) or when the fetus is under the stress of uterine activity during labor, continuous fetal heart rate monitoring is indicated. The combination of fetal heart rate accelerations and the absence of late decelerations in response to contractions excludes the possibility of fetal hypoxia or acidosis. For a thorough discussion of the issues of fetal heart rate monitoring, the reader is referred to standard texts (48).

Obstetrical Management of the Pregnant Asthmatic Patient

Optimally, care of the pregnant asthmatic patient begins with an assessment before conception. At this point, the severity of the patient's asthma and the level of control of asthma can be assessed and projected risk and interventions during pregnancy can be discussed. The conventional medications used to treat asthma—β-sympathomimetic drugs, corticosteroids, theophylline and cromolyn are not contraindicated during pregnancy (see Chapters 7, 8, and 13).

Once the patient becomes pregnant, we perform an ultrasound examination between week 16 and 20 of the pregnancy to confirm gestational age and to assess for structural defects of the fetus.

For patients with mild or well-controlled asthma, obstetric management is similar to routine pregnancy care. The patient is seen at monthly intervals until 32 weeks, then at 34 and 36 weeks, and weekly until term. Kick counts are recommended to the patient from 26-weeks gestation onward, and the fundal height is measured at each visit. Sonography is performed for these patients only if the fundal height falls behind gestational age or for other obstetrical indications. Routine fetal monitoring is not performed, but is reserved for those patients who have either fetal growth disturbances, as demonstrated by sonography, or abnormal fetal movement.

For the patient with severe or poorly controlled asthma, fetal surveillance is more intensive. We perform sonography for serial assessment of fetal growth at 26 weeks, and then at 4- to 6-week intervals throughout the pregnancy. As long as fetal growth is normal and maternal perception of fetal movement is normal, fetal monitoring is initiated at 32 weeks with twice-weekly nonstress testing. If fetal growth is impaired or if maternal perception of fetal movement is abnormal, fetal heart rate monitoring is initiated earlier, as early as 26-weeks gestation.

In the patient with normal fetal growth and amniotic fluid volume, the pregnancy is allowed to proceed to term and no other obstetrical interventions are necessary. If intrauterine growth retardation is diagnosed, but amniotic fluid volume and nonstress testing remain normal, the pregnancy is generally allowed to proceed. However, if the growth impairment is progressive, early delivery following demonstration of a mature lung profile is often considered.

As mentioned previously, the fetus with reduced amniotic fluid volume is at particular risk for adverse outcomes. For these cases, intensive antenatal surveillance is required, and therapy is individualized; often, oligohydramnios will prompt consideration of early delivery for fetal indications.

When a pregnant patient develops an acute exacerbation of asthma, management of the asthmatic episode per se is as for the nonpregnant patient, with use of inhaled bronchodilators, corticosteroids, and aminophylline (see Chapters 13 and Appendix). However, careful monitoring of maternal oxygenation, particularly during the third trimester, is essential. Since the placenta is perfused by an admixture of maternal venous and arterial blood, the fetal oxygenation is relatively protected from changes in maternal arterial oxygenation so long as maternal cardiac output and mixed venous oxygenation are maintained. Declines of maternal oxygenation saturation to the 90–92% range ordinarily are not reflected in abnormal fetal heart rate tracings or adverse fetal outcomes. However, if the maternal arterial oxygen saturation falls below the 90% level, continuous fetal monitoring is recommended if intervention on behalf of the fetus would be performed. Furthermore, in such situations, maternal intubation for fetal indications might be required.

Management of labor in the pregnant asthmatic varies little from such management in nonasthmatic women. The stress of labor may occasionally precipitate an exacerbation of asthma, which is medically treated in the usual way. However, in our experience, serious exacerbations of asthma during labor are uncommon.

One important concern for the pregnant patient in labor is that oral medications are relatively poorly absorbed; gastric emptying slows during labor (49). Thus, in the patient with severe asthma or the patient on a regimen of multiple medications, parenteral administration of antiasthmatic medications (e.g., aminophylline) during labor may occasionally be required. Parenteral hydrocortisone (100 mg every 8 hr) is recommended in corticosteroid-dependent patients to prevent asthma exacerbations and to provide steroid coverage for the physiological stress of labor and delivery.

Finally, betamimetic drugs, when given systemically, may hamper uterine contractions (50). Although betamimetic drugs are, in fact, used to treat preterm labor because of their uterine relaxant effect, impaired uterine contractility during term labor is not a commonly encountered clinical problem. When encountered, it is usually overcome readily with oxytocin augmentation. None of the usual medications or therapeutic modalities that are used during labor itself are contraindicated in the presence of asthma. Narcotics for pain relief and epidural and spinal anesthesia are well tolerated.

General anesthesia is seldom required in obstetrics today, as regional techniques, such as epidural and spinal anesthesia, are readily available and adequate for cesarean delivery (51). If general anesthesia is required, the technique must be carefully considered. In the nonpregnant asthmatic patient who requires general anesthesia, the anesthesiologist may choose to use a halogenated anesthetic gas as the induction agent to maintain bronchodilatation before intubation. This can be done during pregnancy, but will have two potential adverse effects. First, the anesthetic agents will reach the fetus and may cause depression at delivery (52). Second and perhaps more importantly, halogenated anesthetic gases, particularly halothane, are potent relaxants of uterine muscle, and substantial hemorrhage from uterine atony can occur in women anesthetized with halothane (53).

Prostaglandins (PG)

Prostaglandins may be used for labor induction, cervical ripening, or postpartum bleeding (54). In general, prostaglandins should be avoided during pregnancy in asthmatic women if possible (see Chapter 13). If required, PGE_2 would be preferable to PGF derivatives, which are potent bronchoconstrictors. Ergonavine derivatives for treatment of postpartum hemorrhage should also be avoided, if possible, in patients with asthma (see Chapter 13).

ACKNOWLEDGMENT

The authors gratefully acknowledge the valuable assistance of Ms. Terry Esler in the preparation of this manuscript.

REFERENCES

1. Gordon M, Niswander KR, Berendes H, Kantor AG. Fetal morbidity following potentially anoxogenic obstetric conditions. Am J Obstet Gynecol 1970; 106:421–429.
2. Weinstein AM, Dubin BD, Podleski WK, Spector S, Farr R. Asthma in pregnancy. JAMA 1979; 241:1161–1165.
3. Hernandez E, Angell CS, Johnson JWC. Asthma in pregnancy: current concepts. Obstet Gynecol 1980; 55:739–743.
4. Meschia G. Supply of oxygen to the fetus. J Reprod Med 1979; 23:160–165.
5. Weinberger SE, Weiss ST, Cohen WR, Weiss JW, Johnson TS. Pregnancy and the lung. Am Rev Respir Dis 1980; 121:559–579.

6. Prowse CM, Gaensler EA. Respiratory and acid–base changes during pregnancy. Anesthesiology 1965; 26:381–392.
7. Knuttgen HG, Emerson K. Physiological response to pregnancy at rest and during exercise. J Appl Physiol 1974; 36:549–553.
8. Pernoll ML, Metcalfe J, Kovach PA, Wachtel R, Dunham MJ. Ventilation during rest and exercise in pregnancy and postpartum. Respir Physiol 1975; 25:295–310.
9. Pernoll ML, Metcalfe J, Schlenker TL, Welch JE, Matsumoto JA. Oxygen consumption at rest and during exercise in pregnancy. Respir Physiol 1979; 25:285–293.
10. Wulf KH, Kunzel W, Lehmann V. Clinical aspects of placental gas exchange. In: Longo LD, Bartels H, eds. Respiratory gas exchange and blood flow in the placenta. Proceedings of a symposium in conjunction with XXV International Congress of Physiological Sciences, Hanover, Germany 1971. Bethesda, Md: US Department of Health Education and Welfare, National Institutes of Health, National Institute of Child Health and Human Development, 1972:Publ (NIH) 73–361.
11. Andersen GH, Walker J. The effect of labor on the maternal blood–gas and acid–base status. J Obstet Gynaecol Br Commonw 1970; 77:289–293.
12. Templeton A, Kelman GR. Maternal blood-gases, (Pao_2-Pao_2), physiological shunt and VD/VT in normal pregnancy. Br J Anaesth 1976; 48:1001–1004.
13. Meschia G. Placental respiratory gas exchange in fetal oxygenation. In: Creasy R, Resnik R, eds. Maternal–fetal medicine: principles and practice. 2nd ed. Philadelphia: WB Saunders, 1989:303–313.
14. Levinson G, Shnider S, deLorimier AA, Steffenson JL. Effects of maternal hyperventilation on uterine blood flow and fetal oxygenation and acid–base status. Anesthesiology 1974; 40:340–347.
15. Awe RJ, Nicotra MB, Newsom TD, Viles R. Arterial oxygenation in alveolar–arterial gradients in term pregnancy. Obstet Gynecol 1979; 53:182–186.
16. Lees M, Scott D, Kerr M, Taylor S. The circulatory effects of recumbent postural change in late pregnancy. Clin Sci 1967; 32:453–461.
17. Kelman G, Nunn J, Pryse-Roberts C, Greenbaum R. The influence of cardiac output on arterial oxygenation: a theoretical study. Br J Anaesth 1967; 39:450–457.
18. Cousins LM. Obstetrical management and fetal surveillance in the pregnant diabetic. In: Brody S, Ueland K, eds. Endocrine disorders in pregnancy. Norwalk, CT: Appleton-Century-Crofts, 1989:345–361.
19. Lorijn RHW, Longo LD. Clinical and physiologic implications of increased fetal oxygen consumption. Am J Obstet Gynecol 1980; 136:451–457.
20. Longo L, Hill E, Power G. Factors effecting placental oxygen transfer. In: Longo L, Bartels H, eds. Respiratory gas exchange blood flow in the placenta. Bethesda, Md: Public Health Service, DHEW Publication No. [NIH] 73-361, 1972:345–391.

21. Motoyama E, Rivard G, Acheson F, Cook CD. The effects of changes in maternal pH and P_{CO_2} on the P_{O_2} of fetal lambs. Anesthesiology 1967; 28:891–903.
22. Robson J, Schilid H. Effect of drugs on the blood flow and activity of the uterus. J Physiol 1938; 92:9–22.
23. Ahlquist R, Woodbury R. Influence of drugs in uterine activity upon uterine blood flow. Fed Proc 1947; 6:305–314.
24. Rosenfeld C, Barton M, Meschia G. Effects of epinephrine on distribution of blood flow in the pregnancy ewe. Am J Obstet Gynecol 1976; 124:156–163.
25. Adamson K, Mueller-Heubach E, Myers R. Production of fetal asphyxia in the rhesus monkey by administration of catecholamines to the mother. Am J Obstet Gynecol 1971; 109:248–262.
26. DiMarco AF. Asthma in the pregnant patient: a review. Ann Allergy 1989; 62:527–533.
27. Huff RW. Asthma in pregnancy. Med Clin North Am 1989; 73:653–660.
28. Bochner B, Lichenstein L. Anaphylaxis. New Eng J Med 1991; 324:1895–1901.
29. Entman SS, Moise KJ. Anaphylaxis in pregnancy. South Med J 1984; 77:402.
30. Ladner C, Brinkman C, Weston P, Assali N. Dynamics of uterine circulation in pregnant and nonpregnant sheep. Am J Physiol 1970; 218:257–263.
31. Catanzarite V. Obstetrics and gynecology—antepartum care. In: Rakel R, ed. Conn's current therapy. Philadelphia: WB Saunders, 1991:931–939.
32. Campbell S, Warsof S, Little D, Cooper DJ. Routine ultrasound screening for the prediction of gestational age. Obstet Gynecol 1985; 65:613–620.
33. Peeters LLH, Sheldon RE, Jones MD Jr, Makowski EL, Meshia G. Blood flow of fetal organs is a function of arterial oxygen content. Am J Obstet Gynecol 1979; 135:637–646.
34. Crane JP, Kopta MM. Comparative newborn anthropometric data in symmetric versus asymmetric intrauterine growth retardation. Am J Obstet Gynecol 1980; 138:518–522.
35. Hobbins JC, Berkowitz RL, Grannum P. Diagnosis and antepartum management of IUGR. J Reprod Med 1978; 21:319–325.
36. Mintz MC, Landon MB. Sonographic diagnosis of fetal growth disorders. Clin Obstet Gynecol 1988; 31:44–52.
37. Ott WJ, Doyle S, Flamm S. Accurate ultrasonic estimation of fetal weight. Am J Perinatal 1985; 2:178–182.
38. Hadlock FP, Deter RL, Rossavik I. Detection of abnormal fetal growth patterns. In: Athey PA, Hadlock FP, eds. Ultrasound in obstetrics and gynecology, 2nd ed. St Louis: CV Mosby 1985:60–83.
39. Rutherford SE, Phelan JP, Smith CV, Jacobs N. The four quadrant assessment of amniotic fluid volume: an adjunct to antepartum fetal heart rate testing. Obstet Gynecol 1987; 70:353–356.

40. Rochelson B. The clinical significance of absent end-diastolic velocity in the umbilical artery waveforms. Clin Obstet Gynecol 1989; 32:692–702.
41. Chervenak FA, Berkowitz GS, Thornton J, Kreiss C, Youcha S, Ehrenkranz RA, Hobbins JC, Berkowitz RL. A comparison of sonographic estimation of fetal weight and obstetrically determined gestational age in the prediction of neonatal outcome for the very low-birth weight fetus. Am J Obstet Gynecol 1985; 152:47–50.
42. Jobe A. Amniotic fluid tests of fetal lung maturity. In: Creasy R, Resnik R, eds. Maternal–fetal medicine: principles and practice, 2nd ed. Philadelphia: WB Saunders, 1989:426–433.
43. Moore T, Piaquadio K. A prospective evaluation of fetal movement screening to reduce the incidence of antepartum fetal death. Am J Obstet Gynecol 1989; 160:1075–1080.
44. Rochard F, Schifrin BS, Goupil F, Legrand H, Blottiere J, Sureau C. Nonstressed fetal heart rate monitoring in the antepartum period. Am J Obstet Gynecol 1976; 126:699–706.
45. Manning FA, Morrison I, Lange IR, Harman CR, Chamberlain PF. Fetal assessment based on fetal biophysical profile scoring: experience in 12,620 referred high-risk pregnancies. 1. Perinatal mortality by frequency and etiology. Am J Obstet Gynecol 1985; 151:343–350.
46. Freeman RK. The use of the oxytocin challenge test for antepartum clinical evaluation of uteroplacental respiratory function. Am J Obstet Gynecol 1975; 121:481–489.
47. Finberg HJ, Clewell WH. Ultrasound-guided interventions in pregnancy. In: Sander RC, Hill MC, eds. Ultrasound quarterly. New York: Raven Press, 1990:197–226.
48. Freeman RK, Garite TJ, Nageotte MP, eds. Fetal heart rate monitoring, 2nd ed. Baltimore: Williams & Wilkins, 1991.
49. Albright GA, Joyce TH III, Ferguson JE II, Jones MM, eds. Physiology and pharmacology. Physiology of pregnancy. In: Anesthesia in obstetrics—maternal, fetal, and neonatal aspects, 2nd ed. Woburn, MA: Butterworth Publishers, 1986:41–79.
50. Caritis SN, Darby MJ, Chan L. Pharmacologic treatment of preterm labor. Clin Obstet Gynecol 1988; 31:635–651.
51. Shnider SM, Levinson G, eds. Anesthesia for the pregnant patient with asthma. In: Anesthesia for obstetrics, 2nd ed. Baltimore: Williams & Wilkins, 1987:382–391.
52. Shnider SM, Levinson G, eds. Anesthesia for cesarean section. In: Anesthesia for obstetrics, 2nd ed. Baltimore: Williams & Wilkins, 1987:159–178.
53. Gilstrap LC, Hauth JC, Henkins GDJ, Patterson AR. Effect of type of anesthesia on blood loss at cesarean section. Obstet Gynecol 1987; 69:328.
54. Catanzarite V, Aisenbrey G. Prostaglandins: mundane and visionary applications. Contemp Obstet Gynecol 1987; Oct:21–41.

3

Pulmonary Function During Pregnancy in Health and in Asthma

Brita Stenius-Aarniala

University Central Hospital, Helsinki, Finland

The literature on the effect of pregnancy on pulmonary physiology is extensive, and several comprehensive review articles have been published (1–3). For the present reader, the asthmatic patient holds most interest. A major question concerning pregnancy-induced changes in lung physiology involves whether these changes are likely to be of clinical importance in the asthmatic patient during pregnancy. The normal physiological pulmonary alterations which will be considered in this context include changes in ventilatory function, especially a decrease in residual volume (RV) and functional residual capacity (FRC), potentially resulting in premature airway closure during expiration; dyspnea of pregnancy; hyperventilation of pregnancy; and breathing during sleep.

CHANGES IN PULMONARY STRUCTURE AND FUNCTION DURING PREGNANCY

By examining chest roentgenograms of pregnant women in 1938, Thomson and Cohen found an elevation in the level of the diaphragm during pregnancy, along with an increase in the transverse diameter of the chest, and an increase of the subcostal angle in late pregnancy (4). The observed changes in chest wall configuration could not be explained by direct pressure of the uterus against the diaphragm, since the enlargement of the subcostal angle occurred early in pregnancy before any increase occurred in the abdominal girth. Moreover, the pressure of the uterus on the abdominal cavity does not impair diaphragmatic movement, even in late pregnancy (1,5).

Ventilatory function during pregnancy has been investigated in many studies, with largely similar findings (6–9). Alaily and Carrol, employing serial lung function tests in 38 primigravidas, noted a progressive increase in the minute ventilation at rest, and an increase in tidal volume (TV) (6). The respiratory frequency was decreased by a mean of 1.75/min. The mean inspiratory capacity (IC) increased progressively to about 10% above the nonpregnant mean. There was little variation in vital capacity during pregnancy and after delivery. The mean functional residual capacity (FRC) showed a progressive fall during pregnancy, being 21% less at term than in the nonpregnant state. The mean residual volume at term was decreased by 22%, compared with the nonpregnant state. Total lung capacity (TLC) was also reduced during pregnancy by a mean of 5.5%. These changes are summarized in Figure 1. The increase in the minute ventilation is probably a result of a progesterone-induced stimulation of the respiratory drive and of an increase in oxygen consumption.

Milne et al. measured specific airways conductance and forced expiratory volume in 1-sec (FEV_1) monthly from the first trimester until term in 30 subjects in the course of a normal pregnancy and in the postpartum period (7). According to their results there were no significant changes in these measurements throughout pregnancy or compared with postpartum values. The authors concluded that the function of the large airways is not altered in healthy women during normal pregnancy. In addition, maximum midexpiratory flow rates apparently do not change significantly during pregnancy in normal women (10,11).

AIRWAY CLOSURE, BODY POSITION, AND SLEEP

Closing capacity (CC) denotes the lung volume at which dependent small airways close or narrow significantly by gravity. Closing volume (CV) denotes the difference between FRC and CC. In a study by Craig, a reduced CV was found in pregnant women, compared with postpartum values (8). Controversy exists between different studies concerning whether airway closure occurs above the FRC and thus during tidal breathing. In one study, airway closure during tidal breathing was shown

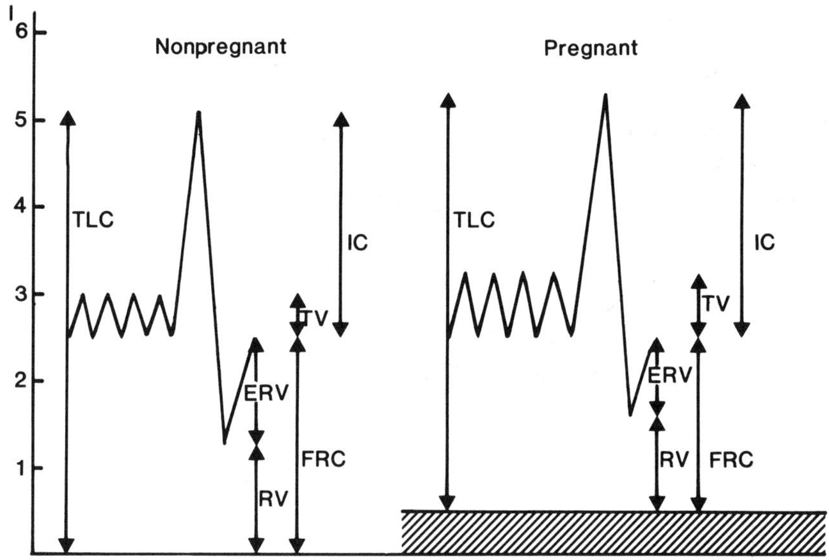

Figure 1 Summary of principal changes in ventilatory function in pregnancy, based on values for 36–38 weeks of gestation and 2–3 months after delivery. ERV, expiratory reserve volume. For other abbreviations see text. (Modified from Ref. 6.)

to occur in 50% of healthy young women when lying down at the end of the pregnancy (12).

It seems clear that airway closure during late pregnancy occurs closer to FRC than in the nonpregnant state. If closing capacity would exceed the FRC, dependent airways would close during tidal breathing. As a rule, this has no clinically significant adverse effect in the healthy pregnant woman. In obstructive lung disease, an increase in FRC helps keep the airways open. In such a patient the reduction in FRC during pregnancy could augment premature airway closure during expiration and, thereby, contribute to hypoxemia caused by ventilation–perfusion mismatching (Figure 2). It has actually been shown that there was a significant fall in FEV_1, peak expiratory flow (PEF), and maximal expiratory flow at 50% of VC during pregnancy in emphysema patients, but not in patients with valvular heart disease or pulmonary sarcoidosis (13). Also, even in the symptom-free asthmatic, the airways may be slightly narrowed because of intraluminal secretion, swelling of the mucosa, and increased smooth-muscle tone. The latter counteracts the elastic recoil of the peribronchial tissue, which normally helps keep

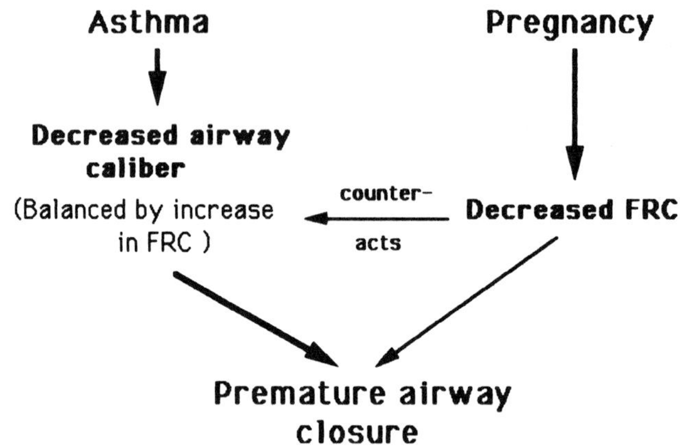

Figure 2 Both asthma and pregnancy contribute to premature airway closure. In the pregnant asthmatic, the decrease in FRC induced by pregnancy counteracts one of the balancing factors in maintaining airway patency.

the airways open during expiration. Thus, in the pregnant asthmatic, several mechanisms may contribute to premature airway closure, including the pregnancy-induced changes in lung volumes and the asthma-induced changes in the airways (see Figure 2).

Norregaard et al. found that the supine position in healthy pregnant women resulted in a reduction in FRC, PEF, and FEV_1, in addition to the decrease produced by the pregnancy itself (14). These changes were not reflected in any change in arterial oxygen saturation nor in the sensation of dyspnea. However, due to premature airway closure, the pregnant asthmatic woman should sleep sitting up if troubled with symptoms. These findings also give some support to the view that delivery, in general, should be conducted with the parturient sitting up (13), and especially so if she has asthma.

Brownell et al. investigated the breathing during sleep in six pregnant women at the end of pregnancy and again postpartum (15). They found that oxygenation was well maintained during sleep in pregnancy. There was no significant change in mean or minimal arterial oxygen saturation during pregnancy, compared with the postpartum period. The frequency of apnea and hypopnea and total apnea–hypopnea time were significantly reduced during pregnancy. A possible explanation for the preservation of nocturnal oxygenation during late pregnancy involves the increased gestational levels of progesterone.

DYSPNEA OF PREGNANCY

Dyspnea is reported by 50–70% of pregnant women (16). Dyspnea usually occurs during the first or second trimester, before any significant increase occurs in abdominal volume. The progesterone-induced increase in respiratory drive causes hyperventilation and a decrease in arterial P_{CO_2}. However, the exact temporal relation between hormone status, functional change, and the development of symptoms is not yet clearly defined (16). According to Gilbert et al., the dyspnea correlates with a low arterial P_{CO_2} (17,18), and women likely to experience dyspnea are those with a relatively high prepregnancy arterial P_{CO_2} (in whom a large difference exists between prepregnancy and pregnancy arterial P_{CO_2} values). The dyspnea is most marked during the first part of pregnancy and improves later, suggesting a gradual acclimatization as pregnancy progresses. It has also been shown that dyspneic pregnant subjects were more sensitive to CO_2 than nondyspneic subjects in that they exhibited an inappropriately large ventilatory response, which may be experienced as dyspnea.

During the last part of pregnancy, increasing body weight and abdominal volume may reduce exercise tolerance; this may be described by some women as dyspnea. Without objective measurements, such as peak flow monitoring, it may be difficult to separate pregnancy-related dyspnea from breathlessness as a symptom of asthma.

ARTERIAL BLOOD GASES AND ACID–BASE BALANCE

The increase in minute ventilation during pregnancy is out of proportion to the elevation in basal metabolic rate that occurs during pregnancy. The minute ventilation at rest increases up to 48% above the nonpregnant level during pregnancy, whereas oxygen consumption and basal metabolic rate are elevated by only 14%. This hyperventilation causes arterial P_{O_2} to increase and arterial P_{CO_2} to decrease during pregnancy, with a concomitant decrease in renal tubular hydrogen ion excretion which partially counteracts this increase in arterial pH (Table 1). The net effect of the respiratory alkalosis and the metabolic compensation is a normal or slightly elevated pH in arterial blood (19). The remaining slight alkalosis is of no clinical importance in the healthy individual. However, respiratory alkalosis in combination with hypoxemia is typical during an attack of asthma. As a result, the alkalosis in a pregnant patient with an exacerbation of asthma may be more pronounced than in the nonpregnant woman with the same degree of asthmatic obstruction.

Pronounced alkalosis and low P_{CO_2} may adversely affect fetal oxy-

Table 1 Recent Studies of Blood Gases in Normal Pregnancy[a]

	Fadel et al.[26]	Liberatore et al.[27]		Templeton and Kelman[28]		
Trimester	Third	First	Third	First	Third	Postpartum
Number of patients	59	17	21	20	20	20
P_{O_2} (mm Hg)	99.3 ± 7.8	105.3 ± 6.0	106.0 ± 5.9	106.4 ± 1.1	101.8 ± 1.0	94.7 ± 1.5
P_{CO_2}	28.8 ± 3.7	28.0 ± 2.2	26.4 ± 3.3	29.4 ± 0.4	30.4 ± 0.6	35.3 ± 0.7
pH	7.42 ± 0.03	7.42 ± 0.02	7.43 ± 0.02	7.46 ± 0.006	7.43 ± 0.006	7.41 ± 0.003
Bicarbonate (mEq/L)	19.0 ± 2.8	18.2 ± 1.3	17.1 ± 1.3			
Base deficit (mmol/L)				2.10 ± 0.3	3.10 ± 0.2	1.24 ± 0.4

[a]Mean ± standard deviation.

Source: Ref. 29.

genation through causing (a) a decrease in uterine and placental perfusion and (b) an increase in oxygen affinity to the fetal hemoglobin, thereby impairing release of oxygen from blood to tissue in the fetus (19). The experimental evidence for this is based on animal studies and on fetuses of mothers hyperventilating during labor (20). No human experimental study has examined the effect of maternal alkalosis combined with hypoxemia such as occurs in acute asthma. In theory, during an attack of asthma, the hypoxia of the fetus might be out of proportion to the hypoxemia in the mother. Indeed, a recent case has been reported in which a pregnant woman manifesting alkalosis after a severe asthmatic exacerbation delivered a stillborn infant (21). It thus becomes especially important to avoid exacerbations of asthma during pregnancy and to monitor blood gas concentrations and acid–balance carefully should such an exacerbation occur.

DIFFUSING CAPACITY

Milne reported a slight increase in carbon monoxide diffusing capacity (DLCO) during early pregnancy (22). The DLCO subsequently started to decrease until 24–27 weeks of pregnancy; thereafter, it remained unchanged until term. These changes appear to be of little clinical significance.

LUNG FUNCTION MEASUREMENTS AS A RISK FACTOR IN PREGNANCY

Lung functions in most asthmatics of childbearing age are usually normal or near normal between asthmatic exacerbations. However, the physician is occasionally faced with the problem of treating the pregnant asthmatic woman with irreversible obstruction. In these instances, it would be helpful if one could identify some limits for acceptable lung function during pregnancy, preferably allowing some reserve for exacerbations of asthma. However, no such recommendations that are based on follow-up of patients with asthma exist in the literature. Some tentative guidelines could perhaps be suggested on the basis of published case reports of women with other chronic pulmonary diseases (23,24). Given the limited information from these case histories, one might postulate that the prerequisites for an uneventful pregnancy may be an arterial PO_2 of 60 mmHg or more and an FEV_1 of greater than 40% of predicted. If the prospective mother exhibits lower values, pregnancy probably should not be recommended.

A potentially difficult situation arises when conception has already occurred in an asthmatic woman with abnormal pulmonary function. Termination of pregnancy because of the asthma should not be recommended solely on the basis of lung function tests, but rather based on the entire clinical picture. After having seen about 700 cases of pregnancy in asthmatics, I have only once recommended termination of pregnancy because of the asthma. A 42-year-old woman who smoked heavily until the present pregnancy experienced during the first trimester a severe lengthy exacerbation of asthma with hypoxemia and alkalosis, but not hypercarbia. The symptoms responded poorly to intensive medication, including systemic steroids (up to 120 mg of methylprednisolone daily) continuously during the 10th–15th weeks of pregnancy. The lowest measured arterial Po_2 was 66 mgHg; however, no values were available during the most severe asthma attacks. The highest measured arterial pH was 7.46. The patient's prepregnancy FEV_1 was 33% of predicted. In the 14th week a decision to terminate the pregnancy was made. A few days before the abortion was due, the patient's symptoms started to improve. The maximal post-medication PEF rose from 26 to 66% and the FEV_1 rose to 43% of predicted. Fortunately, the pregnancy termination was canceled. The pregnancy was then succesfully conducted until the 38th week, when a healthy girl of 2420 g was delivered by cesarean section.

In 11 other severe asthmatics observed in the period 1983–1990, the best FEV_1 values obtained during pregnancy ranged from 33 to 70% of predicted, with a mean of 61% of predicted. The asthma in all patients was monitored carefully, and exacerbations were promptly treated. No major complications occurred relative to pregnancy, delivery, or infant outcomes. Twelve healthy infants were born, with a mean gestation of 275 days. The mean absolute birth weight was 3486 g, and the mean relative birth weight (RBW) was −0.3 SD, two infants being small for dates. Seven cesarean sections were performed, four of which were performed because of poor maternal lung function. No congenital malformations occurred.

These data suggest that the presence of fixed airway obstruction in asthmatic women does not preclude a favorable outcome of pregnancy when the asthma is carefully managed. However, a recent study has shown that asthmatic women manifesting lower mean FEV_1 values during pregnancy are at increased risk of delivering infants with evidence of asymmetric intrauterine growth retardation (25).

SUMMARY

Normal pregnancy is associated with a partially compensated respiratory alkalosis, leading to higher Po_2 and lower Pco_2 levels than in the nongravid state. Although no significant changes in flow rates occur during normal pregnancy, the normal gestational decrease in FRC may exacerbate hypoxemia because of premature airway closure when acute asthma complicates pregnancy.

REFERENCES

1. Weinberger SE, Weiss ST, Cohen WR, Weiss JW, Johnson TS. Pregnancy and the lung. Am Rev Respir Dis 1980; 121:559–580.
2. Noble PW, Lavee AE, Jacobs MM. Respiratory disease in pregnancy. Obstet Gynecol Clin North Am 1988; 15:391–428.
3. Fishburne JI. Physiology and disease of the respiratory system in pregnancy. J Reprod Med 1979; 22:177–189.
4. Thomson KJ, Cohen ME. Studies on the circulation in pregnancy. II. Vital capacity observations in normal pregnant women. Surg Gynecol Obstet 1938; 35:237–248.
5. Gilroy RJ, Mangura BT, Lavietes MH. Rib cage and abdominal volume displacements during breathing in pregnancy. Am Rev Respir Dis 1988; 137:668–672.
6. Alaily AB, Carrol KB. Pulmonary ventilation in pregnancy. Br J Obstet Gynaecol 1978; 85:518–524.
7. Milne JA, Mills RJ, Howi AS, Pack AI. Large airways function during normal pregnancy. Br J Obstet Gynaecol 1977; 84:448–451.
8. Craig DB, Toole MA. Airway closure in pregnancy. Can Anaesth Soc J 1975; 22:665–672.
9. Berry MJ, McMurray RG, Katz VL. Pulmonary and ventilatory responses to pregnancy, immersion, and exercise. J Appl Physiol 1989; 66:857–862.
10. Gazioglu K, Kaltreider NL, Rosen M, Yu PN. Pulmonary function during pregnancy in normal women and in patients with cardiopulmonary disease. Thorax 1970; 25:445–450.
11. Baldwin GR, Moorthin DS, Whelton JA, MacDonell KR. New lung functions and pregnancy. Am J Obstet Gynecol 1977; 127:235.
12. Russell IF, Chambers WA. Closing volume in normal pregnancy. Br J Anaesth 1981; 53:1043–1047.
13. Ang CK, Tan TH, Walters WAW, Wood C. Postural influence on maternal capillary oxygen and carbon dioxide tension. Br Med J 1969; 4:201–203.
14. Norregaard O, Schultz P, Ostergaard A, Dahl R. Lung function and postural changes during pregnancy. Respir Med 1989; 83:467–470.
15. Brownell LG, West P, Kryger MH. Breathing during sleep in normal pregnant women. Am Rev Respir Dis 1986; 133:38–41.
16. Milne JA. The respiratory response to pregnancy. Postgrad Med J 1979; 55:318–324.
17. Gilbert R, Epifano L, Auchincloss JH Jr. Dyspnea of pregnancy, a syndrome of altered respiratory control. JAMA 1962; 182:1073–1077.

18. Gilbert R, Auchincloss JH Jr. Dyspnoea of pregnancy: clinical and physiological observations. Am J Med Sci 1966; 252:270–276.
19. Prowse CM, Gaensler EA. Respiratory and acid–base changes during pregnancy. Anesthesiology 1965; 26:381–392.
20. Huch R. Maternal hyperventilation and the fetus. J Perinat Med 1986; 14:3–17.
21. Sachs BP, Brown RS, Yeah J, Acker D, Niaraki M. Is maternal alkalosis harmful to the fetus? Int J Gynaecol Obstet 1987; 25:65–68.
22. Milne JA, Mills RJ, Coutts JRT, Macnaughton MC, Moran F, Pack AI. The effect of human pregnancy on the pulmonary transfer factor for carbon monoxide as measured by the single-breath method. Clin Sci Mol Med 1977; 53:271–276.
23. Giesler CF, Buehler JH, Depp R. $Alpha_1$-Antitrypsin deficiency. Severe obstructive lung disease and pregnancy. Obstet Gynacol 1977; 49:31–34.
24. Sawicka EH, Spencer GT, Branthwaite MA. Management of respiratory failure complicating pregnancy in severe kyphoscoliosis: a new use for an old technique. Br J Chest 1986; 80:191–196.
25. Schatz M, Zeiger RS, Hoffman CP et al. Intrauterine growth is related to gestational pulmonary function in pregnant asthmatic women. Chest 1990; 98:389–391.
26. Fadel HE, Northrup G, Misenhimer HR, Harp RJ. Normal pregnancy: a model of sustained respiratory alkalosis. J Perinat Med 1979; 7:195.
27. Liberatore SM, Pistelli R, Patalono R, et al. Respiratory function during pregnancy. Respiration 1984; 46:145.
28. Templeton A, Kelman GR. Maternal blood-gasses (P_{AO_2} – Pa_{O_2}) physiological shunt and V_P/V_T in normal pregnancy. Br J Anaesth 1976; 48:1001.
29. Schatz M, Hoffman CP, Zeiger RS, Falkoff R, Mellon M. The course and management of asthma and allergic diseases during pregnancy. In: Middleton E Jr, Reed CE, Ellis EF, et al., eds. Asthma: principles and practice, St Louis: CV Mosby, 1988:1097.

4

Maternal Immunological Changes in Pregnancy

Gillian M.P. Galbraith and Robert Michael Galbraith

Medical University of South Carolina, Charleston, South Carolina

In some respects, pregnancy represents a stable allograft of the genetically dissimilar fetus in the mother, without the need for formal immunosuppressive therapy. Numerous explanations have been advanced to explain this apparent immunological paradox. These fall into two broad categories: reduced immunogenicity of the fetus and impaired immunocompetence of the mother. The latter notion has prompted a huge number of relevant studies in an attempt to demonstrate a state of relative maternal immunosuppression, and several abnormalities have been found. For example, in vitro tests of immune mechanisms have indicated a wide variety of abnormalities. In addition, it has been reported that the frequency of certain infections is increased in pregnancy. Each of these aspects will now be considered in turn.

ABNORMALITIES OF IMMUNOLOGICAL MECHANISMS

As discussed in the following sections, abnormalities both in the number and function of immunocytes have been reported (Table 1). It is worth mentioning at the outset that many of the earlier studies employed technical approaches that we now know to be flawed, and these methodological limitations must be taken into consideration in interpreting the results and conclusions reached in such studies.

Table 1 Summary of Maternal Immunological Changes During Pregnancy

Parameter	Change during pregnancy
Cell counts	
Total white count	Increased
Neutrophils	Increased
Lymphocytes	No change (absolute count)
Monocytes	Increased
T/B cell ratio	No change
CD4/CD8 ratio	No change
Immunoglobulins	
IgG	Decreased
IgA	Some decrease (hemodilution)
IgM	Some decrease (hemodilution)
IgE	No consistent change
Antigen-specific antibody response	No change
Autoantibodies	
Rheumatoid factor	No change in titer
Immune complexes	No increase in titer
In vivo lymphocyte responsiveness	
Allograft rejection	No change
Delayed skin tests	No change
In vitro lymphocyte responsiveness	
PHA	Unchanged in majority of studies
Antigen	Conflicting data
Mixed lymphocyte	No change
In vitro functional changes	
Suppressor cell activity	Increased
Interleukin-2 production	Decreased in some studies
Natural killer function	Decreased
Pregnancy serum	
Effect on lymphocyte responsiveness	Decreased (to PHA, viral antigens, alloantigens)
Effect on monocyte responsiveness	Decreased

Source: Modified from Ref. 83.

Immunocyte Number

A relative leukocytosis and neutrophilia have long been known to be concomitants of pregnancy and may be interpreted as signs of sepsis by the unwary (1,2). The circulating monocyte count is also elevated, but the absolute lymphocyte count is not significantly changed (1–5). Examination of lymphocyte populations and subpopulations have provided more ambiguous results. Initially, T cells were enumerated by their ability to form rosettes with sheep erythrocytes (E-rosettes), and B cells were recognized by surface immunoglobulin. However, several shortcomings were identified, including difficulties with the stability of E-rosettes, causing underestimation of T cells, and binding of antisera recognizing membrane immunoglobulin to Fc receptors, leading to overestimates of B cell number. In addition, the variable contamination of mononuclear cell preparations with monocytes, which are increased in pregnancy (1–5), further emphasized these inaccuracies.

More recently, the introduction of monoclonal antibodies recognizing certain defined cell membrane molecules, and particularly the burgeoning CD series, has provided a relatively simple means of investigating lymphocyte subsets (6). These studies have shown that, although the percentage of lymphocytes in the blood falls during pregnancy, the absolute count may not in fact change that much (1–5). Moreover, T/B-cell ratios appear to be unaffected, and reported decreases in T-cell numbers may largely reflect an artifact of the methods employed for quantitation (7).

Monoclonal antisera have also been employed for evaluation of the CD4/CD8 ratio in pregnancy (4,8–13). Measurement of this "helper/suppressor" ratio was popularized during early studies of acquired immunodeficiency syndrome (AIDS), when it was used as a surrogate test before the introduction of human immunodeficiency virus (HIV) antibody testing. With some exceptions (4,8,9), studies in pregnancy have not revealed any reproducible abnormalities in the distribution of $CD4^+$ and $CD8^+$ cells (7,10–12). Although significant reductions in $CD4^+$ populations have been described in patients whose pregnancies were complicated by preeclamptic toxemia (13) and in those infected with *Toxoplasma gondii* (14), it remains unclear whether such changes are relevant to the physiology of normal pregnancy. Earlier studies used the ability of T cells to form rosettes with IgM and IgG Fc receptors as indices, respectively, of helper and suppressor T cells. Despite some indications of possible differences between pregnant women and nonpregnant controls (15,16), it is now known that Fcμ and Fcγ receptors do not correlate well with expression of CD4 and CD8 antigens or, for that matter, with functional evidence of helper and suppressor activity (17,18). The quantitation of such Fc receptors is further complicated because they are labile (17).

Functional Abnormalities

A wide variety of abnormalities have been reported in vitro, but the correlation with phenomena in vivo remains to be documented. As with assays of immunocyte number, the tests employed, particularly in earlier studies, have not always been reproducible or discriminating. An additional difficulty with monoclonal antisera is that functional properties are frequently, and rather indiscriminately, ascribed or quantitated purely on the basis of the percentage of cells positive for the surface markers, such as CD antigens, that they define. For example, there remains little definitive proof that $CD4^+$ T cells are uniformly helper or inducer in functional terms, or, for that matter, that all $CD8^+$ cells are suppressor–cytotoxic in function (19). With these provisos in mind, existing data will now be briefly summarized.

The function of B cells, namely production of immunoglobulin (Ig) of given antibody specificity, is well established. Consequently, functional abnormalities can be viewed in the contexts of production of immunoglobulin or of specific antibody, or both. Most such studies have been undertaken in vivo, because of both the relative ease of such measurements and the technical demands of quantitating levels of immunoglobulin and specific antibody in vitro. [For the uninitiated, obtaining human B cells of adequate purity and in sufficiently large numbers to measure precisely the minute amounts of antibody produced remains a technological tour de force].

Determinations of serum immunoglobulin in pregnancy have shown some decrease in levels of all major classes, IgG, IgA, and IgM (20–23). The demonstration of a concomitant increase in IgG production in vitro in response to pokeweed mitogen, a T-dependent B-cell mitogen, has prompted the suggestion that defective humoral regulation occurs in pregnancy (24). However, reductions in serum immunoglobulin levels are explicable, in large part, on the basis of hemodilution for IgA and IgM, whereas the larger decrease in IgG levels probably reflects in addition the substantial amounts of this immunoglobulin that are actively transferred across the placenta to the fetus during pregnancy. On the other hand, although allergic phenomena are frequently different in severity or frequency during pregnancy (see Chapters 11 and 14), there are no consistent changes reported for serum IgE levels (21,25).

Measurement of specific antibody production in vivo (e.g., following immunization with tetanus toxoid) provides a simple and effective test of specific B-cell function. No consistent abnormalities in tetanus antibody production have been found (26–28), or in antibody response to influenza vaccine (29). This approach is limited by the potential dangers of immunization with live vaccines during pregnancy. However, antibody to viruses such as Epstein–Barr virus (EBV), herpes, and rubella can be measured directly following natural exposure, and normal serological responses have been found during pregnancy (23,30).

One other index of antibody production is the titer of autoantibodies, and it has been postulated that the presence of high titers during pregnancy could indicate defective immunoregulatory mechanisms. However, no detectable alterations have been found in the titer of rheumatoid factor (31), and despite earlier indications of circulating immune complexes, levels are probably no higher than in nonpregnant subjects (32).

The testing of T-cell function is more complex than for B cells, in large part because T cells are not as clearly monofunctional as B cells, and there is no single generally accepted determinant of T-cell function in vivo. However, several observations indicate that T-cell immunity is grossly intact in vivo. For example, pregnant patients with organ allografts can clearly mount vigorous rejection responses in a fashion comparable with nonpregnant transplant patients (33–35). Furthermore, although the precise role of immunological mechanisms in the control of malignant proliferation remains undetermined, pregnancy does not feature an unusual predisposition to cancer (36). In addition, no substantial change in delayed hypersensitivity to purified protein derivative (PPD) or other standard skin test antigens has been established (37,38).

In vitro alterations in T-cell function have been a popular target for study of putative immunoincompetence in pregnancy. One of the abnormalities most commonly described is reduced T-cell proliferative response to polyclonal mitogens such as phytohemagglutinin (PHA). However, although this was a clear finding in some studies (39–41), others failed to reveal such abnormalities (38,42,43). It is important to note that these results were not generally corrected for the increased levels of circulating monocytes found in pregnancy (1,2). These cells may constitute up to 30% of the mononuclear cell preparations used for blast transformation studies. Their presence may not only "dilute out" otherwise normal T-cell responses, but may also actively inhibit such responses (44). In addition, polyclonal mitogens, such as PHA, are crude and nonselective stimuli, and the biological significance of the effects they stimulate is unclear.

Investigations of lymphocyte proliferative responses to specific microbial antigens in pregnancy have also yielded evidence both of normal function (38) and of depressed responsiveness (43,45). In one recent study, impaired T-cell activation by PPD was normalized by removal of adherent monocytes (46). Cell-mediated reactivity to alloantigens has also been extensively examined and found to be generally unimpaired (42,47).

Although most studies of cell-mediated immunity in pregnancy have focused on proliferative responses, others have addressed the immunoregulatory functions of the system. There is some evidence that in vitro suppressor cell activity is increased in pregnancy (48,49); however, the cell populations involved remain ill-defined and the physiological relevance of the assays employed has not been established. In contrast, deficient cytokine production has been postulated to account for the putative immunoincompetence of pregnancy, and evidence of reduced interleukin-2 production has been presented (50,51), although, again, conflicting data have been reported (52). It is of interest to note that natural killer function appears to be attenuated in pregnancy, but is normalized by the addition of interleukin-2 in vitro (50,53,54).

A possible explanation for the variable results of cell-mediated immune function in vitro is the presence of circulating immunosuppressive factors in maternal serum, which may or may not be included in the reaction mixture, depending on the technique employed. Several investigators have demonstrated an immunosuppressive effect of maternal serum or plasma on the function of normal cells derived from nonpregnant individuals. These effects were observed in a variety of functions, including responses to PHA, viral antigens, and alloantigens (55–57), and also monocyte responsiveness (58). The identity of such factors remains to be proved, although several candidates have been considered. These "pregnancy-specific" factors are generally derived from the fetoplacental unit and include human chorionic gonadotropin, human placental lactogen, pregnancy-associated plasma protein A, α-fetoprotein, and pregnancy-specific β_1-glycoprotein; however, although such proteins may play a local role in immunomodulation at the maternofetal interface, there is little evidence to suggest a generalized immunosuppressive effect attributable to these factors (59), with the possible exception of pregnancy-specific β_1-glycoprotein (60). Similarly, although plasma levels of estradiol, progesterone, and cortisol are increased during pregnancy, immunosuppressive levels are not apparently attained (61): however, lymphocytes from pregnant subjects have increased susceptibility to the suppressive effects of progesterone (62). Finally, a suppressive factor of placental origin that fractionates with IgG has been described, but remains to be characterized (55).

FREQUENCY OF INFECTIONS IN PREGNANCY

The concept of maternal immunoincompetence during pregnancy, when invoked to explain the mother's acceptance of her genetically dissimilar fetus, depends on laboratory evidence of immune dysfunction and clinical evidence of increased susceptibility to infection. However, unlike patients with clear-cut immunodeficiency disorders, there is little evidence that the pregnant woman is more susceptible to opportunistic infections, to common bacterial or viral infections, or to disseminated fungal disease, than is the nonpregnant subject and, with few exceptions, normal pregnancy appears to predispose toward a very narrow spectrum of infectious diseases. Furthermore, the increased incidence of certain localized infections during pregnancy, such as urinary tract infection and cholangitis, is thought to be due to the profound anatomical, mechanical, and hormonal changes of gestation, and should not be assumed to reflect poorly on maternal immunological status. Finally, the pregnant woman receiving antenatal care is subject to relatively intense medical scrutiny, and a mild, nonspecific illness in the mother is more likely to be investigated if there is a possibility of severe fetal consequences, as discussed in the following. This inevitably leads to a higher frequency of diagnosis of certain infections than in the rest of the population.

The exceptions to this general observation are found historically during epidemics of poliomyelitis and influenza, when pregnancy was associated with increased morbidity and mortality from these infections (63,64). However, the increased incidence of gestational poliomyelitis may be attributed to increased exposure, whereas the excess maternal mortality in influenza appeared to be mainly a function of age and cardiopulmonary status, with no increased frequency of infection per se (65). Furthermore, more recent studies found no increased susceptibility to the complications of influenza (66), although it must be appreciated that the virulence of influenza may change over the years owing to the high rate of mutation of the viruses. Similarly, the possible effects of maternal nutrition causing impaired immunocompetence have not been adequately addressed. Otherwise, the range of infections reported to be associated with pregnancy fall into the major groups of latent viruses, intracellular bacteria, and protozoa.

Latent Viruses

Certain latent viruses appear to reactivate during pregnancy, frequently without clinical symptoms in the mother, and rarely with the dissemination typical of cell-mediated immunodeficiency. These include cytomegalovirus (CMV), Epstein–Barr virus (EBV) and herpes simplex type 2 virus (HSV-2) (67–69). Large cohort studies have shown that primary infection with HSV-2 is uncommon in pregnancy (70), and evidence of viral reactivation was found in only 0.2% of asymptomatic patients (71). In contrast, cervical shedding of CMV is common and increases toward the end of pregnancy (67). The immunological (and other) mechanisms underlying reactivation of latent viruses are not completely understood (72); although transient reduction in T-cell responsiveness to CMV antigen in vitro has been observed in seropositive pregnant patients (73), viral shedding is strongly correlated with other factors, including younger age and race (67).

It is also of interest to speculate that, if the pregnant subject is indeed immunocompromised, then infection with human immunodeficiency virus (HIV) might demonstrate increased aggression during gestation. Indeed, retrospective studies tended to support such a contention (74), and the perinatal transmission rate of HIV is high (75). In contrast, data derived from a recent prospective study suggest that pregnancy has no substantial effect on the disease course in the HIV-infected patient (76).

Intracellular Bacteria

Susceptibility of pregnant leprosy patients to increased mycobacterial load may reflect decreased delayed-type hypersensitivity to the organism (77); similar reports of reactivation and dissemination of tuberculosis in pregnancy are difficult to confirm in the current era of antituberculous therapy, but may correlate with delay in diagnosis and treatment (78). Listeriosis during pregnancy has catastrophic effects on the fetus and neonate (79) and has been assumed to show increased prevalence in pregnancy. However, although this has been supported by studies of animal models (80), a large study of reported cases in humans revealed that only 4% occurred during pregnancy, when mild or subclinical disease generally occurred, in contrast with the high morbidity in infected nonpregnant subjects (79). Whether the severe effects on the fetus are due to an unusual affinity of the organism for human placental tissue remains to be determined.

Protozoa

In third-world countries, pregnancy appears to be associated with increased severity of certain endemic diseases, such as malaria and amebiasis (81,82). However, the relative contributions of immune function, nutritional status, and level of antenatal care to the outcome of these infections have not been determined.

SUMMARY

A large body of conflicting data has been accumulated in the attempt to explain the immunological paradox of pregnancy. In terms of in vitro immune function, the weight of the evidence appears to fall equally between support for and against gestational immune dysfunction. However, "the proof of the pudding is in the eating," and the pregnant subject displays few if any of the infections and immunological abnormalities characteristic of an immunodeficient patient. If, indeed, pregnancy imposes an immunological disadvantage, then this is a light burden. Obviously, the occurrence of clinically significant immunosuppression would make little sense from an evolutionary viewpoint, since it would be highly detrimental to the species to lose a large percentage of its pregnant females to overwhelming disease. Whether or not a minor modification of immune reactivity might influence or modify the possibility of fetal rejection is open to argument. It appears far more likely that local alterations in recognition or effector mechanisms at the maternofetal interface would play a more important role. The paradox remains unresolved.

REFERENCES

1. Andrews WC, Bonsnes RW. The leucocytes during pregnancy. Am J Obstet Gynecol 1951; 61:1129–1135.
2. Valdimarsson H, Mulholland C, Fridriksdottir V, Coleman DV. A longitudinal study of leucocyte blood counts and lymphocyte responses in pregnancy: a marked early increase of monocyte–lymphocyte ratio. Clin Exp Immunol 1983; 53:437–443.
3. Plum J, Thiery M, Sabbe L. Distribution of mononuclear cells during pregnancy. Clin Exp Immunol 1978; 31:45–49.
4. Sridama V, Pacini F, Yang S, Moawad A, Reilly M, DeGroot LJ. Decreased levels of helper T cells. A possible cause of immunodeficiency in pregnancy. N Engl J Med 1982; 307:352–355.

5. Moore MP, Carter NP, Redman CWG. Lymphocyte subsets defined by monoclonal antibodies in human pregnancy. Am J Reprod Immunol 1983; 3:161–164.
6. Reinherz EL, Haynes BF, Nadler LM, Bernstein ID. Leukocyte typing II, vol 2. New York: Springer-Verlag, 1986:3–550.
7. Lucivero G, Selvaggi L, Dell'osso A, Antonaci S, Iannone A, Bettocchi S, Bonomo L. Mononuclear cell subpopulations during normal pregnancy. I. Analysis of cell surface markers using conventional techniques and monoclonal antibodies. Am J Reprod Immunol 1983; 4:142–145.
8. Bailey K, Herrod HG, Younger R, Shaver D. Functional aspects of T-lymphocyte subsets in pregnancy. Obstet Gynecol 1985; 66:211–214.
9. Castilla JA, Rueda R, Vargas ML, Gonzalez-Gomez F, Garcia-Olivares E. Decreased levels of circulating $CD4^+$ T lymphocytes during pregnancy. J Reprod Immunol 1989; 15:103–111.
10. Layward L, Brenchley PEC, Coupes BM, Ellis CM, Pumphrey RSH. Decreased levels of helper T cells in pregnancy [letter]. N Engl J Med 1982; 307:1582.
11. Vanderbeeken Y, Vlieghe MP, Delespesse G, Duchateau J. Characterization of immunoregulatory T cells during pregnancy by monoclonal antibodies. Clin Exp Immunol 1982; 48:118–120.
12. Bolis PF, Franchi M, Guaschino S, Sampaolo P, Maccario R. T-lymphocyte subpopulations in pregnancy. Biol Res Pregnancy Perinatol 1983; 4:107–109.
13. Bardeguez AD, McNerney R, Frieri M, Verma UL, Tejani N. Cellular immunity in preeclampsia: alterations in T-lymphocyte subpopulations during early pregnancy. Obstet Gynecol 1991; 77:859–862.
14. Hohlfeld P, Forestier F, Marion S, Thulliez P, Marcon P, Daffos F. *Toxoplasma gondii* infection during pregnancy: T lymphocyte subpopulations in mothers and fetuses. Pediatr Infect Dis J 1990; 9:878–881.
15. Sumiyoshi Y, Gorai I, Hirahara F, Tanaka K, Minaguchi H. Cellular immunity in normal pregnancy and abortion: subpopulations of T lymphocytes bearing Fc receptors for IgG and IgM. Am J Reprod Immunol 1981; 1:145–149.
16. Ong KS, Grieco MH, Goel Z. Increased "T lymphocyte" bearing Fc receptors for IgG in pregnancy. Int Arch Allergy Appl Immunol 1983; 70:220–224.
17. Moretta L, Moretta A, Canonica GW, Bacigalupo A, Mingari MC, Cerottini JC. Receptors for immunoglobulins on resting and activated human T cells. Immunol Rev 1981; 56:141–162.
18. Hayward AR, Layward L, Lydyard PM, Moretta L, Dagg M, Lawton AR. Fc-receptor heterogeneity of human suppressor T cells. J Immunol 1978; 121:1–5.
19. Bottomly K. A functional dichotomy of $CD4^+$ T lymphocytes. Immunol Today 1988; 9:268–274.

20. Maroulis GB, Buckley RH, Younger JB. Serum immunoglobulin concentrations during normal pregnancy. Am J Obstet Gynecol 1971; 109:971–976.
21. Amino N, Tanizawa O, Miyai K, Tanaka F, Hayashi C, Kawashima M, Ichihara K. Changes of serum immunoglobulins IgG, IgA, IgM, and IgE during pregnancy. Obstet Gynecol 1978; 52:415–420.
22. Ostensen M, Lundgren R, Husby G, Rekvig OP. Studies on humoral immunity in pregnancy: immunoglobulins, alloantibodies and autoantibodies in healthy pregnant women and in pregnant women with rheumatoid disease. J Clin Lab Immunol 1983; 11:143–147.
23. Baboonian C, Griffiths P. Is pregnancy immunosuppressive? Humoral immunity against viruses. Br J Obstet Gynaecol 1983; 90:1168–1175.
24. Bisset LR, Fiddes TM, Gillett WR, Wilson PD, Griffin JF. Altered humoral immunoregulation during human pregnancy. Am J Reprod Immunol 1990; 23:4–9.
25. Knobloch VV, Jouja V, Sternova H. IgE im Serum von schwangeren Frauen. Zentralbl Gynaekol 1974; 96:1190–1192.
26. Rao VR, Raman I. Antibody response to tetanus toxoid during pregnancy. Indian J Med Res 1980; 72:840–842.
27. Gill TJ, Repetti CF, Metlay LA, Rabin BS, Taylor FH, Thompson DS, Cortese AL. Transplacental immunization of the human fetus to tetanus by immunization of the mother. J Clin Invest 1983; 72:987–996.
28. Brabin BJ, Nagel J, Hagenaars AM, Ruitenberg E, van Tilborgh AMJC. The influence of malaria and gestation on the immune response to one and two doses of adsorbed tetanus toxoid in pregnancy. Bull WHO 1984; 62:919–930.
29. Murray DL, Imagawa DT, Okada DM, St Geme JW. Antibody response to monovalent A/New Jersey/8/76 influenza vaccine in pregnant women. J Clin Microbiol 1979; 10:184–187.
30. Icart J, Didier J, Dalens M, Chabanon G, Boucays A. Prospective study of Epstein Barr virus (EBV) infection during pregnancy. Biomedicine 1981; 34:160–163.
31. Pope, RM, Yoshinoya S, Rutstein J, Persellin RH. Effect of pregnancy on immune complexes and rheumatoid factors in patients with rheumatoid arthritis. Am J Med 1983; 74:973–979.
32. Pope RM, Yoshinoya S, Persellin RH. The detection of circulating immune complexes and IgG and IgM rheumatoid factors in normal human pregnancy. Am J Reprod Immunol 1982; 2:208–211.
33. Sciarra JJ, Toledo-Pereyra LH, Bendel RP, Simmons RL. Pregnancy following renal transplantation. Am J Obstet Gynecol 1975; 123:411–425.
34. Penn I, Makowski EL, Harris P. Parenthood following renal transplantation. Kidney Int 1980; 18:221–233.
35. Whetham JCG, Cardella C, Harding M. Effect of pregnancy on graft function and graft survival in renal cadaver transplant patients. Am J Obstet Gynecol 1983; 145:193–197.

36. Donegan WL. Cancer and pregnancy. CA 1983; 33:194–214.
37. Lichtenstein MR. Tuberculin reaction in tuberculosis during pregnancy. Am Rev Tuberc 1942; 46:89–92.
38. Hawes CS, Kemp AS, Jones WR, Need JA. A longitudinal study of cell-mediated immunity in human pregnancy. J Reprod Immunol 1981; 3:165–173.
39. Purtilo DT, Hallgren HM, Yunis EJ. Depressed maternal lymphocyte response to phytohemagglutinin in human pregnancy. Lancet 1972; 1:769–771.
40. Yamamoto T, Hirata H, Taniguchi H, Kawai Y, Uematsu A, Sugiyama Y. Lymphocyte transformation during pregnancy: an analysis using whole-blood culture. Obstet Gynecol 1980; 55:215–219.
41. Baboonian C, Grundy JE, O'Brien PMS, Griffiths PD. Responses to mitogenic stimulation of lymphocytes taken during and after pregnancy. FEMS Microbiol Immunol 1989; 47:199–204.
42. Birkeland SA, Kristoffersen K. Cellular immunity in pregnancy: blast transformation and rosette formation of maternal T and B lymphocytes. Clin Exp Immunol 1977; 30:408–412.
43. Gehrz RC, Christianson WR, Linner KM, Conroy MM, McCue SA, Balfour HH. A longitudinal analysis of lymphocyte proliferative responses to mitogens and antigens during human pregnancy. Am J Obstet Gynecol 1981; 140:665–670.
44. Goodwin JS, Webb DR. Regulation of the immune response by prostaglandins. Clin Immunol Immunopathol 1980; 15:106–122.
45. Riley EM, Schneider G, Sambou I, Greenwood BM. Suppression of cell-mediated immune responses to malaria antigens in pregnant Gambian women. Am J Trop Med Hyg 1989; 40:141–144.
46. Bjercke S, Bertheussen K, Maltau JM. Increased relative frequency of suppressor monocytes in peripheral blood in early pregnancy. APMIS 1989; 97:125–130.
47. Vanderbeeken Y, Vlieghe MP, Duchateau J, Delespesse G. Suppressor T lymphocytes in pregnancy. Am J Reprod Immunol 1984; 5:20–24.
48. Fiddes TM, O'Reilly DB, Cetrulo CL, Miller W, Rudders F, Osband M, Rocklin RE. Phenotypic and functional evaluation of suppressor cells in normal pregnancy and in chronic aborters. Cell Immunol 1986; 97:407–418.
49. Castilla, JA, Vargas L, Garcia-Tortosa C, Garcia-Pacheco M, Gonzalez-Gomez F, Garcia-Olivares E. Short-lived suppressor cell activity during normal human pregnancy. J Reprod Immunol 1990; 18:139–145.
50. Vaquer S, De La Hera A, Jorda J, Martinez C, Escudero M, Alvarez-Mon M. Diminished natural killer activity in pregnancy: modulation by interleukin-2 and interferon. Scand J Immunol 1987; 26:691–698.
51. Nicholas NS, Panayi TS, Nouri AME. Human pregnancy serum inhibits interleukin-2 production. Clin Exp Immunol 1984; 58:587–595.

52. Hauser GJ, Lidor A, Zakuth V, Rosenberg H, Bino T, David MP, Spirer Z. Immunocompetence in pregnancy: production of interleukin-2 by peripheral blood lymphocytes. Cancer Detect Prevent Suppl 1987; 1:39–42.
53. Baley JE, Schacter BZ. Mechanisms of diminished natural killer cell activity in pregnant women and neonates. J Immunol 1985; 134:3042–3047.
54. Gonik B, Loftin KC, Tan NS, Crump J. Immune modulation of natural killer cell cytotoxicity against herpes infected target cells in pregnancy. Am J Reprod Immunol 1990; 24:95–98.
55. Vanderbeeken YE, Duchateau J, Collet H, Van Boogaert L, Desseilles P, Lucasi A. Functional modifications of the $CD4^+$ and the $CD8^+$ subset due to maternal serum. Immunopharmacol Immunotoxicol 1989; 11:397–420.
56. Baboonian C, Grundy JE, Lever AM, Griffiths PD. Effect of pregnancy plasma upon in vitro parameters of cell mediated immunity. FEMS Microbiol Immunol 1989; 1:189–198.
57. Park MI, Edwin SS, Scott JR, Branch DW. Interpretation of blocking activity in maternal serum depends on the equation used for calculation of mixed lymphocyte culture results. Clin Exp Immunol 1990; 82:363–368.
58. Levy R, Latzer S, Sachs J, Insler V, Alkan M. Host defense during pregnancy: monocyte adherence and killing. Isr J Med Sci 1990; 26:361–366.
59. Bischof P, Lauber K, Girard JP, Herrmann WL, Sizonenko PC. Circulating levels of pregnancy proteins and depression of lymphoblastogenesis during pregnancy. J Lab Clin Immunol 1983; 12:93–96.
60. Harris SJ, Anthony FW, Jones DB, Masson GM. Pregnancy specific β_1-glycoprotein: effect on lymphocyte proliferation in vitro. J Reprod Immunol 1984; 6:267–270.
61. Stites DP, Siiteri PK. Steroids as immunosuppressants in pregnancy. Immunol Rev 1983; 75:117–138.
62. Szekeres-Bartho J, Hadnagy J, Pasca AS. The suppressive effect of progesterone on lymphocyte cytotoxicity: unique progesterone sensitivity of pregnancy lymphocytes. J Reprod Immunol 1985; 7:121–128.
63. Siegel M, Greenberg M. Incidence of poliomyelitis in pregnancy. N Engl J Med 1955; 253:841–847.
64. Greenberg M, Jacobziner H, Pakter J, Weisl BAG. Maternal mortality in the epidemic of Asian influenza, New York City, 1957. Am J Obstet Gynecol 1958; 76:897–902.
65. Eickhoff TC, Sherman IL, Serfling RE. Observations on excess mortality associated with epidemic influenza. JAMA 1961; 176:776–782.
66. Amstey MS. Up-to-the-minute observations on influenza in pregnancy. Contemp Obstet Gynecol 1984; 24:43–51.
67. Chandler SH, Alexander ER, Holmes KK. Epidemiology of cytomegaloviral infection in a heterogeneous population of pregnant women. J Infect Dis 1985; 152:249–256.
68. Fleisher G, Bolognese R. Persistent Epstein–Barr virus infection and pregnancy. J Infect Dis 1983; 147:982–998.

69. Ng ABP, Reagan JW, Yen SSC. Herpes genitalis. Obstet Gynecol 1970; 36:645.
70. Boucher FD, Yasukawa LL, Bronzan RN, Hensleigh PA, Arvin AM, Prober CG. A prospective evaluation of primary genital herpes simplex virus type 2 infections acquired during pregnancy. Pediatr Infect Dis J 1990; 9:499–504.
71. Brown ZA, Benedetti J, Ashley R, Burchett S, Selke S, Berry S, Vontver LA, Corey L. Neonatal herpes simplex virus infection in relation to asymptomatic maternal infection at the time of labor. N Engl J Med 1991; 324:1247–1252.
72. Croen KD. Latency of the human herpesviruses. Annu Rev Med 1991; 42:61–67.
73. Gehrz RC, Christianson WR, Linner KM, Conroy MM, McCue SA, Balfour HH. Cytomegalovirus-specific humoral and cellular immune responses in human pregnancy. J Infect Dis 1981; 143:391–395.
74. Landesman SH. Human immunodeficiency virus infection in women: an overview. Semin Perinatol 1989; 13:2–6.
75. Rogers MF. Pediatric HIV infection: epidemiology, etiopathogenesis, and transmission. Pediatr Ann 1988; 17:324–330.
76. Selwyn PA, Schoenbaum EE, Davenny K, Robertson VJ, Feingold AR, Shulman JF, Mayers MM, Klein RS, Friedland GH, Rogers MF. Prospective study of human immunodeficiency virus infection and pregnancy outcomes in intravenous drug users. JAMA 1989; 261:1289–1294.
77. Duncan ME, Pearson JMH, Ridley DS, Melson R, Bjune G. Pregnancy and leprosy: the consequences of alterations of cell-mediated and humoral immunity during pregnancy and lactation. Int J Lepr 1982; 50:425–435.
78. Kingdom JC, Kennedy DH. Tuberculous meningitis in pregnancy. Br J Obstet Gynaecol 1989; 96:233–235.
79. McLaughlin J. Human listeriosis in Britain, 1967–85, a summary of 722 cases. Epidemiol Infect 1990; 104:181–189.
80. Redline RW, Lu CY. Role of local immunosuppression in murine fetoplacental listeriosis. J Clin Invest 1986; 79:1234–1241.
81. McGregor IA. The significance of parasitic infections in terms of clinical disease: a personal view. Parasitology 1987; 94:S159–S178.
82. Abioye AA. Fatal amoebic colitis in pregnancy and puerperium: a new clinico-pathological entity. J Trop Med Hyg 1973; 76:97–100.
83. Schatz M, Hoffman CP, Zeiger RS, Falkoff B, Mellon M. The course and management of asthma and allergic diseases during pregnancy. In: Middleton E, Reed CE, Ellis EF, et al, eds. Allergy: principles and practice. St Louis, CV Mosby, 1988:1101.

5

Immunological Diagnosis and Therapy During Pregnancy

Janet Kershaw-McLennan

Cedars-Sinai Medical Center, Los Angeles, California

Sheldon L. Spector

University of California, Los Angeles, California

Allergic disorders, including asthma, are the most common medical conditions to complicate pregnancy. Studies have recently documented that proper management of asthma during pregnancy can minimize complications such as prematurity, low birth weight, and perinatal morbidity (1). Obviously, the aim of medical management during pregnancy is to reduce symptoms while using the least potentially harmful medications to both mother and fetus whenever possible. Often medications can be completely avoided with careful allergy assessment, strict adherence to avoidance programs, and proper use of allergen immunotherapy.

Allergen immunotherapy has been shown to be effective and safe for treatment of allergic rhinitis, allergic asthma, and insect-sting anaphylaxis (2,3). Pregnant women have been receiving immunotherapy since its first introduction by Noon and Freeman in 1911; however, the safety of this practice was documented only somewhat recently (4).

This chapter will review the use of skin testing and in vitro testing for diagnosis of allergic rhinitis and asthma and the use of allergen immunotherapy as it pertains to the pregnant patient. Avoidance therapy guidelines will also be presented as the first-line approach to immunological therapy.

IMMUNOLOGICAL DIAGNOSIS

The first step toward diagnosis of allergic disease involves demonstration of specific IgE. Immediate hypersensitivity or specific IgE can be assayed by either skin testing or by one of several in vitro laboratory methods. When used in conjunction with a careful history, one may determine if there is an allergic basis for symptoms.

Rhinitis of Pregnancy

The rhinitis of pregnancy (see Chapter 14) may be multifactorial. Hormonal changes may induce changes in vascular tone that result in vasomotor instability. The most common form of rhinitis, however, is preexisting allergic rhinitis (5). This must be distinguished from vasomotor instability, rhinitis medicamentosa, and infectious rhinitis, all of which can occur in the pregnant patient. Diagnosis may be obvious from the patient's history and physical examination, but demonstration of specific IgE can be helpful in confirming the diagnosis of allergic rhinitis. A nasal smear may be useful, since an allergic basis is suggested bv a preponderance of eosinophils.

Asthma

The diagnosis of asthma is often more complicated (see Chapter 13). Symptoms of cough, dyspnea, and chest constriction may predominate. The basis for such symptoms is the airway hyperresponsiveness to a variety of triggers, such as pollens, dust mites, animal antigen, or nonspecific inhalants, such as cigarette smoke or environmental pollutants. Measurements of pulmonary function, response to pharmacologic therapy, and response to avoidance of triggers are modalities used in diagnosis. Asthma in the pregnant patient not only endangers the life of the woman, but also that of the developing fetus. Schatz et al. (6) and Spector (7) have reviewed the relation between asthma and pregnancy and, from this work, conclude that uncontrolled asthma is more dangerous than virtually all of its therapy. Especially important during gestation is an attempt to define the contribution of IgE-mediated triggers, as these potentially may be avoided, thereby reducing the need for medications.

Skin Testing

The most commonly used method for detection of specific IgE is the skin test. Allergenic extracts are used according to techniques well described in standard allergy texts (8). Immediate hypersensitivity skin testing is not without danger, but its general safety has been well established (9,10). The prime reason for concern is the small risk of anaphylaxis which, in the pregnant patient, could result in spontaneous abortion, fetal death, or infant abnormalities (see Chapter 15). Consequently, skin testing is not routinely performed during pregnancy. However, there are situations for which the knowledge gained will assist in better patient management.

From the many studies on safety of skin testing, several conclusions can be made that may affect the physician's judgment on how to use this technique during pregnancy. Fatal reactions have occurred more commonly with intradermal testing than with epicutaneous testing. Potent allergens, such as penicillin, nuts, cottonseed, and flaxseed, are more often associated with complications. Finally, patients with subjective or objective symptoms of respiratory distress are at greater risk for respiratory complications and death and should not be tested during respiratory difficulties (9–11). During pregnancy, if skin testing is to be performed, several precautions are suggested. Antigens should be carefully selected on the basis of clinical relevance (i.e., batteries of antigens should be avoided). Epidermal prick or puncture (not intradermal) tests are recommended; a more comprehensive evaluation can be undertaken after completion of pregnancy, should it be needed. In summary, the risk of systemic reaction is small enough that selected tests need not be delayed until after pregnancy. Alternatively, and certainly obviating clinical reactions, in vitro serological tests could be employed.

Serological Testing

The alternative method of detection of specific IgE is by in vitro testing, such as the radioallerogosorbant test (RAST) and others. These tests measure allergen-specific IgE with a solid-phase immunoassay. Such serological assays are sensitive, specific, and reproducible, but entail considerably greater cost and are generally less sensitive than results obtained by skin testing (12,13). Nonetheless, there is no danger of anaphylaxis, making pregnancy one of the times in which in vitro testing is indicated as an appropriate diagnostic tool of primary choice. To avoid excessive costs with use of in vitro testing, one should select antigens according to the patient's history.

Immunological testing methods are bioassays that indicate only the presence of specific IgE. Although they are vital for establishing an avoidance program and for prescribing allergen immunotherapy, they are not diagnostic of allergy in and of themselves. Positive reactions on skin prick testing or in vitro testing may be true positives, yet may not represent clinically relevant antibody (8). A correlation of clinical findings with the specific IgE is necessary to establish the diagnosis of clinical disease caused by IgE-mediated hypersensitivity.

INHALANT IMMUNOTHERAPY

Immunotherapy is an important modality of treatment in the overall care of the allergic patient. Several studies document the efficacy of high-dose immunotherapy in double-blinded controlled trials in the treatment of asthma and allergic rhinitis (14,15). Its efficacy is dependent on both dose and duration of treatment and, with most individuals, it will take several months before there is a clinically significant reduction in patient symptoms. During pregnancy, immunotherapy has been cautiously continued, as an interruption in therapy for 9 months would necessitate starting over. It is usually not initiated in the pregnant woman, as the response to therapy is not always predictable, and the tendency toward systemic reactions is undefined; furthermore, the delay in efficacy would not eliminate the use of medications during the pregnancy (4,16).

The issue of safety of immunotherapy was addressed most recently by Metzger et al. (4) They retrospectively analyzed data from 121 pregnancies in 90 women who received immunotherapy. When compared with a control population of 147 pregnant atopic women not receiving immunotherapy, they concluded that there were no increases in prematurity, toxemia, abortion, or neonatal death. The rate of congenital malformation was consistent with expected rates for the general population. They also tried to assess the effect of immunotherapy on the developing fetus relative to its potential for developing atopy. From these data, it appeared that the fetus was not protected from developing allergic disease if the mother received immunotherapy nor were these children at a greater risk for atopy. Further studies addressing this issue remain to be done.

Earlier studies that addressed the issue of safety of immunotherapy during pregnancy are difficult to interpret. Extract doses were often low, different types of extracts were used, data recording was poor, and often no controls were used. However, Metzger et al. have reviewed these studies and found them to support the use of immunotherapy during pregnancy (4,16). The major risk of immunotherapy during pregnancy is maternal anaphylaxis which has been associated with spontaneous abortion (17). In addition, as noted earlier, maternal anaphylaxis from other causes has been associated with fetal mortality or infant abnormalities (see Chapter 15).

It is now considered standard practice to recommend cautious continuation of allergen immunotherapy during pregnancy, provided it is being given for the appropriate medical conditions. Individuals with a prior history of anaphylaxis or frequent severe local reactions associated with immunotherapy are poor candidates for gestational immunotherapy. As in any population, carelessness of administration is the most frequent cause of systemic reactions. This must be prevented by a system of clearly marking vials so that concentrated extracts cannot be mistaken for starting dilutions.

Patients should not be symptomatic from asthma at the time of their injection. Spirometry or measurement of peak expiratory flows can quantitate the degree of obstruction. A significant reduction in flow rates should be reason to skip an injection or to cut back the dose. This holds true for pregnant asthmatics as well as for the general asthmatic population.

During pregnancy, it is generally recommended that patients receiving a maintenance dose be cut back to half their usual dose. In those patients on the buildup phase, the dose can be increased with caution or, probably safer, no further increase in dose made until pregnancy is completed. Anaphylaxis is always an unpredictable outcome, but these measures may help reduce its occurrence to a level that is generally acceptable, given the risks of uncontrolled asthma on pregnancy outcome. It is important to note that there are no prospective controlled studies that clarify the proper dosage; therefore, careful judgment by the physician must be relied on.

Other measures to be taken to minimize complications of immunotherapy are the avoidance of certain concomitant medications. β-adrenergic antagonists have been associated with more severe and protracted systemic reactions, as well as the potential for severe bronchospasm. Similarly, drugs used for depression, such as monoamine oxidase (MAO) inhibitors, may complicate treatment of systemic reactions with epinephrine, should it be needed (18,19), and these are best avoided in patients on immunotherapy.

An experienced physician must be available with resuscitative equipment in the event of a systemic reaction. A pregnant woman should be treated immediately and vigorously with epinephrine if needed (see Chapter 15). Clinically the risk of severe anaphylaxis is probably greater than the risk of giving epinephrine (16), which may cause uterine contractions and decreased uterine blood flow (20).

In summary, allergen immunotherapy is considered to be safe for both mother and fetus during pregnancy. With immunotherapy, airway hyperreactivity and late-phase responses can be diminished, reducing the need for potentially harmful pharmacologic agents. During pregnancy, modifications of the dosage schedule are advised to prevent systemic reactions.

VENOM IMMUNOTHERAPY

The pregnant patient with stinging-insect hypersensitivity poses a special problem. It is generally accepted that adults with histories of systemic reactions and positive immediate hypersensitivity skin tests should be given venom immunotherapy to prevent anaphylaxis from a subsequent sting. However, venom immunotherapy per se carries with it a risk of anaphylaxis of 5% during the buildup phase and 0.1% during maintenance (21).

Recently, Schwartz et al. (21) compared the risk of anaphylaxis from an insect sting during pregnancy versus the risk of venom immunotherapy. They analyzed data obtained from questionnaires in 26 women with 43 pregnancies. All the women received venom immunotherapy during their pregnancy. The results revealed that 1 patient had sting anaphylaxis, but a normal outcome of pregnancy. Two other patients developed mild adverse reactions from therapy, but had normal pregnancy outcome. The remaining pregnancies ended normally. From these data it appears that the safety and efficacy of venom immunotherapy is similar to that of inhalant allergen immunotherapy, which is accepted to be safe. With an estimated risk of sting anaphylaxis of 4–6%, it was felt that a pregnant patient already receiving maintenance venom immunotherapy should continue with this therapy. Still undefined is the benefit/risk ratio of starting venom immunotherapy during pregnancy.

AVOIDANCE OF ANTIGENS: ENVIRONMENTAL CONTROL

Allergic disease is a result of the interaction between antigen and specific IgE antibody that elicites the release of potent mediators that act on target organs. One of the primary approaches in the treatment of allergic disease is to reduce exposure to environmental antigens when possible. This action may often diminish symptoms such that medication need is reduced and sometimes eliminated. During pregnancy this form of treatment takes on an extremely valuable role, as it may increase patient well-being while avoiding substances that are potentially harmful to the fetus. For an avoidance program to be successful, patient education is paramount. Along with the patient's clinical history, skin testing or serological test results provide a guideline to likely sensitivities. The physician must spend time elaborating specific measures that can be undertaken efficiently and simply by the patient.

Asthmatics must be strongly discouraged from cigarette smoking, particularly during pregnancy. Smoking has been shown to be an independent nonspecific trigger of asthma, in addition to its known contribution to perinatal morbidity (22,23).

There are five major categories of allergenic triggers for asthma and rhinitis that can be reduced by environmental control. These are pollen, house dust mites, cockroach allergen, mold, and animal dander. Eradication regimens for these allergens will be addressed.

Inhalant Pollens

Pollen allergens, such as grass, weeds, and trees, known to trigger asthma and rhinitis are predominantly from wind-borne pollens. In very general terms, tree pollen predominates in early spring, grasses in late spring and early summer, and weeds in late summer and early fall. Pollen-sensitive patients often demonstrate a striking rise in symptoms of asthma, allergic rhinitis, and conjunctivitis during their particular seasons of pollen prevalence.

It is virtually impossible to avoid completely inhalation of pollens, particularly in some portions of the country in which the seasons are prolonged. To reduce exposure, patients should be educated about their sensitivities, pollen seasons, and pollen counts. One can recommend closing windows in the home or car, and using air-conditioning, which reduces pollen exposure.

House Dust Mites

The most important source of allergen in home dust allergy, as first described by Voorhorst, is the dust mite, which belongs to the genus of *Dermatophagoides*. In Europe and North America, both *D. pteronyssinus* and *D. farinae* are important (24). The allergenic portion of the dust mite is its body parts and fecal residue, which can be the provocateur in perennial symptoms of asthma and rhinitis (25).

Climate, season, humidity, and types of home furnishings, all affect the population of house dust mite in one's dwelling (25). Recently introduced are commercially available assays to detect and quantify the amount of dust mite in an area. Preliminary evaluations of their usefulness appear promising (26,27). As patients spend approximately 8 hr in the bedroom, this site is usually chosen for sampling.

After skin tests or in vitro tests confirm the presence of IgE to dust mites, and if symptoms are correlative, one can either sample the bedroom or empirically begin modifications.

The following modifications have been suggested to reduce mite exposure (28):

1. Cover mattresses and box springs with zippered vinyl or plastic encasing. Remove old mattresses, comforters, and pillows.
2. Remove bedroom and family room carpeting. Wooden or vinyl flooring is most desirable.

3. Wash all bedding in 60°C (130°F) every 10–15 days. Cold water will not kill live dust mites.
4. Reduce home humidity to preferably less than 40% with air-conditioning or dehumidifier.
5. Vacuum at least once a week. Patients with sensitivity should have someone else perform this task.

Several acaricides have been developed recently and include benzyl benzoate, pirimiphos methyl, liquid nitrogen, pyrethroids, and polyphenol-benzyl derivates (26,29–31). Benzyl benzoate has been evaluated in controlled studies and has been effective (26,30). However, the safety of this compound and others will have to be demonstrated before it can be advised for use in pregnancy.

Tannic acid 3% is not an acaricide, as it does not kill mites, but rather denatures their allergenic proteins (25). It has been effective in reducing allergen concentration if used repeatedly, but has the drawback of causing stains on light-colored carpets and materials. Its safety for use in the environment of a pregnant woman has not been determined.

Mold Allergy

The most important indoor molds are *Aspergillus*, *Penicillium*, and *Rhizopus* species. Mold growth is encouraged by dark, humid, and poorly ventilated areas. Bathrooms, kitchens, and basements are common sites. By following guidelines for reduction of mite antigen, the conditions for mold growth are usually also addressed.

Dehumidifiers, bathroom ventilation, and electronic air filters may be employed to reduce mold growth (28). There are several mold inhibitor cleaning products on the market; however, their toxicity during pregnancy is unknown, and use of such products is best avoided.

Animal Dander

Control of animal allergen is best achieved by avoiding contact with the offending animal. Even if a pet is eliminated from a home, the level of animal dander declines slowly (32). For patients who are unwilling to eliminate pets from their environment, modifications can be suggested to minimize their exposure to the animal and its dander. Most important is to emphasize the need to restrict animals from the bedroom at all times. This will help create a dander-reduced sanctuary (28). Some relief may be obtained by regular bathing of pets. Finally, use of an air purifier of the high-efficiency particulate air (HEPA) filter type has been shown to effectively reduce airborne particles and allergens. Animal-derived allergens remain airborne longest and are most susceptible to filtration (33).

SUMMARY

The primary goal of treatment during pregnancy is to reduce symptoms and need for medications. Avoidance programs are the most logical recommendations during pregnancy and include avoidance of exposure to cigarette smoke, animal dander, home dust mites, and molds. Medication and immunotherapy are alternatives when foregoing methods prove insufficient.

REFERENCES

1. Schatz M, Hoffman C. Interrelationships between asthma and pregnancy: clinical and mechanistic considerations. Clin Rev Allergy 1987; 5:301–315.
2. American Academy of Allergy and Immunology. Position statement on immunotherapy. J Allergy Clin Immunol 1989; 84:129–130.
3. Malline HJ. Indications for immunotherapy. Allergy 1988; 43(suppl):9–33.
4. Metzger WJ, Turner E, Patterson R. The safety of immunotherapy during pregnancy. J Allergy Clin Immunol 1978; 61:268–272.
5. Incaudo GA. Diagnosis and treatment of rhinitis during pregnancy and lactation. Clin Rev Allergy 1987; 5:325–327.
6. Schatz M, Hoffman CP, Zeiger RS. The course and management of asthma and allergic disease during pregnancy. In Middleton E, Reed CE, Ellis EF, et al, eds. Allergy principles and practice, 3rd ed. St Louis: CV Mosby, 1988:1093–1155.
7. Spector, SL. The treatment of the asthmatic mother during pregnancy and lactation. Ann Allergy 1983; 51:173–178.
8. Bosquet J. In vivo methods for study of allergy: skin tests, techniques, and interpretation. In Middleton E, Reed CE, Ellis EF, et al, eds. Allergy principles and practice, 3rd ed. St Louis, CV Mosby, 1988:419–436.
9. Van Arsdel PP, Larson EB. Diagnostic tests for patients with suspected allergic disease: utility and limitations. Ann Intern Med. 1989; 110:304–312.
10. Lockey RF, Benedict LM, Turkeltaub PC, Bukantz SC. Fatalities from immunotherapy and skin testing. J Allergy Clin Immunol 1987; 79:660–677.
11. Turkeltaub PC, Gergen PJ. The risk of adverse reactions from percutaneous prick-puncture allergenic skin testing, venipuncture and body movements: data from the second National Health and Nutrition Examination

Survey, 1976–1980 (NHANES 11). J Allergy Clin Immunol 1989; 84:886–890.
12. Council on Scientific Affairs. In vitro testing for allergy: report II of the allergy panel. JAMA 1987; 258:1639–1643.
13. Yunginger JW. Clinical significance of IgE. In: Middleton E, Reed CE, Ellis EF, et al, eds. Allergy principles and practice, 3rd ed. St Louis, CV Mosby, 1988:850–857.
14. Pienkowski MM, Norma PS, Lichtenstein LM. Suppression of late-phase skin reaction by immunotherapy with ragweed extract. J Allergy Clin Immunol 1985; 76:729–734.
15. Aas K. Adequate clinical trials of immunotherapy. Allergy 1982; 37:xx.
16. Metzger WJ. Indications for allergen immunotherapy during pregnancy. Comp Ther 1990; 16:17–26.
17. Francis N. Abortion after grass pollen injection. J Allergy 1941; 12:559.
18. Toogood JH. β-Blocker therapy and the risk of anaphylaxis. Can Med Assoc J 1987; 136:929–933.
19. Position Statement. β-Adrenergic blockers and immunotherapy and skin testing. J Allergy Clin Immunol 1989; 84:129–130.
20. Griess FC, Varwilkas D. Effect of sympathomimetic drugs and angiotensin on the uterine vascular bed. Obstet Gynecol 1964; 23:925–926.
21. Schwartz HJ, Golden D, Lockey R. Venom immunotherapy in the hymenoptera-allergic pregnant patient. J Allergy Clin Immunol 1990; 85:702–712.
22. Shiono PH, Klebanof MA, Rhoads GG. Smoking and drinking during pregnancy: their effects on preterm birth. JAMA 1986; 255:82–84.
23. Cnattinquis S, Haglund B, Merik O. Cigarette smoking as a risk factor for late fetal and early neonatal deaths. Br Med J 1988; 297:255–261.
24. Voorhorst R, Spieksma F, Vanekamp H, Keupen MJ, Lykleman W. The house dust mite (*Dermatophagoides pteronyssinus*) and the allergies it produces: identity with the house dust mite. J Allergy 1967; 39:325.
25. Platts-Mills TAE, Chapman MD. Dust Mites: immunology, allergic disease, and environmental control. J Allergy Clin Immunol 1987; 80:755–777.
26. Kersten W, Musken H, Moers FRG. A clinical study on the effectiveness of the acaricide acarosan in treating house-dust mite allergy. J Allergy Clin Immunol 1989; 83:263.
27. Mao JL, Pauli G, Tekara F, Hoyet C, Bischoff E, David B. Guanine content and *Dermatophagoides pteronyssinus* allergens in house dust samples. J Allergy Clin Immunol 1989; 83:926–933.
28. Conner B. Allergy proofing your home without losing your mind. In: Spector S, Sander N, eds. Understanding asthma—a blueprint for breathing. Am Coll Allergy Immunol 1989:147–154.
29. Green WF, Nicholas NR, Salome CM, Woolcock AJ. Reduction of house dust mites and mite allergens: effects of spraying carpets and blankets with Allersearch DMS, and acaricide combined with an allergen reducing agent. Clin Exp Allergy. 1989; 19:203–207.

30. Lau S, Rusche A, Weber A, Bischoff E, Wahn U. Short term efficacy of benzylbenzoate on mite allergen concentrations in house dust. J Allergy Clin Immunol 1989; 83:263.
31. Dietemann A, Hoyet C, Bessot JC, Blay DE, Pauli G. Effects of acaricide application on mite allergen levels and on symptoms of *Dermatophagoides pteronyssinus*. J Allergy Clin Immunol 1989; 83:263.
32. Wood RA, Chapman MD, Adkinson NF Jr, Eggliston PA. The effect of cat removal on allergen content in household-dust samples. J Allergy Clin Immunol 1989; 83:730–734.
33. Nelson HS, Hirsch R, Ohman JL, *et al*. Recommendations for the use of residential aircleaning devices in the treatment of allergic respiratory disease. J Allergy Clin Immunol 1988; 82:661–669.

6

Psychological Changes During Pregnancy: Implications for Medical Care

Andrea B. Stone

University of Massachusetts Medical School, Worcester, Massachusetts

Walter A. Brown

Brown University School of Medicine, Providence, Rhode Island

Pregnancy is a psychological as well as a physical event. The physiological and social role changes associated with pregnancy and pregnancy's particular meaning to a woman produce psychological changes. These changes vary from the mild forgetfulness of pregnancy to a sense of well-being, from the "adaptive anxiety" of the third trimester to the emotional lability of the puerperium. The extent to which these psychological events affect pregnancy outcome and, particularly, the expression of physical illness during pregnancy is unclear. What is clear is that medical care during pregnancy can be usefully informed by awareness of these psychological changes. In this chapter, we will review the changes in anxiety, mood, and cognition that occur throughout pregnancy and the postpartum period, with an emphasis on normal pregnancy. We will also discuss the special experience of pregnant women who suffer from psychiatric disorders, substance abuse, and physical abuse. Finally, we will discuss the effect of these psychological changes on medical care and will suggest diagnostic and therapeutic interventions for the clinician who cares for pregnant women.

OVERVIEW

Early psychoanalytic theories about emotional adjustment during pregnancy emphasized the importance of reproductive function in fulfilling a woman's development. Helene Deutsch saw pregnancy as a psychologically satisfying stage of life when a woman could devote herself entirely to the developing fetus and home life (1). As research on women's attitudes toward pregnancy began to reveal feelings of disappointment, anxiety, and ambivalence, the conflicts associated with pregnancy and its attendant social role changes became more central to theories about the psychology of pregnancy (2). Bibring proposed that the emotional disturbance found during pregnancy reflected a normative crisis that needed to be resolved for women to successfully proceed with adult development (3). For a while, conflict resolution during pregnancy was considered so important that lack of conflict was viewed as pathological. Zajicek explained the limitations of these early formulations:

> Theories about pregnancy and cultural expectations of women's behaviour during this period have often been unrealistic and linked more to the generalized attitude towards women prevalent at the time than to the real experiences of pregnant women (2, p. 33).

Finally, as theories became more informed by research findings, the crises and conflicts of pregnancy were seen as part of the adjustment to motherhood and not confined to the 9 months of pregnancy.

Contemporary research has taken two general approaches: (a) large, naturalistic surveys of psychological symptoms during or after pregnancy and (b) studies of the effect of psychological factors on pregnancy outcome. The survey studies find little distress or differences between patients with and without symptoms if the sample population is selected to accurately represent the general population (2,4). Studies of the connection between adverse pregnancy experiences and psychological condition find greater psychological distress during pregnancy in women with poor outcomes (e.g., low birth weight) (5).

One consistent finding in pregnancy research is that physiological, social, and historical events all seem to affect the psychological experience (Table 1). Few studies, however, control adequately for these factors. Sociocultural variables, including age, parity, employment, marital status, national origin, and whether the pregnancy was planned, affect psychological processes (2,4). Perceived support from partners or parents is important (4). Psychiatric history, medical problems, and previous pregnancy experience are all meaningful (6). Normal pregnancy phenomena, such as fatigue and changes in appetite and sleep, can confound the assessment of depression. The timing of measurement is also important. The psychological experience of pregnancy varies

Table 1 Factors That Affect the Psychological Experience of Pregnancy

Age
Parity
Employment status
Marital status
National origin
Planned vs unplanned pregnancy
Perceived social support
Psychiatric history
Medical problems
Previous pregnancy experience

Table 2 Normal Psychological Changes of Pregnancy

Mild, transient, first-trimester anxiety
Third-trimester anxiety that increases as labor and delivery nears
Moderate, brief, first-trimester depression
Mild forgetfulness, confusion, and distractability

with trimester and awareness of the fetus. In addition, the role of positive psychological changes during pregnancy is unknown.

Taking all of these variables into consideration is a monumental task often overlooked in pregnancy research. Studies that consider these variables most conscientiously find that, although many women report some emotional symptoms (e.g., crying) during pregnancy, most do not have disabling psychological difficulties (Table 2). No study has evaluated women before they become pregnant and followed them through pregnancy and the postpartum period. This approach would provide the most accurate data on pregnancy-specific changes.

Most studies have been done on European populations and may not be generalizable to North American women. Since cultural factors, such as expectations for employment after giving birth, have been shown to be relevant to psychological symptoms, the existing data may not be applicable beyond the culture studied. Furthermore, the few relevant pathophysiological studies of the effects of endogenous steroids on the brain and behavior are hindered by an even more obvious limit to generalizability: almost all of them have been done on rats. Notably absent from existing research are studies examining the psychological implications of pregnancy-related alterations in neurotransmission, despite the wide availability of urine and blood tests to evaluate psychiatrically relevant neurochemicals.

ANXIETY

Mild, transient anxiety is a part of most pregnancies. The infrequency of disabling anxiety symptoms is notable, given the risks of pregnancy and delivery to both the woman and fetus; the uncertainties about the health of the baby and the ability to assume the parental role; and the financial, career, and interpersonal consequences of having a baby.

Although the pathophysiology of anxiety has not been specifically studied during pregnancy, several changes in endocrine function occurring during pregnancy may be pertinent. Progesterone has sufficient sedating and hypnotic properties to have been used as an anesthetic (7). Also, two progesterone metabolites have barbituratelike modulating properties at γ-aminobutyric acid (GABA) receptors (7). [GABA, an inhibitory neurotransmitter, appears to play a fundamental role in the regulation of anxiety.] Rauramo et al. demonstrated that β-endorphin levels show a more prolonged increase in response to stress in pregnant women than in nonpregnant controls exposed to the same stress (8). These endocrine changes may contribute to the lack of significant anxiety symptoms in most pregnant women, despite the obvious stress of pregnancy. β-Endorphin and progesterone's central nervous system activities may enable women to handle the demands accompanying pregnancy without disruptive anxiety symptoms.

Anxiety appears to vary during the course of pregnancy. Some, but not all, researchers have found that women may be most vulnerable to symptoms of anxiety during the first and third trimesters (9,10). Somatic symptoms appear to be associated with anxiety levels (11). The first and third trimesters are usually associated with the most uncomfortable physical symptoms of pregnancy. Third-trimester anxiety may be an adaptive phenomenon (11,12); it appears to increase as delivery nears, may predict a positive-birthing experience (12), and seems to reflect a realistic attitude toward labor and delivery. Third-trimester anxiety alone has not been associated with adverse pregnancy outcome (11).

The consequences of anxiety earlier in pregnancy, especially during the first trimester, are less clear. In a prospective study, Cox and Reading found an increase in anxiety before the onset of complications such as hypertension, intrauterine growth retardation, and edema (13).

Other researchers have also found an association between higher anxiety levels early in pregnancy and adverse outcome (11,14). These and other studies of the relation between anxiety and outcome have come under considerable criticism owing to their methodological limitations (5). For example, the clinical relevance of the anxiety levels found in these studies is rarely determined. Robinson et al. found a decrease in maternal anxiety after prenatal testing (15). The "high levels of anxiety" before testing, however, were only at the 70th percentile of anxiety levels for a nonclinical control group. The follow-up levels were at the 28th percentile. Lubin et al. also detected changes in anxiety levels during pregnancy, but the pooled means for each trimester were within the normal range for the psychometric instruments employed (9). The use of a control group suggests that, although levels of anxiety change during pregnancy, pregnant women in general have, at most, average levels of anxiety.

Certain women appear to be more at risk for developing symptoms of anxiety during pregnancy (Table 3). Women who were younger, unmarried, and smoked, with lower education levels, financial difficulties, and poor social supports were more anxious and had babies with a lower gestational age at birth than older women with fewer socioeconomic stressors (14). Previous pregnancy experience affects anxiety as well. Women who have a history of both live births and spontaneous abortion have higher anxiety levels than women who have

Table 3 Features Associated With Psychological Difficulties During Pregnancy

Age
Marital status
Marital discord
Smoking
Alcohol or drug abuse
Unemployment
Financial difficulties
Poor social supports
Educational level
Doubts about the pregnancy
History of major mental illness
History of postpartum psychosis
Family history of depression or mania
Physical abuse

not had a spontaneous abortion (9). When more average populations (e.g., married, without a history of miscarriage, or significant socioeconomic distress) are studied, anxiety levels are low (15,16).

The diverse results from these studies reflect the fundamental difficulty of studying pregnancy and, especially, pregnancy outcome. Physiological, demographic, and personal matters contribute to each variable, and many variables determine outcome. Significant early-pregnancy anxiety might reflect problematic aspects of a woman's life that may be more directly relevant to pregnancy outcome than the emotional symptom. Late-pregnancy anxiety appears to be a productive adaptation to cope with labor, delivery, and impending motherhood.

MOOD CHANGES DURING PREGNANCY

Dysphoric or low mood is the most investigated mood symptom during pregnancy. As with anxiety, there is little consensus concerning the frequency, significance, or cause of this symptom.

All of the steroid hormones have been shown to have powerful influences on brain activity (17). Estrogen and progestins can alter neurotransmitter synthesis, degradation, release, uptake, and receptor activity (18). In rats, estradiol interacts with both the serotonergic and noradrenergic systems, the leading targets of antidepressant treatment (19,20). The brain structures that contain the greatest concentration of intracellular steroid receptors, the limbic system and the hypothalamus, are probably central to the regulation of mood (18). Therefore, brain exposure to the high levels of circulating hormones of pregnancy might be expected to affect mood.

Progesterone can function as a central nervous system depressant. Estrogens, on the other hand, have effectively been used as antidepressant therapy and to potentiate the action of other antidepressants (21). Oral contraceptives usually do not produce a measurable effect on mood. However, one-sixth of women describe an elevation in mood while taking oral contraceptives; other subgroups experience depressed mood. For example, women with a history of premenstrual symptoms complain of more depression while taking high-dose estrogen compounds (22). This suggest that individuals differ in their susceptibility to the mood-altering properties of gonadal steroids.

In a well-designed study of emotional disorders in pregnancy, Kumar and Robsom found that, among women who were not depressed before pregnancy, 10% experienced moderate, brief depressions during the first trimester (6) (see Table 2). Nearly all new cases of depression remitted by the second or third trimester. They found that depressive symptoms were correlated with marital difficulties, doubts about the pregnancy, a previous history of induced abortion, bereavement during pregnancy, preterm delivery, and cigarette smoking. Other researchers have found an association between depressive symptoms and being unmarried, older, and unemployed (23) (see Table 3). Depressed, pregnant women have been found to be more likely to smoke cigarettes, drink alcohol, abuse cocaine and marijuana, and to have less weight gain than nondepressed pregnant women (23).

In contrast with anxiety, psychological factors, such as perceived social support, appear to be more important than variables, such as age or income, in the development of depressive symptoms during pregnancy. Kendell describes the importance of cultural factors in his review of suicide rates during pregnancy (24). He found that the suicide rate among pregnant women is very low and has dropped significantly in the second half of this century. Most of the earlier suicides were among unmarried women. He attributes both the low rate and the drop over the last 40 years to social values. The influence on mood of other psychological factors, such as the desirability of the pregnancy, attitudes toward motherhood, and self-esteem, are unknown and probably differ greatly among women. For example, Zajicek found that women with high self-esteem during pregnancy had lower self-esteem during the first 4 months postpartum; women with medium self-esteem during pregnancy did not change throughout pregnancy and the first year postpartum; and women with low self-esteem during pregnancy had improved self-images between 4 and 14 months postpartum (2).

Most women do not experience serious, lasting depressive symptoms during or after pregnancy. The first trimester appears to be a time of increased symptoms. Psychological factors related to previous pregnancy experiences play a role in the development of symptoms during subsequent pregnancies. Substance abuse may complicate depression during pregnancy.

COGNITIVE CHANGES

During pregnancy, many women complain of cognitive difficulties, such as forgetfulness, but little systematic investigation has been devoted to this topic (25). Theoretical explanations for this difficulty come from the concept of pregnancy as a developmental crisis: women were having trouble thinking because they were unable to resolve their conflicts about having a baby (26).

Although pathophysiological mechanisms underlying cognitive changes during pregnancy have not been studied, Hampson has found that women's abilities to perform certain cognitive tests vary across the menstrual cycle (27). She found that women performed optimally when estradiol levels were in the midrange. These cognitive differences were not secondary to mood changes. Jarrahi-Zadeh et al. propose that the 2.5-fold increase in corticosteroid levels during pregnancy may be responsible for both mood and cognitive changes (28).

Attentional deficits, such as forgetfulness, confusion, and distractability, are reported consistently during pregnancy (25,28,29) (see Table 2). Reasoning and judgment are not impaired (25,26). Condon and Ball found that a pregnant woman's complaints of cognitive impairment were highly correlated with her partner's report (25), but women perceived a greater magnitude of difficulty than did their partners. Poser et al., in a study inspired by one of the author's pregnancy experiences, asked 51 health professionals who had 79 pregnancies to complete a questionnaire about conditions associated with pregnancy (29). Twenty-one women with 28 pregnancies had at least one of four symptoms of cognitive dysfunction: forgetfulness, disorientation, confusion, or reading difficulty. Symptom onset occurred during all three trimesters. They also found that cognitive deficits did not correlate with either depressed mood or sleep disturbance. They termed the cognitive dysfunction a *benign encephalopathy of pregnancy*. All cognitive difficulties resolved after delivery.

Psychotherapists have also noted changes in women's thinking during pregnancy. They have described a "shift toward primary process thinking," meaning that pregnant women appear to use more intuitive than rational modes of thinking (30). Systematic investigations have failed to support these observations (26,28).

Although it is the least-studied psychological change of pregnancy, pregnant women complain of difficulties with attention and concentration more frequently than they complain of depression or anxiety. These symptoms are independent of mood or sleep difficulties and may be secondary to the central nervous system effects of estradiol or corticosteroids. They remit after pregnancy.

SPECIAL ISSUES

Normal pregnancy does not appear to produce significant emotional disturbance. However, women with psychiatric disorders, substance abuse disorders, and those who are victims of physical abuse are at special psychological risk (see Table 3).

Preexisting Psychiatric Disorders

Approximately two-thirds of women with serious psychiatric disorders will have symptoms during pregnancy (31,32). These symptoms may reflect deterioration, improvement, or no change from their prepregnancy state (33). The remaining one-third experience pregnancy as a respite from chronic symptoms. Psychiatric diagnosis and age explain most of this variation (34). Younger women tend to encounter more difficulty during pregnancy than older women with the same diagnoses (34).

Women with psychotic disorders, such as schizophrenia, manic or depressive psychoses, or schizoaffective disorders, often have less difficulty with their psychiatric symptoms during pregnancy; they often require less medication (35), have fewer hospitalizations (36), have lower rates of illness than nonchildbearing control subjects (37) and report improved symptoms (33). Estrogen's antidopaminergic effect may explain this phenomenon (38). In rats, extended estrogen treatment has affected dopamine receptors similarly to haloperidol (39). The high levels of estrogen during pregnancy may be "treating" psychotic disorders, allowing women to require less medication, have fewer relapses, and feel better. Psychological factors, such as the need to care for a fetus and baby, may play a role in improved mental health for these women as well, but this has not been studied.

Women who suffer from recurrent, nonpsychotic depressive disorders may have depressive episodes during or after pregnancy (40). Those who were younger at the onset of their depressive disorder are more susceptible to pregnancy-related symptoms and also have more severe depressive symptoms than women who do not have pregnancy-related depressive episodes (40).

Women with panic attacks tend to be less symptomatic during pregnancy, but symptoms return or worsen after delivery (41). Progesterone's sedative–hypnotic properties may inhibit panic symptoms.

There is tremendous individual variation in the experience of pregnancy among women with psychiatric disorders that is not explained by demographic factors, personality style, life stressors, or mental health at the time of pregnancy (34). Despite the existence of serious psychiatric symptoms in over two-thirds of these women, most are not evaluated by a psychiatrist during pregnancy (32). The effects of pregnancy on personality disorders, generalized anxiety disorders, and obsessive–compulsive disorder, have not been studied.

Nausea and Vomiting

As detailed earlier, women with no previous psychiatric history do not usually suffer from serious psychiatric symptoms during pregnancy. Despite this, the search for psychological components to the diverse experiences of pregnancy continues. Nausea and vomiting during pregnancy have inspired considerable research and speculation on their psychological origins. They have been seen as both normal or pathological, acceptance or rejection of pregnancy, and wholly psychological or wholly physiological (42). In Wolkind and Zajicek's prospective, psychosocial study of 247 pregnant women, they found that nausea and vomiting after the first trimester were generally associated with social, but not psychiatric, problems (42). Nausea and vomiting that leads to dehydration and ketosis and that cannot be explained medically occasionally heralds an underlying eating disorder, such as bulimia nervosa, that would require psychiatric intervention (43). In general, nausea and vomiting during pregnancy appears to be a manifestation of physiological, not psychological processes.

Postpartum Disorders

In contrast with pregnancy, the first 3 months postpartum is a time of increased vulnerability to serious psychiatric symptoms, especially psychoses (36,44). Since Pitt first described an atypical depression occurring after childbirth, a tremendous volume of medical literature has been devoted to the subject of postpartum depressive symptoms (45). Syndromes as different as emotional lability for a few days after delivery to psychotic disorders, all have been characterized as "postpartum depression." Postpartum "blues," a mild, transient depressive phenomenon, occurs 2–4 days after delivery in 50–80% of women (46). Postpartum psychotic illness develops in 0.2% of women (46). These two syndromes appear to be specific to the postpartum period. The underlying pathophysiological mechanism may be related to the tremendous drop in estrogen and progesterone that occurs after parturition. The blues do not appear to be related to demographic or obstetric variables or to have lasting psychiatric importance (44).

The only obstetric variable associated with postpartum psychosis is primiparity. A personal or family history of affective disorders, especially bipolar disorder, is the single best predictor of postpartum psychosis (44). Women with bipolar illness may have a rate of postpartum recurrences as high as 50% (47). The onset is usually within the first month and often within the first 2 weeks postpartum. The syndrome is characterized by an extremely volatile course. Women may be asymptomatic at one moment and severely disturbed a short time later. Prominent symptoms include agitation, confusion, hallucinations, delusions, disrupted sleep, and occasionally, violent behavior (48). The risk of suicide or infanticide is serious enough to warrant hospitalization or constant observation. The treatment is the same as for any acute psychotic episode. Mood-stabilizing agents, such as lithium or carbamazepine, may be necessary. Premenstrual relapses and relapses after subsequent pregnancies are common (44,49). A postpartum psychosis may also herald the onset of bipolar illness with recurrences unrelated to pregnancy (50).

The consistent timing of the onset of postpartum psychosis implicates the tremendous drop in reproductive hormones that takes place immediately after delivery. Estrogen is known to modulate dopamine receptor sensitivity (39). The rapid withdrawal of estrogen after delivery may lead to psychotic symptoms in vulnerable individuals owing to supersensitive dopamine receptors (51). Prophylactic, high-dose estrogen treatment beginning within 24 hr of delivery in women with a history of postpartum psychosis has been effective in preventing relapses (48; Sichel DA, personal communication).

Some women will develop other serious psychiatric illnesses for the first time during the postpartum period. Depression, panic disorder, and obsessive–compulsive disorder, all have had their onset postpartum (44,52,53). Once again, family history or a history of other psychiatric disorders have been associated with the development of these postpartum syndromes.

The significance of moderate to severe nonpsychotic depressive episodes occurring after pregnancy is controversial. These syndromes are characterized by more severe and persistent symptoms than the blues. Women may be markedly depressed, hopeless, and anhedonic, and have disturbances in appetite and sleep, but they are not psychotic. The onset of symptoms may coincide with the blues or may be weeks to months later. The average prevalence rate for postpartum depressive episodes that begin within 3 months of delivery is 12% (44). Many women remain symptomatic for more than 6 months. Depressive symptoms during pregnancy, a personal or family history of mood disorder, and marital difficulties, or poor social support may increase the likelihood of a depressive episode occurring at this time. Recent, well-controlled studies have shown that the prevalence rate of nonpsychotic depressive episodes postpartum does not differ from the rate of depressive episodes in well-matched, nonpregnant control subjects (54). The main difference between the childbearing and the nonchildbearing groups was that postpartum subjects had more severe symptoms when depressed than the nonchildbearing women. O'Hara suggests "... that childbirth and the demands of the postpartum period constitute a nonspecific stress which increases the likelihood of a depressive episode in an already vulnerable woman" (44).

Substance Abuse

Other than documentation of the negative consequences to the fetus, there is little information about substance abuse during pregnancy. Nevertheless, women do abuse alcohol and drugs during pregnancy (43,55). In a recent evaluation of urine drug screens in low-income clinics serving minority women and private obstetrical settings serving middle-class white women, the incidence of positive drug screens was approximately 15% in both groups (56). Substance abuse has serious negative health consequences for both the fetus and mother. Alcohol and other recreational drugs can be teratogenic (55). Many women substance abusers do not receive adequate antenatal care. Undiagnosed substance abuse poses hazards to the mother and fetus at delivery owing to unanticipated withdrawal syndromes and interactions with both anesthesia and pain management. Women with depressive symptoms and those who are victims of physical abuse or other forms of violence are more likely to abuse substances than other women (57).

Physical Abuse

Pregnant women, compared with nonpregnant women, are at increased risk for physical abuse (58). Gelles reported that pregnant women were at greater risk than nonpregnant women for all types of violence: overall, minor, and severe (58). Previous abuse is the best predictor of abuse during pregnancy, although abuse may begin in pregnancy (59,60). Preexisting battering may increase, decrease, or stay the same during pregnancy. Perpetrators are usually male partners, but pregnant adolescents and young adults may be abused by their parents (59). A male partner's substance abuse also predicts a pregnant woman's susceptibility to violent victimization (61).

Nearly half of abused, pregnant women report emotional symptoms, especially depression. Many have a history of suicide attempts (59,61). Abused, pregnant women are more likely to drink alcohol and smoke cigarettes than do nonabused pregnant women (59). Although there have been no studies looking at physical violence as a specific risk factor for adverse pregnancy outcome, its associations with alcohol abuse, smoking, and suicidality suggest that it increases the likelihood of adverse outcome.

Women with psychiatric disorders, substance abuse, or physical abuse may have significant psychopathology during pregnancy or in the postpartum period. Although psychotic disorders are often improved during pregnancy, the postpartum period presents a time of increased vulnerability both for women with preexisting conditions and for women with a predisposition to developing major psychiatric disorders.

Depressions that occur postpartum may be more severe than depressions occurring at other times of life. Depressive symptoms during pregnancy often coexist with substance abuse and physical abuse. When left untreated these instances of serious psychiatric difficulties clearly have a negative effect on mothers and infants. Unfortunately, more often than not they are undiagnosed and untreated.

IMPLICATIONS FOR MEDICAL CARE

Routine Interventions

Most psychological changes during pregnancy are mild and transient. They do not need treatment by a mental health professional. Support, education, allowing a patient to discuss her concerns (ventilation), and providing reassurance are effective approaches for many mild difficulties (62). The challenge for the medical practitioner is to recognize serious symptoms that require further evaluation and care (Table 4).

Perceived social support and continuing employment have both been associated with less psychological distress during pregnancy. Therefore, the involvement of a woman's partner or parent in her medical care may provide "emotional prophylaxis." Also, unless medically contraindicated, a physician may recommend continued employment during pregnancy for the same purpose.

Table 4 General Principles for Psychological Management During Pregnancy

Ventilation
Support
Education
Reassurance
Referral to mental health professional when symptoms are severe or prolonged

Pregnancy also provides a unique time in many women's lives in that they come for medical care more routinely than at any other time of life. Medical practitioners are afforded the opportunity of educating women in a consistent, nonconfrontational way on the health effects of smoking, drinking, substance abuse, noncompliance with prescribed medical regimens, and other health risk behaviors. Women have been shown to be highly motivated toward behavior change during pregnancy; they decrease both smoking and drinking (63,64). Diagnostic tests, such as ultrasound, that enable a woman to see the fetus, can lead to improved health behaviors (63). These changes can be long-term (64).

Reassuring and educating women about the "normal" range of psychological experiences during pregnancy is helpful, even before psychological symptoms have developed. Anxiety, especially in the third trimester; mild, transient depressive symptoms; forgetfulness; and confusion; all can be a part of the normal pregnancy. These symptoms can be quite distressing if women do not realize that they often accompany pregnancy, are usually transient, and do not reflect any profound, underlying deficiencies. Ultrasound examinations and other genetic testing may decrease anxiety in women who are especially concerned about the well-being of the fetus (15,65). Writing instructions for medical treatment may improve compliance with treatment and may help alleviate the frustration and anxiety caused by memory difficulties. Learning to make lists also may help accomplish this (29).

Significant anxiety during the first trimester and depressive symptoms that are persistent require further evaluation. Detailed investigation of a women's stressors, including financial difficulties, perception of social support, substance abuse, and the presence of physical abuse, may point to the source of a pregnant woman's symptoms. Women with protracted depressive symptoms, such as low mood, inability to enjoy normally pleasurable activities, diminished appetite, hopelessness, and suicidal ideation, should be referred for evaluation by a mental health professional.

Certain medical presentations may arise from underlying psychological distress. For example, anxious pregnant patients often present with somatic symptoms that cannot be explained by their medical status (9). Battered women often come to the emergency room with a confusing array of physical symptoms and injuries (60). Alcohol use and cigarette smoking that continue unchanged during pregnancy may suggest underlying depressive pathology or ongoing physical violence (57,61).

Although there is no data on how psychological changes during pregnancy may modify the psychology of asthma and allergic symptoms, pregnancy may exacerbate these conditions in women whose symptoms tend to worsen with stress. Schatz et al. have adapted the general principles of psychological management during pregnancy (ventilation, education, support, and reassurance) to this patient population (66). A woman should be given the opportunity to express her fears and concerns about her pregnancy. Education should include information concerning the effects of asthma and allergies on pregnancy and the infant, the effects of pregnancy on asthma and allergic symptoms, the effects of medications, the likelihood of having a baby with asthma or allergies, and how to decrease the possibility of allergies developing in the infant. Providing support means scheduling regular visits and being available to handle unanticipated problems. Applying these principles is reassuring, as is the knowledge that the medical physician, the obstetrician, and the patient are collaborating to maximize the chances of a good outcome for the woman and her child.

Since the pharmacokinetics of most drugs during pregnancy are unknown, drugs taken during pregnancy may cause unexpected psychological symptoms. A drug's metabolism and effects are altered by gender, blood volume, and circulating hormones (67). If new psychological symptoms develop in a pregnant woman receiving medication, the possibility of a drug-induced side effect should be included in the differential diagnosis.

Psychiatric Disorders and Substance Abuse

Women with a history of a previous psychotic episode, manic episode, or major depressive episode, especially one that occurred postpartum, should probably be referred for psychiatric evaluation (43). This permits assessment of baseline mental status and education of the patient about risks of recurrence of symptoms; it establishes a relationship with a psychiatric practitioner and facilitates prophylactic interventions. Women with a family history of major affective illness should be carefully monitored for the development of affective symptoms, especially postpartum.

Women with chronic psychiatric disorders such as schizophrenia, bipolar disorder (manic–depressive illness), or recurrent depression should be referred for psychiatric evaluation if they are not already involved in treatment. They can be safely treated for most symptoms of major mental illness, particularly after the first trimester. Untreated mental illness is needlessly distressing to the patient and potentially dangerous. Changes in existing psychiatric medication should be done in consultation with the treating psychiatrist. When necessary, a psychiatric hospitalization may provide the safest means for treating a pregnant woman during the first trimester.

Since the risk of an untreated postpartum psychosis, obsessional disorder, or major depression includes danger to both the mother and infant, all women should be asked about psychological symptoms early in the postpartum period, especially 1–3 weeks postpartum. Any woman who appears to have developed symptoms that are disruptive or interfere with her functioning, even if they wax and wane, should be referred for psychiatric evaluation.

The task of making a diagnosis of ongoing substance abuse may be made more difficult by the advent of legal prosecution of women who use drugs and alcohol during pregnancy as child abusers. Asking women about substance abuse routinely, establishing an open, nonjudgmental relation, and education about risks may help uncover substance abuse difficulties. When substance abuse is suspected, the evaluation should include urine testing, especially since many drug abusers use multiple substances. Ideally, treatment should take place in a setting experienced in treating pregnant women, since detoxification is not always safe toward the end of pregnancy.

SUMMARY

Psychological symptoms cannot be treated if they are unrecognized. Most women experience mild, transient psychological symptoms during pregnancy that respond to support, reassurance, and education. The first trimester has the highest incidence of anxious and depressive symptoms. Reassurance that these symptoms are normal and transient will alleviate associated anxiety. The postpartum period is a time of particular vulnerability to psychological symptoms. Women with persistent, disturbing symptoms should be referred for further evaluation.

Pregnancy provides a unique opportunity for physicians to initiate preventive medical care. Pregnant women are especially motivated for behavior change. Physicians can take advantage of this by providing health education and intervention for alcohol and substance abuse, cigarette smoking, and physical abuse.

REFERENCES

1. Deutsch H. The psychology of women. New York: Grune & Stratton, 1947.
2. Zajicek E. The experience of being pregnant. In: Wolkind S, Zajicek E, eds. Pregnancy: a psychological and social study. New York: Grune & Stratton, 1981:31–56.

3. Bibring GL. Some consideration of the psychological processes in pregnancy. Psychoanal Study Child 1959; 14:113–121.
4. Nilsson A. Para-natal emotional adjustment: a prospective investigation of 165 women. Acta Psychiatr Scand Suppl 1970; 220:1–61.
5. Istvan J. Stress, anxiety, and birth outcomes: a critical review of the evidence. Psychol Bull 1986; 100:331–348.
6. Kumar R, Robson KM. A prospective study of emotional disorders in childbearing women. Br J Psychiatry 1984; 144:35–47.
7. Cowley DS, Roy-Byrne PP. Panic disorder during pregnancy. J Psychosom Obstet Gynaecol 1989; 10:193–210.
8. Rauramo I, Salminen K, Laatikainen T. Release of β-Endorphin in response to physical exercise in nonpregnant and pregnant women. Acta Obstet Gynecol Scand 1986; 65:609–612.
9. Lubin B, Gardener SH, Roth A. Mood and somatic symptoms during pregnancy. Psychosom Med 1975; 37:136–146.
10. Elliott SA, Watson JP, Brough DI. Mood changes during pregnancy and after the birth of a child. Br J Clin Psychol 1983; 22:295–308.
11. Gorsuch RL, Key MK. Abnormalities of pregnancy as a function of anxiety and life stress. Psychosom Med 1974; 36:352–362.
12. Crowe K, von Baeyer C. Predictors of a positive childbirth experience. Birth 1989; 16:59–63.
13. Cox DN, Reading AE. Fluctuations in state anxiety over the course of pregnancy and the relationship to outcome. J Psychosom Obstet Gyneacol 1989; 10:71–78.
14. Pagel MD, Smilkstein G, Regen H, Montano D. Psychosocial influences on newborn outcomes: a controlled prospective study. Soc Sci Med 1990; 30:597–604.
15. Robinson GE, Garner DM, Olmsted MP, Shime J, Hutton EM, Crawford BM. Anxiety reduction after chorionic villus sampling and genetic amniocentesis. Am J Obstet Gynecol 1988; 159:953–956.
16. Reading AE, Cox DN. The effects of ultrasound examination on maternal anxiety levels. J Behav Med 1982; 5:237–247.
17. Pfaff DW, McEwen BS. Actions of estrogens and progestins on nerve cells. Science 1983; 219:808–814.
18. McEwen BS. Gonadal and adrenal steroids and the brain: implications for depression. In: Halbreich H, ed. Hormones and depression. New York: Raven Press, 1987:239–253.
19. Biegon A, McEwen BS. Modulation by estradiol of serotonin$_1$ receptors in brain. J Neurosci 1982; 2:199–205.
20. Sar M, Stumpf WE. Central noradrenergic neurones concentrate ^{3}H-oestradiol. Nature 1981; 289:500–502.
21. Duman KS, Enna SJ. On the relationship between hormones, depression and neurotransmitter receptor responses to antidepressants. In: Halbreich U, ed. Hormones and depression. New York: Raven Press, 1987:279–296.

22. Glick ID, Quitkin FM, Bennett SE. The influence of estrogens, progestins and oral contraceptives on depression. In: Halbreich U, ed. Hormones and depression. New York: Raven Press, 1987:339–356.
23. Zuckerman B, Amaro H, Bauchner H, Cabral H. Depressive symptoms during pregnancy: relationship to poor health behaviors. Am J Obstet Gyecol 1989; 160:1107–1111.
24. Kendell RE. Suicide in pregnancy and the puerperium. Br Med J 1991; 302:126–127.
25. Condon JT, Ball SB. Altered psychological functioning in pregnant women: an empirical investigation. J Psychosom Obstet Gynaecol 1989; 10:211–220.
26. Bailey LA, Bailey BJ. The psychological experience of pregnancy. Int J Psychiatry Med 1986; 16:263–274.
27. Hampson E. Estrogen-related variations in human spatial and articulatory-motor skills. Psychoneuroendocrinology 1990; 15:97–111.
28. Jarrahi-Zadeh A, Kane FJ, Van De Castle RL, Lachenbruck PA, Ewing JA. Emotional and cognitive changes in pregnancy and early puerperium. Br J Psychiatry 1969; 115:797–805.
29. Poser CM, Kassirer MR, Peyser JM. Benign encephalopathy of pregnancy. Acta Neurol Scand 1986; 73:39–43.
30. Condon JT. Altered cognitive functioning in pregnant women: a shift towards primary process thinking. Br J Med Psychol 1987; 60:329–334.
31. Zajicek E. Psychiatric problems during pregnancy. In: Wolkind S, Zajicek E, eds. Pregnancy: a psychological and social study. New York: Grune & Stratton, 1981:57–73.
32. McNeil TF, Kaij L, Malmquist-Larsson A. Women with nonorganic psychosis: mental disturbance during pregnancy. Acta Psychiatr Scand 1984; 70:127–139.
33. McNeil TF, Kaij L, Malmquist-Larsson A. Women with nonorganic psychosis: pregnancy's effect on mental health during pregnancy. Acta Psychiatr Scand 1984; 70:140–148.
34. McNeil TF, Kaij L, Malmquist-Larsson A. Women with nonorganic psychosis: factors associated with pregnancy's effect on mental health. Acta Psychiatr Scand 1984; 70:209–219.
35. Krener P, Simmons MK, Hansen RL, Treat JN. Effect of pregnancy on psychosis: life circumstances and psychiatric symptoms. Int J Psychiatry Med 1989; 19:65–84.
36. Pugh TF, Jerath BK, Schmidt WM, Reed RB. Rates of mental disease related to childbearing. N Engl J Med 1963; 268:1224–1228.
37. Paffenbarger RS. Epidemiological aspects of mental illness associated with childbearing. In: Brockington IF, Kumar R, eds. Motherhood and mental illness. New York: Grune & Stratton, 1982:19–36.
38. Euvrard C, Oberlander C, Boissier JR. Antidopaminergic effect of estrogens at the striatal level. J Pharmacol Exp Ther 1980; 214:179–185.

39. Di Paolo T, Poyet P, Labrie F. Effect of chronic estradiol and haloperidol treatment on striatal dopamine receptors. Eur J Pharmacol 1981; 73:105–106.
40. Frank E, Kufper DJ, Jacob M, Blumenthal SJ, Jarrett DB. Pregnancy-related affective episodes among women with recurrent depression. Am J Psychiatry 1987; 144:288–293.
41. Cowley DS, Roy-Byrne PP. Panic disorder during pregnancy. J Psychosom Obstet Gynaecol 1989; 10:193–210.
42. Wolkind S. Nausea and vomiting of pregnancy. In: Wolkind S, Zajicek E, eds. Pregnancy: a psychological and social study. New York: Grune & Stratton, 1981:75–88.
43. Oppenheim GB. Psychological disorders in pregnancy. In: Priest RB, ed. Psychological disorders in obstetrics and gynaecology. London: Butterworths, 1984:93–146.
44. O'Hara MW. Postpartum "blues", depression, and psychosis: a review. J Psychosom Obstet Gynecol 1987; 7:205–227.
45. Pitt B. "Atypical" depression following childbirth. Br J Psychiatry 1968; 114:1325–1335.
46. Harding JJ. Postpartum psychiatric disorders: a review. Compr Psychiatry 1989; 30:109–112.
47. Reich T, Winokur G. Postpartum psychosis in patients with manic–depressive disease. J Nerv Ment Dis 1970; 151:60–68.
48. Hamilton JA. Postpartum psychiatric syndromes. Psychiatr Clin North Am 1989; 12:89–103.
49. Brockington IF, Kelly A, Hall P, Deakin W. Premenstrual relapse of puerperal psychosis. J Affective Disord 1988; 14:287–292.
50. Akiskal HS, Walker P, Puzantian VR, King D, Rosenthal TL, Dranon M. Bipolar outcome in the course of depressive illness. J Affective Disord 1983; 5:115–128.
51. Seeman MV. Interaction of sex, age, and neuroleptic dose. Compr Psychiatry 1983; 24:125–128.
52. Metz A, Sichel DA, Goff DC. Postpartum panic disorder. J Clin Psychiatry 1988; 49:278–279.
53. Sichel DA, Cohen LS, Driscoll GA, Rosenbaum J. Postpartum obsessive compulsive disorder. Psychosomatics (in press).
54. O'Hara MW, Zekoski EM, Philipps, LH, Wright EJ. Controlled prospective study of postpartum mood disorders: comparison of childbearing and nonchildbearing women. J Abnorm Psychol 1990; 99:3–15.
55. Brockington IF, Kumar R. Drug addiction and psychotropic drug treatment during pregnancy and lactation. In: Brockington IF, Kumar R, eds. Motherhood and mental illness. New York: Grune & Stratton, 1982:239–255.
56. Chasnoff IJ, Barrett ME, Landress HJ. [Letter]. N Engl J Med 1990; 322:1202.
57. Zuckerman B, Amaro H, Bauchner H, Cabral H. Depressive symptoms during pregnancy: relationship to poor health behaviors. Am J Obstet Gynecol 1989; 160:1107–1111.

58. Gelles RJ. Violence and pregnancy: are pregnant women at greater risk of abuse? J Marriage Fam 1988; 50:841–847.
59. Hillard PJA. Physical abuse in pregnancy. Obstet Gynecol 1985; 66:185–190.
60. Helton AS, McFarlane J, Anderson ET. Battered and pregnant: a prevalence study. Am J Public Health 1987; 77:1337–1339.
61. Amaro H, Fried LE, Cabral H, Zuckerman B. Violence during pregnancy and substance use. Am J Public Health 1990; 80:575–579.
62. Brown WA. Psychological care during pregnancy and the postpartum period. New York: Raven Press, 1979.
63. Reading AE, Campbell S, Cox DN, Sledmere CM. Health beliefs and health care behaviour in pregnancy. Psychol Med 1982; 12:379–383.
64. Fingerhut LA, Kleinmen JC, Kendrick JS. Smoking before, during and after pregnancy. Am J Public Health 1990; 80:541–544.
65. Reading AE, Cox DN. The effects of ultrasound examination on maternal anxiety levels. J Behav Med 1982; 5:237–247.
66. Schatz M, Hoffman CP, Zeige RS, et al. The course and management of asthma and allergic diseases during pregnancy. In: Middleton E, Reed CE, Ellis EF, et al, eds. Allergy: principles and practice. St Louis: CV Mosby, 1988:1106.
67. Kato R. Sex-related differences in drug metabolism. Drug Metab Rev 1974; 3:1–32.

7

Use of Medication During Pregnancy and Lactation: General Considerations

Richard S. Abrams

Rose Medical Center and University of Colorado School of Medicine, Denver, Colorado

INTRODUCTION

Risk versus Benefit

Less than a generation ago physicians reassured expectant mothers that their fetuses enjoyed complete protection within the uterus. Tragic experiences with substances such as thalidomide and alcohol have now swung public perception to the commonly held belief that nothing is safe to take during pregnancy; thus, relagating pregnant women to the status of "therapeutic orphans." Few clinical settings dramatize the delicate balance between risk and benefit better than pregnancy. Even though it is true that most drugs do not harm the developing fetus, clearly some do. The use of any drug during pregnancy entails acceptance of risks. These risks require careful communication between health care professional and patient. Indications for the use of any drug during pregnancy must be carefully considered, ideally before conception. The standard caveat about risks and benefit in the *Physician's Desk Reference* provides little help to the clinician faced with the need to care for a patient with a significant medical disorder. To ensure the well-being of the fetus, its mother must remain healthy.

It is now clear that medical conditions, such as asthma, can jeopardize the health of both mother and fetus. When drug therapy is indicated, it is important to use the drug as effectively as possible. Medications must be given in effective doses and patients monitored for therapeutic effect, drug level, or both. Whenever possible, drugs with which there has been some experience in pregnancy should be used. Patients must be encouraged to actively participate in their own medical care by providing them with a clear understanding of their medical disorder and its effect on pregnancy, what is known and not known about the proposed treatment, possible alternatives to drug therapy, and continuing access to care to assess therapeutic effect and any adverse effects.

Clearly, choosing appropriate drug therapy for pregnant women with asthma and allergies must include an understanding of altered pharmacokinetics during gestation and an appreciation for possible developmental toxicity in the fetus. This chapter briefly highlights current knowledge about drug therapy and human reproduction. Information about specific drug therapy for the management of asthma will be discussed in subsequent chapters.

Major Causes of Human Developmental Defects

Developmental defects in humans are broadly divided into those resulting from known genetic causes, approximately 20%; chromsomal aberrations, 3–5%; environmental causes (drugs, chemicals, infections, maternal metabolic imbalance, and radiation), 4–6%; and unknown causes, 65–70%. Thus, the cause of almost all congenital anomalies remains unknown. These unknown causes of birth defects may include unrecognized interactions among drugs, chemicals, and genetic causes. Simply avoiding known teratogens could result in prevention of anomalies in up to 7500 newborns each year.

Evaluating Drug Risk

Perhaps the greatest impediment to ensuring the safety of drugs during pregnancy is the inability to prospectively test them in humans. For obvious practical and ethical reasons, experimental animals are used to test pharmaceutic products before obtaining Food and Drug Administration (FDA) approval. Animal studies have the advantages of being inexpensive, avoiding unnecessary human exposure, and providing the ability to test one variable at a time. With the exception of coumarin-type anticoagulants, almost every chemical known to be teratogenic in humans is also teratogenic in one or more laboratory species. It thus appears that positive animal teratology studies are at least suggestive of potential human harm. Moreover, the more animal species in which a compound is teratogenic, the more likely it is to have a human effect, albeit not the same effect as in animals (1). Clinicians should not ignore developmental toxicity tests in animals merely because laboratory rats are not like humans (1). Unfortunately, animal models are far from perfect. It must always be remembered that before its release in the 1950s, thalidomide was tested in rats and mice and determined to be free of teratogenic effects.

Other sources of information on the reproductive safety of drugs include case reports and epidemiological studies. Case reports of variable detail and quality are submitted by clinicians to registries and for journal publication. Their major benefit is to identify rare events. Case reports provided the first awareness of teratogenesis following maternal use of thalidomide. The obvious disadvantage of case reports lies in their inability to establish causation.

The epidemiological techniques of case–control studies and cohort studies are often used to further explore possible links between drugs and adverse reproductive outcome. *Case–control studies* begin with a specific outcome and examine medical records for exposure to a drug. Records of a control group of nonaffected children are searched to arrive at an odds ratio for a drug producing a specific effect. Confidence intervals must be presented to indicate whether a relation is statistically significant. Such retrospective studies are always fraught with potential bias from the researcher. Moreover, studies often require numerous subjects to achieve meaningful confidence intervals.

Cohort studies are the opposite of case–control studies. They begin with a group of subjects exposed to a drug and a control group of nonexposed subjects. These groups are followed prospectively to determine the frequency of adverse outcomes and to calculate a risk ratio. If an adverse outcome is rare, cohort studies need even more subjects than are required for case–control studies.

To help overcome the difficulty and bias of aggregating results of multiple independent studies, the mathematical technique of meta-analysis was developed (2). By using meta-analysis, studies of varying sample size can be combined by giving more weight to larger studies. Reviews using this statistical technique can be extremely helpful for evaluating the risk of specific drugs and for counseling patients.

Epidemiological studies of drug risks during pregnancy have clearly grown in importance. It is essential, however, to remember the pitfalls in interpreting them and to be cautious in advising patients on the basis of studies that purport to show only weak associations between exposures and adverse pregnancy outcomes. An important reason for being concerned about the size of the effect is that unknown or inadequately accounted for confounding variables can easily produce artifactual small effects. It is far less likely that confounding variables account for large effects (3).

The Food and Drug Administration Use-in-Pregnancy Ratings

The FDA has established categories for the use of drugs during pregnancy (Table 1) (4). Categories are based on the degree to which available information has ruled out risk to the fetus, balanced against the drug's potential benefits to the patient. Ratings range from *A*, for the drugs that have been tested for teratogenicity under controlled conditions without showing evidence of damage to the fetus, to *D* and *X* for drugs that are definitely teratogenic. The *D* rating is generally reserved for drugs with no safer alternatives. The *X* rating means there is absolutely no reason to risk using the drug during pregnancy. This classification tends to oversimplify a very complex problem. Most drugs are assigned to categories *B* and *C* where safety cannot be ensured. In addition the rating system does not apply to adverse effects of drugs during breast-feeding.

DEVELOPMENTAL TOXICITY OF DRUGS

Teratogens

A *teratogen* is defined as an agent that induces structural malformations, metabolic or physiological dysfunction, or psychological deficits,

Table 1 Key to FDA Use-in-Pregnancy Ratings

Category	Interpretation
A	Controlled studies show no risk. Adequate, well-controlled studies in pregnant women have failed to demonstrate risk to the fetus.
B	No evidence of risk in humans. Either animal findings show risk, but human findings do not; or, if no adequate human studies have been done, animal findings are negative.
C	Risk cannot be ruled out. Human studies are lacking, and animal studies are either positive for fetal risk, or lacking as well. However, potential benefits may justify the potential risk.
D	Positive evidence of risk. Investigational or postmarketing data show risk to the fetus. Nevertheless, potential benefits may outweigh the potential risk.
X	Contraindicated in pregnancy. Studies in animals or humans, or investigational or postmarketing reports have shown fetal risk that clearly outweighs any possible benefit to the patient.

either at birth or in a defined postnatal period. In an estimated 65–70% of all cases the cause of birth defects is unknown. The large "unknown" category, however, does not exclude the possibility that drugs or chemicals have contributed to these defects, especially because information on the hazards of drugs and chemicals is largely based on case reports, rather than epidemiological studies.

Since the thalidomide tragedy of the early 1960s, teratology has emerged as a discipline of great interest to the scientific and medical community, as well as to regulatory agencies, industry, lawyers, and the public at large. Congenital malformations and low birth weight remain the leading causes of infant deaths in the United States today. Malformations account for over one-half of infant deaths as well as reduced life expectancy in survivors.

Malformations

Malformations constitute structural abnormalities of prenatal origin that are present at birth and that seriously interefere with viability or physical well-being. A *major malformation* is defined as one that is incompatible with survival or one that requires major surgery for correction, such as cleft palate or congenital heart disease. Numerous studies have concluded that approximately 3% of all newborn children are affected by major malformations. Inclusion of all minor malformations, such as ear tags or extra digits, increases the overall malformation rate to approximately 7–10%. This figure constitutes the so-called background incidence of malformations. To understand the additional risk of malformation after exposure to a drug or chemical, the background incidence of anomalies in the general population must always be considered.

Abnormal Growth

It is now clear that important development continues beyond the classic teratogenic period of the first trimester. Drugs capable of causing malformations are also capable of inducing other abnormalities of development as well. From 12-weeks gestation until term the fetus undergoes significant growth and organization of the central nervous system. Adverse effects of drugs during this time can be expected to manifest in abnormalities of fetal growth and brain function. Perhaps no drug illustrates this point more tragically than alcohol. In humans, other agents known to cause intrauterine growth retardation include cigarette smoking, warfarin, phenytoin, heroin, methadone, and trimethadione.

Fetal Death

If given in a sufficiently high dose, virtually any drug or chemical is capable of causing intrauterine death. When toxicity occurs during early gestation, the embryo dies and is resorbed. When intrauterine death occurs during late gestation the fetus cannot be completely resorbed and a stillborn or dead, and often, macerated fetus results. Mortality may be due to direct toxic action on the conceptus or it may be due to the combined effect of toxicity and a developmental malformation. It is usually impossible to distinguish between the two. It has been suggested that, in humans, spontaneous abortion may serve as a selective means of terminating abnormal conception.

Functional Impairment

The effect of drugs on the developing fetus is not limited to structural abnormalities or fetal death. It is now known that a medication administered during pregnancy may produce long-term neurobehavioral effects. Examples of human behavioral effects of antenatal drug toxicity include hyperactivity, brief attention span, and temper outbursts observed in offspring of narcotic-addicted mothers; mental retardation in the offspring of women treated with anticonvulsants, alcohol, and lead; and the abnormal reflexes seen in children born to mothers who ingested methyl mercury.

PRINCIPLES OF TERATOGENESIS

Whether or not a drug or chemical can potentially cause abnormal fetal development is governed by several fundamental principles of teratogenesis. Paraphrasing Karnofsky (5), Schardein (6) illustrated these principles by the following axiom, ". . . a teratogenic response depends upon the administration of a specific treatment of a particular dose to a genetically susceptible species when the embryos are in a susceptible stage of development."

Species Variability

The current basis of the FDA's risk categories for drug use during pregnancy relies largely on extrapolation of data from animal studies to humans. Unfortunately, not all species are equally susceptible or sensitive to the teratogenic effect of a drug or chemical. A study by Jelovsek et al. demonstrated that 75% of positive human teratogens can be predicted on the basis of animal study results alone (1). However, false-negative results in this study remained high, reaching 25%.

Human experience reminds us of the fallibility of animal studies. Before its release, thalidomide was tested in rats and mice and was thought to be safe. It was subsequently noted to be a serious human teratogen. Conversely, certain strains of mice are extremely sensitive to various substances that have not been shown to cause adverse effects in humans. For example, in mice, corticosteroids cause cleft lip, but there is no current evidence to suggest that therapeutic doses of corticosteroids produce congenital anomalies in humans (7).

Some species variability can be explained on the basis of genetic factors. However, variable teratogenicity occurs even within litters of inbred animals. Other factors that may account for differing effects in strain susceptibility include maternal parity and weight, fetal weight, number of young, placental transfer, rate of drug metabolism, fetal and maternal production of hormones, vitamin supplements, and other environmental factors, such as diet, season, and temperature.

Another important difference among species is the portion of gestation devoted to organogenesis when drugs can exert their teratogenic effects. Of the 280 days of human gestation, approximately 40 days (31–71 days after the last menstrual period) constitute the teratogenic period (approximately 14% of human gestation). In the rat, the teratogenic period comprises 10 days of its total 21-day gestation (approximately 50%). The teratogenic effect of a substance depends on timing as well as the nature of the teratogen, its dose, and host variability.

Critical Periods of Gestation

Preconception

Drugs remain pharmacologically active throughout gestation, and their cellular actions will affect the developing fetus differently at different stages of development. Even before conception, drugs can have a profound effect on fertility and gametogenesis. This point can be easily illustrated by the fact that ovulation can be pharmacologically stimulated or prevented. While awaiting ovulation, the oocyte may be exposed to potentially cytotoxic or mutagenic chemicals. It is also now recognized that mutagenic effects of drugs taken by a woman before conception may not become manifest until subsequent generations.

Recently, attention has been directed to the reproductive effects of drugs on men. Soyka and Joffe summarized the possible mechanisms involved in the effect of paternal ingestion of drugs on the fetus as follows: (a) an indirect effect on the normal metabolic and endocrine function of the male, (b) direct damage to spermatozoa, and (c) the potential of the drug within the ejaculate to affect either the intrauterine environment or the newly fertilized ova (8). Nevertheless, drug effects on spermatogenesis may be transient, since new spermatocytes are produced every 78 days. There are now several reports of the return of normal fertility following treatment with cytotoxic chemotherapeutic agents.

Preimplantation

The first 2 weeks after conception are referred to as the *preimplantation period*. During this time the blastocyst is formed before implantation. There is little association between drug exposures during this time and congenital anomalies. The common explanation for the apparent lack of association between congenital anomalies and drug exposure during preimplantation holds that any adverse effects produced during this period are likely to be devastating to the pregnancy, resulting in spontaneous abortion. Survival of the pregnancy implies that totipotential cells will continue to divide normally. Because the fate of early embryonic cells is not irrevocably determined, if one cell is destroyed another can resume its function. This effect is usually referred to as all-or-none. There is new evidence, however, that drug exposure during the preimplantation period can produce adverse effects manifest at birth. Intrauterine growth retardation has been observed in the offspring of pregnant rabbits given a cocktail of ethanol, nicotine, caffeine, sodium salicylate, and dichlorodiphenyltrichloroethane (DDT) during preimplantation (9). It is, therefore, inappropriate to conclude that adverse effects of drugs during preimplantation will necessarily conform to an all-or-none effect.

Organogenesis

The time of greatest teratogenic potential corresponds to the period during which a particular organ is developing most rapidly. The classic teratogenic period in humans occurs from 4 weeks through 10 weeks after the last menstrual period (LMP). Adverse pharmacologic effects during this time can lead to irreversible malformations, many of which are still compatible with continued growth and live birth. If a pregnant woman is exposed to a teratogen during the early portion of the teratogenic period, a defect in the heart or central nervous system is likely. Exposure near the end of organogenesis is likely to result in a defect of the ear or palate. An understanding of embryology and the precise timing of exposure is obviously important. For example, a teratogen given at the end of organogenesis or later will not result in an anomaly of the heart because the heart has already completed its development. The relative timing for several birth defects in humans is presented in Table 2.

Table 2 Relative Timing of Various Malformations in Humans

Malformation	Time of induction before week
Meningomyelocele	4
Esophageal atresia	4
Tracheoesophageal fistula	4
Transposition of great vessels	5
Cleft lip	5
Diaphragmatic hernia	6
Ventricular septal defect	6
Syndactyly	6
Cleft palate	8–9
Malrotation of gut	10
Meckel's diverticulum	10
Omphalocele	10
Bicornuate uterus	10
Hypospadias	12

Fetal Development

The fetal period from approximately 12 weeks after the LMP until term is characterized by growth and functional maturation of the conceptus. Adverse drug effects during this period of gestation can be expected to result in abnormalities of intrauterine growth and brain function. The fetal alcohol syndrome is largely a disorder of the fetal period. Emerging interest in behavioral teratology has focused on the period of fetal development. Functional maturation of liver, lung, gonads, and other organs may also be affected during this period of gestation.

In recent years, it has also become apparent that there can be delayed effects of drugs given during fetal development. The concept of long-term latency was illustrated by the discovery that female fetuses exposed to diethylstilbestrol (DES) are at an increased risk for adenocarcinoma of the vagina, not discovered until after puberty. Nor have male offspring been spared the long-term effects of DES. Some have abnormalities of the reproductive system, such as epididymal cysts, hypotrophic testes, capsular induration, and pathological semen.

Perinatal Period

There has been a rapid increase in the use of medications during the immediate perinatal period. Drugs used during this time may have profound maternal effects in addition to their effects on the fetus and the newborn's immediate adjustment to extrauterine life. Since the neonate clears drugs slowly, effects of maternally administered drugs may last for several hours or days, during a time when the neonate must make major cardiorespiratory adjustments and become metabolically independent.

Prevention of preterm birth has become a major goal of perinatologists. Awareness of β-adrenergic action on uterine smooth muscle provided one of the first means of inhibiting preterm labor, but not without other significant maternal and fetal effects. Maternal cardiovascular, pulmonary, and metabolic effects include hypotension, tachycardia, arrhythmias, bronchodilatation, and hyperglycemia. Moreover, placental transfer of these tocolytic agents is rapid and potentially causes similar β-adrenergic effects in the fetus.

Another group of drugs currently employed during the perinatal period comprises prostaglandins and prostaglandin synthetase inhibitors. Perhaps the most common use of prostaglandins in obstetric practice is for ripening of an unfavorable cervix or induction of labor with a favorable cervix. These drugs can cause clinically significant maternal bronchoconstriction. Prostaglandin synthetase inhibitors are used to inhibit labor. However, they are also capable of prematurely closing the ductus arteriosus and have been associated with primary pulmonary hypertension in some infants.

Birth may also mean sudden discontinuation of transplacentally acquired drugs. It is now well recognized that the newborn may suffer withdrawal symptoms from maternally ingested narcotics, barbiturates, and even antihistamines.

Finally, drugs administered to mothers during the immediate peripartum period can be expected to diffuse into breast milk. Concerns about drugs during lactation include both inhibition of milk production and direct effects on the newborn.

Dose–Response

The effect of most teratogens lies within a narrow range between that which will kill the fetus and that which has no discernible effect. Dose–response relations imply a quantitative correlation between embryopathy and the dose of a drug or chemical. Such a relation has been repeatedly demonstrated in animal models. For example, the number of fetuses affected with cleft palate in a litter of mice can be predicted by the dose of corticosteroid given at a critical period of gestation.

Dose is not, however, the only determinant of fetal toxicity. Another important variable is duration of treatment. In general, short-term dosage schedules are of greater teratogenic insult to the developing embryo than extended administration. The vehicle, carrier, or suspending agent, either by delaying absorption or by prolonging blood concentrations of a drug or chemical may also be a confounding factor in determining embryopathy. Finally, drug interactions may influence teratogenicity. For example, cyclophosphamide and fluorouracil given individually to rats produce malformations in rats in frequencies of 26 and 10%, respectively. Given together, however, in the same dose they produce malformations in 100% of offspring (10).

Drug Specificity and Interaction

It is a basic principle of teratogenesis that some agents have greater teratogenic potential than others. From animal studies, as well as human experience, it is apparent that some drugs must be given in extremely high doses, often producing severe maternal toxic effects, before any adverse effect on the fetus can be observed. Although it is commonly held that any drug given in sufficient quantity may be teratogenic, this may not, in fact, be true. Short of severe maternal toxicity or death, many drugs have never been linked to adverse fetal effects. On the other hand, drugs such as thalidomide, retinoic acid, warfarin (Coumadin), and many anticonvulsants are capable of causing malformations in doses commonly held to be within the therapeutic range.

It is also true that two teratogens administered simultaneously may not have the same effect as either administered individually. Possible mechanisms for the adverse effects of drug interactions include induction or inhibition of enzyme systems and competition for binding sites that could influence concentrations of unbound and active teratogen.

PHARMACOKINETIC ALTERATIONS DURING PREGNANCY

Absorption

Gastric emptying time during gestation has been demonstrated to diminish from an average of 30 min in nonpregnant individuals to between 80 and 130 min (11). The clinical significance of this change would be expected to be a delay in the attainment of peak drug concentrations. Small-intestinal transit time is also prolonged, but the clinical significance of this observation remains poorly understood. There is little clinical information about the absorption of drugs in pregnant women.

Pregnancy-associated changes in drug absorption are not confined to the gastrointestinal tract. Because of increases in respiratory minute volume, alterations have been demonstrated in the absorption of drugs administered as volatile gases (anesthetic agents) and as aerosols (bronchodilators) (12). It might be anticipated that highly lipid-soluble anesthetic agents would be absorbed and cleared more rapidly during pregnancy. Moreover, an increase might be expected to occur in the absorption rate of inhaled bronchodilators during pregnancy.

Distribution

After absorption, drugs distribute into body fluids and tissues. Changes in blood volume, tissue perfusion, drug lipid solubility, and protein binding affect drug distribution and the rate at which equilibrium between tissue and plasma concentration is achieved. During pregnancy plasma volume increases by approximately 50% (13) and cardiac output by 30% (14). Total body water increases by 8 L, or more if edema is present. The implications of this physiological increase in volume include lower plasma concentration of a single dose of a drug, and a decrease in drug elimination (i.e., a prolonged half-life) unless there is a simultaneous increase in drug metabolism or excretion (discussed later).

Distribution of any drug also depends on its lipid solubility and the total body fat content. The property of lipid solubility allows drugs to cross biological barriers, such as cell membranes, the blood–brain barrier, and the placenta, whereas highly water-soluble drugs usually cross such membranes poorly. Total body fat increases during pregnancy by 3–4 kg (12). Thus, not only will fat-soluble drugs have an increased volume of distribution, but increased serum lipids may compete for protein-binding sites, leading to a greater fraction of unbound drug.

Protein binding also plays a major role in the pharmacokinetics of gestation. Plasma albumin concentration falls approximately 10 g/L by the third trimester. The effect of this decrease is particularly significant for highly protein-bound, acidic drugs. Since only the unbound fraction of a drug is biologically active, reduced-binding capacity may change the ratio of unbound/bound drug and alter the therapeutic effect. Alterations in protein binding must be considered when interpreting the clinical significance of plasma measurements of highly protein-bound drugs.

Excretion and Metabolism

There is a 50% increase in glomerular filtration rate during pregnancy that results in a creatinine clearance of 150–200 mL/min, compared with approximately 100 mL/min in nongravid individuals. At 26-weeks gestation renal plasma flow increases by 80%. It then falls at term, but remains 60% higher than in nonpregnant women (15). The result of these changes is an increased clearance of drugs excreted by the kidneys.

Water-soluble drugs are excreted mainly unchanged by the kidneys, but lipid-soluble drugs must be metabolized by the liver before they are excreted in bile or urine. Pregnancy increases the rate of hepatic metabolism through a greater concentration of progesterone, which enhances the activity of hepatic microsomal oxidation (16). For drugs that require hepatic metabolism, the net effect is a decrease in plasma drug concentration relative to dose.

The complex interrelation of drug distribution and elimination can be illustrated by the fate of theophylline. Studies have demonstrated that the volume of distribution for theophylline increases as gestation progresses. Moreover, clearance is reduced approximately 20–50%, and its half-life is prolonged by about 30% (17–19). These pharmacokinetic changes during pregnancy may result in increased plasma theophylline concentration, especially during the third trimester, with the potential for clinical drug toxicity. Patients should be observed for toxicity, and theophylline serum concentrations should be measured more frequently during the last half of gestation.

Placental Transport

The properties of drugs that permit them to be absorbed and to distribute across biological membranes also allow them to cross the placenta. There is, in fact, no placental barrier to most medications. The question, therefore, should not be if a drug crosses the placenta, but rather, what concentration does it achieve in the fetus. Differences in steady-state drug concentrations reflect factors such as molecular weight, lipid solubility, ionization, and protein binding. Most drugs are simple chemical compounds of low molecular weight that diffuse easily across the placenta. Chemicals of molecular weight less than 100 will readily cross biological membranes, regardless of their lipid solubility, whereas those the molecular weights of which exceed 1000 generally do not cross the placenta, even if they are highly lipid-soluble.

Differences in pH between maternal blood (pH 7.35–7.40) and fetal blood (pH 7.20–7.25) can lead to unequal drug concentrations in the two compartments. Nonionized molecules cross biological membranes more readily than ionized molecules. Drugs that are weak bases with pK_a values near blood pH are mainly nonionized and, therefore, easily cross the placenta. After crossing the placenta, weak bases become more acidic in fetal blood; accordingly, the concentration of nonionized drug diminishes in the fetal compartment. This mechanism is commonly referred to as *ion trapping*. In contrast with weak bases, ion trapping induced from fetal to maternal circulations is likely to occur with weak acids (20).

The degree of protein binding is another determinant of a drug's ability to cross the placenta. Throughout pregnancy there is a gradual decrease in the concentration of maternal albumin and an increase in fetal concentration. Since only the free fraction of a drug crosses the placenta, highly protein-bound drugs (e.g., dicloxacillin, 96%) achieve higher maternal concentrations, whereas the least protein-bound drugs (e.g., digoxin, ampicillin, 20%) reach high concentrations in the fetus and amniotic fluid.

Placental transport can be summarized by stating that the fetus receives unbound, nonionized, lipid-soluble molecules of low molecular weight. Of course, most drugs fulfill these criteria, since it is these very properties that allow them to cross all biological membranes.

Intermediate Metabolites

It is now recognized that many adverse fetal effects result not from parent drugs, but from their metabolism to more active or toxic compounds. Oxidative intermediates, such as epoxides, are highly reactive and capable of covalently binding to embryonic or fetal nucleic acids, which at critical periods of embryogenesis are theoretically capable of disrupting normal development.

The metabolism of thalidomide to a toxic metabolite only in certain species, including humans, has been proposed as the explanation for why the drug causes birth defects in some animals and not others (21). The well-known teratogenicity of several anticonvulsant medications has now been linked to toxic intermediary metabolites produced during the biotransformation of the parent compound. Drug combinations may be potentially even more toxic. Recent epidemiological data suggest that when combinations of anticonvulsant drugs (e.g., phenytoin, carbamazine) that form oxidative metabolites are administered during pregnancy, the risk of an adverse outcome is approximately eight times as high as with single-drug therapy (22). A recent study suggested that enzymatic markers exist that permit determination of which fetuses are at increased risk for congenital malformations induced by anticonvulsant medications (23).

DRUGS AND LACTATION

With the capability to detect minute concentrations of drugs, it has been shown that virtually all maternally ingested drugs will enter breast milk, usually in amounts less than 2% of the maternal dose (24). The ability of any drug to enter breast milk depends on its molecular size, binding to milk proteins, lipid solubility, and ionization (25).

The molecular size of most drugs is not an impediment to passage into breast milk. All but the very largest molecules, such as insulin and heparin, are able to cross the alveolar acini in the mammary gland. Only the fraction of drug that is not protein-bound can leave the maternal circulation and enter breast milk. Thus, drugs that are highly protein-bound are less likely to enter breast milk when compared with drugs that are less protein-bound (26). Lipid solubility is also important for the concentration of drugs in breast milk. Highly lipid-soluble drugs enter breast milk to a greater extent than less lipid-soluble drugs. Finally, drug ionization must be considered. The average pH of breast milk is 7.08, which is lower than that of maternal blood. Therefore, the pKa of a drug will affect the amount that enters breast milk. Weak acids are likely to be ionized in the maternal circulation, thereby reducing their transfer into breast milk. Weak bases are likely to be nonionized in maternal circulation, increasing both their lipid solubility and passage into milk. Once reaching the relatively acidic milk, weak bases will be ionized, leading to ion trapping in the milk.

RISK COUNSELING

The use of any drug during pregnancy entails acceptance of risks. Equally important is the understanding that failure to treat an important medical problem may jeopardize the health of both a mother and her unborn child. These risks require careful communication between physician and patient.

The indications for any prescribed medication must be clearly explained and alternatives to pharmacologic therapy considered. The potential effects of the drug on both mother and fetus need to be considered. Important background information essential for counseling includes known teratogenic risks of a particular drug, drug dose, and gestational age at exposure. Since the specific response of the conceptus will depend on genetic factors, in addition to dose-dependent pharmacologic effects, information about genetic background should be included. Taking a careful family history may identify individuals at unusually high risk. For example, a family history of neural tube defects, congenital heart disease, or other birth defects suggests that the risk of any drug may be theoretically greater than it might be for the general population. Although this increased risk may not be quantifiable, its theoretical presence may influence decisions, and patients must be aware that they are accepting higher than average risks.

Three common scenarios will help illustrate the kinds of problems encountered while counseling patients about the use of medications during pregnancy (27). First, the most frequently asked question is, "Is any medication safe to take during pregnancy?" Patients should be counseled that, technically, drugs are not determined to be safe. Some have been proved harmful, and others are presumed to be safe when no evidence of harm can be demonstrated. The difference is subtle, but it means that no drug can be guaranteed to be 100% safe. The standard warning about risks and benefits in the *Physicians' Desk Reference* is of little help to the clinician faced with the need to manage a pregnant patient whose medical disorder itself is capable of jeopardizing both her fetus and herself. The best approach to this problem is for the physician to obtain all the information available about the particular drug and, then, help the patient decide if the drug is necessary. It is important to remind patients that even if a drug is in no way teratogenic, 3% of the women who take it will have an abnormal baby. This risk constitutes the background incidence of birth defects in the general population.

A second commonly asked question is, "Since I took this drug before I knew I was pregnant, should I terminate the pregnancy?" It is unreasonable either to reassure the patient that no risk is associated with the drug or, conversely, to recommend termination of a pregnancy solely because of exposure to a drug about which only limited information is available. Once an attempt has been made to gather all current information about the known risks of a drug, patients must play an active role in the decision process. They should also be informed that contemporary techniques of prenatal diagnosis can be effectively employed before 18 weeks gestation to detect many, if not most, major congenital anomalies.

Finally, we are often confronted by a woman who has given birth to an infant with an anomaly who asks, "Did any of the medications I took cause the birth defect?" Implicit in this question is the assignment of responsibility to oneself or one's physician. We need not be reminded of the medicolegal implications of this question. Discussions need to be open and direct. Counseling requires an understanding of the process of disbelief, anger, and guilt that characterizes parents' adaption to this crisis. It will be useful to help parents understand the basic principles of teratology and to remind them of the relatively brief period of gestation during which the fetus is vulnerable to a teratogen. They should be reminded that all of the major organ systems have been formed before the completion of the first trimester. Therefore, it is generally true that exposure to a drug during the second or third trimester is unlikely to cause a major structural defect.

A complete examination by an expert in dysmorphology may often provide a clue to the cause of a major anomaly that would otherwise be overlooked. It is always appropriate to obtain an autopsy in cases of intrauterine fetal death or neonatal death. The findings may have significant bearing on the patient's perception and plans for future pregnancy. It is also important to schedule a counseling session a month or more after the birth of an anomalous child or a neonatal death. This allows the family to voice their concerns and ask questions that may affect future family planning. At this time it is also essential to explore the effect of the tragic event on the psychological health of each member of the family.

REFERENCES

1. Jelovsek FR, Mattison DR, Chen JJ. Prediction of risk for human developmental toxicity: how important are animal studies for hazard identification? Obstet Gynecol 1989; 74:624–636.
2. Wolf FM. Meta-analysis. N Engl J Med 1987; 317:576.
3. Angell M. The interpretation of epidemiologic studies. N Engl J Med 1990; 323:823–825.
4. Physician's Desk Reference. Oradell, NJ: Medical Economics Company, 1990:336.
5. Karnofsky DA. Drugs as teratogens in animals and man. Annu Rev Pharmacol 1965; 5:447–472.
6. Schardein JL. Chemically induced birth defects. New York: Marcel Dekker, 1985:1–48.
7. Schatz M, Patterson R, Zeitz S, O'Rourke J, Melam H. Corticosteroid therapy for the pregnant asthmatic patient. JAMA 1975; 233:804–807.
8. Soyka LF, Joffe JM. Male mediated drug effects on offspring. Prog Clin Biol Res 1980; 36:49–66.
9. Fabro S, McLachlan JA, Dames NM. Chemical exposure of embryos during the preimplantation stages of pregnancy; mortality rate and intrauterine development. Am J Obstet Gynecol 1984; 148:929–938.
10. Wilson JG. Teratogenic interaction of chemical agents in the rat. J Pharmacol Exp Ther 1964; 144:429–436.

11. Shaw SJ, Brooks PM, McNeil JJ, Moulds RFW, Ravenscroft PJ, Smith AJ. The effects of pregnancy on drug pharmacokinetics. Med J Aust 1988; 149:675–677.
12. Krauer B, Krauer F, Hytten FE. Pregnancy and its effect on drug handling: the influence of physiological changes in pregnancy. In: Lind T, Singer A, eds. Current reviews in obstetrics and gynaecology. Edinburgh: Churchill-Livingstone, 1984:19–50.
13. Pirani BKK, Campbell DM, MacGillivray I. Plasma volume in normal pregnancy. J Obstet Gynaecol Br Commonw 1973; 80:884–887.
14. Katz R, Karliner JS, Resnik R. Effects of a natural volume overload (pregnancy) on left ventricular performance in normal human subjects. Circulation 1978; 58:434–441.
15. Dunlop W. Serial changes in renal haemodynamics during normal human pregnancy. Br J Obstet Gynaecol 1981; 88:1–9.
16. Davis M, Simmons CJ, Dordoni B, Maxwell JD. Induction of hepatic enzymes during normal human pregnancy. J Obstet Gynaecol Br Commonw 1973; 80:690–694.
17. Gardner MJ, Schatz M, Cousins L, et al. Longitudinal effects of pregnancy on pharmacokinetics of theophylline. Eur J Clin Pharmacol 1987; 32:289–295.
18. Frederiksen MC, Ruo TI, Chow MJ, Atkinson AJ Jr. Theophylline pharmacokinetics in pregnancy. Clin Pharmacol Ther 1986; 40:321–328.
19. Carter BL, Driscoll CE, Smith GD. Theophylline clearance during pregnancy. Obstet Gynecol 1986; 68:555–559.
20. Mucklow JC. The fate of drugs in pregnancy. Clin Obstet Gynecol 1986; 13:161–175.
21. Gordon GB, Spielberg SP, Blake DA, Balasubramanian V. Thalidomide teratogenesis: evidence for a toxic arene oxide metabolite. Proc Natl Acad Sci USA 1981; 78:2545–2548.
22. Lindhout D, Hoppener RJ, Meinardi H. Teratogenicity of antiepileptic drug combinations with special emphasis on epoxidation (of carbamazepine). Epilepsia 1984; 25:77–83.
23. Buehler BA, Delimont D, Van Waes M, Finneli RH. Prenatal prediction of risk of the fetal hydantoin syndrome. N Engl J Med 1990; 322:1567–1572.
24. Rivera-Calimlim L. The significance of drugs in breast milk. Clin Perinatol 1987; 14:51–70.
25. Rieder MJ. Drugs and breastfeeding. In: Koren G, ed. Maternal–fetal toxicology. A clinicians' guide. New York: Marcel Dekker, 1990: 63–85.
26. Wilson JT. Determinants and consequences of drug excretion in breast milk. Drug Metab Rev 1983; 14:619–652.
27. Coustan DR, Carpenter MW. The use of medications in pregnancy. Med Times 1984; 112:45–51.

8

The Reproductive Effects of Specific Medications for Asthma and Allergy

Anthony R. Scialli

Georgetown University Medical Center and
Columbia Hospital for Women Medical Center
Washington, D.C.

Armand Lione

Associated Pharmacologists and Toxicologists
Washington, D.C.

INTRODUCTION

Developmental Toxicity

Although birth defects are the most dramatic evidence of embryogenesis gone amiss, other endpoints of abnormal development are equally significant. These include spontaneous abortion (miscarriage), fetal death (stillbirth), and functional abnormalities, such as impairments in the nervous or immune systems. In addition, growth retardation, preterm labor, and other obstetric complications are developmental problems of clinical importance. The incidence of adverse pregnancy outcome in the general population should be considered when evaluating possible effects of a disease or of medications on pregnancy. For example, congenital anomalies are recognized in 3–8% of liveborn infants, miscarriage occurs in 20–25% of clinically diagnosed pregnancies, and severe mental retardation occurs in 1–2% of individuals. The challenge is to determine whether an exposure increases the incidence of adverse outcome over the background incidence.

How Therapies Are Evaluated

It is understood that experimental animals differ from humans in many ways, including drug handling, sensitivities to drug effects, and embryonic timetables. These differences notwithstanding, animal teratology experiments can be useful in evaluating human drug risks. Animal studies are designed to maximize the response of the system to potential toxic effects of test agents. This is accomplished by using large doses, with the highest dose customarily being chosen as one that induces maternal toxicity. It is believed that a testing scheme using appropriate doses in at least two species, one of which is a nonrodent, will be sufficient to raise a suggestion of human developmental risk. There are, in fact, no known human developmental toxicants that would not be identified in this manner. It follows that if an agent is appropriately tested in animals and found not to be a developmental toxicant, its potential for developmental toxicity in humans is low. Positive data in animal studies are not as informative, because it may not be possible to know whether maternal toxicity or the high doses used were responsible for the effects of the offspring.

Human reports, when available, are reassuring supplements to negative animal data. By themselves, human studies rarely include sufficient numbers of exposed individuals to rule out a low-order increase in adverse pregnancy outcome. One of the largest studies conducted in this area was the Collaborative Perinatal Project (1). In this investigation, women were enrolled as early as possible during pregnancy. Histories included exposures to medications and other agents. As the pregnancies went forward, women continued to be asked about exposures. The outcomes for more than 50,000 children were evaluated, and associations between exposures and birth defects were identified. As the investigators of this study noted, the many different exposures and the numerous different adverse outcomes made it likely that some exposures and outcomes would be associated by chance alone. Therefore, all positive data from the Collaborative Perinatal Project should be viewed as preliminary until independently confirmed.

ANTIHISTAMINES*

Brompheniramine

Brompheniramine, an antihistamine, is commonly used in cold and allergy medications, many of which are available without a prescrip-

*Only antihistamines for which published human gestational data exists are included in this review.

tion. The reproductive and developmental toxicity of this and other antihistamines have not been investigated in great detail. The data collected in the Collaborative Perinatal Project did suggest a significant association between the use of brompheniramine during pregnancy and an increase in the incidence of birth defects. Of the 50,000+ mother–child pairs examined in this study, only 65 fetuses were exposed to brompheniramine. Of these children, 10 had detectable malformations at birth (1, pp 322–327). Syndactyly was observed in 3 of the brompheniramine-exposed children. This incidence of malformations yielded a relative risk of 2.34 for brompheniramine. The relative risk values for the five other antihistamines investigated in the Perinatal Project ranged from 0.81 to 1.25, and averaged 1.10. Although these data might appear to suggest that brompheniramine is a teratogen, the authors correctly cautioned that the number of cases collected was too small to establish the drug as a developmental toxicant. We did not locate additional investigations that addressed this question. In light of this finding, however, it would appear prudent to avoid the use of brompheniramine during pregnancy and to use an alternative antihistamine, if one is needed.

Brompheniramine and other antihistamines may, in theory, inhibit lactation. One case report described a 3-month-old nursing infant who became irritable, cried excessively and had difficulty sleeping shortly after its mother began ingesting a medication containing 6 mg of dexbrompheniramine and 120 mg of *d*-isoephedrine (2). The symptoms resolved spontaneously, within 12 hr, when breast-feeding was stopped. Although the observed symptoms were not definitively related to brompheniramine exposure, concern is raised that this antihistamine, like others (3), may be excreted in breast milk and adversely affect the nursling.

Chlorpheniramine

Chlorpheniramine is an antihistamine commonly used in numerous prescription and nonprescription nasal medications. No teratogenic effects were detected in mice that received this antihistamine during gestation (4). The Collaborative Perinatal Project identified 1070 women who were exposed to chlorpheniramine during the first trimester, but no significant increase in overall birth defects was detected in this population (1, pp 322–327). There was, however, an increased relative risk of eye and ear malformations and of inguinal hernia associated with chlorpheniramine use. In view of the "fishing expedition" design of the Collaborative Perinatal Project, these findings should be viewed as requiring independent confirmation.

The use of chlorpheniramine is under investigation in the management of the ovarian hyperstimulation syndrome, which infrequently complicates ovulation induction procedures. The fluid shifts that may produce significant illness or fatality with this syndrome have been controlled with chlorpheniramine in a rabbit model (5). A similar success was reported in a human case of ovarian hyperstimulation syndrome (6).

The notion that H_1 blockers, such as chlorpheniramine, may reduce menstrual loss in some women has been investigated in a few reports (7–9). The available data are not convincing, however, that this or other antihistamines are effective at reducing total menstrual blood loss.

It has been recommended that antihistamines be avoided by nursing mothers due to largely theoretical concerns about their inhibition of lactation and the possibility that the infant may experience sedation and even convulsions because of this exposure (10; p 84). However, there are no data establishing adverse effects due to the lactational use of these drugs. Chlorpheniramine and other antihistamines are considered compatible with breast feeding by the American Academy of Pediatrics (19).

Diphenhydramine

Diphenhydramine was one of the first antihistamines sold in the United States (11). It is now used in many prescription and nonprescription drugs, including some over-the-counter (OTC) hypnotic products. Teratogenicity testing in rats, mice, and rabbits has not suggested an association between diphenhydramine and congenital malformations (4, 12).

As a class, antihistamines are not considered to be teratogenic (13,14), although some antihistamines have been associated with birth defects in retrospective studies. For example, Saxen (15) found that first-trimester use of diphenhydramine was more common among mothers of 599 children born with oral clefts (20 exposures), than among mothers of 590 controls without clefts (6 exposures). In contrast, however, no significant increase in the incidence of major or minor malformations was uncovered by Heinonen et al. (1, pp 322–327), who studied the outcomes of 595 births that included first-trimester use of diphenhydramine, and 2948 pregnancies that included the use of this drug at some time during pregnancy. Data from another study indicated that significantly fewer infants with malformations were exposed to antihistamines while in utero than were controls (16). Diphenhydramine was the second most commonly used antihistamine in the study population (16).

The placental transfer of diphenhydramine has been demonstrated in sheep (17), and a comparable fetal distribution of this compound in humans is likely. Although there is no compelling evidence that antihistamines are dangerous in pregnancy, there is concern that the physiologic role of histamine in the fetus may be compromised by these agents. Histamine, for example, is felt to be important in the cardiovascular response to stress in the newborn. Also, infants and young children may convulse when given antihistamines, raising the concern that third-trimester use of these drugs may cause adverse nonteratogenic effects that have yet to be characterized.

Diphenhydramine withdrawal has been reported in one infant who was exposed in utero (18). In this report, generalized tremulousness and diarrhea began on the fifth day of life of an infant whose mother had taken 150 mg/day of diphenhydramine throughout pregnancy. The infant was treated with phenobarbital until the symptoms disappeared (18).

Considerations regarding antihistamines and lactation are discussed in the section on chlorpheniramine. Diphenhydramine is classified as compatible with breast-feeding by the American Academy of Pediatrics (19).

Hydroxyzine

Hydroxyzine, a benzhydrylpiperazine antihistamine, is used as a sedative and antianxiety agent as well as an antipruritic. In rats, hydroxyzine and related antihistamines, such as meclizine and buclizine, are teratogenic, producing malformations of the palate and skeleton when administered during sensitive periods of gestation (20,21). Hydroxyzine has been associated with teratogenesis in beagle puppies (22) and doses of 5.5 mg/kg have been associated with a high frequency of abortions in pigs and monkeys (23). Metabolic studies indicate that a metabolite of hydroxyzine, norchlorcyclizine, is the active form of this antihistamine that is transferred to the rat fetus (24). Rodents may not be suitable species for studying the human teratogenicity of this and other histamine antagonists, because histamine constricts arterioles in rodent tissues, but dilates them in human tissues (25). Fetal edema caused by the antihistamines in rats has been suggested as the mechanism by which this and related compounds induce orofacial malformations (26).

Data on the gestational effects of hydroxyzine exposure during the first trimester may be derived from 50 pregnancies identified in the

Collaborative Perinatal Project. The use of hydroxyzine in this study was associated with an incidence of anomalies not statistically different from a control incidence, and no clear pattern of malformations was evident (1; pp 328, 335–337, 341, 438). In addition, the incidence of congenital malformations in the infants of 74 women using hydroxyzine as an antiemetic in early pregnancy in another study was not increased compared with controls (27). Although the findings in animals are of concern, available epidemiologic data do not suggest there is a substantial risk of human teratogenesis from first-trimester exposures to hydroxyzine.

The use of hydroxyzine as a sedative during labor and delivery has been effective and relatively safe (28). Like many sedatives, hydroxyzine can decrease the response rate of the fetal heart to stress, but this effect has not been associated with clinical import in terms of fetal well-being (29). One case of neonatal withdrawal syndrome was associated with hydroxyzine after maternal use of this compound as an antipruritic throughout pregnancy. This pregnancy also included prenatal exposure to phenobarbital during the 3 weeks before delivery (30). Respiratory depression in the neonate is a theoretical consequence of hydroxyzine administration to the laboring woman. This problem would not be amenable to treatment with an opioid antagonist such as naloxone. Hydroxyzine is considered to be compatible with breast feeding (19).

Tripelennamine

Tripelennamine is an antihistamine. This agent has been found to be mildly genotoxic in cultured human hepatocytes (31); however, it is unknown if this in vitro effect is relevant to an estimate of reproductive hazard. Use of this agent during early pregnancy was not associated with an increase in birth defects in 100 women reported by the Collaborative Perinatal Project (1; pp 323–324). Negative findings were also reported in an older survey of drug use during pregnancy (32). Tripelennamine is encountered as a drug of abuse (along with pentazocine) as a substitute for heroin. The combination of tripelennamine and pentazocine is known as "T's and blues." When pregnant rats are treated with tripelennamine–pentazocine by gavage, reduced body weights and minor behavioral abnormalities are seen in the offspring (33). The use of T's and blues during human pregnancy has been reported (34–37). Adverse effects have included prematurity, growth retardation, and a neonatal withdrawal syndrome. Interactive behavioral deficits have also been described in the infants exposed antenatally to this combination (36). Although such adverse effects may be due to the pentazocine or other aspects of the life-style of drug-abusing women, a role for tripelennamine cannot be ruled out.

Tripelennamine is not considered contraindicated during nursing (19). Considerations regarding antihistamines and lactation are discussed in the section on chlorpheniramine.

Cimetidine

Cimetidine can selectively block histamine-induced acid secretion in the stomach and has become a very popular drug in the treatment of duodenal ulcers. Clinical data on the use of cimetidine during the first trimester are quite limited. Experiments in animals suggest that cimetidine is not teratogenic in rats, rabbits, and mice (38). Rat studies have also shown, however, a delay in development of the prostate and seminal vesicles (38,39) and an impairment of sexual maturation in male offspring exposed antenatally to this drug (39,40). Some concern exists, therefore, that prolonged fetal exposure to this agent may inhibit normal masculization in a male fetus. A study performed by the manufacturer, however, showed that cimetidine administered during pregnancy in the rat does not have demasculinizing effects on the offspring (41). Other researchers recently reported that they did not detect a delay in sexual development in cimetidine-exposed rats (42), but they did not monitor the possible effects on prostate and seminal vesicle formation that were reported previously. Although clinical reports on fetal antiandrogenic effects were not located, cimetidine has been clearly associated with antiandrogenic effects in adult humans. These effects include the occasional development of gynecomastia and a decline in sperm count (without loss of fertility) among men treated with this drug (43), as well as the use of this drug to reduce hair growth in hirsute women (44). In rat experiments, large doses administered over a period of 6 months reduced the size of the testes, prostate gland, and seminal vesicles (45).

In contrast with the use of cimetidine in early pregnancy, the use of this drug before cesarean section as preanesthetic prophylaxis against gastric acid aspiration (Mendelson's syndrome) has been investigated extensively, without demonstrable adverse effects on exposed neonates (46–49). These studies have demonstrated, however, that cimetidine does cross the placenta. In late pregnancy, a maximum fetal/maternal ratio of serum cimetidine was calculated as 0.84 and occurred 1.5–2 hr after maternal ingestion (50). Excretion of this drug by both mother and neonate is apparently rapid. The plasma half-life for cimetidine in adults is approximately 2 hr. Most of the drug is excreted in the urine unchanged. Neonates exposed to cimetidine during cesarean section had no detectable drug in their blood samples 2 hr after delivery (46). In one case report, however, a mother who took 1200 mg cimetidine daily for treatment of an ulcer during the ninth month of gestation gave birth to a child with transient liver impairment (51). A variety of other clinical reports on the use of cimetidine in late pregnancy have not uncovered additional indications of hepatic impairment among exposed offspring (46–49).

Cimetidine is concentrated and excreted in breast milk. A lactating woman who ingested a typical daily dose of this drug (1200 mg) could transfer 6 mg (1.5 mg/kg) to her infant each day (52). Although no adverse effects have been reported among infants exposed to cimetidine, the Committee on Drugs of the American Academy of Pediatrics classified this drug as contraindicated during breast-feeding. Theoretical concerns cited by the committee included the suppression of gastric acidity in exposed infants, an inhibition of drug metabolism, and possible central nervous system (CNS) stimulation (53).

ADRENERGIC AGONISTS

Oxymetazoline

Oxymetazoline is an α-adrenergic agonist used in nonprescription topical nasal decongestants. Because nasal congestion is relatively common during pregnancy and oxymetazoline is available for use without medical supervision, it is of concern that some gravidas may overdose themselves with this drug. The excessive use of oxymetazoline nasal sprays has been associated with bradycardia and hypotension in an elderly patient (54) and a diverse group of adverse reactions in young children, including sedation, epileptiform convulsive attacks, and insomnia (55). When studied in 12 uncomplicated pregnancies, a single dose of a 0.05% oxymetazoline nasal spray did not significantly alter blood flow velocity in the uterine arcuate artery, fetal aorta, or umbilical artery (56). The authors of this study concluded that the use of oxymetazoline nasal sprays, in recommended doses, appears to be safe for healthy pregnant patients, but they point out that they could not expand their findings to conditions during which the absorption of oxymetazoline might be increased (e.g., rhinitis), nor could they recommend the use of this medication in pregnancies with signs of uteroplacental insufficiency (56). In one case report, the excessive use of an oxymetazoline nasal spray by a woman in her 41st week of pregnancy was associated with a nonreactive nonstress test and late decelerations in fetal heart rate, suggesting that uterine perfusion may have been impaired (57). Uterine blood vessels contain only α-adrenergic receptors, which are capable of causing constriction when stimulated. Normally, these vessels are maximally dilated (58). A dose of another α-agonist, phenylephrine, equivalent to the content of one "cold" tablet, decreased uterine blood flow by 40% in pregnant sheep (59) (see section on phenylephrine). A more recent investigation, also performed in pregnant ewes, indicated that the uterine vascular bed is substantially more responsive to the vasoconstrictive effects of α-agonists than the overall systemic vasculature (60). The decongestant, pseudoephedrine, which is also available in OTC products, normally will not produce adverse effects until more than four times its therapeutic dose is consumed (61). Because of its favorable therapeutic index, pseudoephedrine appears to be the preferred decongestant for use during pregnancy (see section on pseudoephedrine).

Phenylephrine

Phenylephrine is a sympathomimetic drug used as a decongestant in many nonprescription cold medicines. The Collaborative Perinatal Project included more than 4000 women exposed to this agent during pregnancy, 1249 of whom were exposed during the first 4 lunar months (1; pp 345–346, 439, 476, 491). Possible associations were found between first-trimester exposure and ear and eye defects, syndactyly, and clubfoot, and between pregnancy use in general and hip dislocation, musculoskeletal deformities, and umbilical hernia. It is important to recognize, however, that these associations are based on the appearance of small numbers of children with malformations. For example, for abnormalities associated with first-trimester exposure to phenylephrine, the largest group consisted of eight children with eye and ear defects. Critical statistical analysis of these data has not been performed, and it is not currently known whether, in fact, phenylephrine increases the incidence of any birth defect.

Perhaps of greater concern than the Collaborative Perinatal Project report is the potential for phenylephrine, and other α-adrenergic agonists, to induce maternal hypertension and to reduce uterine blood flow at doses comparable to those used to produce therapeutic effects. Uterine blood vessels contain only α-adrenergic receptors, which are capable of causing constriction when stimulated. Normally, these vessels are maximally dilated (58). A dose of phenylephrine equivalent to the content of one "cold" tablet has been shown to decrease uterine blood flow by 40% in pregnant sheep (59). More recent investigations, also performed in pregnant ewes, indicated that the uterine vascular bed is substantially more responsive to the vasoconstrictive effects of α-agonists than the overall systemic vasculature (60), and sensitivity to phenylephrine increased during pregnancy (62). Because of their vasoconstrictive effects, phenylephrine, and the related agent, phenylpropanolamine, can produce a rapid increase of diastolic blood pressure at doses only two to three times their recommended therapeutic dose (61,63). In contrast, the decongestant, pseudoephedrine, requires a dose larger than four times its therapeutic dose to affect blood pressure. Because of its favorable therapeutic index, pseudoephedrine appears to be the preferred decongestant for use during pregnancy.

Phenylpropanolamine

Phenylpropanolamine is a sympathomimetic drug very commonly used in nonprescription cold pills and diet pills. As many as 5 billion doses of phenylpropanolamine were sold in the United States in 1980 (64).

The Collaborative Perinatal Project found a possible association between use of this agent during the first 4 months of pregnancy and hypospadias, eye and ear malformations, polydactyly, and pectus excavatum (1; pp 345–356). The number of malformations in this study was small (seven cases in the largest of the groups), and the retrospective design does not permit the conclusion that phenylpropanolamine was the causative agent in these abnormalities. A retrospective study with a similar design was unable to find an association between this agent and an increased incidence of birth defects (14).

In the United States, the Food and Drug Administration (FDA) regulations permit the sale of phenylpropanolamine in maximum unit doses of 37.5 mg, or 75 mg in a timed-release formulation (61). The administration of 50–75 mg phenylpropanolamine can produce hypertension in previously normotensive subjects. Horowitz et al. (63) recorded peak supine diastolic blood pressures of 100 mmHg or higher in 12 of 37 healthy medical students who ingested 85 mg phenylpropanolamine. A lower incidence of hypertension was also observed in medical students who ingested 50 mg phenylpropanolamine in a timed-release form.

Uterine blood vessels contain only α-adrenergic receptors, which are capable of causing constriction when stimulated. Normally, these vessels are maximally dilated (70). A dose of phenylephrine equivalent to the content of one "cold" tablet decreased uterine blood flow by

40% in pregnant sheep (59). A more recent investigation, also performed in pregnant ewes, indicated that the uterine vascular bed is substantially more responsive to the vasoconstrictive effects of α-agonists than the overall systemic vasculature (60).

A growing number of cases have been reported suggesting that myocardial injury (65) and intracranial hemorrhage (66,67) have been associated with the ingestion of recommended doses of phenylpropanolamine. One case of intracerebral hemorrhage occurred in a patient 3 weeks after childbirth (67). This patient had used phenylpropanolamine as a dieting aid without incident for an extended period before pregnancy. The hypertensive effects of phenylpropanolamine may be particularly troubling for patients with preexisting high blood pressure or for those who are ingesting other medications that may enhance the effects of phenylpropanolamine, such as monoamine oxidase inhibitors (61). The use of phenylpropanolamine as a diet aid during pregnancy is particularly inappropriate in the light of clinical observations that it lacks effectiveness for this indication (68) and the belief that weight loss during pregnancy is contraindicated. Some observers do not consider phenylpropanolamine safe enough for sale to the general public as a nonprescription medication (69,70).

In contrast to phenylpropanolamine, the decongestant, pseudoephedrine, which is also available in OTC products, has a much more favorable therapeutic index and normally will not increase blood pressure until more than four times its therapeutic dose is consumed (61). Because of its favorable therapeutic index, pseudoephedrine appears to be the preferred decongestant for use during pregnancy.

Pseudoephedrine

Pseudoepherine (Sudafed) is a sympathomimetic used in nonprescription (OTC) cold medications as a decongestant. There is one case report describing a woman who consumed 480–840 mL/day of a cough syrup that contained pseudoephedrine throughout pregnancy. Her daily intake of drugs from this source included 5 g pseudoephedrine, 16.8 g guaifenesin, 1.68 g dextromethorphan, and 79.8 mL of ethanol. The infant had features of fetal alcohol syndrome, and displayed irritability, tremors, and hypertonicity (71). Although the available data are quite limited, other observations on related sympathomimetic amines do not indicate that they are human developmental hazards (1, pp 345–356; 72).

Pseudoephedrine has mixed α- and β-agonist properties. Although the use of some OTC α-agonists, such as phenylephrine and phenylpropanolamine, has been associated with the impairment of uterine blood flow in sheep (59,60), ephedrine, an optical isomer of pseudoephedrine, does not alter intervillus blood flow (73,74). When ingested by healthy pregnant subjects in the third trimester, a single 60-mg dose of pseudoephedrine did not significantly alter blood pressure or blood flow velocities in the uterine or fetal circulation (75). The dose of pseudoephedrine likely to alter blood pressure is roughly four times the usual therapeutic dose. This "therapeutic index" is much higher for pseudoephedrine than for any of the other OTC decongestants (61). For this reason, as well as from the available clinical data, pseudoephedrine appears to be the preferred decongestant for use during pregnancy.

Pseudoephedrine is excreted in breast milk (76). The reported milk/plasma ratio for this agent was approximately 3.0. A nursing neonate may ingest about 0.6% of the maternal dose (76). The use of this drug during lactation has not been associated with adverse effects in exposed newborns. The American Academy of Pediatrics categorized pseudoephedrine as compatible with breast feeding (19).

Epinephrine

Epinephrine (adrenalin) is an endogenous sympathomimetic catecholamine. Direct injection of rat fetuses with 1–50 μg of epinephrine on day 17 of gestation produced limb defects (77). Administration of similar doses to rabbit fetuses on days 18–22 induced hemorrhages, edema, and necrosis of the distal extremities (78). The injection of pregnant mice with epinephrine produced a 14% frequency of cleft palate (99). In the chick embryo a variety of abnormalities were produced by the direct application of epinephrine to the chorioallantoic membrane; these included hemorrhages of the head, skin, and extremities (80), and malformations of the cardiovascular system (81). The latter have been attributed to catecholamine-induced dysrhythmias that are blocked by metoprolol (82). In placental animals, it is also possible that epinephrine's adverse effects are mediated by uterine vascular constriction (83).

The placental transfer of epinephrine has been reported (84). There is only one report that suggests epinephrine might be associated with human teratogenesis. The Collaborative Perinatal Project found a significant association between first-trimester exposure to epinephrine and an increased risk of major and minor malformations (1; pp 345–356, 439, 477, 492). Inguinal hernia was the only specific anomaly that was associated with epinephrine both after first-trimester exposures or anytime during pregnancy (1; pp 345–356, 439, 477, 492). Further investigation is needed to demonstrate that these findings reflect specific teratogenic effects of this endogenous sympathomimetic, and not the consequences of the severe maternal disorders for which epinephrine is often given.

Ephedrine

Ephedrine is a sympathomimetic used in cold and allergy preparations and used in the treatment of hypotension after spinal or epidural block. The drug was found by one group to be associated with cardiovascular anomalies in the chick, even when very small doses were used (85). This teratogenic effect was potentiated by caffeine (86). There is a case report of a human abortus with a major congenital heart defect who was exposed at embryonic day 30 to ephedrine (87). The exposure also included other medications (theophylline and phenobarbital). The Collaborative Perinatal Project was unable to identify an association between ephedrine exposure in the first trimester and an increase in any kind of birth defect (1; pp 345–356). This report included 373 exposed pregnancies. Near term, ephedrine may be given to treat or avoid hypotension associated with epidural analgesia or with anaphylactic reactions (88–92). No adverse effects of such therapy have been documented, and ephedrine has been found not to alter intervillous blood flow (91, 92).

It is unknown whether ephedrine therapy contraindicates nursing. There is one case report of a baby with disturbed behavior who was exposed through breast milk to ephedrine and to an antihistamine. The child's symptoms resolved when nursing was discontinued (2).

Isoproterenol

Isoproterenol is the isopropyl analogue of epinephrine. It is a β-adrenergic agonist used in the therapy of asthma. Injection of this agent into incubating chick eggs resulted in abnormal cardiovascular development involving cardiomegaly, coronary artery maldevelopment, fatty degeneration of muscle, ventricular septal defect, aortic arch anomalies, and hypoplasia of right-sided structures (93–97). The developmental toxicity of isoproterenol in the chick can be antagonized by pretreatment with β-blocking agents (94–96). It is believed that catecholamine-induced alterations in blood flow in the embryonic cardiovascular system are responsible for isoproterenol-associated toxicity (97,98). This agent has also been found to cause hepatotoxicity (99) and limb malformations in a small percentage of chick embryos (100). Teratogenic effects have also been noted after administration of isoproterenol to mice (101) and hamsters (102). Experiments in rats (103,104) and rabbits (104,105) have not shown teratogenic effects, although hemodynamic effects of the drug are evident in several experimental animals (106–109).

There are no available studies that enable a prediction of possible human developmental toxicity of isoproterenol. The Collaborative Perinatal Project included 31 women who used this agent during the first trimester. No increase in birth defects was shown (1; pp 346–347).

Isoproterenol is similar to other β-adrenergic agents in decreasing uterine muscle contractility in animals and humans (110–112). This agent is not in clinical use for premature labor because cardiovascular side effects in the mother, and perhaps the fetus, would be more prominent than those associated with more selective β-adrenergic agonists. We have been unable to locate data on the possible effects of isoproterenol in nursing women.

Male and female gonads are innervated by sympathetic nerves, and it is possible that isoproterenol would affect gonadal function. Ovarian progesterone secretion, for example, was increased by isoproterenol in a cat preparation (113). Injection of isoproterenol into immature rats resulted in Leydig cell hypertrophy (114). Isoproterenol treatment of Leydig cells in culture resulted in increased testosterone production in the mouse (115–117) and rat (117). Human sperm exposed to isoproterenol in vitro showed increased motility after 2 hr of incubation (118). It is not possible from available data, however, to estimate whether clinical use of isoproterenol would affect gonadal function or fertility in men or women.

Metaproterenol

Metaproterenol (orciprenaline) is a selective β_2-adrenergic agent that has been used as an inhalant to produce bronchodilation and administered intravenously to delay delivery in premature labor (119,120) or to alleviate fetal bradycardia during parturition (120,121). Experiments using mice, rats, and rhesus monkeys have not associated metaproterenol with teratogenic activity (122,123); however, a study in mice found metaproterenol administration to be associated with an increase in maternal serum corticosterone and consequent induction of cleft palate in the offspring (124). This mechanism of teratogenicity would not be expected to be effective in human pregnancy. Rabbit studies have produced conflicting results, ranging from the induction of multiple defects (123) to no discernible effects on the offspring (125). A third rabbit study examined effects on aortic arch structures, particularly the ductus arteriosus, and found no anomalies attributable to metaproterenol treatment of the doe (126).

In a large-scale study of 259 women with asthma who used inhaled bronchodilators (primarily metaproterenol) during pregnancy, no significant increases were found in the incidence of perinatal mortality, congenital malformations, preterm births, low-birth-weight infants, Apgar scores, labor or delivery complications, or postpartum bleeding (127). Increased incidences of maternal hypertension and transient tachypnea of the neonate were observed in the women using inhaled bronchodilators, but these outcomes seemed more clearly associated with the severity of the mother's asthmatic condition than with the use of bronchodilators (127). Since severe, uncontrolled asthma carries significant risk of gestational complications, the authors concluded that the available data support the intermittent or regular use of this agent, when indicated, in the management of asthma in pregnancy (127). A long-term follow-up of infants who were exposed to a related β-agonist (ritodrine) in utero during the third trimester did not uncover any association with harmful effects (128).

Like other β-agonists, metaproterenol in sufficient doses will cause a variety of side effects in the mother, including tachycardia, hyperglycemia, nervousness, and tremor (119, 121). Comparable symptoms may also be found in exposed neonates (119, 121).

Albuterol

Albuterol (salbutamol) is a β-sympathomimetic used in the treatment of asthma. This agent has also been used to treat preterm labor. In one preliminary report, teratogenic effects were found when albuterol was administered to pregnant mice, but similar effects were not found in rats or rabbits (129). We have not identified any studies that suggest the β-sympathomimetics, including albuterol, are teratogenic in humans: however, experience with them in early pregnancy is limited. For example, no abnormalities were found in the offspring of three women who received albuterol continuously, beginning early in the second trimester (130–132). In contrast to these reports, there is a great deal of data available on the use of albuterol as a tocolytic agent in late pregnancy (133–142). Typically, albuterol will increase maternal cyclic-AMP, glycogenolysis, lipolysis, and insulin levels, but will decrease serum potassium levels (134, 139–41). The overall effects on the circulatory system include an increase in heart rate and a drop in blood pressure (134, 135, 137). Although these effects are more prominent in the mother, the fetus may be expected to show a similar response. The placental transfer of albuterol has been demonstrated in an in vitro system using perfused human placentas (143). In contrast with the available reports on intravenously administered albuterol, one recent report suggests that no significant improvement in pregnancy outcome was associated with the extended oral administration of albuterol in patients with preterm labor (142). Long-term adverse effects in the offspring have not been noted with β-sympathomimetics as a group (128,144).

Terbutaline

Terbutaline is a sympathomimetic drug with predominantly β_2-activity. In the United States, it is approved for use only in the treatment of asthma; however, clinical reports from several European nations, as well as the United States, indicate it is frequently used as a tocolytic agent (145–149).

No reports were located that specifically investigated the possible developmental effects of terbutaline when used early in gestation. Reports comparing the tocolytic effectiveness of terbutaline with magnesium sulfate (147) and ritodrine (147,148), an FDA approved tocolytic, indicated that terbutaline may be comparable with or superior to other available compounds. As with other sympathomimetics in large doses, maternal and fetal side effects can be expected (150). These side effects may include hyperglycemia, cardiovascular complications, and pulmonary edema in the gravida (148,149,151), and a reactive postnatal hypoglycemia in the neonate (159). Main et al. (153) have suggested that pregnant patients on long-term terbutaline therapy had a more severe impairment of glucose tolerance than those treated with ritodrine. Stubblefield and Heyl (146) reported on the use of subcutaneous, rather than intravenous, terbutaline in the treatment of premature labor, and successfully prolonged labor using lower doses of terbutaline. Short-term dosing with terbutaline has also been used successfully to relieve fetal bradycardia associated with labor (121,154,155).

Isolated clinical reports have described cases in which tocolytic therapy with terbutaline may have been associated with sudden, unforeseen fetal death (156), maternal liver impairment (157), and a paradoxical induction of uterine hypertonus (158). We cannot tell from these reports whether a causal relation existed between drug therapy and adverse outcome.

Isoetharine

Isoetharine is a sympathomimetic amine with predominant β_2-activity. It is used as a bronchodilator. We have been unable to locate references on possible reproductive effects of this agent. Isoetharine has structural and pharmacologic similarity to terbutaline, discussed in the previous section.

Bitolterol

Bitolterol is a β_2-adrenergic drug used in inhalation therapy of asthma. Bitolterol is metabolized by lung esterases to colterol, the active bronchodilator (159). According to the manufacturer, inhalation of radiolabeled bitolterol is followed by detection of small amounts of label in blood and urine, suggesting that colterol or its metabolites are absorbed from the lung. We have found no published studies on possible reproductive effects of bitolterol. Studies reported by the manufacturer suggest no mutagenic potential in bacterial and mouse cell culture assays and no impairment of fertility in male or female rats after high doses of bitolterol. The drug was reported not to be teratogenic in rats and rabbits. A small increase in frequency of cleft palate was seen in mice receiving subcutaneous injections of high-dose bitolterol. There are no data available on possible effects of this agent on nursing.

Pirbuterol

Pirbuterol, a β-sympathomimetic, is an analogue of albuterol and is used as a bronchodilator. Administration of pirbuterol at 300 mg/kg per day to pregnant rats and rabbits did not result in an increase in birth defects in the offspring (159). The highest dose was associated with fetal growth impairment in the rats and with abortion in some of the rabbits. We have been unable to locate references on possible human reproductive effects of this agent.

MAST CELL INHIBITORS

Cromolyn

Cromolyn inhibits the release of histamine and other mediators from mast cells. It may be used in the management of allergic rhinitis (Nasalcrom) or asthma (Intal). Intravenous and subcutaneous injections of cromolyn or closely related compounds did not produce fetal malformations in mice, rats, or rabbits (160). A report on 296 pregnant women who used cromolyn during their pregnancies did not uncover any indication of fetal abnormalities directly associated with the use of this drug (161). Less than 10% of an inhaled dose of cromolyn is believed to be absorbed systemically (10; pp 92–93). No information was located on the transfer of cromolyn across the placenta or its excretion into breast milk.

METHYLXANTHINES

Theophylline

Theophylline is a methylxanthine stimulant that occurs naturally in teas and cocoa. In its purified form it has been used medicinally as a diuretic, cardiac stimulant, and bronchodialator. In teratogenesis experiments, theophylline administration to pregnant mice produced cleft palate and digit defects (162,163). Similar teratogenic effects were not observed, however, in rat experiments (164–166). When determined in mice and rats, the no-observable adverse effect level (NOAEL) for developmental toxicity was approximately 10- to 30-fold greater than doses required to maintain clinically useful serum levels of theophylline (166). Extended administration of high doses of theophylline does produce adverse effects on reproduction in male and female rodents (167), but there is no indication that data from such studies has direct application to the human use of this compound.

Theophylline is commonly used in the treatment of asthma and chronic obstructive pulmonary disease in pregnant patients (168–171). Thus, numerous pregnancies have included exposure to this agent without an observable increase in congenital defects. Specific investigations on the human teratogenicity of theophylline did not uncover any association with malformations or stillbirth (1, pp 361–370; 172). A collection of case reports recently described three pregnant asthmatics who used theophylline and other drugs throughout gestation and gave birth to offspring with cardiovascular anomalies (173). These reports are not sufficient, however, to establish a cause-and-effect relation, but they do suggest a focus for additional investigations. The induction of sister chromatid exchange and chromosomal breakage were significantly elevated in cell cultures by concentrations of theophylline that correspond to serum levels attained during the clinical use of this drug (174). Further studies of the possible clastogenic effects of theophylline in whole animals have been called for (174). A much more relevant concern in the clinical use of this drug is its toxicity to the mother, fetus, and neonate. The volume of theophylline distribution increases in pregnancy, but the renal clearance of this drug may decrease (175–177). Because it is difficult to predict how pregnancy may alter the dose requirements of an individual woman, serum theophylline levels should be used to guide therapy. This drug readily crosses the placenta

(178–182). Theophylline concentrations in the fetus are likely to be equal to or slightly higher than those in the mother (180,181). Some investigations indicate that theophylline is metabolized to caffeine in the fetal liver (183,184); however, the clinical significance of this observation has not been established.

Newborns who were exposed to theophylline in utero have shown signs of theophylline intoxication, including jitteriness, tachycardia, and vomiting (178,179). Generally, these symptoms have been observed in neonates with blood theophylline levels of more than 10 μg/mL (180,181). Because levels attained in the mother may be 8–20 μg/mL (182), it should be anticipated that the newborn may show drug effects. In one case, exposure to theophylline throughout gestation resulted in severe apneic spells in a newborn, requiring therapy with theophylline until the spells resolved (180).

Methylxanthines, including theophylline, can depress lipid synthesis in developing neural systems, raising the concern that theophylline exposure during gestation may induce neurologic deficits in some offspring (185). Investigations into the neurologic development of infants treated with theophylline for apnea have not uncovered any abnormalities at 9 through 27 months of age (186,187). Additional, long-term investigations will be necessary to determine if any significant alterations in human brain development are induced by methylxanthine exposure.

Theophylline is excreted into breast milk (177,188–190); and a milk/plasma ratio of 0.73 has been reported (190). Theophylline, administered orally at a dose of 1 mg/kg per day, did not significantly affect the milk volume and composition or the growth of rat pups (10, p 283; 192). Although less than 1% of the maternal dose of theophylline may be transferred to the neonate (188,189), increased sensitivity to this drug may produce toxic effects in the newborn, including vomiting, feeding difficulties, jitteriness, and cardiac arrhythmias. Some clinicians suggest that breast-feeding women nurse their infants just before ingesting their regular dose of theophylline to minimize neonatal exposure to the drug (10; p 283).

Aminophylline

Aminophylline is a methylxanthine derived from complexing theophylline and ethylenediamine. The methylxanthines are used in the therapy of asthma and are similar in action and toxicity. Aminophylline given in high doses in pregnant rats resulted in a small number of digit deformities in the offspring (193). Human experience with this drug has not resulted in a measurable increase in birth defects in exposed pregnancies (1,32). Data from a rabbit model suggested that aminophylline treatment during pregnancy may increase fetal pulmonary phospholipids and decrease the incidence of the respiratory distress syndrome of prematurity (194); however, agreement with this conclusion is not universal (195). Improvement in pulmonary function in preterm rabbits in which the does had been treated with aminophylline has been attributed to accelerated fetal body growth and improved postnatal regulation of breathing, rather than to an increase in surfactant phospholipids (196). A comparison between glucocorticoids and aminophylline in preterm human pregnancy showed no difference between the two in the induction of fetal lung maturity, suggesting that aminophylline may be useful for this indication (197). The smooth-muscle relaxant effect of aminophylline extends also to the uterus (198). This drug compares favorably with ritodrine as a tocolytic agent (199), although not all studies agree that aminophylline is effective for this indication (200). Aminophylline crosses the placenta readily and cord blood levels of the drug are similar to levels in maternal blood (181). This may result in signs of methylxanthine toxicity in the newborn, including jitteriness and a possible withdrawal syndrome (180). Methylxanthines are present in breast milk and may theoretically affect the nursling (201).

ANTICHOLINERGICS

Atropine

Atropine is an anticholinergic agent that has been formulated into several prescription and nonprescription sedatives, cold medications, and antidiarrheal agents. It is also commonly used as one of the preanesthetic medications before cesarean sections and may be utilized by inhalation for asthma. Animal experiments have not suggested that atropine readily induces congenital abnormalities. Relatively high doses of atropine did not cause developmental abnormalities in rats, chicks, or dogs (202–204). The skeletal abnormalities detected after atropine was administered to pregnant mice on day 9 of gestation may have resulted from the maternal toxicity of the atropine and not from a selective teratogenic effect (205). An attempt to reproduce these findings was unsuccessful (206).

The systemic absorption of atropine from ophthalmic solutions can be minimized by compressing the lacrimal sac during and for 1 min following the eye drops. Although atropine readily crosses the placenta (207,208) and may alter fetal heart rate (209) or inhibit fetal breathing (210), fetal exposure to this drug has not been associated with adverse developmental effects or significant fetotoxicity, when it occurred early in pregnancy (1, pp 346–353; 32), or shortly before delivery (211–213). Concern has been expressed concerning the possibility that fetal atropine exposures during cesarean section may decrease the resistance in the lower cardioesophageal sphincter and predispose a newborn to the aspiration of food (10; pp 31–33). Atropine can be used to block the bradycardia produced by vagal stimulation of the heart, but this use of atropine in the fetus and neonate is not commonly recommended (10; pp 31–33).

Although the elimination of atropine is reduced in children younger than 2 years of age, atropine exposures through breast milk have not been widely associated with neonatal toxicity (214). The American Academy of Pediatrics considers the use of atropine compatible with breast-feeding (19).

Ipratropium

Ipratropium is *n*-isopropylatropine, a quarternary ammonium anticholinergic used as a bronchodilator. Systemic anticholinergic effects of inhaled ipratropium are infrequent (215). The manufacturer reports negative reproductive studies in mice, rats, and rabbits, and negative teratogenicity studies in rats and rabbits at doses several hundred to several thousand times the recommended human dose. Published teratology studies have also been negative in rats and rabbits (216,217). We have been unable to locate references on possible reproductive effects of this agent in humans; however, the potential for developmental hazard associated with maternal inhalation therapy is believed to be low.

GLUCOCORTICOIDS

Prednisone and Prednisolone

Prednisone is a glucocorticoid used in collagen–vascular and other disorders. Prednisolone is its active metabolite. High doses of prednisone consistently cause teratogenic effects in rodents that have not been associated with the use of this drug during human pregnancies. For example, prednisone and prednisolone, similar to the naturally occurring glucocorticoid, cortisone, cause cleft palate in mice and rats (218,219). Also, fetal mice exposed to prednisone antepartum show behavioral changes, suggesting an androgenic orientation in females (220). Data available from both animal experiments and human observations suggest prenatal exposure to prednisone may retard fetal growth and be associated with an increased incidence of low birth weight offspring (221,222). Occasionally, this outcome has been attributed to the underlying disease for which the corticosteroids were given (often a collagen–vascular disease) (223). Other investigators, however, have observed a high prevalence of fetal growth retardation in the offspring of renal transplant patients treated with glucocorticoids, despite good graft function and normal or only slightly elevated blood pressure (224). Although one report has suggested an increase in stillbirths among women treated with prednisolone (225), and a second describes an infant born with hydrocephalus to a mother treated with 100 mg/day of prednisone (226), a substantial number of additional reports have described successful pregnancies among women exposed to these agents before pregnancy and throughout gestation (227). A compilation by Schatz et al. of 216 reported corticosteroid-exposed pregnancies in asthmatic women found no increase in adverse outcome associated with treatment (228).

A male transplant patient, treated for several years with prednisone, fathered a child with multiple deformities (229), but a possible relation with prednisone treatment seems unlikely. High doses of corticosteroids can damage spermatogenesis, and recovery may require as long as 6 months (230), but these drugs do not seem to affect chromosome number or sperm morphology (231).

Aside from possible teratogenic risks, there have been concerns that some of the toxicity associated with glucocorticoids in adults might be manifested in exposed fetuses. Cataracts are occasionally observed in adults receiving corticosteroids, and congenital cataracts were reported in one infant exposed to prednisone throughout pregnancy (232). Suppression of the immune system is a common effect of glucocorticoids. Although immunosuppression lasting 15 weeks after birth was observed in one infant born of a woman receiving high doses of prednisone and azathioprine (233), lymphopenia and reduced immunoglobulin levels have not been commonly observed in similarly treated infants (234).

When administered to lactating women, small amounts of prednisone and its active metabolite, prednisolone, will enter breast milk (235–237). For maternal doses of prednisolone larger than 20 mg/day, some clinicians recommend that mothers wait at least 4 hr before nursing (237). Even at 80 mg/day, however, the amount secreted in breast milk would be equivalent to less than 10% of nursing infant's endogenous cortisol production, and it is unlikely that such a dose could produce clinically significant effects (237). The American Academy of

Pediatrics considers prednisone and prednisolone compatible with breast-feeding (19).

Hydrocortisone

The reproductive effects of the corticosteroids appear to be well represented by those of prednisone, discussed in the foregoing. We have not identified other considerations peculiar to hydrocortisone.

Beclomethasone

Beclomethasone dipropionate is a steroidal anti-inflammatory agent given by inhalation to control the symptoms of asthma (Beclovent or Vanceril) and by the intranasal route to treat allergic rhinitis or nasal polyps (Vancenase or Beconase). When administered by inhalation approximately 10–25% of the inhaled drug will enter the respiratory tract, where it is hydrolyzed to the monopriopionate analogue. The parent compound and this metabolite are absorbed into the general circulation and transformed in the liver to inactive metabolites. In the systemic circulation, beclomethasone and its metabolites are tightly bound to proteins, which minimizes their systemic effects (238). Evidence of adrenal suppression has been shown with beclomethasone only when recommended doses have been exceeded (16 inhalations per day) (239,240).

The developmental toxicity of beclomethasone in mice and rabbits is similar to that associated with other corticosteroids, consisting of increased fetal resorptions and cleft lip/palate (241,242). High-dose inhalation studies in pregnant monkeys and feeding studies in rats have demonstrated that a decrease in fetal survival and weight is associated with the maternal toxicity of this agent, but without an observable increase in fetal malformations in these species (243–246).

Two clinical studies have investigated the outcome of 101 pregnancies in which women received beclomethasone or prednisone, or both, for severe asthma (247,248). The prevalence of congenital malformations in this population was within the normal range for all births, although the incidence of premature deliveries and low-birth-weight infants was slightly increased (248). Because status asthmaticus during pregnancy may be deleterious to both mother and fetus (247), the possible risks of beclomethasone use by a gravida must be compared with the risks associated with asthma attacks that lead to hospitalizations, as well as the possible toxic effects of alternative, systemic corticosteroids. Inhaled beclomethasone is as effective as oral prednisone in controlling the symptoms of patients with mild to moderate asthma

(249). A daily dose of 400 μg of the inhaled drug (two puffs four times daily) is approximately equal to 7.5 mg of prednisone in its effect on asthma. In mild to severe asthma, the use of beclomethasone has decreased the required dose of prednisone needed to control asthma attacks (250).

Data from one study suggest that the incidence of side effects with inhaled beclomethasone is significantly less than that observed when systemic corticosteroids are used in the treatment of asthma (251). However, a high proportion of patients (45–77%) using beclomethosone develop oropharnygeal candidiasis. Rinsing the mouth and gargling with water after each inhalation may reduce colonization with *Candida* (251). Use of a spacer device reduces mouth and throat deposition of drug and concomitantly the incidence of thrush (252) and may decrease systemic effects of the drug as well (253).

Flunisolide

Flunisolide is a synthetic glucocorticoidlike drug that is active by intranasal administration in the treatment of allergic rhinitis (Nasalide) and by inhalation for asthma (AeroBid). Nasal or inhalational administration of glucocorticoid medications may result in significant systemic absorption (254); however, flunisolide may be particularly poorly absorbed. According to the manufacturer, administration of nasal flunisolide does not result in suppression of endogenous cortisol, even when the drug is used at higher-than-recommended doses. Although we have been unable to identify published reproductive studies on this agent, the manufacturer reports that flunisolide has teratogenic and embryotoxic effects in experimental animals similar to those seen with other glucocorticoids (see earlier discussion of prednisone).

Triamcinolone

Triamcinolone is a synthetic corticosteroid. It has been associated with cleft palate in the offspring when given to pregnant mice, rats, rabbits, and hamsters (255–258). It also caused central nervous system, craniofacial, and other abnormalities in the offspring of three different nonhuman primates (259–263). It has been noted that triamcinolone is 200 times more potent in producing palatal clefts in mice than is cortisone (255). In avian experiments, triamcinolone produces inhibition of scale and feather development, as do other corticosteroids; however, triamcinolone is 10,000 times more potent a teratogen in this model than is hydrocortisone (264). The potent teratogenic effects seen in several species are cause for concern that this agent may also be a developmental toxicant in humans. A recent case report has suggested that the topical use of 40 mg triamcinolone per day for atopic dermatitis, from 12–29 weeks of gestation, may have produced severe intrauterine growth retardation in an exposed offspring (265). Triamcinolone is best avoided during pregnancy in favor of corticosteroids, such as prednisone, for which there are more data on human pregnancy effects. It should be noted, however, that inhaled triamcinolone (Azmacort), used for asthma, is likely to be associated with reduced systemic exposure. Possible adverse pregnancy outcome after inhaled triamcinolone has not been studied.

ANTIMICROBIALS

Penicillin

Penicillins have been formulated with a variety of substituents added onto the fundamental β-lactam thiazolidine nucleus. Benzylpenicillin (penicillin G) and phenoxymethylpenicillin (penicillin V) are two of the oldest and most commonly used derivatives. High-dose animal experiments in mice (266) and rabbits (267) did not reveal any indications of adverse reproductive effects.

The pharmacokinetics of the penicillins during pregnancy have been studied in detail (268–271), and the placental transfer of these antibiotics has been well characterized (268–272). Penicillins accumulate in amniotic fluid in large amounts during maternal ingestion (270). This is caused by fetal urinary excretion of the antibiotic into the amniotic fluid, which continues until the mother stops ingesting the drug. Thereafter, the fetus gradually reabsorbs the antibiotic (probably by swallowing the amniotic fluid) and clears the drug by passage across the placenta to the mother. No adverse fetal effects have been associated with this process. In general, the penicillins have not been teratogenic in humans and their widespread use in pregnancy has not yet produced recognized adverse effects (1, pp 297–313; 273).

All penicillins may produce anaphylaxis during pregnancy or immediately postpartum (274). If anaphylaxis is severe and uncontrolled, it may compromise the placental circulation and cause fetal damage or death (275).

Penicillins are excreted into breast milk in small amounts (276). This exposure is unlikely to have detectable effects in the newborn, but such exposure to penicillins may be sufficient to cause allergic sensitization in the infant.

Ampicillin and Pivampicillin

Ampicillin is a penicillin antibiotic. Maternal and fetal exposure to this drug will also occur when the antibiotic, pivampicillin, is administered. Pivampicillin is readily transformed to ampicillin (277).

In rat experiments, there are two reports in which high doses of ampicillin, administered orally, did not produce teratogenic effects (278,279). In a third report, high doses of ampicillin were associated with limb defects (72). The pharmacokinetics of ampicillin during pregnancy have been studied in detail (268,280), and the placental transfer of ampicillin has been well characterized, similar to that for penicillins in general (as just discussed) (269,280–282).

Despite the widespread use of ampicillin, only one case report was located that suggested the use of this antibiotic may have been associated with congenital malformations (283). In general, the penicillins have not been shown to be teratogenic in humans and their relatively common use in pregnancy has not yet produced recognized adverse effects (1, pp 297–313, 435). Women taking these drugs will show a decrease in urinary estriol secretion, probably owing to alterations in intestinal flora in the mother (284–286). There is no evidence that decreases in measurable urinary estriol in patients taking ampicillin correlate with impaired fetal well-being (285,286). An interaction between ampicillin and oral contraceptives has been suggested to cause a decrease in the effectiveness of these contraceptives (287,288), but detailed investigations of this question did not confirm the suggested interaction (289,290).

Ampicillin, similar to other penicillins, may produce anaphylaxis during pregnancy or immediately postpartum (274), which, if severe and uncontrolled, may compromise the placental circulation and cause fetal brain damage or death.

Ampicillin is excreted in breast milk in small amounts. The milk/plasma ratio for this drug was measured in 14 lactating mothers and found to vary between 0.01 and 0.58 (277). The maximum dose of ampicillin likely to be ingested by a nursing neonate was estimated as 0.5 mg/day (277). This dose is unlikely to have detectable effects in the newborn, but may be sufficient to cause allergic sensitization in the infant (277).

Cephalexin

Cephalexin is a cephalosporin antibiotic. It is well absorbed after oral administration and readily crosses the placenta (291,292); the cord blood level after maternal ingestion of the drug at term is about one-third that found in the maternal serum (292). This drug was not teratogenic when tested in rats and mice (293,294). Use of cephalexin during human pregnancy without adverse consequences has been described (291,295–297).

Cephalexin reaches breast milk in small amounts (298). This is not considered a contraindication to nursing.

Cefaclor

Cefaclor is an oral cefalosporin antibiotic. This drug was not teratogenic when tested in rats, mice, rabbits, or ferrets at up to 2 g/kg per day (299–301). We have been unable to locate human studies on reproductive effects of this agent.

Cefixime

Cefixime, an analogue of cefotaxime, is an orally active third-generation cephalosporin. Studies in rats show this drug capable of crossing the placenta and of entering breast milk; however, the levels found in the offspring after exposure by either route are very low (302). We have been unable to locate references on possible human reproductive effects of this agent.

Clavulanate

Clavulanate is a β-lactam that impedes the action of bacterial β-lactamases on coadministered antibiotics. The administration of clavulanic acid, in combination with amoxicillin, produced no teratogenic effects when tested in rats (303,304) or pigs (305). The use of this combination in 80 women with bacteriuria of pregnancy was not associated with any detectable adverse effects in the exposed offspring (297). The principal maternal side effect of amoxicillin–clavulanic acid was vaginal irritation or discharge, which may have been caused by an overgrowth of *Candida* or other opportunistic organisms (297).

Erythromycin

Erythromycin is an orally effective macrolide antibiotic. One report suggested that erythromycin increased the incidence of urogenital abnormalities in rats (306). Human case reports on anomalies in newborns exposed in utero to erythromycin did not indicate that this drug produced a consistent pattern of defects (307,308). The Collaborative Perinatal Project monitored 79 pregnancies with first-trimester exposure to this antibiotic and 230 exposures to it at any time during pregnancy, but did not uncover evidence to suggest a relation with major or minor malformations (1, pp 297–313).

The treatment of chlamydial and mycoplasmal infections with erythromycin during pregnancy has been investigated by several clinicians. This use of erythromycin has been associated with improved gestational outcomes (i.e., increased birth weight) and reduced infant morbidity (309–312). One group of researchers reported that women with histories of spontaneous pregnancy wastage who were mycoplasma-positive in the urogenital tract experienced significant decreases in their pregnancy loss rate after treatment with erythromycin (313). The estolate ester of erythromycin has been associated with a relatively high incidence of subclinical, reversible hepatotoxicity when used during pregnancy (314); therefore, the use of other derivatives of erythromycin is preferred.

Erythromycin crosses the placenta in small quantities (315–317), but maternal dosing with this antibiotic has not proved effective in suppressing the growth of fetal pathogens (318).

Erythromycin is excreted into the breast milk in small quantities (317). These would not be expected to be clinically significant.

Troleandomycin

Troleandomycin is the triacetylated ester of oleandomycin, an antibiotic derived from *Streptomyces antibioticus*. We have been unable to locate references on possible reproductive effects of troleandomycin.

Tetracyclines

Tetracyclines are a group of antimicrobials that act by inhibiting protein synthesis. They were commonly used during pregnancy after first being introduced in the 1950s (319). Animal teratology studies on these agents give conflicting results. Exposure of gestating rats to tetracycline in one study resulted in an increase in cleft palate and limb abnormalities (320); however, three other studies were unable to document any teratogenic effect of this agent in rats (321–323), and a fourth showed only an increased frequency of hydroureter in exposed animals (324). Oxytetracycline was teratogenic in dogs (325), but not in mice, rats, and rabbits (326,327). There have been a few studies suggesting that tetracycline treatment of pregnant rats results in abnormal development of lymphatic and thymic tissues (328,329). This raises the possibility of altered immunoregulation related to antenatal drug exposure. Staining of the cornea and lens of the eye has also been observed in rat fetuses exposed to tetracycline (330), but there are no controlled clinical investigations to indicate that such effects may occur in humans.

Although there are several case reports of abnormalities in human pregnancies following tetracycline use by the mother, the Collaborative Perinatal Project (1, pp 297–313, 435, 472, 486) was not able to identify the tetracyclines as causes of major birth defects. Possible associations with minor defects were suggested; however, the few cases (most of which involved inguinal hernia as the only defect) do not permit the conclusion that these agents are human teratogens. Administration of tetracyclines in the second or third trimesters of pregnancy can cause staining of the teeth of the child and up to a 40% depression of bone growth (especially of the fibula in preterm pregnancies (331–333)). Tetracycline, given intravenously, may result in hepatic necrosis in pregnant women (334,335). Many women reported to have developed this complication had been treated for pyelonephritis, and it is possible that renal impairment is an important contributor to this toxic effect. The mobilization of tetracycline from bone during pregnancy has been suggested as a possible toxicologic mechanism for some cases of fatty liver during pregnancy (336). This scenario would be possible among women who had been treated extensively with tetracycline for dermatologic conditions (336).

Tetracycline is excreted into breast milk in low concentrations. The reported milk/plasma ratios have ranged from 0.25 to 1.5 (319,337,338). Serum levels of breast-fed infants exposed to maternal tetracycline in their milk were unmeasurably low (319). The American Academy of Pediatrics considers tetracycline compatible with breast-feeding (19).

Sulfamethoxazole

Sulfamethoxazole is frequently administered in combination with trimethoprim in the oral treatment of urinary tract infections, chronic bronchitis, and gonorrhea (339). Much concern over the administration of this drug combination in pregnant women has been focused on the folate antagonist in the mixture, trimethoprim.

Sulfamethoxazole, similar to other sulfonamides, can cross the placenta in humans (339,340) and shares the potential problems of this class of antimicrobials, including the induction of idiosyncratic sulfonamide reactions and the displacement of other compounds from plasma proteins. In the fetus and newborn, sulfonamides, such as sulfamethoxazole, may displace bilirubin from plasma-binding sites and cause kernicterus to develop at lower bilirubin levels. Such a complication is currently theoretical, but it is a predominant reason for withholding sulfonamide therapy in the third trimester of pregnancy. Human birth defects have not been associated with this group of drugs, even when administered during the first trimester (1, p 458; 341–343). The number of human case studies available for sulfamethoxazole and other sulfonamides is still small, however, and animal data suggesting sulfonamide-induced malformations in some species (344,345) cannot be totally discounted.

Sulfamethoxazole and other sulfonamides are excreted into breast milk (346,347). Exposure to this group of anti-infectives should be avoided in premature infants and in infants with hyperbilirubinemia or glucose-6-phosphate dehydrogenase deficiency. Except for the preceding conditions, the American Academy of Pediatrics considers sulfonamides compatible with breast-feeding (53).

Trimethoprim

Trimethoprim is a folic acid antagonist used as an antimicrobial agent. Although trimethoprim is now available for use as a single agent (Trimpex), it is commonly administered in combination with a sulfonamide because together they produce a synergistic antimicrobial effect. The use of trimethoprim during pregnancy is generally avoided because of the concern that it may limit the availability of folic acid to the fetus and impair normal growth (348,349).

Trimethoprim is well absorbed orally and readily transferred across the placenta to the fetus (339,340). Rats exposed to high doses of trimethoprim and sulfamethoxazole on days 8 through 15 of gestation developed cleft palate, micrognathia, and limb shortening (350). Similar doses of sulfamethoxazole alone were not embryotoxic. Of the available reports on several hundred women exposed to trimethoprim during pregnancy (341–343,351,352), only one infant was born with a birth defect, which consisted of mental and growth retardation and craniofacial malformations (Niikawa–Kuroki syndrome). In addition to any adverse drug effect in this case, the combined viral and bacterial infections that afflicted the mother during the second month of pregnancy may have played a role in the etiology of the infant's birth defects (353).

Trimethoprim is excreted into breast milk in small amounts (354,355). No adverse effects have been observed in exposed infants (354), and available estimates of the potential risk to the suckling infant suggest that trimethoprim use is compatible with breast-feeding (19,355).

EXPECTORANTS AND ANTITUSSIVES

Iodine

Iodine-containing medications have been used as expectorants and topical antiseptics during pregnancy. Because maternal iodine can be readily transferred to the fetus (356), extended exposure to iodine-containing medications can lead to hypothyroidism and goiter in the fetus and newborn (357). When goiter is severe enough, it may cause tracheal compression and asphyxiation. Most of the reported fatalities caused by iodine intoxication resulted from the use of iodine-containing expectorants during pregnancy. An analysis of these cases suggested that cardiomegaly may also be associated with excessive iodine exposure during gestation (357). The use of iodides as expectorants is now contraindicated by the American Academy of Pediatrics (358). In contrast, the administration of iodine for several days before maternal thyroid surgery has not been associated with fetal hypothyroidism or goiter (359–361).

A second major source of maternal iodine exposure is the use of topical antiseptics and vaginal anti-infectives containing povidone (polyvinylpyrrolidone) and iodine. Both douching and perineal use of povidone–iodine products have increased maternal serum iodine levels in pregnancy (362–365) and alter maternal (362,363) and fetal (363) thyroid function. Although iodine exposure from these products has not been associated with clinical symptoms of hypothyroidism or goiter in exposed infants, concern exists that continued use of povidone–iodine products could lead to iodine intoxication (366,367).

Iodine is transferred to breast milk (363,368). In one case report, a mother who had used a povidone–iodine vaginal gel for 6 days without douching became concerned when she noted an iodine odor coming from her 7-month-old breast-fed baby. Serum and urine iodine levels in the newborn were elevated, but no signs of thyroid dysfunction were detected in the baby (368).

Given these observations, the repeated or routine use of iodine-containing products is not recommended during pregnancy or lactation (358,362,363,365,368).

Guaifenesin

Guaifenesin is used as an expectorant. The FDA Panel on Cough and Cold Products recently classified this compound as an effective expectorant in patients with chronic bronchitis; however, the small study used as the basis for this classification has not yet been published in a refereed journal (369). Other studies have not produced data that indicate this agent is effective as an expectorant. For example, Hirsch et al. (370) found guaifenesin was ineffective as an expectorant in patients with chronic bronchitis. Kuhn et al. (371) reported guaifenesin did not significantly reduce cough frequency and demonstrated only a decrease in sputum thickness in the subjective reports made by patients with colds (371). The dose of guaifenesin used in this study was approximately two times higher than that recommended by the manufacturer (372).

The Collaborative Perinatal Project found that the incidence of inguinal hernias was increased in a group of 197 offspring who were exposed to guaifenesin during the first trimester (1, p 478). No significant association was identified in the same study when pregnancy outcomes were evaluated after exposures any time during gestation. A separate study involving 241 women exposed to guaifenesin during the first trimester did not identify an increase in congenital defects (14).

Because guaifenesin has a reputed effect on fluid secretion in the respiratory tract, one research group investigated whether the administration of this drug could alter the characteristics of cervical mucus and improve sperm survival and fertility (373). Although this brief report did suggest guaifenesin improved fertility in 80% of the cases in whom the cause of infertility was believed to be primarily the cervical mucus, additional studies, both larger in scale and improved in design, will be needed to determine the significance of this isolated report.

Dextromethorphan

Dextromethorphan is used as an antitussive in nonprescription products. Although dextromethorphan is the *d*-isomer of the opioid, levorphanol, it is not active as an analgesic and retains only the antitussive properties of these agents. Dextromethorphan was not found by the Collaborative Perinatal Project to be associated with an increase in birth defects when used in the first 4 months of pregnancy (1). We have been unable to locate other reports on possible reproductive effects of this agent.

Codeine

Codeine is a widely used narcotic analgesic and antitussive. Teratogenicity studies in hamsters and mice have associated codeine administration with skeletal abnormalities (324,325). In contrast, no adverse effects were uncovered when codeine was administered to pregnant rats or rabbits (376). Retrospective studies of human pregnancies that involved the first-trimester use of codeine have associated this compound with a variety of anomalies, including respiratory tract malformation, pyloric stenosis, inguinal hernia, cardiac and circulatory system defects, and cleft lip and palate (1, pp 287–295; 377–379). The absence of a consistent pattern in these retrospective associations, however, as well as criticisms of possible bias in the data collected for these observations, make it currently impossible to consider codeine a human teratogen. The available data do suggest the cautious use of codeine during the first trimester, until adequate data from human pregnancies are compiled.

Neonatal withdrawal, characterized by tremor, jitteriness, diarrhea, and poor feeding, has been seen in babies born to both addicted and nonaddicted women when the women had been taking codeine-containing medications in the days before delivery (380,381). If present during labor, codeine can produce respiratory depression in the newborn, which can be alleviated by naloxone administration.

Small amounts of codeine are transferred to breast milk (382), but the quantities are not considered sufficient to contraindicate breastfeeding (19).

MISCELLANEOUS

Acetaminophen

Acetaminophen (paracetamol) is an analgesic that appears to work by inhibiting prostaglandin synthesis in the central nervous system. This drug was not teratogenic in mice (383) and did not cause intrauterine growth abnormalities in rats (384). In high doses, acetaminophen is toxic to the rat testis (385).

Human case reports of malformed babies born after use of acetaminophen exist (386–392); however, many of these cases feature exposure to numerous other agents. In addition, the lack of uniformity of abnormalities among these cases make less likely their association with a single causative agent. The Collaborative Perinatal Project did not find an association between use of acetaminophen during pregnancy and congenital anomalies in the offspring (1, pp 286–295). Another retrospective study on congenital heart disease similarly found no association between this group of abnormalities and maternal acetaminophen use during pregnancy (393). There has been concern about possible nonmalforming toxicity of acetaminophen during pregnancy. Although hepatotoxicity of this drug appears to be less in young animals than in adults (394), there has been at least one case report of a human stillbirth with evidence of hepatic toxicity after maternal ingestion of 30 g of acetaminophen in a 24-hr period (395). Other cases of acetaminophen overdose during pregnancy with normal outcomes for the offspring have been reported (396–400).

Acetaminophen therapy near term has raised concern because other prostaglandin synthetase inhibitors have been associated with neonatal hemorrhage, inhibition of labor, and premature closure of the ductus arteriosus. Although these complications have not been documented in humans, there are few data to establish the safety of acetaminophen therapy. One study on neonatal intracranial hemorrhage found a significant association with maternal aspirin use, but not with use of acetaminophen (401). Studies in rats (402) and in sheep (403) have demonstrated that acetaminophen, like aspirin, can be associated with premature closure of the ductus arteriosus. In spite of these potential adverse consequences, acetaminophen is still considered by many to be the analgesic and antipyretic of choice during all trimesters of pregnancy (404).

Aspirin

Aspirin, an oral analgesic and antipyretic, is one of the most frequently used drugs in pregnancy. In very large doses, aspirin is teratogenic in rodents (405,406). In even larger doses, aspirin produces similar embryotoxicity in rhesus monkeys (406). The anomalies observed include neural tube defects, skeletal malformations, and facial clefts. Some case–control studies have reported associations between congenital malformations and aspirin use early in gestation, but the various studies have not uncovered a consistent outcome attributable to drug use. One study, for example, reported an increase in cleft palate among offspring of aspirin users (378); a second found an increase in stillbirth rate and reduced birth weight among women who used aspirin intermittently during pregnancy, but no congenital malformations (407). A large prospective study of 50,000 pregnancies did not uncover any evidence of aspirin-induced teratogenicity (408). A retrospective, case–control study suggested that aspirin use during pregnancy might increase the risk of certain heart defects in the offspring (393). However, another case–control study of children with congenital heart defects found no association between these abnormalities and maternal use of aspirin during pregnancy (409).

Near term, use of aspirin and other prostaglandin synthetase inhibitors may cause closure or constriction of the fetal ductus arteriosus with resultant pulmonary hypertension (410,411). Aspirin also decreases platelet adhesiveness and aggregation, which may explain the finding that premature babies whose mothers take aspirin within 1 week of delivery have an increased frequency of intracranial bleeding (412). Thus, the available reports suggest analgesic doses of aspirin may complicate delivery and adversely affect the newborn. Therefore, aspirin use is not recommended in late pregnancy (413).

Several studies have indicated that the use of small daily doses of aspirin (60–100 mg) by women at high risk of preeclampsia may significantly reduce the incidence of pregnancy-induced hypertension (414–418). Additional findings from these studies have suggested a significant increase in fetal birth weight among high-risk patients who do not become hypertensive (414,418). In a separate but related study, low-dose aspirin therapy was associated with a significant increase in birth weight, fetal head circumference, and placental weight in women with moderate hypertension (415). Aspirin did not have significant effects on pregnancy outcome in women with indications of extreme hypertension. Newborns exposed to low-dose aspirin in utero have not had an excessive incidence of bleeding abnormalities (414,415). Detailed biochemical investigations have indicated that exposed newborns had significantly reduced levels of platelet cyclooxygenase (63%), but enzyme levels were not completely suppressed (418–420). These findings have been interpreted to suggest that low doses of aspirin may permit normal hemostatic competence in the fetus and newborn (418,419). Despite all this optimism, proponents of the use of low-dose aspirin recommend that treatment be stopped at least 5 days before the estimated date of delivery to avoid possible hematologic abnormalities in the newborn (414,420). A consistent and unresolved criticism of the available studies has centered on the reliable identification of pregnant women who would be suitable for treatment with low-dose aspirin. For example, the use of angiotensin infusion to identify women at high risk for pregnancy-induced hypertension (417) is considered by some as invasive, and sometimes dangerous (414). The rollover test, which is much simpler and safer to perform, has also been used to identify potential hypertensives (414), but it is likely to produce false-positive results in a large percentage of pregnant women (421). Because of these considerations and the relatively few pregnancies studied, the available findings on this use of aspirin must be considered preliminary, until the current large-scale clinical trials to evaluate the efficacy and safety of this treatment have been completed (422).

Immunotherapy

"Allergy shots" contain small doses of allergens and are used to desensitize individuals. Most of these allergens are environmental, and it may be assumed that all pregnant women are exposed to many such allergens. No specific teratogenic allergens have been shown to be causes of abnormal pregnancy in humans. Published studies demonstrate no increase in incidence of birth defects in women receiving allergy shots (1, 423–428). Desensitization to penicillin has been used successfully during pregnancy to permit the use of this drug for the treatment of syphilis (429).

Amantadine

Amantadine is an antiviral drug that is also used in parkinsonianlike disorders. It was teratogenic in rats in one study (430), but not in a second (431). Neither of these reports found amantadine to have teratogenic activity in rabbits. One case report of amantadine use during human pregnancy described cardiovascular malformations in the offspring (432); however, this case does not provide sufficient information for any conclusion as to the developmental toxicity of amantadine.

Influenza Vaccine

Influenza is a respiratory tract infection caused by a group of myxoviruses. Experimental infection of pregnant mice is associated with maternal and neonatal mortality and depressed neonatal growth, but no evidence of transplacental transmission or an increase in congenital anomalies (433,434). Several early reports on pregnancy outcome in humans following influenza infection have been summarized (435). Although some reports link a history of influenza (given by the mother) with an increased incidence of neural tube defects and other anomalies in the offspring, studies using serological evidence of infection have failed to confirm this (436–438).

The influenza vaccine is a killed virus vaccine. There has been a case report of a baby born with severe brain abnormalities following a pregnancy in which the mother was vaccinated at 6 postconception weeks (439). The authors believed that the timing of vaccination might explain the development of the brain abnormalities. There have been two reports, which together include 245 women vaccinated just before or during pregnancy. No adverse outcomes were attributable to the vaccine (440,441).

REFERENCES

1. Heinonen OP, et al. Birth defects and drugs in pregnancy, Littleton, MA: Publishing Sciences Group, 1977.
2. Mortimer EA Jr. Drug toxicity from breast milk? Pediatrics 1980; 60:780–781.
3. O'Brien TE. Excretion of drugs in human milk. Am J Hosp Pharm 1974; 31:844–854.
4. Naranjo P, deNaranjo E. Embryotoxic effects of antihistamines. Arzneimittelforschung 1968; 18:188–195.
5. Pride SM, et al. Clinical, endocrinologic, and intraovarian prostaglandin F responses to H-1 receptor blockade in the ovarian hyperstimulation syndrome: studies in the rabbit model. Am J Obstet Gynecol 1984; 148:670–674.
6. Kirshon B, et al. Management of ovarian hyperstimulation syndrome with chlorpheniramine maleate, mannitol, and invasive hemodynamic monitoring. Obstet Gynecol 1988; 71:485–487.
7. McCain J, Olley J. The effects of an oral nasal decongestant upon menstrual cycle. Am J Obstet Gynecol 1963; 87:354–362.
8. Bedi P, et al. Preliminary report of a trial of a long acting antihistaminic buclizine hydrochloride in patients with bleeding after insertion of an intrauterine device. Indian J Med Res 1968; 56:884.
9. Pendergrass PB, et al. The effect of an H_1 blocker, chlorpheniramine maleate, on total menstrual loss. Gynecol Obstet Invest 1984; 18:238–243.
10. Berkowitz R, et al. Handbook for prescribing medications during pregnancy, 2nd ed. Boston: Little, Brown & Co, 1986:84.
11. Lowe ER, et al. The antihistamine properties of Benadryl, beta-dimethylaminoethyl benzhydryl ether hydrochlorides. J Pharmacol Exp Ther 1946; 86:229–238.
12. Schardein JL, et al. Teratogenesis studies with diphenydramine HCl. Toxicol Appl Pharmacol 1971; 18:971–916.
13. Greenberger P, Patterson R. Safety of therapy for allergic symptoms during pregnancy. Obstet Gynecol Surv 1979; 34:284–286.
14. Aselton PA, et al. First-trimester drug use and congenital disorders. Obstet Gynecol 1985; 65:451–455.
15. Saxen I. Cleft palate and maternal diphenhydramine intake. Lancet 1974; 1:407–408.
16. Nelson MM, Forfar JO. Associations between drugs administered during pregnancy and congenital abnormalities of the fetus. Br Med J 1971; 1:153–157.
17. Yoo SD, et al. Placental transfer of diphenhydramine in chronically instrumented sheep. J Pharm Sci 1986; 75:685–687.
18. Parkin DE. Probable Benadryl withdrawal manifestations in a newborn infant. J Pediatr 1974; 85:580.

19. Committee on Drugs, American Academy of Pediatrics. The transfer of drugs and other chemicals into human breast milk. Pediatrics 1989; 84:924–936.
20. King CTG, Howell J. Teratogenic effect of buclizine and hydroxyzine in the rat and chlorcyclizine in the mouse. Am J Obstet Gynecol 1966; 95:109–111.
21. Walker BE, Patterson A. Induction of cleft palate in mice by tranquilizers and barbiturates. Teratology 1974; 10:159.
22. Earl FL, et al. Teratogenic research in beagle dogs and miniature swine. Lab Anim Drug Test Symp Int Comm Lab Anim, 5th, Stuttgart: Fischer, 1973:233–247.
23. Steffek AJ, et al. Abortive effects and comparative metabolism of chlorcyclizine in various mammalian species. Teratology 1968; 1:399–406.
24. Narrod SA, et al. Metabolism of meclizine in the rat. J Pharmacol Exp Ther 1965; 147:380–384.
25. Douglas WW. Histamine and 5-hydroxytryptamine (serotonin) and their antagonists. In: Gilman AG, et al., eds. The pharmacological basis of therapeutics, 7th ed. New York: Macmillan, 1985:611.
26. Posner HS, Darr A. Fetal edema from benzhydroylpiperizines as a possible cause of oral–facial malformations in the rat. Toxicol Appl Pharmacol 1970; 17:67–75.
27. Erez S, et al. Double-blind evaluation of hydroxyzine as an antiemetic in pregnancy. J Reprod Med 1971; 7:57–59.
28. Zsigmond EK, Paterson RL. Double-blind evaluation of hydroxyzine hydrochloride in obstetric anesthesia. Anesth Analg 1967; 46:275.
29. Petrie RH, et al. The effect of drugs on fetal heart rate variability. Am J Obstet Gynecol 1978; 130:294.
30. Prenner BM. Neonatal withdrawal syndrome associated with hydroxyzine hydrochloride. Am J Dis Child 1977; 131:529.
31. Robbiano L, et al. DNA-damaging activity of tripelennamine in primary cultures of human hepatocytes. J Cancer Res Clin Oncol 1986; 111:71–74.
32. Mellin GW. Drugs in the first trimester of pregnancy and fetal life of *Homo sapiens*. Am J Obstet Gynecol 1964; 90:1169–1180.
33. Driscoll CD, et al. Behavioral and developmental effects of prenatal exposure to pentazocine and tripelennamine combinations. Neurobehav Toxicol Teratol 1986; 8:605–613.
34. von Almen WF 2nd, Miller JM Jr. "T's and blues" in pregnancy. J Reprod Med 1986; 31:236–239.
35. Schaffer MI, et al. Spontaneous live birth with a maternal history of intravenous use of pentazocine and tripelennamine (T's and blues). J Forensic Sci 1983; 28:489–495.
36. Chasnoff IJ, et al. Pentazocine and tripelennamine ("T's and blue's"): effects on the fetus and neonate. Dev Pharmacol Ther 1983; 6:162–169.

37. Dunn DW, Reynolds J. Neonatal withdrawal symptoms associated with "T's and blues" (pentazocine and tripelennamine). Am J Dis Child 1982; 136:644–645.
38. Leslie GB, Walker TF. A toxicological profile of cimetadine. In: Burkland WA, Simkins ML, eds. Cimetadine. Amsterdam: Excerpta Medica, 1977:24–33.
39. Anand S, Van Thiel DH. Prenatal and neonatal exposure to cimetidine results in gonadal and sexual dysfunction in adult males. Science 1982; 218:493–494.
40. Parker S, et al. Prenatal and neonatal exposure of male rat pups to cimetidine but not ranitidine adversely affects subsequent adult sexual functioning. Gastroenterology 1984; 86:675–680.
41. Walker TF, et al. Cimetidine does not demasculinize male rat offspring exposed in utero. Fundam Appl Toxicol 1987; 8:188–197.
42. Shipiro BH, et al. Prospective study on the sexual development of male and female rats perinatally exposed to maternally administered cimetidine (TXL 02073). Toxicol Lett 1988; 44:315–330.
43. Sawyer D, et al. Cimetidine: adverse reactions and toxicity. Am J Hosp Pharm 1981; 38:188–197.
44. Vigersky RA, et al. Treatment of hirsute women with cimetidine: a preliminary report. N Engl J Med 1980; 301:1042.
45. Finkelstein W, Isselbacher KJ. Cimetidine. N Engl J Med 1978; 299:992–996.
46. Qvist N, et al. Cimetidine as pre-anesthetic agent for cesarean section. J Perinat Med 1985; 13:179–183.
47. Okasha AS, et al. Cimetidine–antacid combination as premedication for elective caesarean section. Can Anaesth Soc J 1983; 30:593–597.
48. Frank M, et al. Comparison of the prophylactic use of magnesium trisilicate mixture B.P.C., sodium citrate mixture or cimetidine in obstetrics. Br J Anaesth 1984; 56:355–362.
49. McAuley DM, et al. Cimetidine in labour: absence of adverse effect on the high-risk fetus. Br J Obstet Gynaecol 1985; 92:350–355.
50. Howe JP, et al. The placental transfer of cimetidine. Anaesthesia 1981; 36:371–375.
51. Glade G, et al. Cimetidine in pregnancy: apparent transient liver impairment in the newborn. Am J Dis Child 1980; 134:87–88.
52. Somogyi A, Gugler R. Cimetidine excretion into breast milk. Br J Clin Pharmacol 1979; 7:627.
53. Committee on Drugs, American Academy of Pediatrics. The transfer of drugs and other chemicals into human milk. Pediatrics 1983; 72:375–383.
54. Glazener F, et al. Bradycardia, hypotension, and near-syncope associated with Afrin (oxymetazoline) nasal spray. New Engl J Med 1983; 309:731.
55. Soderman P, et al. CNS reactions to nose drops in small children. Lancet 1984; 1:573.

56. Rayburn WF, et al. Uterine and fetal Doppler flow changes from a single dose of a long-acting intranasal decongestant. Obstet Gynecol 1990; 76:180–182.
57. Baxi LV, et al. Fetal heart rate changes following maternal administration of a nasal decongestant. Am J Obstet Gynecol 1985; 153:799–800.
58. Smith NT, Corbascio AN. The use and misuse of pressor agents. Anesthesiology 1970; 33:58–101.
59. Cottle MKW, et al. Effects of phenylephrine and sodium salicylate on maternal and fetal cardiovascular indices and blood oxygenation in sheep. Am J Obstet Gynecol 1982; 143:170–176.
60. Magness RR, et al. Systemic and uterine responses to alpha-adrenergic stimulation in pregnant and nonpregnant ewes. Am J Obstet Gynecol 1986; 155:897–904.
61. Pental P. Toxicity of over-the-counter stimulants. JAMA 1984; 252:1898–1903.
62. McLaughlin MK, et al. Vascular catecholamine sensitivity during pregnancy in the ewe. Am J Obstet Gynecol 1989; 160:47–53.
63. Horowitz JD, et al. Hypertensive responses induced by phenylpropanolamine in anorectic and decongestant preparations. Lancet 1980; 1:60–61.
64. Lasagna L. Phenylpropanolamine and blood pressure. JAMA 1985; 253:2491–2492.
65. Pentel PR, et al. Myocardial injury after phenylpropanolamine ingestion. Br Heart J 1982; 47:51–54.
66. Kase CS, et al. Intracerebral hemorrhage and phenylpropanolamine use. Neurology 1987; 37:399–404.
67. Maher LM. Postpartum intracranial hemorrhage and phenylpropanolamine use. Neurology 1987; 37:1686.
68. Med Lett. Phenylpropanolamine for weight reduction. 1984; 26:55–56.
69. Lee KY, et al. Severe hypertension after ingestion of an an appetite suppressant (phenylpropanolamine) with indomethacin. Lancet 1979; 1:1110–1111.
70. Bennett WM. Hazards of the appetite suppressant phenylpropanolamine. Lancet 1979; 2:42–43.
71. Chasnoff IJ, Diggs G. Fetal alcohol effects and maternal cough syrup abuse. Am J Dis Child 1981; 135:968.
72. Nishimura H, Tanimura T. Clinical aspects of the teratogenicity of drugs. Amsterdam: Excerpta Medica, 1976:231.
73. Hollmen AI, et al. Intervillous blood flow during caesarean section with prophylactic ephedrine and epidural anaesthesia. Acta Anaesth Scand 1984; 28:396–400.
74. Hollmen AI, et al. Regional anaesthesia and uterine blood flow. Ann Chir Gynaecol 1984; 73:149–52.
75. Smith CV, et al. Effect of a single dose of oral pseudoephedrine on uterine and fetal Doppler blood flow. Obstet Gynecol 1990; 76:803–806.

76. Findlay JWA, et al. Pseudoephedrine and triprolidine in plasma and breast milk of nursing mothers. Br J Clin Pharmacol 1984; 18:901–906.
77. Jost A. Degenerescence des extremites du foetus de rat provoquée par l'adrenaline. CR Acad Sci (Paris) 1953; 236:1510–1512.
78. Jost A, et al. Congenital amputations determined by the *br* gene and those induced by adrenalin injection in the rabbit fetus. In: Swinyard CA, ed. Limb development and deformity: problems of evaluation and rehabilitation. Springfield: CC Thomas, 1969:187–199.
79. Loevy H, Roth BF. Induced cleft palate development in mice: comparison between the effect of epinephrine and cortisone. Anat Rec 1968; 160:386.
80. Gatling RR. The effect of sympathomimetic agents on the chick embryo. Am J Pathol 1962; 40:113–127.
81. Hodach RJ, et al. Aortic arch anomalies associated with administration of epinephrine in chick embryos. Teratology 1974; 9:203–210.
82. Rajala GM, et al. Ventricular blood pressure and cardiac output changes in epinephrine- and metoprolol-treated chick embryos. Teratology 1988; 38:291–296.
83. Rosenfeld CR, Bortan MD, Meschia G. Effects of epinephrine on distribution of blood flow in the pregnant ewe. Am J Obstet Gynecol 1976; 124:156.
84. Morgan CD, et al. Placental transfer of catecholamines in vitro and in vivo. Am J Obstet Gynecol 1972; 112:1068–1075.
85. Nishikawa T, et al. Cardiovascular teratogenicity of ephedrine in chick embryos. Toxicol Lett 1985; 29:59–63.
86. Nishikawa T, et al. Potentiating effects of caffeine on the cardiovascular teratogenicity of ephedrine in chick embryos. Toxicol Lett 1985; 29:65–68.
87. Matsuoka R, et al. An aborted human fetus with truncus arteriosus communis—possible teratogenic effect of Tedral. Heart Vessels 1985; 1:176–178.
88. Hughes SC, et al. Placental transfer of ephedrine does not affect neonatal outcome. Anesthesiology 1985; 63:217–219.
89. Entman SS, Moise KJ. Anaphylaxis in pregnancy. South Med J 1984; 77:402.
90. Stalder JB, et al. Cesarean section under peridural anesthesia and hypotension: value of preventative intravenous ephedrine. Rev Med Suisse Romande 1983; 103:867–870.
91. Hollmen AI, et al. Intervillous blood flow during caesarean section with prophylactic ephedrine and epidural anaesthesia. Acta Anaesth Scand 1984; 28:396–400.
92. Hollmen AI, et al. Regional anaesthesia and uterine blood flow. Ann Chir Gynaecol 1984; 73:149–52.
93. Dusek J, Ostadal B. Ultrastructure of isoproterenol-induced myocardial damage in chick embryos. Physiol Bohemoslov 1985; 34:297–302.

94. Ostadal B, et al. Different effect of propranolol and verapamil on isoprenaline-induced changes in the chick embryo heart. Physiol Bohemoslov 1987; 36:301–311.
95. Janatova T, et al. The effect of oxidized isoprenaline on the chick embryonic heart. Can J Physiol Pharmacol 1986; 64:897–903.
96. Kuhlmann RS, et al. Reduction of catecholamine-induced cardiovascular malformations in the chick embryo with metoprolol. Teratology 1983; 28:9–14.
97. Cheung MO, et al. Chronotropism and blood flow patterns following teratogenic doses of catecholamines in 5-day-old chick embryos. Teratology 1977; 16:327–343.
98. Clark EB, et al. The effect of isoproterenol on cardiovascular function in the stage 24 chick embryo. Teratology 1985; 31:41–47.
99. Dusek J, Ostadal B. Isoproterenol-induced damage to the liver of chick embryos. Physiol Bohemoslov 1984; 33:67–73.
100. Bruyere HJ Jr, et al. External malformations in chick embryos following concomitant administration of methylxanthines and beta-adrenomimetic agents. I. Gross pathologic features. Teratology 1983; 28:257–269.
101. Robson JM, et al, eds. Embryopathic activity of drugs. Boston: Little, Brown & Co, 1965:110.
102. Geber WF. Comparative teratogenicity of isoproterenol and trypan blue in the fetal hamster. Proc Soc Exp Biol Med 1969; 130:1168–1170.
103. Jones–Price C, et al. Teratologic evaluation of isoproterenol hydrochloride (CAS No. 51-30-9) in CD rats. Gov Rep Announce Index Iss 9, 1983.
104. Vogin EE, et al. Teratology studies in rats and rabbits exposed to an isoproterenol aerosol. Toxicol Appl Pharmacol 1970; 16:374–381.
105. Hollingsworth RL, et al. Fetal rabbit ductus arteriosus assessed in a teratologic study on isoproterenol and metaproterenol. Toxicol Appl Pharmacol 1969; 14:641.
106. Robkin MA, et al. Autonomic receptors of the early rat embryo heart: growth and development. Proc Soc Exp Biol Med 1976; 151:799–803.
107. Tweed WA, et al. Effects of isoproterenol-induced tachycardia on myocardial blood flow and glycogen in the fetal lamb. Biol Neonate 1987; 52:104–14.
108. Van de Walle AF, Martin CB Jr. Effect of isoproterenol on uterine blood flow and cardiac output distribution in pregnant guinea pigs. Am J Obstet Gynecol 1985; 152:1058–1062.
109. Macdonald AA, et al. Effects of adrenergic agonists and antagonists on the blood pressure and heart rate of the pig fetus. Res Vet Sci 1984; 36:61–65.
110. Legrand C, et al. Rat myometrial adrenergic receptors in late pregnancy. Biol Reprod 1987; 37:641–650.
111. Maruta K, et al. Changes in action potential and beta-adrenergic effects of the circular muscle of postpartum rat uterus. Jpn J Physiol 1985; 35:567–579.

112. Ke R, et al. Prolonged inhibition of human myometrial contractility by intermittent isoproterenol. Am J Obstet Gynecol 1984; 149:841–844.
113. Wheeler AG, et al. Influence of adrenergic receptors on ovarian progesterone secretion in the pseudopregnant cat and oestradiol secretion in the oestrous cat. J Reprod Fertil 1987; 79:195–205.
114. Bergh A, et al. The effect of long-term variation in sympathetic activity on testicular morphology in immature rats. Andrologia 1987; 19:448–451.
115. Pointis G, Latreille MT. Catecholamine-induced stimulation of testosterone reproduction of Leydig cells from fetal mouse testis. J Reprod Fertil 1987; 80:321–326.
116. Pointis G, Latreille MT. β-Adrenergic stimulation of androgen production by fetal mouse Leydig cells in primary culture. Experientia 1986; 42:617–619.
117. Anakwe OO, Moger WH. Ontogeny of rodent testicular androgen production in response to isoproterenol and luteinizing hormone in vitro. Biol Reprod 1984; 30:1142–1152.
118. Semczuk M. The effects of beta-adrenergic drugs on the human sperm motility in vitro. I. The effects of propranolol and isoprenaline. Andrologia 1987; 19:256–261.
119. Baillie P, et al. Treatment of premature labour with orciprenaline. Br Med J 1970; 4:154–155.
120. Zilianti M, Aller J. Action of orciprenaline on uterine contractility during labor, maternal cardiovascular system, fetal heart rate, and acid–base balance. Am J Obstet Gynecol 1971; 109:1073–1079.
121. Mendez-Bauer C, et al. Treatment of acute intrapartum fetal distress by β_2-sympathomimetics. Am J Obstet Gynecol 1987; 156:638–642.
122. Banerjee BN, Woodard G. Teratologic evaluation of metaproterenol in the rhesus monkey (*Macaca mulatta*). Toxicol Appl Pharmacol 1971; 20:562–564.
123. Rx Bull. Orciprenaline sulphate. 1971; 2:25–28.
124. Iida H, et al. Corticosterone induction of cleft palate in mice dosed with orciprenaline sulfate. Teratology 1988; 38:15–27.
125. Matsuo A, et al. Teratology study with orciprenaline sulfate in rabbits. Arzneimittelforschung 1982; 32:808–810.
126. Hollingsworth RL, et al. Fetal rabbit ductus arteriosus assessed in a teratologic study on isoproterenol and metaproterenol. Toxicol Appl Pharmacol 1971; 18:231–234.
127. Schatz M, et al. The safety of inhaled beta-agonist bronchodilators during pregnancy. J Allergy Clin Immunol 1988; 82:686–695.
128. Freysz H, et al. A long term evaluation of infants who received a beta-mimetic drug while in utero. J Perinat Med 1977; 5:94–99.
129. Szabo KT, et al. Effects of several beta-receptor agonists on fetal development in various species of laboratory animals: preliminary report. Teratology 1975; 12:336–337.

130. Lind T, et al. Continuous salbutamol infusion over 17 weeks to pre-empt premature labour. Lancet 1980; 2:1165–1166.
131. Addis GJ. Long-term salbutamol infusion to prevent premature labour. Lancet 1981; 1:42–43.
132. Edmonds DK, Letchworth AT. Prophylactic oral salbutalmol to prevent premature labour. Lancet 1982; 1:1310–1131.
133. Gummerus, M. The management of premature labor with salbutamol. Acta Obstet Gynecol Scand 1981; 60:375–377.
134. Hastwell G, et al. A study of 208 patients in premature labor treated with orally administered salbutamol. Med J Aust 1978; 1:465–469.
135. Korda AR, et al. The treatment of premature labor with intravenously administered salbutamol. Med J Aust 1974; 1:744–746.
136. Liggins GC, Vaghan GS. Intravenous infusion of salbutamol in the management of premature labor. J Obstet Gynaecol Br Commonw 1973; 80:29–33.
137. Ng KH, Sen DK. Hypotension with intravenous salbutamol in premature labour. Br Med J 1974; 3:257.
138. Pincus R. Salbutamol infusion for premature labour—the Australian trials experience. Aust NZ Obstet Gynaecol 1981; 21:1–4.
139. Thomas DJB, et al. Metabolic effects of salbutamol infusion during premature labour. Br J Obstet Gynaecol 1977; 84:497–499.
140. Lunell NO, et al. The immediate effect of a beta-adrenergic agonist (salbutamol) on carbohydrate and lipid metabolism during the third trimester of pregnancy. Acta Obstet Gynecol Scand 1977; 56:475–478.
141. Wager J, et al. Metabolic and circulatory effects of oral salbutamol in the third trimester of pregnancy in diabetic and non-diabetic women. Br J Obstet Gynaecol 1981; 88:352–361.
142. Gummerus M, Halonen O. Prophylactic long-term oral tocolysis of multiple pregnancies. Br J Obstet Gynaecol 1987; 94:249–251.
143. Sodha RJ, Schneider H. Transplacental transfer of beta-adrenergic drugs studied by an in vitro perfusion method of an isolated human placental lobule. Am J Obstet Gynecol 1983; 147:303–310.
144. Wallace RL, et al. Inhibition of premature labor by terbutaline. Obstet Gynecol 1978; 51:387–392.
145. Haller DL. The use of terbutaline for premature labor. Drug Intell Clin Pharm 1980; 14:757–764.
146. Stubblefield PG, Heyl PS. Treatment of premature labor with subcutaneous terbutaline. Obstet Gynecol 1982; 59:457–462.
147. Beall MH, et al. A comparison of ritodrine, terbutaline, and magnesium sulfate for the suppression of preterm labor. Am J Obstet Gynecol 1985; 153:854–859.
148. Kosasa TS, et al. Ritodrine and terbutaline compared for the treatment of preterm labor. Acta Obstet Gynecol Scand 1985; 64:421–426.

149. Ingemarsson I, Bengtsson B. A five-year experience with terbutaline for preterm labor: low rate of severe side effects. Obstet Gynecol 1985; 66:176–180.
150. Berg G, Ryden G. Ritodrine or terbutaline—the optimal dosage in the treatment of preterm labor. Am J Obstet Gynecol 1987; 156:260–261.
151. Katz M, et al. Cardiovascular complications associated with terbutaline treatment for preterm labor. Am J Obstet Gynecol 1981; 139:605–608.
152. Epstein MF, et al. Neonatal hypoglycemia after beta-sympathomimetic tocolytic therapy. J Pediatr 1979; 94:449–453.
153. Main EK, et al. Chronic oral terbutaline tocolytic therapy is associated with maternal glucose intolerance. Am J Obstet Gynecol 1987; 157:644–647.
154. Patriarco MS, et al. A study on intrauterine fetal resuscitation with terbutaline. Am J Obstet Gynecol 1987; 157:384–387.
155. Ingemarsson I, et al. Single injection of terbutaline in term labor. I. Effect on fetal pH in cases with prolonged bradycardia. Am J Obstet Gynecol 1985; 153:859–865.
156. Lenke RR, Trupin S. Sudden, unforeseen fetal death in a woman being treated for premature labor. J Reprod Med 1984; 29:872–874.
157. Suzuki M, et al. Maternal liver impairment associated with prolonged high-dose administration of terbutaline for premature labor. Obstet Gynecol 1985; 66:14S–15S.
158. Bhat N, et al. Paradoxical response to intravenous terbutaline. Am J Obstet Gynecol 1985; 153:310–311.
159. Sakai T, et al. Reproduction studies of pirbuterol hydrochloride. Yakuri to Chiro 1980; 8:731–743, cited in Shepard TH. Catalog of teratogenic agents. Baltimore: Johns Hopkins University Press, 1989:512.
160. Cox JSG, et al. Disodium cromoglycate (Intal). Adv Drug Res 1970; 5:115–196.
161. Wilson J. Use of sodium cromoglycate during pregnancy. Acta Ther Med 1982; 8[suppl]:45–51.
162. Fujii T, Nishimura H. Teratogenic actions of some methylated xanthines in mice. Okajimas Folia Anat Jpn 1969; 46:167–175.
163. Tucci SM, Skalko RG. The teratogenic effects of theophylline in mice. Toxicol Lett 1978; 1:337–341.
164. Maren TH, Ellison AC. The teratological effect of certain thiadiazoles related to acetazolamide, with a note on sulfanilamide and thiazide diuretics. Johns Hopkins Med J 1972; 130:95–104.
165. Fujii T, et al. Rat fetal edema by methylated xanthines. Teratology 1972; 6:106.
166. Lindstrom P, et al. The developmental toxicity of orally administered theophylline in rats and mice. Fundam Appl Toxicol 1990; 14:167–178.
167. Morrissey RE, et al. Reproductive effects of theophylline in mice and rats. Fundam Appl Toxicol 1988; 10:525–536.

168. Greenberger P, Patterson R. Safety of therapy for allergic symptoms during pregnancy. Ann Intern Med 1978; 89:234–237.
169. Hernandez E, et al. Asthma in pregnancy: current concepts. Obstet Gynecol 1980; 55:739–743.
170. Lalli CM, Raju L. Pregnancy and chronic obstructive pulmonary disease. Chest 1981; 80:759–761.
171. Turner ES, et al. Management of the pregnant asthmatic patient. Ann Intern Med 1980; 93:905–918.
172. Neff RK, Leviton A. Maternal theophylline consumption and the risk of stillbirth. Chest 1990; 97:1266–1267.
173. Park JM, et al. Cardiovascular anomalies associated with prenatal exposure to theophylline. South Med J 1990; 83:1487–1488.
174. Day P, et al. Effects of theophylline on chromosomal breakage and sister-chromatid exchange. Mutat Res 1989; 224:409–413.
175. Carter BL, et al. Theophylline clearance during pregnancy. Obstet Gynecol 1986; 68:555–559.
176. Frederiksen MC, et al. Theophylline pharmacokinetics in pregnancy. Clin Pharmacol Ther 1986; 40:321–318.
177. Gardner MJ, et al. Longitudinal effects of pregnancy on the pharmacokinetics of theophylline. Eur J Clin Pharmacol 1987; 31:289–295.
178. Arwood LL, et al. Placental transfer of theophylline: two case reports. Pediatrics 1979; 63:844–846.
179. Yeh TF, Pildes RS. Transplacental aminophylline toxicity in a neonate. Lancet 1977; 1:910.
180. Horowitz DA, et al. Apnea associated with theophylline withdrawal in a term neonate. Am J Dis Child 1982; 136:73–74.
181. Ron M, et al. Maternal–fetal transfer of aminophylline. Acta Obstet Gynecol Scand 1984; 63:217–218.
182. Labovitz E, Spector S. Placental theophylline transfer in pregnant asthmatics. JAMA 1982; 247:786–248.
183. Aranda JV, et al. Metabolism of theophylline to caffeine in human fetal liver. Science 1979; 206:1319–1321.
184. Bory C, et al. Metabolism of theophylline to caffeine in premature newborn infants. J Pediatr 1979; 94:988–993.
185. Volpe JJ. Effects of methylxanthines on lipid synthesis in developing neural systems. Semin Perinatol 1981; 5:395–405.
186. Aranda JV, Dupone C. Metabolic effects of methylxanthines in premature infants. J Pediatr 1976; 89:833–834.
187. Nelson RM, et al. Developmental outcome of premature infants treated with theophylline. Dev Pharmacol Ther 1980; 1:274–280.
188. Yurchak AM, Jusko WJ. Theophylline secretion into breast milk. Pediatrics 1976; 57:518–525.
189. Stec GP, et al. Kinetics of theophylline transfer to breast milk. Clin Pharmacol Ther 1980; 28:404–408.

190. Berlin CM. Excretion of methylxanthines in human milk. Semin Perinatol 1981; 5:389–394.
191. Hart AD, Grimble RF. Effect of methylxanthines on lactational performance of rats. Ann Nutr Metab 1990; 34:297–302.
192. Hart AD, Grimble RF. Effect of methylxanthines on milk volume and composition, and growth of rat pups. Br J Nutr 1990; 64:339–350.
193. Georges A, Denef J. Les anomalies digitale: manifestations teratogeniques des derives xanthique chez le rat. Arch Int Pharmacodyn Ther 1968; 172:219–222.
194. Patterson CE, et al. Fatty acid synthesis in the fetal lung: relationship to surfactant lipids. Biochim Biophys Acta 1986; 878:110–126.
195. Landers S. Effect of aminophylline and caffeine on total and surfactant phospholipid in fetal rabbit lung. Am Rev Respir Dis 1984; 130:204–208.
196. Cosmi EV, et al. Effect of aminophylline on lung maturation in preterm rabbit fetuses. Am J Obstet Gynecol 1986; 154:436–439.
197. Granati B, et al. The prevention of respiratory distress syndrome in premature infants: efficacy of antenatal aminophylline treatment versus prenatal glucocorticoid administration. Pediatr Pharmacol 1984; 4:21–24.
198. Laifer SA, et al. The effect of aminophylline on uterine smooth muscle contractility and prostaglandin production in the pregnant rat uterus in vitro. Am J Obstet Gynecol 1986; 155:212–215.
199. Melis GB, et al. Aminophylline treatment of preterm labor. Acta Eur Fertil 1984; 15:357–361.
200. Lipshitz J. Uterine and cardiovascular effects of aminophylline. Am J Obstet Gynecol 1978; 131:716–718.
201. Berlin CM. Excretion of methylxanthines in human milk. Semin Perinatol 1981; 5:389–394.
202. Back KC, et al. A toxicopathologic study of endobenzyline bromide, a new cholinergic blocking agent. Toxicol Appl Pharmacol 1961; 3:422–430.
203. Maeda H, Yasuda M. Induction of digital malformations in rat fetuses by combined administration of papeverine hydrochloride and atropine sulfate. Teratology 1979; 20:157.
204. Beuker ED, Platner WS. Effect of cholinergic drugs on development of chick embryo. Proc Soc Exp Biol Med 1956; 91:539–543.
205. Arcuri PA, Gautieri RF. Morphine—induced fetal malformations: III Possible mechanisms of action. J Pharm Sci 1973; 62:1616–1634.
206. Zellers JE. Influence of atropine and diphenhydramine on the teratogenic capability of codeine in CF-1 mice. Diss Absts Int [B] 1979; 39:5870.
207. Kivalo I, Saarikoski S. Placental transmission of atropine at full-term pregnancy. Br J Anaesth 1977; 49:1017–1021.
208. Kanto J, et al. Placental transfer and pharmacokinetics of atropine after a single maternal intravenous administration.

209. Onnen I, et al. Placental transfer of atropine at the end of pregnancy. Eur J Clin Pharmacol 1979; 15:443–446.
210. Roodenburg PJ, et al. Effect of maternal intravenous administration of atropine (0.5 mg) on fetal breathing and heart pattern. Contrib Gynecol Obstet 1979; 6:92–97.
211. Abboud T, et al. Fetal and maternal cardiovascular effects of atropine and glycopyrrolate. Anesth Analg 1983; 62:426–430.
212. Diaz DM, et al. Cardiovascular effects of glycopyrrolate and belladonna derivatives in obstetric patients. Bull NY Acad Med 1980; 56:245–248.
213. Janz D, Fuchs U. Are anti-epileptic drugs harmful when given during pregnancy? Ger Med Monatsschr 1964; 9:20–22.
214. Stewart JJ. Gastrointestinal drugs. In: Wilson JT, ed. Drugs in breast milk. Balgowlah, Australia: ADIS Press, 1981:65–71.
215. Anderson WM. Hemodynamic and non-bronchial effects of ipratropium bromide. Am J Med 1986; 81:45–53.
216. Nishimura M, et al. Reproduction studies of ipratropium bromide (SCH 1000) on rats and rabbits. Iyakuhin Kenkyu 1978; 9:393–416.
217. Niggeschulze A, Palmer AK. [Reproductive toxicological investigations with ipratropium bromide]. Arzneimittelforschung 1976; 26:989–992.
218. Walker B. Induction of cleft palate in rats with antiinflammatory drugs. Teratology 1971; 4:39–42.
219. Pinsky L, DiGeorge AM. Cleft palate in the mouse: a teratogenic index of glucocorticoid potency. Science 1965; 147:402–403.
220. Reinisch JM, et al. Prenatal exposure to prednisone permanently alters fighting behavior of female mice. Pharmacol Biochem Behav 1980; 12:213–216.
221. Reinisch JM, et al. Prenatal exposure to prednisone in humans and animals retards intrauterine growth. Science 1978; 202:436–438.
222. Scott JR. Fetal growth retardation associated with maternal administration of immunosuppressive drugs. Am J Obstet Gynecol 1977; 128:668–676.
223. Fine LG, et al. Systemic lupus erythematosus in pregnancy. Ann Intern Med 1981; 94:667–677.
224. Pirson Y, et al. Retardation of fetal growth in pateints receiving immunosuppressive therapy. N Engl J Med 1985; 313:328.
225. Warrell DW, Taylor R. Outcome for the foetus of mothers receiving prednisolone during pregnancy. Lancet 1968; 1:117–118.
226. Lancet. Are sex hormones teratogenic? 1974; 2:1107–1108.
227. Schardein JL. Chemically induced birth defects. New York: Marcel Dekker, 1985:310.
228. Schatz M, Hoffman CP, Zeiger RS, Falkoff R, Mellon M. The course and management of asthma and allergic diseases during pregnancy. In: Middleton E Jr, Reed CE, Ellis EF, et al, eds. Allergy: principles and practice, 3rd ed. St Louis: CV Mosby, 1988:1124–1125.

229. Tallent MB, et al. Birth defects in child of male recipient of kidney transplant. JAMA 1970; 211:1854–1855.
230. Mancini RE, et al. Effect of prednisolone upon normal and pathologic human spermatogenesis. Fertil Steril 1966; 17:500–513.
231. Jensen MK. Chromosome studies in patients treated with azathioprine and amethopterin. Acta Med Scand 1967; 182:445–455.
232. Kraus AM. Congenital cataract and maternal steroid injection. J Pediatr Ophthalmol 1975; 12:107–108.
233. Cote CJ, et al. Effects on the neonate of prednisone and azathioprine administered to the mother during pregnancy. J Pediatr 1974; 85:324–328.
234. Cederqvist LL, et al. Fetal immunoglobin synthesis following maternal immunosuppression. Am J Obstet Gynecol 1977; 129:687–690.
235. Katz FH, Duncan BR. Entry of prednisone into human milk. N Engl J Med 1975; 293:1154.
236. McKenzie SA, et al. Secretion of prednisone into breast milk. Arch Dis Child 1975; 50:894–896.
237. Ost L, et al. Prednisolone excretion in human milk. J Pediatr 1985; 106:1008–1011.
238. Glaxo Group. Beclovent inhaler: a product monograph. Fort Lauderdale: 1980:7–9.
239. Toogood JH, et al. A graded dose assessment of the efficacy of beclomethasone diproprionate aerosol for severe asthma. J Allergy Clin Immunol 1977; 59:298–308.
240. Toogood JH, et al. Minimum dose requirements of steroid-dependent asthmatic patients for aerosol beclomethasone and oral prednisone. J Allergy Clin Immunol 1978; 61:355–364.
241. Esaki K, et al. Effects of inhalant administration of beclomethasone dipropionate on the reproduction in mice. CIEA Preclin Rep 1976; 2:213–222.
242. Oguro Y, et al. Pharmacological and toxicological studies on beclomethasone dipropionate. Yamaguch Igaku 1970; 19:65–86.
243. Tanioka Y. Teratogenicity test on beclomethasone dipropionate by inhalation in rhesus monkeys. CIEA Preclin Rep 1976; 2:155–164.
244. Sudon S, et al. Teratological and fertility studies on beclomethasone dipropionate: 1. Fertility studies in rats by oral administration. Oyo Yakuri 1979; 18:1003–1019.
245. Furuhashi T, et al. Teratologic and fertility studies on beclomethasone dipropionate: 2. Teratological studies by oral administration. Oyo Yakuri 1979; 18:1021–1038.
246. Hasegawa T, et al. Teratological and fertility studies on beclomethasone dipropionate: 3. Perinatal and postnatal study in rats by oral administration. Oyo Yakuri 1979; 18:1039–1054.
247. Greenberger PA, et al. Beclomethasone dipropionate for severe asthma during pregnancy. Ann Intern Med 1983; 98:478–480.

248. Fitzsimons R, et al. Outcome of pregnancy in women requiring corticosteroids for severe asthma. J Allergy Clin Immunol 1986; 78:349–353.
249. British Thoracic and Tuberculosis Association. Inhaled corticosteroids compared with oral prednisone in patients starting long-term corticosteroid therapy for asthma. Lancet 1975; 2:469–473.
250. Cameron SJ, et al. Substitution of beclomethasone aerosol for oral prednisolone in the treatment of chronic asthma. Br Med J 1973; 4:205–207.
251. Brompton Hospital/Medical Research Council collaborative trial. Double-blind trial comparing two dosage schedules of beclomethasone dipropionate aerosol in the treatment of chronic bronchial asthma. Lancet 1974; 2:303–307.
252. Newhouse MT, Dolovich MG. Control of asthma by aerosols. N Engl J Med 1986; 315:870–874.
253. Brown PH, Blundell G, Gruring AP, Crompton GK. Do large volume spacer devices reduce the systemic effects of high dose inhaled corticosteroids. Thorax 1990; 45:736–739.
254. Kimmerle R, Rolla AR. Iatrogenic Cushing's syndrome due to dexamethasone nasal drops. Am J Med 1985; 79:535–537.
255. Walker BE. Cleft palate produced in mice by human-equivalent dosage with triamcinolone. Science 1965; 149:862–863.
256. Walker BE. Induction of cleft palate in rabbits by several glucocorticoids. Proc Soc Exp Biol Med 1967; 125:1281–1284.
257. Walker BE. Effects of glucocorticoids on palate development in the rat. Anat Rec 1969; 163:281.
258. Shah RM, Kilistoff A. Cleft palate induction in hamster fetuses by glucocorticoid hormones and their synthetic analogues. J Embryol Exp Morphol 1976; 36:101–108.
259. Hendrickx AG, et al. Teratogenic effects of triamcinolone on the skeletal and lymphoid systems in nonhuman primates. Fed Proc 1975; 34:1661–1665.
260. Hendrickz AG, et al. Craniofacial and central nervous system malformations induced by triamcinolone acetonide in nonhuman primates. 1. General teratogenicity. Teratology 1980; 22:103–114.
261. Parker RM, Hendrickz AG. Craniofacial and central nervous system malformations induced by triamcinolone acetonide in nonhuman primates. 2. Craniofacial pathogenesis. Teratology 1983; 28:35–44.
262. Tarara RP, et al. Central nervous system malformations induced by triamcinolone acetonide in nonhuman primates: pathogenesis. Teratology 1988; 38:259–270.
263. Jerome CP, Hendrickx AG. Comparative teratogenicity of triamcinolone acetonide and dexamethasone in the rhesus monkey (*Macaca mulatta*). J Med Primatol 1988; 17:195–203.
264. Fisher CJ, Sawyer RH. A comparison of hydrocortisone and triamcinolone inhibition of scale and feather development. Teratology 1986; 33:37–45.

265. Katz VL, et al. Severe symmetric intrauterine growth retardation associated with the topical use of triamcinolone. Am J Obstet Gynecol 1990; 162:396–397.
266. Boucher D, Delost P. Developpement post-natal des descendents issus de mères traitées avec la penicilline au cours de la gestion chez la souris. CR Soc Biol (Paris) 1964; 158:528–532.
267. Brown DM, et al. Effects of antibiotics upon pregnancy in the rabbit [abstr]. Toxicol Appl Pharmacol 1968; 12:295.
268. Philipson A. Pharmacokinetics of ampicillin during pregnancy. J Infect Dis 1977; 136:370–376.
269. Bray R, et al. Transfer of ampicillin into fetus and amniotic fluid from maternal plasma in late pregnancy. Am J Obstet Gynecol 1966; 96:9328–9342.
270. Hutter A, Parks J. The transmission of penicillin through the placenta. A preliminary report. Am J Obstet Gynecol 1945; 49:663–665.
271. Woltz J, Zintel H. The transmission of penicillin to the previable fetus. JAMA 1946; 131:969–970.
272. Wasz-Hockert O, et al. Transplacental passage of azidocillin, ampicillin, amipicillin and penicillin G during early and late pregnancy. Acta Paediatr Scand Suppl 1970; 206:109–110.
273. Ravid R, Toaff R. On the possible teratogenicity of antibiotic drugs administered during pregnancy—a prospective study. In: Klingber M, et al. eds. Drugs and fetal development. New York: Plenum Press, 1972; 505–510.
274. Gallagher JS. Anaphylaxis in pregnancy. Obstet Gynecol 1988; 71:491–493.
275. Kosim H. Intrauterine fetal death as a result of ananphylactic reaction to penicillin in a pregnant woman. Dapim Refuiim 1959; 18:136–137.
276. Greene H, et al. Excretion of penicillin in human milk following parturition. Am J Obstet Gynecol 1946; 51:732–733.
277. Branebjerg PE, Heisterberg L. Blood and milk concentrations of ampicillin in mothers treated with pivampicillin and in their infants. J Perinat Med 1987; 15:555–558.
278. Bachev S, et al. Experimental studies on the teratogenic effect, acute and chronic toxicity of ampicillin. Suvrem Med 1974; 25:28–32.
279. Korzhova VV, et al. Effect of ampicillin and oxacillin on fetal and neonatal development. Bull Exp Med (USSR) 1981; 91:169–170.
280. Jordhein O, Hagen AG. Study of ampicillin levels in maternal serum, umbilical cord serum and amniotic fluid following administration of pivampicillin. Acta Obstet Gynecol Scand 1980; 59:315–317.
281. MacAulay M, et al. Placental transfer of ampicillin. Am J Obstet Gynecol 1966; 96:943–950.
282. Kraybill EN, et al. Transplacental ampicillin: inhibitory concentrations in neonatal serum. Am J Obstet Gynecol 1980; 138:793–796.

283. New Zealand Committee on Adverse Drugs Reactions. Sixth annual report. NZ Med J 1971; 74:623–627.
284. Willman K, Pulkkinen M. Reduced maternal plasma and urinary estriol during ampicillin treatment. Am J Obstet Gynecol 1971; 109:893–896.
285. Aldercreutz H, et al. Effect of ampicillin administration on plasma conjugated and unconjugated estrogen and progesterone levels in pregnancy. Am J Obstet Gynecol 1977; 128:266–271.
286. Van Look PFA, et al. Effect of ampicillin or amoxicillin administration on plasma and urinary estrogen levels during normal pregnancy. Eur J Obstet Gynecol Reprod Biol 1981; 12:225–233.
287. Dossetor J. Drug interactions with oral contraceptives. Br Med J 1975; 4:467–468.
288. DeSano EA Jr, Hurley SC. Possible interactions of antihistamines and antibiotics with oral contraceptive effectiveness. Fertil Steril 1980; 37:853–854.
289. Friedman CI, et al. The effect of ampicillin on oral contraceptive effectiveness. Obstet Gynecol 1980; 55:33–37.
290. Back DJ, et al. The effects of ampicillin on oral contraceptive steroids in women. Br J Clin Pharmacol 1982; 14:43–48.
291. Peterson ML, et al. Transplacental transfer of cephalexin. Clin Med 1972; 79:23–24.
292. Creatsas G, et al. A study of the kinetics of cephapirin and cephalexin in pregnancy. Curr Med Res Opin 1980; 7:43–46.
293. Aoyama T, et al. Teratologic studies of cephalexin in mice and rats. Oyo Yakuri 1969; 3:249–263.
294. Welles JS, et al. Toxicology and pharmacology of cephalexin in laboratory animals. Antimicrob Agents Chemother 1968, cited in Schardein JL. Chemically induced birth defects. New York. Marcel Dekker, 1985:365.
295. ChuChen K, Sabeti S. L'evaluation clinique de la cephalexin orale. Int J Clin Pharmacol 1970; 2(suppl):124–128.
296. Mizuno S, et al. Clinical evaluation of cephalexin in obstetrics and gynaecology. In: Proceedings Symposium Clinical Evaluation of Cephalexin. London: Royal Society of Medicine, 1969.
297. Pedler SJ, Bint AJ. Comparative study of amoxicillin–clavulanic acid and cephalexin in the treatment of bacteriuria during pregnancy. Antimicrob Agents Chemother 1985; 27:508–510.
298. Kafetzi D, et al. Passage of cephalosporins and amoxicillin into the breast milk. Acta Paediatr Scand 1981; 70:285–288.
299. Markham JK, et al. Reproduction studies on cefaclor (Lilly cephalosporin 99638) in four species. Toxicol Appl Pharmacol 1978; 45:292.
300. Nomura A, et al. Reproduction study of cefaclor. I. Teratological study in mice, rats, and rabbits. Chemotherapy 1979; 27(suppl 7):846–864.
301. Furuhashi T, et al. Fertility and perinatal study of cefaclor in rats. Chemotherapy 1979; 27:865–880.

302. Halperin-Walega E, et al. Disposition of cefixime in the pregnant and lactating rat. Transfer to the fetus and nursing pup. Drug Metab Dispos 1988; 16:130–134.
303. Baldwin JA, et al. Reproduction studies of BRL 14151K and BRL 25000. Teratology and peri- and postnatal studies in rats. Chemotherapy 1983; 31:238–262.
304. Hirakawa T, et al. Reproduction studies in rats. Chemotherapy 1983; 31:263–272.
305. James PA, et al. Reproduction studies of BRL 25000. Teratology studies in the pig. Chemotherapy 1983; 31:274–279.
306. Takaya M. [Teratogenic effects of antibiotics]. J Osaka City Med Center 1965; 14:107–115.
307. Liban E, Abramovici A. Fetal membrane adhesions and congenital malformations. In: Klingberg MA, Abramovici A, Chemke J, eds. Drugs and fetal development. Plenum Press, New York, 198?:337–350.
308. Jaffe P, et al. Incidence of congenital limb-reduction deformities. Lancet 1975; 1:526–527.
309. Schachter J, et al. Experience with the routine use of erythromycin for chlamydial infections in pregnancy. N Engl J Med 1986; 314:276–279.
310. McGregor JA, et al. Adjunctive erythromycin treatment for idiopathic preterm labor: results of a randomized, double-blind, placebo-controlled trial. Am J Obstet Gynecol 1986; 154:98–103.
311. McCormack WM, et al. Effect on birth weight of erythromycin treatment of pregnant women. Obstet Gynecol 1987; 69:202–207.
312. FitzSimmons J, et al. Chlamydial infections in pregnancy. J Reprod Med 1986; 31:19–22.
313. Quinn PA, et al. Efficacy of antibiotic therapy in preventing spontaneous pregnancy loss among couples colonized with genital mycoplasmas. Am J Obstet Gynecol 1983; 45:239–244.
314. McCormack, WM et al. Hepatotoxicity of erythromycin estolate during pregnancy. Antimicrob Agents Chemother 1977; 12:630–635.
315. Kiefer L, et al. The placental transfer of erythromycin. Am J Obstet Gynecol 1955; 69:174–177.
316. Philipson A, et al. Transplancental passage of erythromycin and clindamycin. N Engl J Med 1973; 288:1219–1220.
317. Rothman K, Pochi P. Use of oral and topical agents for acne in pregnancy. J Am Acad Dermatol 1988; 16:431–442.
318. Fenton LJ, Light LJ. Congenital syphilis after maternal treatment with erythromycin. Obstet Gynecol 1976; 47:492–494.
319. Posner AC, et al. Tetracycline in obstetric infections. In: Antibiotics Annual, 1954–55. New York: Medical Encyclopedia, 1956:345–348.
320. Fillippi B. Antibiotics and congenital malformations: evaluation of the teratogenicity of antibiotics. In: Woollam DHM, ed. Advances in teratology, vol 2. New York: Academic Press, 1967:237–256.

321. Bevelander G, Cohlan SQ. The effect on the rat fetus of transplacentally acquired tetracycline. Biol Neonate 1962; 4:365–370.
322. Hurley LS, Tuchmann-Duplessis H. Influence de la tetracycline sur la developpement pre- et post-natal du rat. CR Acad Sci (Paris) 1963; 257:302–304.
323. Cohlan SQ. Drugs and pregnancy. Prog Clin Biol Res 1980; 44:77–96.
324. McColl JD, et al. Effect of some therapeutic agents on the developing rat fetus. Toxicol Appl Pharmacol 1965; 7:409–417.
325. Savini EC, et al. Effets teratogenes de l'oxytetracycline. Therapie 1968; 23:1247–1260.
326. Mela V, Filippi B. Una carenza vitaminica insorta nel corso di un trattamento antibiotico puo avere effetto teratogeno. Minerva Med 1957; 48:2459–2462.
327. Morrissey RE, et al. The developmental toxicity of orally administered oxytetracycline in rats and mice. Fundam Appl Toxicol 1986; 7:434–443.
328. Savitskaia TN. [Features of the structure of the mesenteric and tracheobronchial lymph nodes in rat offspring after exposure to tetracycline]. Arkh Anat Gistol Embriol 1984; 87:66–72.
329. Petrova TB. [Structure of the thymus gland of the rat in the prenatal and early postnatal periods of development after exposure to tetracycline during the period of fetogenesis]. Arkh Anat Gistol Embriol 1984; 87:61–66.
330. Krejci L, et al. Eye changes due to systemic use of tetracycline in pregnancy. Ophthal Res 1980; 12:73–77.
331. Rendle-Short TJ. Tetracycline in teeth and bone. Lancet 1962; 1:1188.
332. Kline AH, et al. Transplacental effect of tetracyclines on teeth. JAMA 1964; 188:178–180.
333. Kutscher AH, et al. Discoloration of deciduous teeth induced by administrations of tetracycline antepartum. Am J Obstet Gynecol 1966; 96:291–292.
334. Schultz JC, et al. Fatal liver disease after intravenous administration of tetracycline in high dosage. N Engl J Med 1963; 269:999–1004.
335. Allen ES, Brown WE. Hepatic toxicity of tetracycline in pregnancy. Am J Obstet Gynecol 1966; 95:12–18.
336. Wenk RE, et al. Tetracycline-associated fatty liver of pregnancy, including possible pregnancy risk after chronic dermatologic use of tetracycline. J Reprod Med 1981; 26:135–141.
337. Knowles JA. Drugs in milk. Pediatr Curr 1972; 21:28–32.
338. Graf VH, Reimann S. Untersuchungen uber die knozentration von pyrrolidino-methyl-tetracycline in der muttermilch. Dtsch Med Wochenschr 1959; 84:1694.
339. Ylikorkala O, et al. Trimethoprim–sulfonamide combination administered orally and intravaginally in the 1st trimester of pregnancy: its ab-

sorption into serum and transfer to amniotic fluid. Acta Obstet Gynecol Scand 1974; 52:229–234.
340. Reid DWJ, et al. Maternal and transplacental kinetics of trimethoprim and sulfamethoxazole, separately and in combination. Can Med Assoc J 1975; 112:67S–72S.
341. Williams JD, et al. The treatment of bacteriuria in pregnant women with sulphamethoxazole and trimethoprim. Postgrad Med J 1969; 45(suppl):71–76.
342. Brumfitt W, Pursell R. Trimethoprim/sulfamethoxazole in the treatment of bacteriuria in women. J Infect Dis 1973; 128(suppl):S657–663.
343. Ochoa AG. Trimethoprim and sulfamethoxazole in pregnancy. JAMA 1971; 217:1244.
344. Bass AD, et al. Mechanism by which sulfadiazine affects the survival of the mammalian embryo. J Pharm Exp Ther 1951; 101:362–367.
345. Kato T, Kitigawa S. Production of congenital anomalies in fetuses of rats and mice with various sulfonamides. Congenital Anom 1973; 13:7–15.
346. Hepburn JS, et al. Secretion of ingested sulfanilamide in breast milk and in the urine of the infant. J Biol Chem 1938; 123:liv–lv.
347. Stewart HL, Pratt JP. Sulfanilamide excretion in human breast milk and effect on breast-fed babies. JAMA 1940; 111:1456–1458.
348. McEwen LM. Trimethoprim/sulfamethoxazole mixture in pregnancy. Br Med J 1971; 4:490–491.
349. Smithells RW. Co-trimoxazole in pregnancy. Lancet 1983; 2:1142.
350. Helm F, et al. Untersuchungen uber den Einfluss der Kombination Sulfamoxol Trimethoprim (CN3123) and Fertilitat und Embryonalentwicklung an Ratten und Kaninchen. Arzneimittelforschung 1976; 26:643–651.
351. Brumfitt W, Pursell R. Double-blind trial to compare ampicillin, cephalexin, co-trimoxazole, and trimethoprim in treatment of urinary infection. Br Med J 1972; 2:673–676.
352. Bailey RR. Single-dose antibacterial treatment for bacteriuria in pregnancy. Drugs 1984; 27:183–186.
353. Koutras A, Fisher S. Niikawa–Kuroki syndrome: a new malformation syndrome of postnatal dwarfism, mental retardation, unusual face and protruding ears. J Pediatr 1982; 101:417–419.
354. Arnauld R, et al. A study of the passage of trimethoprim into the maternal milk. Quest Med 1972; 25:959–964.
355. Miller RD, Salter AJ. The passage of trimethoprim/sulphamethoxazole into breast milk and its significance. In: Daikos GK, ed. Progress in chemotherapy. Proceedings of the 8th International Congress of Chemotherapy, Athens, 1973. Athens: Hellenic Society for Chemotherapy, 1974:687–691.
356. Wolff J. Iodide goiter and the pharmacologic effects of excess iodide. Am J Med 1969; 47:101–124.

357. Mehta PS, et al. Congenital iodide goiter and hypothyroidism: a review. Obstet Gynecol Surv 1983; 38:237–247.
358. Committee on Drugs, American Academy of Pediatrics. Adverse reactions to iodide therapy of asthma and other pulmonary diseases. Pediatrics 1982; 57:272–274.
359. Herbst AL, Selenkow HA. Hyperthyroidism during pregnancy. N Engl J Med 1965; 273:627–633.
360. Selenkow HA, Herbst AL. Hyperthyroidism during pregnancy. N Engl J Med 1966; 274:165–166.
361. Pritchard JA, et al. Williams obstetrics, 17th ed. Norwalk, CT: Appleton-Century-Crofts, 1985:605.
362. Jacobson JM, et al. Changes in thyroid function and serum iodine levels after prepartum use of a povidone–iodine vaginal lubricant. J Reprod Med 1984; 29:98–100.
363. l'Allemand D, et al. Iodine-induced alteration of thyroid function in newborn infants after prenatal and perinatal exposure to povidone iodine. J Pediatr 1983; 102:935–938.
364. Bachrach LK, et al. Maternal–fetal absorption of povidone–iodine. J Pediatr 1984; 104:158–159.
365. Vorherr H, et al. Vaginal absorption of povidone–iodine. JAMA 1980; 244:2628–2629.
366. Chabrolle JP, Rossier A. Goitre and hypothyroidism in the newborn after cutaneous absorption of iodine. Arch Dis Child 1978; 53:495–498.
367. Galina MP, et al. Iodides during pregnancy: an apparent cause of neonatal death. N Engl J Med 1962; 267:1124.
368. Postellon DC, Aronow R. Iodine in mother's milk. JAMA 1982; 247:463.
369. Fed. Reg. Expectorant drug products for over-the-counter human use; final monograph. 1989; (Feb 28):8494–8509.
370. Hirsch SR, et al. The expectorant effect of glyceryl guaiacolate in patients with chronic bronchitis. A controlled in vitro and in vivo study. Chest 1973; 63:9–14.
371. Kuhn JJ, et al. Antitussive effects of guaifenesin in young adults with natural colds. Chest 1982; 82:713–718.
372. Hendley JO, Gwaltney JM. Antitussive effect of guaifenesin. Chest 1983; 84:118–119.
373. Check JH, et al. Improvement of cervical factor with guaifenesin. Fertil Steril 1982; 37:707–708.
374. Geber WF, Schramm LC. Comparative teratogenicity of morphine, heroin, and methadone in the hamster. Pharmacologist 1975; 11:248.
375. Zellers JE, Gautieri RF: Evaluation of teratogenic potential of codeine sulfate in CF-1 mice. J Pharm Sci 1977; 66:1727–1731.
376. Lehmann VH. [Teratologic studies in rabbits and rats with the morphine derivative codeine.] Arzneimittelforschung 1976; 26:551–554.

377. Bracken MB, Holford TR. Exposure to prescribed drugs in pregnancy and association with congenital malformations. Obstet Gynecol 1981; 58:336–344.
378. Saxen I. Associations between oral clefts and drugs taken during pregnancy. Int J Epidemiol 1975; 4:37–44.
379. Rothman KJ, et al. Exogenous hormones and other drug exposures of children with congenital heart disease. Am J Epidemiol 1979; 109:433–439.
380. Van Leeuwen G, et al. Narcotic withdrawal reaction in a newborn infant due to codeine. Pediatrics 1965; 36:635–636.
381. Mangurten HH, Benawra R. Neonatal codeine withdrawal in infants of nonaddicted mothers. Pediatrics 1980; 65:159–160.
382. Horning MG, et al. Identification and quantification of drugs and drug metabolites in human breast milk using GC-MS-COM methods. Mod Probl Paediatr 1975; 15:73–79.
383. Wright HN. Chronic toxicity studies of analgesic and antipyretic drugs and congeners. Toxicol Appl Pharmacol 1967; 11:280–292.
384. Lubawy WC, Burriss Garret RJ. Effects of aspirin and acetaminophen on fetal and placental growth in rats. J Pharm Sci 1977; 66:111–113.
385. Jacqueson A, et al. Effects of daily high doses of paracetamol given orally during spermatogenesis in the rat testes. Arch Toxicol 1984; [Suppl 7]:164–166.
386. Williams DA, et al. Prune perineum syndrome: report of a second case. Teratology 1983; 28:145–148.
387. Harley JD, et al. Aromatic drugs and congenital cataracts. Lancet 1964; 1:472–473.
388. Golden SM, Perman KI. Bilateral clinical anophthalmia: drugs as potential factors. South Med J 1980; 73:1404–1407.
389. General Practitioner Clinical Trials: Drugs in pregnancy survey. Practitioner 1963; 191:775–780.
390. Opitz JM, et al. Congenital effects of bromism? Lancet 1972; 1:91–92.
391. McNeil JR. The possible teratogenic effect of salicylates on the developing fetus. Brief summary of eight suggestive cases. Clin Pediatr 1973; 12:347–350.
392. Golden NL, et al. Propoxyphene and acetaminophen. Possible effects on the fetus. Clin Pediatr 1982; 21:752–754.
393. Zierler S, Rothman KJ. Congenital heart disease in relation to maternal use of Bendectin and other drugs in early pregnancy. N Engl J Med 1985; 313:347–352.
394. Mancini RE, et al. Developmental susceptibility to acetaminophen toxicity. Res Commun Chem Pathol Pharmacol 1983; 27:603–606.
395. Haibach H, et al. Acetaminophen overdose with fetal demise. Am J Clin Pathol 1984; 82:240–242.
396. Roberts I, et al. Paracetamol metabolites in the neonate following maternal overdose. Br J Clin Pharmacol 1984; 18:201–206.

397. Byer AJ, et al. Acetaminophen overdose in the third trimester of pregnancy. JAMA 1982; 247:3114–3115.
398. Stokes IM. Paracetamol overdose in the second trimester of pregnancy. Case report. Br J Obstet Gynaecol 1984; 91:286–288.
399. Ludmir J, et al. Maternal acetaminophen overdose at 15 weeks of gestation. Obstet Gynecol 1986; 67:750–751.
400. Riggs BS, et al. Acute acetaminophen overdosage during pregnancy. Obstet Gynecol 1989; 74:247–253.
401. Rumack CM, et al. Neonatal intracranial hemorrhage and maternal use of aspirin. Obstet Gynecol 1981; 58:52S–56S.
402. Momma K, Takeuchi H. Constriction of fetal ductus arteriosus by nonsteroidal anti-inflammatory drugs. Prostaglandins 1983; 26:631–643.
403. Peterson RG. Consequences associated with nonnarcotic analgesics in the fetus and newborn. Fed Proc 1985; 44:2309–2312.
404. Niederhoff H, Zahradnik HP. Analgesics during pregnancy. Am J Med 1983; 75:117–120.
405. Klein KL, et al. Aspirin-induced teratogenesis: a unique pattern of cell death and subsequent polydactyly in the rat. J Exp Zool 1981; 216:107–112.
406. Wilson JG, et al. Comparative distribution and embryotoxicity of acetylsalicylic acid in pregnant rats and rhesus monkeys. Toxicol Appl Pharmacol 1977; 41:67–78.
407. Turner G, Collins E. Fetal effects of regular salicylate ingestion during pregnancy. Lancet 1975; 2:338–339.
408. Slone D, et al. Aspirin and congenital malformations. Lancet 1976; 1:1373–1375.
409. Werler MM, et al. The relation of aspirin use during the first trimester of pregnancy to congenital cardiac defects. N Engl J Med 1989; 321:1639–1642.
410. Levin DL, et al. Morphologic analysis of the pulmonary vascular bed in infants exposed in utero to prostaglandin synthetase inhibitors. J Pediatr 1978; 92:478–483.
411. Moise KJ, et al. Indomethacin in the treatment of premature labor: effects on the fetal ductus arteriosus. N Engl J Med 1988; 319:327–331.
412. Rumack CM, et al. Neonatal intracranial hemorrhage and maternal use of aspirin. Obstet Gynecol 1981; 58(suppl):52S–56S.
413. Corby DG. Aspirin in pregnancy: maternal and fetal effects. Pediatrics 1978; 62:930–945.
414. Schiff E, et al. The use of aspirin to prevent pregnancy-induced hypertension and lower the ratio of thromboxane A_2 to prostacyclin in relatively high risk pregnancies. N Engl J Med 1989; 321:351–356.
415. Trudinger BJ, et al. Low-dose aspirin therapy improves fetal weight in umbilical placental insufficiency. Am J Obstet Gynecol 1988; 159:681–685.

416. Beaufils M, et al. Prevention of pre-eclampsia by early antiplatelet therapy. Lancet 1985; 1:840–842.
417. Wallenburg HC, et al. Low-dose aspirin prevents pregnancy-induced hypertension and pre-eclampsia in angiotensin-sensitive primigravidae. Lancet 1986; 1:1–3.
418. Benigni A, et al. Effect of low-dose aspirin on fetal and maternal generation of thromboxane by platelets in women at risk for pregnancy-induced hypertension. N Engl J Med 1989; 321:357–362.
419. Ylikorkala O, et al. Maternal ingestion of acetylsalicylic acid inhibits fetal and neonatal prostacyclin and thromboxane in humans. Am J Obstet Gynecol 1986; 155:345–349.
420. Stuart MJ, et al. Effects of acetylsalicyclic acid ingestion on maternal and neonatal hemostasis. N Engl J Med 1982; 307:909–912.
421. Phelan JP, et al. Is the supine pressor test an adequate means of predicting acute hypertension in pregnancy? Am J Obstet Gynecol 1977; 128:173–176.
422. Wallenberg HCS. Idiopathic recurrent fetal growth retardation and aspirin–dipyridamole therapy. Reply. Am J Obstet Gynecol 1989; 160:764.
423. Chester SW. Pregnancy and the treatment of hay fever, allergic rhinitis, and pollen asthma. Ann Allergy 1950; 8:772, 798.
424. Derbes VJ, Sodeman WA. Reciprocal influence of bronchial asthma and pregnancy. Am J Med 1946; 1:367–375.
425. Jensen K. Pregnancy and allergic diseases. Acta Allergol 1953; 6:44.
426. Maietta AL. The management of the allergic patient during pregnancy. Ann Allergy 1955; 13:516–522.
427. Metzger WJ, et al. The safety of immunotherapy during pregnancy. J Allergy Clin Immunol 1978; 61:268–272.
428. Schaefer G, Silverman F. Pregnancy complicated by asthma. Am J Obstet Gynecol 1961; 82:182–189.
429. Ziaya PR, et al. Intravenous penicillin desensitization and treatment during pregnancy. JAMA 1986; 256:2561–2562.
430. Lamar JK, et al. Effects of amantadine hydrochloride on cleavage and embryonic development in the rat and rabbit. Toxicol Appl Pharmacol 1970; 17:272.
431. Vernier VG, et al. The toxicologic and pharmacologic properties of amantadine hydrochloride. Toxicol Appl Pharmacol 1969; 15:642–665.
432. Nora JJ, et al. Cardiovascular maldevelopment associated with maternal exposure to amantadine. Lancet 1975; 2:607.
433. Williams K, Mackenzie JS. Influenza infections during pregnancy in the mouse. J Hyg (Lond) 1977; 79:249–257.
434. Mackenzie JS, et al. Influenza A virus and its influence on the outcome of pregnancy in the mouse. Dev Biol Stand 1976; 39:489–496.
435. Larsen JW. Influenza and pregnancy. Clin Obstet Gynecol 1982; 25:599–603.

436. Brown GC. Maternal virus infection and congenital anomalies. A prospective study. Arch Environ Health 1970; 21:362.
437. Elizan TS, et al. Viral infection in pregnancy and congenital CNS malformations in man. Arch Neurol 1969; 20:115.
438. Warrell MJ, et al. Examination for influenza IgA and IgM antibodies in pregnancies associated with neural tube defects. J Med Microbiol 1981; 14:159.
439. Sarnat HB, et al. Cerebral embryopathy in late first trimester: possible association with swine influenza vaccine. Teratology 1979; 20:93–99.
440. Deinard AS, Ogburn P Jr. A/NJ/8/76 influenza vaccination program: effects on maternal health and pregnancy outcome. Am J Obstet Gynecol 1981; 140:240–254.
441. Sumaya CV, Gibbs RS. Immunization of pregnant women with influenza A/New Jersey/76 virus vaccine: reactogenicity and immunogenicity in mother and infant. J Infect Dis 1979; 140:141–146.

9

Medical–Legal Aspects of Prescribing During Pregnancy

Frederick H. Fern

Lester Schwab Katz & Dwyer
New York, New York

David B. Brushwood

University of Florida
Gainesville, Florida

There are few personal injuries so emotion-laden as those of a defective newborn. Birth defects trigger feelings of surprise, guilt, and disappointment following an event that has been joyfully anticipated as a celebration of life. In times past, parents could be expected to adjust to their child's abnormality, recognizing the blessings of life in whatever form and accepting the additional responsibilities that their new child's special needs might present. But in today's litigious environment, shattered expectations can cause tough questions to be asked: What went wrong? Who is to blame? And, inevitably, is somebody legally liable? The frequency of drug use during pregnancy, and the knowledge that some drugs are teratogens, may focus attention on a drug used by a mother as the possible cause of a newborn's injury.

If it can be shown, with a reasonable degree of scientific certainty, that a drug ingested by a pregnant woman caused harm to the fetus, then the logical conclusion is that the harm could have been avoided through noningestion of the drug. The question then becomes whether ingestion of the drug would have been prevented if somebody along the drug distribution chain had made a better decision about exposing the fetus to the risk of harm. Recent litigation has examined the decisions made by drug manufacturers, physicians, and pregnant women concerning fetal exposure to risk. Since a fetus is in no position to avoid such exposure, that body of litigation has queried to what degree drug manufacturers, physicians, and pregnant women owe a duty to a fetus to avoid exposure of the fetus to an unreasonable risk of harm. The responsibility of the physician to prevent drug-induced birth defects can be evaluated only within the framework of the totality of responsibility, which includes the pharmaceutical manufacturer as well as the patient, and possibly others.

CHARACTERIZING A LEGAL ACTION ON BEHALF OF A FETUS

Types of Actions

In 1946, the case of *Bonbrest v Katz* (1) held that a child born alive may recover for injuries suffered before birth if the fetus was viable at the time of injury. This rule, or variants of it, has now been adopted in all jurisdictions (2). Recent litigation has expanded on the *Bonbrest* rule, and has become complex, both conceptually and semantically. Distinctions are based on whether the lawsuit is brought on behalf of the parents or child, and on whether the child was born healthy or impaired.

A *wrongful pregnancy* action is brought by the parents of a healthy, but unplanned child, where the complaint alleges preconception negligence by a physician, pharmaceutical manufacturer, or pharmacist concerning a contraceptive procedure or medication that did not work (3). In a *wrongful birth* case, the parents of a deformed or handicapped child are suing for alleged postconception negligence of a physician or other party whose failure to act prevented the parents from exercising their option to terminate the pregnancy (4). A *wrongful life* claim is brought by or on behalf of a child who suffers an impairment (5). This action is difficult to distinguish from the parents' wrongful birth claim, because it also alleges that the parents were prevented from terminating the pregnancy. Wrongful life claims have been virtually unanimously rejected by courts because of the difficulty of rationally determining whether the plaintiff has suffered a legally cognizable injury by being born, when the action that allegedly should have occurred would have resulted in no life at all. Courts have steered away from a theory that assumes nonexistence is desirable (6).

Acceptance of the wrongful life theory in a drug-induced birth defect case first occurred in *Harbeson v Parke-Davis Inc.* (7), the court overcoming reservations expressed in prior cases. In an analysis of this case, Furrow used the phrase *diminished life* (8), which he had coined earlier (9). The concept of diminished life, as suggested by Furrow, relates to the difference between a defective child who claims that it would be better not to have been born because accurate genetic counseling would have led to an abortion, as opposed to a defective child who claims that it would be better to have been born without the defect because counseling regarding teratogenicity would have led to a drug not being used by the mother. In the case of the first child, the defendant's alleged negligence is passive, it being a failure to act to prevent the birth of a child whose defect was not caused by the defendant. In the case of the second child, the defendant's alleged negligence is active. By distributing or prescribing a drug without an adequate warning, the action of the defendant has caused the child's defect. Because damages are clear and the value of life is not questioned, diminished life as a theory of recovery is free of the pragmatic and policy concerns that attend the wrongful life action. Thus, a court need not decide whether nonexistence is better than impaired existence.

Fetal Rights

Legal recognition of the fetus as an entity with its own rights occurred first in property law in which the fetus was given the status of a person solely for the purpose of inheritance and subject to the condition that it later be born alive (10). The live birth requirement has also been incorporated into criminal statutes, many of which recognize fetal existence, but impose criminal penalties for harm to the fetus only after the victim has been born (11). Adherence to a live birth requirement limits the right of a fetus because there is no recognition of the fetus as separate from the woman before birth. Here, the early cases in property law and criminal law are more a recognition of the woman's rights during pregnancy than of fetal rights.

A perspective on fetal rights that is consistent with medial principles and that helps clarify duties to the fetus in a drug exposure situation is proposed by Capron within the context of genetic counseling (12). Capron argues that a fetus has the right to have its parents decide what is in its best interests. If one accepts this argument, then effectively the fetus is placed on equal footing with other patients who must have a decision made for them because they lack the capacity to make the decision themselves. Exposure to a drug involves possible benefits and possible detriments that must be weighed when making a decision. By applying Capron's logic to a fetal drug exposure case, it becomes a fetal right to have a decision concerning use of a possibly teratogenic drug made in such a way that consideration is given to the potential detriment to the fetus in light of all relevant factors.

Presumably, the person best able to consider fetal risks is the woman who carries the fetus. Only she can hazard a guess as to how life will be for the child if it is born with an impairment, given the variability of family situations and parenting skills. But her decision can only be as sound as the information she is given, and adequate information must be given by the manufacturer to the physician who can help the woman understand the information and appreciate its significance to her and her fetus. Where the potential benefit to the woman is slight and the potential harm to the child is great, a logical extension of fetal rights is to impose a duty on physicians to carefully consider fetal risk before prescribing, and not to prescribe the drug if fetal risk outweighs maternal benefit.

FOOD AND DRUG ADMINISTRATION REGULATION

Teratogenicity Testing

The recognition of a teratogenic agent in humans is often difficult. Traditional methods of testing drug safety, using clinical trials to compare the incidence of an adverse effect in exposed and unexposed populations, are severely limited in teratogenicity testing for moral reasons. The result is that the most reliable data come either from animal experiments, in which agents are administered at high doses throughout the period of organogenesis, or from epidemiological surveys of women who usually have had low-dose exposure at unknown periods and frequencies.

The regulatory guidelines for animal reproductive studies issued by the Food and Drug Administration (FDA) have become standard as a screen for teratogenicity (13). Two test species are used, most frequently the rat and rabbit. Pregnant females are dosed daily with the test compound during organogenesis and are killed before birth of the offspring. The uterus is removed, and fetuses are examined for external, visual, and skeletal anomalies. Different doses are administered, and a no observable effect level (NOEL) is determined. This dose is then divided by a safety factor to determine a safe dose for humans. Unfortunately, although animal tests may reveal teratogenic activity, they do not necessarily correlate well with risks in humans (14).

After a drug has been marketed for a period, it may be possible to use epidemiologic methods to examine a relationship between exposure and outcome in humans. From prospective cohort studies or retrospective case–control studies, statistical analysis may be used to determine whether chance alone can be ruled out as the reason for an association between exposure and outcome. Only after a significant period of human exposure can there be firm data on which to base a conclusion that a drug poses an appreciable risk of harm to the human fetus. In the interim, the high degree of scientific uncertainty justifies extreme caution in prescribing newly marketed drugs.

Teratogenicity Information

The acquisition of scientific information serves little purpose unless the information is conveyed in an orderly and understandable fashion to those who need it to make decisions. In an effort to increase the amount of information available concerning teratogenicity and to standardize the way the information is expressed to facilitate comparisons, the FDA has adopted a letter-coded categorization of drugs based on their risk to the fetus (15). The letters *A*, *B*, *C*, *D*, and *X* are used, with the fetal risk increasing as the letter goes farther down the alphabet (i.e., *A* equals least risk, *X* equals the highest risk). This system applies only to prescription drugs, so it is included in the labeling directed to the physician, not the patient.

A survey of the 100 most frequently prescribed products disclosed that only 59 conform to the letter code system (16). Most letter-coded products were labeled as category C, which signifies that "Either studies in animals have revealed adverse effects on the fetus (teratogenic or embryocidal or other) and there are no controlled studies in women, or studies in women and animals are not available. Drugs should be given only if the potential benefit justifies the potential risk to the fetus" (17). Another 22 drugs did not follow the letter-coded system, but carried a statement along the lines of "Safety for use in pregnancy has not been established. This drug should be given only if the potential benefit outweighs the potential harm to the fetus" (16).

Ambiguous warnings, such as those presented by the drugs in category C and the 22 minimally labeled drugs, disclose no hard data about fetal risk, but they admonish that this risk should be balanced against the benefit before prescribing. Such warnings place the physician in a quandary. How can the uncertainty of fetal risk be balanced against the certainty of maternal benefit? A caution that discloses no useful information, but instructs that informed decisions should be made, encourages overly conservative decisions. The decision to use a drug carries with it potential responsibility for having caused a birth defect should one occur. Making decisions based on known risk is difficult enough; good decisions based on unexplained uncertainty are impossible.

RESPONSIBILITY TO THE FETUS

The Manufacturer

Traditionally the law has recognized that the duty owed by the drug manufacturer to the patient is to disclose known or knowable information about drug risks to the physician, but not directly to the patient. This prescription drug rule has been criticized generally (18) and specifically for teratogenicity (19). The criticism focused on the responsibility to protect the patient's right to know about material risks. In an attempt to protect the patient, a comprehensive program of direct-to-patient warnings was adopted by the FDA in 1980, but was later rescinded (20). Civil litigation that would modify the prescription drug rule has not been warmly received (21). The problem of inadequate information is a very real one in the area of teratogenicity, where studies indicate that pregnant women want to know the probability that a drug may have adverse fetal effects, but they are not receiving the information (22). Under such circumstances, responsible maternal decision-making is not possible.

As the best expert on its own drug, a manufacturer should also be the best source of information. This means not only that reasonable and state-of-the-art scientific methods be used to obtain information, but also that the information be conveyed on a timely basis to those who need it to make a decision about drug risks. Physicians know the characteristics of their patients, but must rely on manufacturers for information about drug products. Labeling directed to the physician might be made more useful if it had a separate section designated as *fetal toxicity information for the patient* in which specific language was used to describe what is known about teratogenicity and what is reported or suspected, but not yet confirmed. Vague admonitions in drug labeling to consider poorly characterized and ill-defined risks, place a high degree of responsibility on the shoulders of the physician, without effectively equipping the physician to meet the responsibility. Pharmaceutical manufacturers must attempt to ascertain all relevant information about teratogenic effects and effectively disseminate that knowledge to the medical community.

The Physician

For those drugs that are recognized teratogens or fetal toxins, the physician's responsibility is clear: do not prescribe such drugs during pregnancy. But there are several complicating factors. Conception does not immediately cause the occurrence of physiological or psychological changes, so a fertile and sexually active woman faces the constant possibility of being pregnant and not knowing it. The physician has the responsibility of helping a patient during childbearing years manage this problem through contraceptive advice and, if possible, by recommending a waiting period before initiating drug therapy, to either confirm or rule out pregnancy. When a patient contemplates using a drug that is of benefit to her, but potentially harmful to the fetus, she has a right to know the character of the risk. This involves not only the simple disclosure of information by the physician, but also provision of the opportunity for reflection and assistance in reaching a decision (23).

A far greater problem is presented by drugs that are suspected, but unconfirmed, teratogens. It has been suggested that physicians feel particularly uncomfortable dealing with uncertainty in obstetrics (24). A physician's admission to a patient that the teratogenic risk of a recommended drug is unknown is a difficult admission, because it recognizes fallibility. Physicians are unlikely to admit to patients that (a) they are acting with uncertainty; (b) there are multiple decision strategies inherent with uncertainty, ranging from high risk-averse ones to less risk-averse ones; (c) they prefer a strategy that focuses on fetal risk and preventing it; and (d) this strategy may decrease maternal benefit or increase maternal risk (24). Yet the physician's disclosure responsibility is to assist the patient in understanding the information that is available, though it may be limited. No matter what a pharmaceutical manufacturer may do to increase the availability of information, the manufacturer cannot write a warning directed to each individual patient. Only the physician knows the unique characteristics of the patient's life-style, education level, or values, and he or she must tailor the consultation accordingly. It is the physician who can disclose risk-related information and then instruct the patient on the decision-making strategies and options available.

A pregnant woman may make a decision with which her physician disagrees. This will most likely occur when another physician has prescribed a large supply of medication for a woman who then becomes pregnant and continues using the medication, contrary to her obstetrician's advice. It is foreseeable that a woman who is using medication would disregard her physician's advice to avoid pregnancy. Under such circumstances, the physician may attempt to coerce the woman into adopting rational behavior—either through counseling (You don't want to do anything that might hurt your baby, do you?) or by eliminating the availability of the medication, refusing to prescribe it, or canceling previously authorized refills. But patient behavior is not irrational simply because it is contrary to what the physician believes is correct. The physician's responsibility is to inform and assist with a decision; once an informed decision is made by the patient, the physician's responsibility is to treat the patient within the parameters of that decision.

The Pregnant Woman

A pregnant woman has a responsibility to manage her medication use in a way that accounts for the risks and benefits of drugs, both to herself and to the fetus she carries. A woman's responsibility not to cause harm to a fetus, once she has foregone the exercise of her legal right to terminate the pregnancy, must impose certain limitations on her freedom of action. In deciding whether a woman acted improperly by exposing her fetus to an unreasonable risk of harm, it is necessary to evaluate both the magnitude and probability of harm to the fetus posed by hazard exposure and the magnitude and probability of harm to the woman posed by hazard avoidance. Invariably this analysis will occur after the risk to the fetus has materialized, so care must be taken not to overemphasize the reality of fetal harm; for when the woman made her decision, the harm was a theoretical probability and not yet a reality. The result of the analysis will be a comparison of the woman's actual behavior with that of the "reasonable pregnant woman".

Because the relation between mother and fetus is unique among interpersonal relations, the standard for reasonable maternal conduct requires unique analysis. Cherniak develops a realistic model of maternal liability for prenatal injury, limited entirely to gross negligence (25). Within this model, for there to be liability, a conscious disregard for the welfare of the fetus would have to be proved. Only if it could be shown that the woman knew or should have known that her conduct created a substantial risk of serious harm to the fetus and the cost to her of avoiding the risk was minimal, would liability attach. The focus is on the woman's actual or constructive knowledge and on her responsibility to consider the risk to the fetus as well as the risk to herself before engaging in risk behavior. Thus the ingestion of potentially teratogenic medication would not be actionable unless the woman knew or should have known that there was the possibility of harm to the fetus, and she disregarded that knowledge in deciding to use the drug for her benefit. A pregnant woman who has considered fetal risk, has used a drug, and has given birth to a defective child has not acted unreasonably unless the risk is so frequent and so severe that it would be clearly deemed unacceptable when compared with the usual and customary behavior of other pregnant women.

LESSONS FROM LITIGATION

Manufacturer Liability

One of the earliest legal opinions to establish the manufacturer's responsibility in a fetal harm case is *Woodill v Parke-Davis and Co.* (26). The parents of a minor child sought to recover damages for injuries suffered in utero, the injuries having allegedly been caused by the drug oxytocin (Pitocin). The issue of primary concern was whether, in an action seeking to hold a defendant manufacturer liable for failure to warn of a danger attendant to the use of the drug, the plaintiff must allege and prove that the defendant actually knew, or should have known, of the danger. The court held that the imposition of a knowledge requirement is a proper limitation to place on a manufacturer's liability, predicated upon a failure to warn of a danger inherent in a product. The reasoning of *Woodill* was reinforced and updated in *Brown v Superior Court* (29). In this case brought by a number of daughters whose mothers had taken diethylstilbestrol (DES), the court rejected the plaintiff's assertion that a drug manufacturer should be held liable for failure to warn of risks inherent in a drug, even though it did not know and could not have known, by the application of scientific knowledge available at the time of distribution, that the drug could produce the undesirable side effects suffered by the plaintiff. In essence, this approach relieves the drug manufacturer of the burden of the scientific uncertainty that accompanies the distribution of an as yet undocumented teratogen. Yet if the manufacturer does not bear the burden of uncertainty, then that burden must shift to the physician and the patient.

Physician Liability

The case of *Harbeson v Parke-Davis, Inc.* (28) considers the level of knowledge required of physicians when prescribing drugs and when advising patients concerning the use of drugs during pregnancy. When phenytoin (Dilantin) was prescribed for Mrs. Harbeson, none of the doctors knew that the drug could cause fetal hydantoin syndrome (FHS). The lower court found that a search of the medical literature would have revealed several articles concerning the correlation of Dilantin and FHS. In addition, there was evidence that the warning in the *Physicians' Desk Reference* (PDR) was sufficient to put physicians on notice as to the effect of the drug. The court held that it was not unreasonable to expect the doctors in this case to discover the risk.

The *Harbeson* case next considered whether the risks Dilantin posed to the fetus were material. The court applied a two-step test of materiality incorporating an objective standard. The first step is to define the existence and nature of the risk and its likelihood of occurrence. The second step is to decide whether the probability of that type of harm is a risk that a reasonable patient would consider in deciding on treatment. The court referred to expert testimony presented at trial and agreed that this testimony satisfied the first step in the materiality test. The court also concluded that a reasonable patient would have considered the risk of teratogenicity in deciding on treatment. Therefore, the appeals court upheld the finding by the district court that the risks posed by Dilantin were material, noting that the goal of risk disclosure is to make the patient an active participant in the decision-making process. If a risk is material, then it must be disclosed to the patient.

In the unusual case of *Roberts v Patel* (29), the court was asked to decide whether the fetus, as well as the mother, is a patient. The facts of this case disclose that, while the natural mother was in labor, the defendant physicians advised that the labor should be temporarily halted by the use of alcohol and another drug. Allegedly as the result of this treatment, the child suffered permanent spastic quadriplegia. A lawsuit was initiated by the adoptive mother of the child, but the natural mother was not a party to the lawsuit. The defendant argued that the only duty of disclosure owed was to the natural mother, and that the lawsuit should be dismissed because she was not involved in the legal action. The court rejected this argument, citing a line of Illinois fetal rights cases, and concluded:

> In light of the strong Illinois' policy favoring protection of a fetus, and in light of Illinois' recognition of a protectable interest in the fetus in ordinary malpractice claims, even prior to conception, we hold that [the] mother's physicians owed a duty of informed disclosure not only to [the] mother, but to [the child] as well; in this situation the physician had two patients (30).

Obviously, recognizing a duty of disclosure to a fetus is one thing, whereas a realistic way of meeting the duty is an entirely separate matter. In the ensuing discussion, the court indicated that, although there is a duty of disclosure to the fetus, this duty can be met by informing the woman of the risks to the fetus.

Thus, when a physician treats a pregnant woman, there are, in reality, two patients being treated, and both patients may bring an action against the physician based on informed consent. The guide for disclosure is materiality, the presumption being that individuals have a right to determine what shall be done with their bodies. Teratogenicity would appear to be of such a significant character that if teratogenic potential is disclosed to the physician by the manufacturer, it likewise must be disclosed by the physician to the patient. Although theoretically possible, it is difficult to imagine a pregnant woman who would not want to consider the possibility of fetal harm when deciding whether or not to use a drug.

Maternal Liability

The only reported legal opinion squarely on point as to the civil liability of a pregnant woman to her fetus is the case of *Grodin v Grodin* (31). In this case a child, through his father, appealed from a grant of judgment dismissing his mother as a defendant in a lawsuit brought by him. The child had developed brown and discolored teeth as the result of his mother's ingestion of the drug tetracycline during pregnancy. He alleged negligence of his mother in failing to seek proper medical care, failing to request that her physician perform a pregnancy test, and failing to inform her physician that she was taking tetracycline. The lower court granted judgment for the mother, based on parent–child tort immunity, which prevents a child from suing a parent.

The appellate court ruled that parent–child immunity had largely been overruled, but that an exception remained within which the exercise of reasonable parental discretion still shielded a parent from a lawsuit brought by a child. The *Grodin* court acknowledged that a woman's decision to continue taking drugs during pregnancy is an exercise of her discretion; therefore, it should be immunized from litigation. But the court also held that the reasonableness of that exercise of discretion is subject to litigation, and the judgment for the mother was reversed, with the case remanded for a determination of the reasonableness of the alleged negligent conduct. However, the court provided no indication of the parameters for determining the standard of a reasonable pregnant woman.

LEGAL STANDARDS FOR CAUSATION

Causation Defined

The term *proximate cause* is most often used to describe the combination of causation issues that need to be addressed before the imposition of legal liability on the defendant (32). This combination may be divided into two distinct components: (a) causation in fact, and (b) causation in law. Causation in fact, sometimes referred to as "but for" causation, establishes a connection between the defendant and the injury (32). Causation in law determines that the connection is sufficiently substantial that the law will impose liability on the defendant (32). This is a policy decision made by courts based on the evidence set forth in the case.

The threshold issue of causation in fact, specifically whether the defendant caused the plaintiff's injury, is usually a question of fact (37). In drug-induced birth defects litigation, the relation between the defendant's product and the injury is often fiercely disputed, because the mechanism of the injury may not be patent, if present at all. Although definite proof of causation in fact may be impossible to obtain (34), the law requires that it be established by a "preponderance of the evidence" as in all other litigation (32). In other words, the plaintiff must show that exposure to the product was more likely than not the cause of the injury (32). If the plaintiff merely demonstrates that the drug was a possible cause, he or she has failed to prove causation. As stated by the court in *Holbrook v Rose* (35), the "proof must be sufficient to tilt the balance from 'possibility' to 'probability' " (35,36).

To prove causation in fact, most courts require a two-step approach (37). The first step requires the plaintiff to prove that the agent can and does cause birth defects. This is referred to as general causation. The second step requires proof that the agent caused the birth anomaly in the particular plaintiff. This is known as specific causation. Failure to prove general causation is often fatal to establishing causation in the particular case (38). However, courts may permit cases to be decided by the jury based solely on evidence of specific causation in very limited circumstances (39).

Opposing Experts

Expert testimony is crucial in linking plaintiff's injury to the defendant's product. Today, experts in a multitude of fields may testify on the complex medical and scientific issues involved in a drug-induced birth defect case. For example, parties may consult or call as expert or fact witnesses diverse specialists such as geneticists, teratologists, developmental toxicologists, embryologists, biostatisticians, dysmorphologists, epidemiologists, toxicologists, and physicians from various disciplines. Often the primary responsibility of the expert witnesses is to testify that it is more probable than not that either the defendant's product was or was not the cause, in fact, of the birth anomaly. For the defendant to be found liable, this testimony must persuade the jury that the product more likely than not caused the injury (40).

In most cases, both sides present testimony from expert witnesses to support their position, and such testimony often is diametrically opposed. One court eloquently articulated the problem concerning proof of causation by expert witnesses in Bendectin birth defect cases by stating:

> The expert witnesses on each side are often the same, from case to case, and even when different scientific conclusions and theories are based on the same or similar statistical studies and scientific experiments. The cases are variations on a theme, somewhat like an orchestra which travels to different music halls, substituting musicians from time to time but playing essentially the same repertoire (41).

This observation illustrates the issue of determining whether the persons retained and presented to testify by either side are true experts in their respective fields or merely "hired guns," who will present an opinion without any supporting scientific basis (42).

Often, the medical and scientific communities have not determined a causal relation between exposure to the defendant's product and birth defects. In these cases, the jury, generally composed of ordinary citizens with no medical or scientific background, are asked to decide whether a causal link exists between the defendant's product and the birth defects (43). Additionally, jury decisions on the issue of causation may be unduly influenced by the opinion testimony of experts who may not be generally accepted in the medical and scientific communities. Although limitations exist, if expert witnesses can testify that a causal link exists, some courts hold that the credence to be given to such testimony is within the province of the jury (44). Most courts will closely examine the scientific reasoning and basis of the opinions proffered by expert witnesses in reaching their conclusions to avoid the potential of improper causation determinations by the jury (45).

Minimum Requisites for Admissibility

Historically, expert testimony was placed under strict scrutiny by the courts (46). In *Frye v United States* (47), the court excluded testimony based on the results of a polygraph test and enunciated the standard for the admissibility of scientific evidence based on novel theories or techniques as follows:

> [W]hile courts will go a long way in admitting expert testimony, deducted from a well recognized scientific principle or discovery, *the thing from which the deduction is made* must be sufficiently established to have gained general acceptance in the particular field in which it belongs (47). [Emphasis added]

Therefore, if the opinions of expert witnesses as to causation are not based on principles "sufficiently established to have gained general acceptance in the particular field in which it belongs," the evidence is merely speculation and cannot form the basis of a verdict (48).

Although the standard was followed for many years, it fell into disfavor at approximately the same time the Federal Rules of Evidence were codified which authorize the admission of expert testimony, so long as it is rendered by a qualified expert and is helpful to the trier of fact (49). The "helpfulness" standard in Federal Rule 702 implicitly contains the proposition that expert testimony that is based on unreliable methodology is unhelpful and excludable from evidence (50). Many courts abandoned the strict scrutiny standard of *Frye* in ascertaining whether a scientific hypothesis was proved or merely one expert's opinion (46). Consequently, relaxation of the standard permitted an increase in the quantity of expert testimony allowed to be presented to a jury.

Courts have recognized that controlling the expert testimony presented to a jury is becoming a difficult problem under the more relaxed Federal Rules of Evidence and are beginning to exercise greater control over its admissibility to prove causation (51). Causation "requires a complex series of inferences drawn from scientific experiment and observation and statistical comparison" (52). Mere temporal association is not sufficient to establish causation (53). While remaining mindful of their traditional respect for scientific opinions and lack of expertise, courts are examining the medical and scientific information upon which the expert witnesses draw their conclusions (54). It is clear from recent cases that simply because the plaintiff has presented an expert opinion on causation does not mean that the court will allow the jury to reach a verdict based on such opinion if not based on sound scientific proof (51).

Commentators have urged the courts to admit opinions of expert witnesses only when the conclusions are based on credible, reliable medical and scientific data (55,56). Today, the scientific evidence upon which expert witnesses base their causation opinions will be scrutinized by the courts. Their conclusions will likely be excluded from consideration if the basis for their opinions is not based on scientifically valid evidence, rather than unsubstantiated personal beliefs.

PROVED, POSSIBLE, AND UNLIKELY TERATOGENS

Determining the teratogenicity of an agent in humans is extremely difficult. Many scientific and ethical limitations exist in establishing by statistical significance this devastating characteristic of an agent. Proof of teratogenicity was simplified in thalidomide cases by the unique, dramatic, and rare phocomelic effects it caused when taken by women during their early weeks of pregnancy (55). However, this type of definitive causal link has not been duplicated with any scientific certainty between any other agent and any given birth defect (57). Additionally, most teratologists agree with Karnofsky's principle that states that any agent can be shown to be teratogenic in animals providing sufficient quantities are administrated at the appropriate time (58). This principle further complicates the study of teratogenicity.

An amalgamation of criteria assembled by Dr. Thomas Shepard to determine whether an agent has human teratogenic potential is summarized in Table 1. A list of proved, (Table 2) possible, and unlikely (Table 3) teratogens, also compiled by Dr. Shepard, based on data known to date are considered the standard reference for the scientific, medical, and legal communities (68). They should be studied by all physicians prescribing to women of childbearing age.

The foregoing tables are not considered an inclusive catalog of all the human teratogens that exist in our modern world. Many compounds

Table 1 Amalgamation of Criteria for Proof of Human Teratogenicity[a]

1. Proved exposure to agent at critical time(s) in prenatal development (prescriptions, physician's records, dates).
2. Consistent findings by two or more epidemiologic studies of high quality:
   a. Control of confounding factors
   b. Sufficient numbers
   c. Exclusion of positive and negative bias factors
   d. Prospective studies, if possible
   e. Relative risk of 6 or more (?)
3. Careful delineation of the clinical cases. A specific defect or syndrome, if present, is very helpful.
4. Rare environmental exposure associated with rare defect. Probably three or more cases (examples: oral anticoagulants, methimazole and scalp defects (?), and heart block and maternal rheumatism).
5. Teratogenicity in experimental animals important, but not essential (i.e., oral anticoagulants as exception).
6. The association should make biological sense.
7. Proof in an experimental system that the agent acts in an unaltered state. Important information for prevention.

[a]Items 1, 2, and 3 or 1, 3, and 4 are essential criteria. Items 5, 6, and 7 are helpful, but not essential.
Source: Ref. 73.

Table 2 Teratogenic Agents in Human Beings

Radiation	*Drugs and environmental chemicals*
Atomic weapons	Aminopterin and methylaminopterin
Radioiodine	Androgenic hormones
Therapeutic	Busulfan
Infections	Chlorobiphenyls
Cytomegalovirus (CMV)	Coumarin anticoagulants
Herpes virus hominis? I & II	Cyclophosphamide
Parvovirus B-19 (erthema infectiosum)	Diethylstilbestrol
Rubella virus	Diphenylhydantoin and trimethadione
Syphilis	Etretinate
Toxoplasmosis	Lithium
Venezuelan equine encephalitis virus	Mercury, organic
Maternal metabolic imbalance	Methimazole and scalp defects
Alcoholism	Penicillamine
Cretinism, endemic	13-*cis*-Retinoic acid (isotretinoin and Accutane)
Diabetes	Tetracyclines
Folic acid deficiency (following gastric bypass surgery)	Thalidomide
Hyperthermia	Trimethadione
Phenylketonuria	Valproic acid
Rheumatic disease and congenital heart block	
Virilizing tumors	

Source: Ref. 73.

presently used by society have little or no information concerning teratogenicity. New agents that are continuously being developed are added to this roll. With the enormous number of compounds and ethical considerations that preclude testing on human subjects, it is easy to comprehend the immense task researchers face in determining whether products have teratogenic potential. However, these lists serve as guidelines for the physician in assessing questions of teratogenicity and will grow as more scientific research is devoted to this vital assignment (59,60).

PRESCRIBING DURING PREGNANCY

Goals

Clearly, the intention of any physician in managing a pregnant patient is to achieve a healthy mother and a healthy baby (61). A primary goal

Table 3 Possible and Unlikely Teratogens

Possible teratogens	*Unlikely*
?Binge drinking	Agent Orange
?Carbamazepine	Anesthetics
?Cigarette smoking	Aspartame
?Cocaine	Aspirin (but aspirin in the 2nd half of pregnancy may increase cerebral hemorrhage during delivery)
?Disulfiram	Bendectin (antinauseant)
?Folic acid deficiency	Birth control pills
?High vitamin A	Illicit drugs (marihuana, LSD)
?Lead	Metronidazole
?Primidone	Oral contraceptives
?Streptomycin	Rubella vaccine
?Toluene abuse	Spermicides
?Varicella virus	Video display screens
?Zinc deficiency	

Source: Ref. 73.

of prescribing during pregnancy should be to maintain the mother's health to provide a healthy environment for the developing fetus (61). Also, an important consideration in prescribing should be to minimize the risk to the fetus from the medications selected to treat the mother (61,62). An obstacle to this aim is that many medications possess an unknown teratogenic risk (63). To overcome this obstacle, it is essential for the physician to obtain accurate and up-to-date information about the potential teratogenicity of medications being prescribed.

The medical community learned a very valuable lesson from the thalidomide experience of the 1960s: drugs of low toxicity in an adult can present a formidable hazard to a fetus (64). The thalidomide tragedy made an indelible impression on public perception concerning the deleterious effects on a fetus that can result from maternal exposure to medications during pregnancy (65). This heightened awareness has increased the pressure and liability potential on pharmaceutical manufacturers and the medical profession, especially those physicians treating women during childbearing years (64). When medications are prescribed during pregnancy, patients expect their physicians to know that the drugs will not be harmful to the fetus (64). In turn, physicians expect to receive sufficiently reliable information concerning the potential teratogenicity of medications from pharmaceutical manufacturers, governmental agencies, and the scientific community.

The medical profession's need for practical information to meet this expectancy is well recognized. However, some argue that this essential information is not being readily or adequately provided to physicians (64). When the information is available, it is often contradictory or confusing (60,66). Some of the confusion is due to the lack of reliable data on the reproductive toxicology of a drug (64). Dissemination of available information is, at worst, imprecise or, at best, not systematic (67). A more precise and structured method of reporting and providing information about a drug's teratogenic potential to physicians is required to provide practical data for the prescriber on which to base clinical decisions.

Human epidemiological studies, whether prospective or retrospective, are the most reliable means of evaluating teratogenicity and causation (55). Because of state-of-the-art limitations or ethical considerations, human data is not always available to determine causation. Furthermore, reproductive toxicology studies seem to convey protection to the pharmaceutical manufacturer or render political protection to the regulatory body, such as the FDA, rather than produce valuable information for the practitioner (61). Finally, the complex issue of causation makes it extremely difficult to interpret information alleging a link between the medication and the risk to the fetus in definitive scientific terms (61). These barriers need to be removed to enable an informed decision by the practitioner concerning prescribing practices for the pregnant patient.

PRACTICAL CONSIDERATIONS FOR THE PRACTITIONER WHEN PRESCRIBING DURING PREGNANCY

The expanding complexity and potential for legal liability associated with prescribing medications to a pregnant patient may encourage many physicians to engage in "therapeutic nihilism" (60). Although this stance may invoke sympathy owing to the inadequacy of good teratogenic information available to the practitioner, taken together with the current litigious nature of our society, abstaining from prescribing may endanger the health and welfare of both the mother and fetus (60,61). Pharmacologic intervention may be necessary to control a variety of serious medical conditions that the pregnant patient may suffer from such as asthma, diabetes, epilepsy, and hypertension. Fortunately, medicolegal risks associated with prescribing to a pregnant patient may be diminished, but not eliminated, by adhering to reasonable prescribing procedures.

By instituting sensible, well-informed policies for decisions on prescribing, most physicians can avoid being accused of or actually causing harm to the fetus (61). The following nine points are general practical considerations that all practitioners treating patients during childbearing years should consider, before prescribing medications (68):

1. Consult with all female patients of reproductive age who suffer from medical disorders and are taking medications before they conceive. Refer them to or encourage them to seek counseling before embarking on planned pregnancies.
2. Evaluate the need for any drug being prescribed during pregnancy and give careful consideration to alternative modalities of treatment. Document this process in the patient's medical records.
3. Scrutinize all drug regimens in pregnant patients to determine how careful therapeutics and good control can minimize risks. Use the lowest therapeutic dose possible, as fetal risk is likely increased with increased dosage.
4. Prescribe medications that have been widely used by practitioners in pregnancy for years or that have a clearer safety record in human or animal data in preference to medications possessing insufficient teratogenicity information or those recently introduced on the market.
5. Communicate with patients effectively. Studies have shown that decisions whether or not to sue the physician are often decided on the basis of prior communications between the patient and the physician (69). Patients are more hesitant to sue a physician whom they like or with whom they have a good rapport.
6. Document, document, document! A note should be entered into the patient's medical record briefly summarizing the communication between the physician and the patient. The physician should ensure that the patient understands the information being conveyed and provide an opportunity for the patient to ask any questions that arise. The note should reflect the patient's understanding, as well as the final outcome of the discussion. The physician should write the note contemporaneously or soon after the consultation session.
7. *Never* guarantee an outcome of a pregnancy. Truthfully and factually discuss the incidence of malformations with women who are concerned.
8. If the patient is on drug therapy when she becomes pregnant, arrange for a consultation with either a geneticist, medical teratologist, dysmorphologist, high-risk obstetrician, or perinatologist. The physician should ensure that the specialists document their discussions with the patient. The option of a therapeutic abortion should be presented, if deemed necessary.

9. Maintain a file on all drugs or family of drugs that are regularly prescribed to pregnant patients. State-of-the-art knowledge concerning medications may be obtained from a variety of authoritative sources, as discussed in the following. Copies of this information should be placed in the patient's file to demonstrate that the physician was familiar with the product(s) and made an informed decision about the use of the product(s) during pregnancy. Also, this material may be used in communicating with the patient.

There is no guarantee that a physician will not be sued or even found liable for injury to a fetus if he or she follows the above guidelines. However, the guidelines serve as excellent prophylactic measures to avoid harm to the mother or the fetus, or both, and protect against the potential of legal liability. At the very least, a physician following these simple suggestions should possess a more defensible position as opposed to one who cannot demonstrate a reasonable prescribing process for his or her pregnant patients.

Sources of Information

The acquisition of the latest accurate information concerning the teratogenicity of medications is one of the most challenging tasks facing the medical practitioner treating pregnant patients. Fortunately, the computer revolution has enabled the development of sophisticated data bases from which information concerning teratogenicity may be retrieved by the physician. Computers located in a private physician's office or home may be linked to national or international sources of drug information that can provide the latest scientific information on medications. This information may be most beneficial in making prescribing decisions in pregnant patients. Additional avenues of information are being developed and improved to facilitate the exchange of information between researchers and clinicians.

The following are some of the potential sources where information on drugs to be prescribed during pregnancy can be found (57,64,70):

Package Labeling. The FDA has developed letter-coded pregnancy risk categories for prescription medications (15) to facilitate comparisons of medications. The attributes and limitations of this system have been previously discussed.

Pharmacists. Pharmacists possess an extensive knowledge of medications, including teratogenic information. They maintain patient drug profiles as well as a large volume of reference materials concerning the pharmacology and teratogenicity of medications. Additionally, a major responsibility of the profession of pharmacy is communicating information about medications to other health care professionals and patients (72).

Peer-Review Publications. Primary medical and scientific journals publish articles by physicians and researchers concerning the teratogenicity of agents. Although these publications provide the latest information available, a physician may find the tasks of reading all of the journal articles, interpreting the data, and applying the data in his or her own practice too time-consuming, and not worth the time invested.

Newsletters. This format provides a physician with a comprehensive yet simplified discussion on a variety of medical topics. The tasks associated with reviewing and summarizing peer-review publications is assumed by the publisher of the newsletter. Consequently, a physician receives up-to-date information without the burden of extensive literature searches and reading primary material. Two newsletters providing valuable information on medications are *The Medical Letter on Drugs and Therapeutics* and *Reproductive Toxicology.*

Textbooks and Compendia. Several excellent textbooks and compendia are available on teratogenicity and serve as reference works. The *Handbook of Teratology* [Wilson and Frazier, 1977 (72)], *The Catalog of Teratogenic Agents* [Shepard, 1989 (73)], and *Chemically Induced Birth Defects* [Schardein, 1985; 2nd ed. 1992 (74)] serve as valuable resource materials that provide a broad knowledge base. However, a major limitation of this medium is the significant time lapse before publication. Information contained in textbooks may become outdated before publication or shortly thereafter. Therefore, textbooks should not be the sole source of medical information.

Computer-Assisted Services. As the computer revolution continues to grow, more information is becoming available to the medical community. Computers have enabled the storage of large volumes of data on teratogenicity of medications and permit easy access to such information. A physician may contact various services, such as the Reproductive Toxicology Center, or Arizona Teratogen Information Program, which will assist in answering reproductive issues. Also, computerized medical data bases, such as *Reprotox*, the first computerized data base on the reproductive effects of chemical and physical agents, and *TERIS*, which provides summaries and ratings on risk levels, are excellent sources to evaluate teratogenic risk. A summary of the data on the gestational use of specific asthma and allergy medications from Reprotox (as of June, 1992) is found in Chapter 8.

Drug Information Centers. Many hospitals and schools of pharmacy operate drug information centers that provide answers to a variety of medication questions. These centers possess extensive medical references and are usually staffed by specially trained experts on drug information. Health care professionals as well as patients frequently use these centers to obtain practical information on medications.

CONCLUSION

Efforts directed toward reducing fetal exposure to unreasonable teratogenic risk have as their central focus the generation, dissemination, and responsible use of information relating to reproductive toxicology and teratogenicity. Manufacturers generate or obtain information through scientific research and disseminate it through product labeling. Physicians further disseminate the information by interpreting its significance for a particular patient, and encouraging rational decisions by explaining the risks and benefits of drug use for a patient. Pregnant women use the information to weigh the pros and cons of drug therapy, including risks and benefits to the fetus. Despite best efforts by all involved, birth anomalies are inevitable, although careful consideration of available information, and effective therapeutic management can help reduce the incidence of drug-induced birth defects.

ACKNOWLEDGMENT

We gratefully acknowledge the assistance of Christopher P. Orlando in completing the manuscript.

REFERENCES

1. 65 F.Supp. 138 (D.D.C. 1946).
2. *Huskey v Smith*, 265 So.2d 596 (Ala. 1972).
3. *See, Hartke v McKelway*, 526 F.Supp. 97 (D.D.C. 1981), *cert. denied*, 464 U.S. 983 (1983).
4. *See, Turpin v Sortini*, 643 P.2d 954 (Cal. 1980).
5. *See, Curlender v Bio-Sciences Laboratories*, 165 Cal. Rptr. 337 (App. 1980).
6. Morreim. The concept of harm reconceived: a different look at wrongful life Law Philos 1988; 7:3.
7. 656 P.2d 483 (Wash. 1984).
8. Furrow. Impaired children and tort remedies: the emergence of a consensus. Law Med Health Care 1983; 11:148.
9. Furrow. Diminished lives and malpractice: courts stalled in transition. Law Med Health Care 1982; 10:100.
10. *See, e.g., Medlock v Brown*, 136 S.E. 551 (Ga. 1927); *Christian v Carter*, 137 S.E. 596 (N.C. 1927).

11. *See, e. g., People v Greer*, 402 N.E.2d 203 (Ill. 1980); *Keeler v Superior Court*, 470 P.2d 617 (Cal. 1970).
12. Capron. Tort liability in genetic counseling. Columbia Law Rev 1979; 79:618.
13. Palmer. Regulatory requirements for reproductive toxicology: theory and practice. In: Kimmel C, Buelka-Sam J, eds. Developmental toxicology. 1981.
14. Brown, Fabro. The value of animal teratogenicity testing for predicting human risk. Clin Obstet Gynecol 1983; 26:467.
15. 21 C.F.R. § 201.57 (1988).
16. Brushwood. Drug induced birth defects: difficult decisions and shared responsibility. W Va Law Rev 1988; 91:51.
17. 21 C.F.R. § 201.57(f)(6) (1988).
18. Gilhooley. Learned intermediaries, prescription drugs, and patient information. St. Louis Univ. Law J 1986; 30:633.
19. *See* Comment. Drugs during pregnancy: dangerous business—the continued movement to provide adequate warnings for the consumer. Nebr Law Rev 1983; 62:526.
20. 46 Fed Reg 13,193 (1981).
21. Schwartz. Consumer warnings for oral contraceptives: a new exception to the prescription drug rule. Food Drug Cosmet Law J 1986; 41:241.
22. Brackbill, McManus, Doering, Robinson. Exposure to drugs with possible adverse effects during pregnancy and birth. Birth 1982; 9:165.
23. Katz. The silent world of doctor and patient. 1984.
24. Rhoden. Informed consent in obstetrics: some special problems. West N Engl Law Rev 1987; 9:67.
25. Cherniak. Recovery for prenatal injuries: the right of a child against its mother. Suffolk Univ Law Rev 1976; 10:582,607.
26. 402 N.E.2d 194 (Ill. 1980).
27. 751 P.2d 470 (Cal. 1988).
28. 746 F.2d 517 (9th Cir. 1984).
29. 620 F.Supp. 323 (N.D.Ill. 1985).
30. 620 F.Supp. at 326.
31. 301 N.W.2d 869 (Mich. 1980).
32. Woodside. Special problems of birth defect litigation. In: Vinson DE, Slaughter AH, eds. 1988. Products liability: pharmaceutical drug cases 221, 222.
33. Prosser. Law of torts § 41 4th ed., 1971.
34. *See Grinnell v Charles Pfizer & Co.*, 274 Cal.App. 424, 79 Cal.Rptr. 369 (1969); Marder v G.D. Searle & Co., 630 F.Supp. 1087 (D.Md. 1986).
35. 458 S.W.2d 155 (Ky. Ct. App. 1970).
36. *See also Lynch v Merrell-National Laboratories*, 830 F.2d 1190 (1st Cir. 1987).
37. *See, e.g.*, In re Agent Orange Product Liability Litigation, 597 F.Supp. 740 (E.D.N.Y. 1984); *Lawson v G.D. Searle & Co.*, 64 Ill.2d 543, 356 N.E.2d 779 (1976).

38. *See, e.g., Muniz Nunez v American Home Products Corp.*, 582 F.Supp. 459 (D.P.R. 1984).
39. *See, e.g., Basko v Sterling Drug*, 416 F.2d 417 (2d Cir. 1969).
40. *See, e.g., Turpin v Merrell-Dow Pharmaceutical, Inc.*, 959 F.2d 1349 (6th Cir. 1992).
41. *Turpin v Merrell-Dow Pharmaceutical, Inc.*, 959 F.2d 1349 (6th Cir. 1992).
42. *See Turpin v Merrell-Dow Pharmaceutical, Inc.*, 959 F.2d 1349 (6th Cir. 1992) (close judicial analysis necessary since expert witnesses are not always "unbiased scientists").
43. See Weinstein. Improving expert testimony. Univ Rich Law Rev 1986; 20:473,491–492, n.71; Austrian. Expert evidence in toxic tort litigation. For the defense 1989; Feb: 17.
44. *See, e.g., Lanzilotti v Merrell-Dow Pharmaceuticals, Inc.*, No. 82-0183 (E.D. Pa. 1986), following Ferebee v *Chevron Chem. Co.*, 736 F.2d 1529, 1534 (D.C. Cir.), *cert. denied*, 469 U.S. 1062 (1984).
45. *See, e.g., Cadarian v Merrell-Dow Pharmaceuticals, Inc.*, 745 F.Supp. 409 (E.D. Mich. 1989).
46. Gass. Using the Frye rule to control expert testimony abuse. For the defense 1989; Feb: 23.
47. 293 F.2d 1013, 1014 (D.C. Cir. 1923).
48. *See Puhl v Milwaukee Automobile Insurance Co.*, 8 Wis.2d 343, 9 N.W.2d 163 (1959).
49. See Federal Rules of Evidence 702, 703, and 705.
50. *See United States v Downing*, 753 F.2d 1224 (3rd Cir. 1985); *Deluca v Merrell-Dow Pharmaceuticals*, 911 F.2d 941 (3rd Cir. 1990).
51. Austrian. Expert evidence in toxic tort litigation. For the defense 1989; Feb: 17. *See, e.g.*, In re Air Crash Disaster at New Orleans, Louisiana, 795 F.2d 1230 (5th Cir. 1986); *Richardson v Richardson-Merrell, Inc.* 857 F.2d 823 (D.C. Cir. 1988), *cert. denied*, 493 U.S. 882 (1989).
52. *Turpin v Merrell-Dow Pharmaceutical, Inc.*, 959 F.2d 1349 (6th Cir. 1992).
53. In re *Richardson-Merrell, Inc.*, 624 F.Supp. 1212, 1228–29 (S.D. Ohio 1985).
54. *See, e.g., Richardson v Richardson-Merrell, Inc.*, 857 F.2d 823 (D.C. Cir. 1988), *cert. denied*, 493 U.S. 882 (1989); *Turpin v Merrell-Dow Pharmaceutical, Inc.*, 959 F.2d 1349 (6th Cir. 1992).
55. See, Davis, Ivie, Hernandez. Special problems of birth defect litigation. In: Vinson DE, Slaughter AH, eds. 1988. Products liability: pharmaceutical drug cases 655, 681.
56. Shelton. The need for scientific data in chemical exposure litigation. For the defense 1988; Dec: 18.
57. Shepard TH. Human teratology. In: Wilson JG, Fraser FC, eds. Handbook of Teratology. 1977:237, 257, 313.
58. Shepard TH. Human teratogenicity. Adv Pediatr 1986; 225:227.
59. See *generally*, Briggs. Drugs in pregnancy and lactation. In: Young LY, Koda-Kimbie MA, eds. Applied therapeutics: the clinical use of drugs. 1988: 1541, 1547. (table on the effect of drugs on the fetus/neonate).

60. Drug interactions and adverse drug reactions. In: AMA Drug Evaluations. 5th ed. 1983: 71,34–40. (table on adverse drug reactions in pregnancy).
61. Hawkins HF. Prescribing in pregnancy. In: Hawkins HF, ed. Drugs and Pregnancy. 1983: 41–42.
62. *See also* Turner, Milstein. Drug-induced diseases. In: Dipiro JT, et al, eds. Pharmacotherapy: a pathophysiological approach. 1989: 64.
63. *See* McCombs. Pregnancy. In: Dipiro JT, et al., eds. Pathophysiological approach. 1989: 49.
64. Scialli. A clinical guide to reproductive and developmental toxicology. 1992: 231–54.
65. Stewart. *Adverse drug reactions. In: Gennaro AR, ed. Remington's pharmaceutal sciences.* 18th ed. 1990: 1340.
66. *See* Schwartz. The obstetrician's view. In: Schwartz RH, Yaffe SJ, eds. Drugs and Chem risks to the newborn. 1979: 153–156.
67. *See* Smithells. The challenge of teratology. Teratology 1980; 77:22.
68. *See also* Brent. Medicolegal aspects of teratology. In: Sever JL, Brent RL, ed: Teratogen update: environmentally induced birth defect risks. 203, 1986: 203, 290–210.
69. *See generally*, Hickson, et al. Factors that prompted families to file medical malpractice claims following perinatal injuries. JAMA 1992; 267:1359. (Families expressed dissatisfaction with physician-patient communication).
70. Wexler. Information resources in toxicology. 1982.
71. *See* Molzon. What kinds of patient counseling are required?, Am Pharm 1992; 50:NS32 (3).
72. Wilson JG, Frazer FC, eds. Handbook of teratology. 1977.
73. Shepard TH. Catalog of teratogenic agents, 6th ed. Baltimore: Johns Hopkins University Press, 1989.
74. Schardeim JL. Chemically induced birth defects. New York: Marcel Dekker, 1985 (2nd ed, 1992, in press).

10

The Effect of Asthma on Pregnancy and Labor

Joan C. Gluck

Allergy Associates, Miami, Florida

Paul A. Gluck

University of Miami School of Medicine, Miami, Florida

Sami L. Bahna

University of South Florida and All Children's Hospital, St. Petersburg, Florida

Most chronic illnesses impose some risk to the pregnant woman or her fetus. One such illness is bronchial asthma, which occurs in up to 7% of women of childbearing age (1) and complicates at least 1% of pregnancies (2), making it the most common chronic respiratory disease in pregnant women. Recently data has indicated that the presence of asthma can deleteriously affect the course and outcome of pregnancy (Table 1). Awareness of such information should alert the medical profession to the importance of optimal control of asthma in women of childbearing age, in general, and during pregnancy, in particular (3). This chapter will explore the reported adverse effects of maternal asthma on pregnancy and the potential mechanisms involved.

EFFECT ON PREGNANCY

In the past, there were reports of increased *maternal mortality* from severe acute asthma during pregnancy or labor (2,4) but this has become rare in recent years, primarily because of better control of the disease in this vulnerable group (5–7).

In a retrospective study in Norway (8), 381 pregnancies in asthmatic women were compared with 125,423 control pregnancies in women

Table 1 Effect of Asthma on Pregnancy and Labor

	Approximate risk (times control)	Ref.
On pregnancy		
Toxemia of pregnancy/preeclampsia	2–3	8–10
Chronic hypertension	2.5–3.5	11,13
Hyperemesis gravidarum	2.5	8
Antepartum hemorrhage	2	8
Abruptio placentae	3–4	9,10
On labor		
Induction of labor	1.5	14
Cesarean section	1.5–3	9,10,14
Other obstetrical interventions	1.5	8
On fetus/newborn		
Stillbirth	1.5	8
Neonatal mortality	2	8
Perinatal mortality	2	2,8
Preterm births	1.5–3.0	6,8,13
Low-birth-weight infants	1.5–9.0	2,6,7,8,14,20
Hypoxia at birth	2	8
Transient tachypnea of the newborn	4	13,15

Source: Modified from Ref. 3.

who reported no disease from pregnancy. Asthmatics had significantly higher incidences of *toxemia of pregnancy* (10.5 vs 4.7%), *vaginal bleeding* (4.7 vs 2.2%), and *hyperemesis gravidarum* (2.1 vs 0.8%). These patients had easy access to medical care, but information on the degree of control of their asthma was not available.

More recent studies have confirmed an increase in *pregnancy-induced hypertension* (PIH) in the pregnancies of asthmatic women (9,10). The incidence of PIH seems to be especially increased by systemic corticosteroid treatment (10). A report that PIH occurred less frequently in asthmatic women treated with theophylline (11) was not confirmed in a subsequent larger study (10). The exact mechanism of PIH is unknown. Current theories include (a) an enhanced sensitivity to vasopressor, (b) an abnormal maternal immunological response, and (c) an imbalance in production of vasoactive prostaglandins (thromboxane A and prostacyclin), resulting in vasoconstriction of small arteries, platelet activation, and placental insufficiency (12). The possible beneficial effect of theophylline, as a phosphodiesterase inhibitor, may be through reducing vascular reactivity and inhibition of platelet aggregation. An increase in the prevalence of *chronic hypertension* has also been reported in the pregnancies of asthmatic women compared with control women (11,13).

The incidence of *abruptio placenta* in asthmatics has been reported to be 9% (vs 2% in controls) in one small study (9) and 1.5% (vs 0.5% in controls) in a larger study (10), although the difference in the latter study was not statistically significant.

An increased incidence of *hyperemesis gravidarum* in asthmatics has been noted in two studies (2,8). There is no clear explanation for this observation. It is conceivable, however, that asthma and hyperemesis gravidarum can be aggravated by each other and by emotional stress.

EFFECT ON LABOR

A few studies have shown that women with asthma tend to have more difficulties than nonasthmatics at about the time of labor. In a retrospective study (8), *interventions at labor* were slightly more frequent in asthmatics than in controls, including artificial rupture of membranes (2.6 vs 1.4%), forceps or vacuum extraction (2.9 vs 2.4%), cesarean section (1.8 vs 1.1%), and other types of intervention (5.0 vs 3.8%). None of these differences was statistically significant. In another report (14), however, asthmatic women were more frequently subjected than nonasthmatics to induction of labor (25 vs 17%) and cesarean section (25 vs 9%). A significant increase in cesarean section rate in asthmatic women was also noted by others (9,10). On the other hand, a group of 294 satisfactorily controlled asthmatics showed no significant increase in cesarean section rate (20.1 vs 19%) (15).

In one study (10), a prolonged third-stage labor (the duration between delivery of the infant and extrusion of the placenta) and intrapartum hemorrhage tended to be more frequent in asthmatic women who had received oral theophylline at the time of delivery, but the difference was not statistically significant.

EFFECT ON FETUS

Normally, the arterial Po_2 in the fetus is only about one-fourth to one-third that in the adult (16). The fetus receives oxygen through the umbilical vein, where the Po_2 is similar to that in maternal uterine vein blood, and it normally thrives at this low oxygen level because of multiple compensatory mechanisms that are described in other parts of this volume (see Chapter 2).

Table 2 Factors Potentially Related to Increased Perinatal Mortality and Morbidity in the Pregnancies of Asthmatic Women

Factors	Observations
Poor asthma control	Acute asthma associated with hypertension (22) that improves with amelioration of asthma (23).
	Acute asthma may be associated with hypoxia, hypocapnia, alkalosis, and dehydration (24).
	Lower birth weight in infants of mothers hospitalized for asthma during pregnancy (2920 g) vs infants of mothers not requiring emergency therapy for gestational asthma (3354 g) (7).
	Lower gestational pulmonary function associated with lower birth weight and asymmetric intrauterine growth retardation in infants of asthmatic mothers (25).
	No increase in perinatal mortality in recent studies in which asthma was managed by specialists (5,7,10,13,18).
Asthma medication	β-Agonists may cause hypertension (26).[a]
	Epinephrine may cause reduced uteroplacental blood flow (22,28).[a]
	Theophylline may cause vasoconstriction in certain vascular beds (29).[a]
	Increased incidence of low-birth-weight infants and lower mean birth weight in infants of previously infertile mothers who received 10 mg of prednisone daily throughout pregnancy for pregnancy maintenance compared with control pregnancies (30).
	Increased preeclampsia in corticosteroid-treated asthmatic women (10).
Maternal extrapulmonary autonomic nervous system abnormalities	Vascular smooth-muscle β-adrenergic hyporesponsiveness to intravenous isoproterenol (31) and α-adrenergic hyperresponsiveness to intradermal phenylephrine (32) in asthmatic subjects may predispose to hypertension or reduced uteroplacental blood flow.
	Increased bronchial hyperreactivity (to histamine) associated with uterine muscle hyperreactivity (preterm labor) in pregnancies producing premature infants (33).

Table 2 Continued

Factors	Observations
Maternal smoking	Increased incidence of smoking in asthmatic vs. nonasthmatic pregnant women (11).
	Maternal smoking associated with increased perinatal mortality (34), prematurity (35), and lower birth weight (36).
Black race	Increased prevalence of black race in asthmatic subjects (37).
	Increased prevalence of low-birth-weight infants of black mothers (36).

[a]These effects have not been documented to be clinically significant in human pregnancy, but there are no definitive studies.
Source: Ref. 19.

The hallmark of asthma, particularly when symptomatic, is hypoxemia, which, together with released mediators, may substantially jeopardize fetal oxygenation. The fetus can compensate for limited degrees of hypoxia by redistribution of blood to vital organs, decreased gross body movement, and increased oxygen tissue extraction capacity (17). Considering the risk of hypoxemia and the increased incidence of pregnancy and labor complications in asthmatic women, one may expect an increased frequency of problems to the fetus and newborn in the pregnancies of asthmatic women.

The limited available information on early pregnancy in asthmatic women does *not* indicate an increase in *abortion rate* (5). On the other hand, according to one study (8), there were increased rates of *stillbirth* (13.1:1000 vs 7.8:1000), *perinatal death* (26.1:1000 vs 14.6:1000), and *neonatal death* (18.5:1000 vs 8.0:1000). These findings may reflect a disadvantaged intrauterine biological environment, since the post-neonatal mortality (from 4 weeks to 12 months of age) was not increased (2.6:1000 vs 3.4:1000 in controls). Increased perinatal mortality (5.9% vs 3.2%) was also reported in another study (2). Several more recent studies have suggested that perinatal mortality rates are not significantly increased when maternal asthma is adequately controlled (5,7,10,13,14,18).

Increases in the rates of *preterm birth* and *low-birth-weight* infants have been reported in several studies of pregnant asthmatic women (see Table 1). Newborns of asthmatic mothers have also manifested an increased incidence of *hypoxia at birth* (8) and *transient tachypnea* (15).

A major concern of parents, particularly in the presence of a maternal illness, is the possible occurrence of *congenital malformations* in the infant. Fortunately, maternal asthma has not been associated with an increased prevalence of anomalies in the newborn (5–8,18). The potential teratogenicity of medications for asthma and allergy are discussed elsewhere (see Chapter 8).

MECHANISMS

An understanding of the mechanism(s) of maternal asthma's adverse effects on pregnancy should allow institution of optimal intervention for gestational asthma management. Potential mechanism(s) have been summarized elsewhere (19) and include (a) suboptimal asthma control, (b) medication used to treat asthma, (c) extrapulmonary autonomic nervous system abnormalities, (d) increased prevalence of smoking in asthmatic subjects, and (e) increased prevalence of black race in asthmatic subjects. The data supporting these various mechanisms are summarized in Table 2. The available data do not fully define the mechanism(s) of maternal asthma's potential adverse effects on pregnancy and the infant. However, the available information suggests that poor asthma control may be the most important factor. For example, a recent study of a large asthmatic cohort who were actively managed during pregnancy revealed no increases when compared with matched non-asthmatic controls in the frequencies of preeclampsia, antepartum hemorrhage, abruption, cesarean section rate, perinatal mortality, or low-birth weight infants (13).

SUMMARY

Asthma in pregnant women can be associated with increased maternal and fetal risks. In the mother, there may be an approximately 1.5- to 3-fold increase in toxemia of pregnancy, pregnancy-induced hypertension, chronic hypertension, antepartum hemorrhage, abruptio placenta, hyperemesis gravidarum, complicated labor, induction of labor, and cesarean section. In the fetus, there may be a 1.5 to 2-fold increase in stillbirth, neonatal death, and preterm birth as well as an up to ninefold increase in low-birth-weight infants and a fourfold increase in transient tachypnea of the newborn. Congenital anomalies are not increased, however. Recent studies indicate that most such risks are decreased by optimal control of maternal asthma.

ACKNOWLEDGMENT

The authors thank Miss Pam Queen for typing the manuscript.

REFERENCES

1. Turkeltaub PC, Gergen PJ. Prevalence of upper and lower respiratory conditions in the US population by social and environmental factors: data from the second National Health and Nutrition Examination Survey, 1976 to 1980 (NHANES II). Ann Allergy 1991; 67:147–154.
2. Gordon M, Niswander KR, Berendes H, Kantor AG. Fetal morbidity following potentially anoxigenic obstetric conditions. VII. Bronchial asthma. Am J Obstet Gynecol 1970; 106:421–429.
3. Bahna SL. Asthma management: care of the pregnant patient and her newborn. Consultant 1985; 25:75–89.
4. Williams DA. Asthma and pregnancy. Acta Allergol (Copenh) 1967; 22:311–323.
5. Schatz M, Patterson R, Zeitz S, O'Rourke J, Melam H. Corticosteroid therapy for the pregnant asthmatic patient. JAMA 1975; 233:804–807.
6. Fitzsimons R, Greenberger PA, Patterson R. Outcome of pregnancy in women requiring corticosteroids for severe asthma. J Allergy Clin Immunol 1986; 78:349–353.
7. Greenberger PA, Patterson R. The outcome of pregnancy complicated by severe asthma. Allergy Proc 1988; 9:539–543.
8. Bahna SL, Bjerkedal T. The course and outcome of pregnancy in women with bronchial asthma. Acta Allergol 1972; 27:397–406.
9. Gluck JC, Gluck PA. Asthma in pregnancy [abstr]. Presented at the American College of Obstetrics and Gynecology District IV Meeting, Orlando, Florida, Nov 1975.
10. Stenius-Aarniala R, Piirila P, Teramo K. Asthma and pregnancy: a prospective study of 198 pregnancies. Thorax 1988; 43:12.
11. Dombrowski MR, Bottoms SF, Boike GM, Wald J. Incidence of preeclampsia among asthmatic patients lower with theophylline. Am J Obstet Gynecol 1986; 155:265–267.
12. Imperiale TF, Petrulis AS. A meta-analysis of low-dose aspirin for the prevention of pregnancy-induced hypertensive disease. JAMA 1991; 266:261–265.
13. Schatz M, Zeiger RS, Hoffman CP, Harden KM. The outcome of pregnancy in actively managed asthmatic women: a prospective case-control analysis [abstr]. J Allergy Clin Immun 1992; 89:342.
14. Lao TT, Huengsburg M. Labor and delivery in mothers with asthma. Eur J Obstet Gynecol Reprod Biol 1990; 35:183–190.
15. Schatz M, Zeiger RS, Hoffman CP, Saunders BS, Harden KM, Forsythe AB. Increased transient tachypnea of the newborn in infants of asthmatic mothers. Am J Dis Child 1991; 145:156–158.

16. Meschia G. Placental respiratory gas exchange and fetal oxygenation. In: Creasy RK, Resnik R, eds. Maternal–fetal medicine. Philadelphia: WB Saunders, 1984.
17. Rudolph AM. Oxygenation in the fetus and neonate—a perspective. Semin Perinatol 1985; 8:158.
18. Apter AJ, Greenberger PA, Patterson R. Outcome of pregnancy in adolescents with severe asthma. Arch Intern Med 1989; 149:2571–2575.
19. Schatz M. Asthma during pregnancy: interrelationships and management. Ann Allergy 1992; 68:123–133.
20. Schaefer G, Silverman F. Pregnancy complicated by asthma. Am J Obstet Gynecol 1961; 82:182–191.
21. Moore LG, Rounds SS, Jahnigen D, Grover RF, Reeves JT. Infant birth weight is related to maternal arterial oxygenation at high altitude. J Appl Physiol 1982; 52:695–699.
22. Fischl MA, Pitchenik A, Gardner LB. An index predicting relapse and need for hospitalization in patients with acute bronchial asthma. N Engl J Med 1981; 305:783.
23. Fanta CH, Rossing TH, McFadden ER Jr. Treatment of acute asthma. Am J Med 1986; 80:5–10.
24. Nowark RM, Tomlanovich MC, Sarkar DD, et al. Arterial blood gases and pulmonary function testing in acute bronchial asthma. JAMA 1983; 249:2043–2046.
25. Schatz M, Zeiger RS, Hoffman CP. Intrauterine growth is related to gestational pulmonary function in pregnant asthmatic women. Chest 1990; 98:389–392.
26. Huff BB, ed. Physician's desk reference. Oradell, NJ. Medical Economics, 1991.
27. Misenheimer HR, Margolies SI, Panigel M, et al. Effects of vasoconstrictive drugs on the placental circulation of the rhesus monkey. Invest Radio 1972; 7:496.
28. Rosenfeld CR, Barton MD, Meschia G. Effects of epinephrine on distribution of blood flow in the pregnant ewe. Am J Obstet Gynecol 1976; 124:156.
29. Bowton DL, Alford PT, McLees BD, et al. The effect of aminophylline on cerebral blood flow in patients with chronic obstructive pulmonary disease. Chest 1987; 91:874.
30. Reinisch JM, Simon NG, Karow WG, Gandelman R. Prenatal exposure to prednisone in human and animals retards intrauterine growth. Science 1978; 202:436.
31. Larsson K. Studies of sympatho-adrenal activity and adrenoreceptor function in bronchial asthma. Eur J Respir Dis 1985; 66(suppl):1.
32. Kaliner M, Shelhammer JH, David PB, et al. Autonomic nervous system abnormalities and allergy. Ann Intern Med 1982; 96:349.
33. Bertrand JM, Riley SP, Papkin J, Coates AL. The long-term pulmonary sequelae of prematurity: the role of familial airway hyperreactivity and the respiratory distress syndrome. N Engl J Med 1985; 312:742.

34. Cnattingius S, Haglund B, Meirik O. Cigarette smoking as risk factors for late fetal and early neonatal death. Br Med J 1988; 297:258–261.
35. Shiono PH, Klebanoff MA, Rhoades GG. Smoking and drinking during pregnancy: their effect on preterm birth. JAMA 1984; 251:911.
36. Sexton J, Hebel JR. A clinical trial of change in maternal smoking and its effect on birthweight. JAMA 1984; 251:911.
37. Centers for Disease Control. Asthma—United States 1980–1987. MMWR 1990; 39:493.
38. Centers for Disease Control. Low birthweight—United States 1975–1987. MMWR 1990; 39:148.
39. Schatz M, Zeiger RS. The management of asthma, rhinitis and anaphylaxis during pregnancy. Curr Obstet Med 1991; 1:65–97.

11

Effect of Pregnancy on Asthma: A Critical Appraisal of the Literature

Elizabeth F. Juniper and Michael T. Newhouse

McMaster University, Hamilton, Ontario, Canada

The question that we address in this review is: What is the effect of pregnancy on clinical asthma severity?

The earliest reports of the effect of pregnancy on asthma started appearing in the 1930s and, since then, there have been numerous case reports, retrospective and prospective studies, and reviews on the topic. Enormous variance in the results has led to confusion and diversity of opinion. Probably the most important reasons for this discrepancy have been weak study designs, methodological flaws, and nongeneralizable study samples. As a result, many of the conclusions drawn by these studies are, at best, questionable and sometimes invalid.

Since 1953, 14 studies have evaluated the effect of pregnancy on asthma and the results published in accessible journals (1–14). Our approach has been to evaluate each of these studies from the aspects of study design, subjects, sample sizes, outcome measures, whether other factors affecting asthma were considered, and statistical methods. In this review, we critically appraise the literature, discuss the methodological strengths and weaknesses of the studies, and consider how differences in conclusions may have arisen. Table 1 presents a summary of the 14 studies.

EVALUATION OF AN INTERVENTION

To determine the effect of an intervention, usually a drug, on a specific condition, most investigators will agree that the optimum study design

Table 1 Summary of Studies

First author (yr) country	Study design	Source of subjects	Asthma inclusion criteria	Time of enroll-ment	Number of subjects	Number of pregnancies	Outcomes	Other factors affecting outcomes considered
Jensen (1953) Denmark	Case series	Allergy consultation clinic	Married women with bron-chial asthma	0–6 yr postdelivery	61	1–6 per subject	Patient recall	Eosinophils, allergy skin test, vital capacity
Gandevia (1953) Australia	Case control	Allergy clinic	Women with asthma	Unknown	18	25	Patient recall	NIL
Turiaf (1958) France	Case series	General hospital	Women with asthma	Unknown	198	Unknown	Case rec-ords	NIL
Schaefer (1961) USA	Case series	Obstetric–pulmonary clinic	Women with asthma	Unknown	271	Unknown	Patient recall	Seasonal allergens, climate, emotions, respiratory infection
Gammal (1963) Egypt	Case series	Chest service	Women with bronchial asthma	Unknown	112	1–6 per subject	Patient and physician recall, asthma attacks, therapy	Corticosteroids, season, duration of asthma
Wulfsohn (1964) S. Africa	Case series	Unknown	Bantu women with asthma	Postdelivery	18	Unknown	Patient recall	NIL

Hiddlestone (1964) New Zealand	Case series retrospective and prospective	Asthma clinic	Pregnant women with asthma	? During pregnancy	44	83	Case records, asthma assessment each trimester	Atopy, sex of foetus, menstrual asthma, puberty asthma
Williams (1967) UK	Case series	Asthma clinic	Women with asthma	Unknown	100	210 1–6 per patient	Case records, asthma attacks, therapy, hospitalizations	Menstrual asthma, season of delivery, respiratory infection, asthma severity
Sims (1976) UK	During cohort	Maternity hospital	Pregnant women with reversible bronchospasm in previous 3 yr	Pre-20-wk gestation	27	27	Spirometry (FEV, FVC), exercise induced ↓ in spirometry	FEV/VC, <70%
Gluck (1976) USA	During cohort	Prenatal clinic O and G emergency room	All pregnant asthmatics	During pregnancy	47	47	Observer record of asthma severity and therapy (change defined)	Asthma severity, IgE

Table 1 (Continued)

First author (yr) country	Study design	Source of subjects	Asthma inclusion criteria	Time of enroll-ment	Number of subjects	Number of pregnancies	Outcomes	Other factors affecting outcomes considered
Schatz (1988) USA	During–after cohort	Medical care program–prenatal clinic	All women with asthma history and reversible obstructive airway disease	During pregnancy	330	366	Patient recall, physician interpreted symptom and medication diary cards	NIL
Stenius-Aarniala (1988) Finland	During–after cohort	Maternity centers, outpatient practice	ATS and ACCP criteria of asthma	20% 1st trimester, 54% 2nd trimester, 26% 3rd trimester	181	198	Maintenance medication, (spirometry and daily PEFR not reported)	NIL
White (1989) UK	During–after cohort	Antenatal clinic	"Do you have asthma?"	During pregnancy	31	31	Patient recall, symptom and medication diary, daily PEFR	Asthma severity duration of asthma, menstrual asthma, season, smoking
Juniper (1989) Canada	Before–during–after cohort with controls	Asthma clinic, general practice, media	Airway hyperresponsiveness and current asthma symptoms	Preconception	16	16	Airway responsiveness, maintenance medications, asthma severity score, spirometry	Allergens, respiratory infection, reflux, inhaled steroids

is a double-blind, randomized controlled trial (RCT). The strengths of such a design have been well documented and RCTs have become the cornerstone of clinical drug evaluation. In fact, the results from any less rigorous design are usually viewed with extreme caution and awareness of potential biases.

However, in investigating the effect of an intervention, the study architecture alone is insufficient to exclude biases, and it is important that other factors are carefully controlled to ensure the validity of the conclusions. These include random or consecutive subject selection from a well-defined population, validated objective and subjective measures of outcome, control of contaminants and cointerventions, no loss to follow-up, and appropriate statistical analysis.

Pregnancy can be considered an intervention, and the evaluation of the effect of pregnancy on asthma is analogous to determining the effect of a drug on asthma. Although a randomized controlled trial is clearly not possible, the most valid results can be obtained only through use of rigorous study design, with all factors that can affect outcome carefully controlled.

STUDY DESIGN

If the effect of pregnancy on asthma could be evaluated with one or two well-designed randomized controlled trials, much of the current confusion could be resolved very quickly. However, pregnancy cannot be randomized and, therefore, we are left with weaker study designs, ranging in strength of evidence from the prospective cohort (with controls) to the case series (15). As one progresses from the prospective cohort to the case series, there is the potential for more and more of the well-described biases (16) to invalidate the conclusions. We start our critical appraisal of the 14 studies by examining the strengths and weaknesses of the various study designs.

Before-During-After Prospective Cohort With Controls

We conducted a study in which we enrolled asthmatic women who had the potential and were trying to become pregnant (14). They were assessed regularly before conception, throughout their pregnancy, and for 3 months thereafter. Data collected preconception and from the women who failed to conceive within 1 year were used as control data. The design provided strong before, during, and after data in the pregnant women, and the magnitude of change seen during pregnancy could be compared with the natural fluctuations of asthma in women who were not pregnant. A weakness of this design is that if women develop asthma for the very first time as a result of pregnancy, they would not be included.

During-After Prospective Cohort With No Controls

Several of the more recent studies fall into this category (9–13). Asthmatic women were enrolled after conception, followed during pregnancy, and for various time periods thereafter. This allowed objective and subjective measurements to be made and permitted estimation of within-subject changes between pregnancy and after delivery. Unfortunately, none of these studies have matched nonpregnant asthmatic controls, which would have strengthened the inference that the observed changes could be attributed to pregnancy.

If one uses the drug intervention analogy, the during–after study design is equivalent to enrolling patients into a study after starting the drug and making the assumption that recovery after withdrawal returns the patient to the preintervention state. In our study, we showed that this is not a valid assumption, because the patients who required regular inhaled steroids showed a significant improvement in airway responsiveness between preconception and postdelivery, and this systematic change, which was independent of pregnancy, did not occur in the non-steroid-dependent patients (17). Late enrollment into a during-after study may also produce a serious selection bias. Asthmatic patients who become symptom-free during the first months of pregnancy, as a result of the pregnancy, are unlikely to meet the inclusion criteria, thus biasing the results in favor of patients who remain stable or deteriorate during pregnancy.

Two studies included a control cohort of pregnant nonasthmatic women (9,12). For Stenius-Aarniala et al. (12), these were ideal for addressing the primary question of the effect of asthma on pregnancy, but not suitable for the secondary question on the effects of pregnancy on asthma. Sims et al. (9) had a similar control group with the same limitations.

Case Control

Gandevia (2) interviewed 18 athmatic women, who had experienced a total of 25 pregnancies, and 19 nonpregnant asthmatic patients selected at random from the same allergy clinic. The former were asked how their asthma had been during their pregnancies, and the latter were asked to compare the state of their asthma over the previous 9 months with a comparable period over the previous year. The authors acknowledge the limitations of subjective recall in their observation that the number of subjects reporting change in asthma severity during pregnancy tended to be slightly greater than the natural fluctuations in the control group.

Case Series

The remaining studies (1,3–8) we have loosely classified as "case series" because the subjects do not appear to have been enrolled into a formal prospective protocol during their pregnancies. The investigators seem to have either extracted the data from the charts or interviewed the patients after one or more pregnancies. Our uncertainty arises because the methods of data collection often are not clearly described in the manuscripts. Chart reviews by Williams (8), Gammal and Warraki (5), and Hiddlestone (7), in which changes in asthma severity were estimated from medication requirements, symptoms, and hospitalizations before, during, and after pregnancy, may actually provide some quite strong evidence. Chart reviewers are less likely to introduce an expectation bias, because they extract hard data from the charts, and the estimates of change in asthma severity during pregnancy are based on these hard data. More confidence can be placed in data gathered from charts than from subjective patient recall, the technique used by Jensen (1), Schaefer and Silverman (4), and Wulfsohn and Politzer (6). Probably the study providing the weakest evidence is that of Jensen (1), who interviewed patients up to 5 years after pregnancy, at which time errors of recall may have been a serious problem.

SUBJECTS

Sampling Strategies

Some of the differences in results among studies may be attributed to the populations from which the study samples were drawn and the sampling techniques. A random sample of all women with asthma planning a pregnancy, entered consecutively, and with no refusals would provide the best generalizable estimate of outcome in a particular catchment area. However, such sampling would still miss women who develop asthma for the first time during pregnancy and would be unlikely to account for any differences between regions, ethnic background, or culture. Both the place and time of enrollment can affect the generalizability of the results. Patients studied by Jensen (1), Gandevia (2), Schaefer and Silverman (4), Gammal and Warraki (5), Hiddlestone (7), and Williams (8) came from asthma or allergy clinics. These may have been biased toward women with more severe asthma, since the milder cases may not have attended such clinics. Stenius-Aarniala et al. (12) acknowledge that, because asthma patients were referred to their study, they may have tended to capture more severe cases. Jensen (1) actually excluded 22 of his 106 potential subjects because they did not have allergic disease during pregnancy. The generalizability of Wulfsohn and Politzer's (6) sample of Bantu women to other cultures is uncertain. Sims et al. (9), White et al. (13), and Schatz et al. (11) appear to have achieved good generalizable samples by enrolling from obstetrical populations. Sims et al. (9) included consecutive maternity hospital patients who had experienced an asthma attack in the previous 3 years, and White et al. (13) enrolled from an antenatal clinic by asking the question, Do you have asthma? Schatz et al. (11) asked all women from a medical care program who registered for prenatal care whether they had asthma or asthma symptoms. The limitation of this approach is that it is dependent on the patient's knowledge. We (14) enrolled preconception and could not use the unbiased obstetrical source. Thirty percent of our patients came from an allergy clinic and 60% from local family physicians and through advertising in the local media. The latter improved generalizability, but may have introduced a volunteer bias. We may have attracted patients with increased health consciousness and those who experienced notable changes in their asthma during previous pregnancies. Conversely, patients reluctant to be "guinea pigs" would not have come forward. The expectation component of the volunteer bias was minimized by including at least 50% first pregnancies.

Inclusion Criteria

Ideally, one would like to capture a random sample of asthmatic women who will represent the broad spectrum from very mild to very severe asthma. In capturing this sample, it is essential to ensure that all the subjects actually do have asthma. History alone can be inadequate, because there is a risk of including patients who do not have the condition. The point was made recently by Yernault that dyspnea, wheezing, and respiratory insufficiency during pregnancy may be cardiac rather than respiratory in origin (18). Evidence that this may be important is suggested in the study by Schaefer and Silverman (4), who noted that some of their patients did not manifest the classic symptoms of asthma.

Only three studies used objective subject entry criteria. Schatz et al. (11) required subjects to demonstrate variable airflow limitation, and the subjects of Stenius-Aarniala et al. (12) satisfied the criteria for asthma set by the American Thoracic Society and the American College of Chest Physicians. We (14) required subjects to have current symptoms of asthma and airway hyperresponsiveness to methacholine. However, one of the limitation of such stringent criteria is that all of these studies may have missed milder asthmatics who had either only morning dipping of their spirometry or normal responsiveness because they were not currently in contact with a seasonal allergen.

In the remaining studies, inclusion appears to have been based on history alone. This runs the risk of not only including patients who might have an incorrect diagnosis of asthma, but also those currently in remission. Sims et al. (9) acknowledge that they may have included some of the latter in their sample when they set their entry criterion as having had an attack of reversible bronchospasm in the last 3 years.

Exclusion Criteria and Dropouts

Exclusion of eligible subjects frequently does not receive a lot of attention, but it can have an important effect on the generalizability of the results. Exclusion at enrollment may occur because the investigators decide a priori not to include certain patients or because patients refuse to participate. Ideally, both should be kept to a minimum, because excluded patients may experience changes in their asthma during pregnancy that are different from the changes of those who are included. However, it is sometimes necessary to exclude certain potentially eligible patients from studies because they produce so much noise in the outcome measures that the signal being produced by the intervention becomes obscured. For example, this can occur if women with severe illnesses in addition to asthma are included. In these patients, either the illness itself or its treatment may affect the severity of the asthma during pregnancy and contaminate the results. Although it can be argued that all potential subjects should be included in a study, the increased noise that these subjects introduce means that the sample size has to be greatly increased. If increasing the sample size is not feasible, then the study runs an increased risk of incurring a type 2 statistical error. In our study (14), we knew that it was going to be difficult to enroll asthmatic women before conception and, therefore, made the decision to exclude women with other serious illnesses to minimize the noise.

It is also important for the generalizability of the results to ensure that patient dropout during a study is kept to a minimum because, once again, those who drop out may be different from those who complete the study. For instance, if patients drop out because of severe asthma problems, the results would be seriously biased.

Schatz et al. (11) identified 573 potential subjects, of whom 463 entered the study; 330 were included in the final documentation. The reasons for leaving the study were identified as inconvenience, leaving the area, abortion, and not fulfilling the documentation criteria.

In our study (14), 26 women met the inclusion–exclusion criteria but 6 dropped out after one clinic visit. The reasons were dislike of the breathing tests ($n=3$), recommendation of a family doctor ($n=1$), moving from the area ($n=1$), and the decision not to conceive ($n=1$). The remaining 20 patients completed the study.

Other studies do not report how many of their potential subjects were not included in the final analysis; therefore, it is difficult to estimate whether exclusions or dropouts biased the results.

Bias owing to late enrollment in prospective studies has been alluded to already. The requirement that women should have demonstrable clinical asthma at the time of postconception enrollment not only tends to yield a sample of more severe asthmatics, but it runs the risk of excluding asthmatics of all severities who have improved into the normal range since conception.

Sample Size

There is a tendency to consider that the larger the sample size, the more reliable must be the results. As in all clinical trials of an intervention, the sample size should be dictated by the question being asked, and the strength of the conclusion will be based on the inferential probability of the statistical analysis. In the design stage, the investigator defines the magnitude of change to be detected in the primary outcome for it to be considered clinically important (signal) and estimates the variance (noise) associated with the measurement of that clinically important difference. When measurements are being made, either technically or by a standardized questionnaire, it is only a matter of mathematical gymnastics to calculated the sample size necessary to avoid a type 2 error.

In our study (14), we ensured that all our measurement instruments had good reproducibility and were also responsive to clinically important changes (airway responsiveness, the medication-scoring system, spirometry, and the symptom-scoring instrument). We minimized the chance of a type 2 statistical error and, with only 20 subjects, were able to detect statistically significant improvements in airway responsiveness and clinical asthma severity during pregnancy and to show statistically that these changes were greater than the natural fluctuations in asthma when a patient is not pregnant. Increasing a sample size when one has already shown that there is minimal risk of a type 1 error in the primary outcomes is unlikely to alter the conclusions, but it may increase the comfort level of the reader.

Schatz et al. (11) enrolled a much larger sample ($n = 330$), but only used data from 75 of these for inferential statistical analysis of the objective outcomes. Unfortunately, the statistical analysis was broken down into individual 4-week periods, and the overall effect of pregnancy on the objective outcomes in this subgroup of 75 patients was not reported. Stenius-Aarniala et al. (12) also enrolled a large sample ($n = 182$), but did not report any inferential statistical analysis on the effect of pregnancy on objective outcomes.

In the case series studies, statistical analysis was usually only descriptive. Large sample sizes may tend to give the impression of increased credibility, but because outcomes were rarely standardized either within or between studies, the results are very difficult to interpret (see Measures of Outcome).

Single Versus Multiple Enrollment

It is very tempting to enroll an eligible subject into a study twice or more. This may be ideal if one is examining the within-subject reproducibility of a response to an intervention; however, it is unacceptable when the primary question concerns the overall effect of an intervention. Hiddlestone (7) actually included one woman ten times for each of her ten pregnancies. If a multigravid subject was consistently different from the true population mean, she would produce a serious bias. Mixing within and between subject variance for examining the overall effect of pregnancy on asthma should be avoided.

MEASURES OF OUTCOME

Clinical Asthma Severity

Overall clinical asthma severity can be estimated objectively from the combination of (a) severity of airflow limitation (symptoms and spirometry) and (b) medication requirements. If one is held constant, the other may be used to estimate the change in severity. When both change, estimation of severity becomes very complicated, and the data are difficult to interpret.

Sims et al. (9) were the first investigators to report objective data for all subjects from a prospective study. They measured spirometry and were unable to detect any changes caused by pregnancy. However, they acknowledge that medications were altered as necessary and this might have masked potential changes in spirometry (Table 2).

In our study (14), patients were instructed to keep their asthma symptoms well controlled on a minimum of medication, and they were given a definition of "well controlled." They were instructed to increase medications when symptoms deteriorated and decrease them when they ameliorated. The estimate of asthma severity, therefore, was the amount of medication taken to maintain control. We also measured spirometry and asthma symptom scores to ensure that patients were compliant with the instructions. The results showed that there was a significant decrease in medication requirements during pregnancy (Table 3) and that this was not at the expense of good control (Figure 1). In

Table 2 Study Results: Effect of Pregnancy on Asthma

First author (Ref.)	Sample size	Improved % [95%CI]	The same % [95%CI]	Deteriorated % [95%CI]
Jensen (1)	61	41 [29–53]	15 [5–25]	44 [31–57]
Gandevia (2)	25	48 [28–68]	28 [10–46]	24 [7–41]
(control)	(19)	(47 [25–69])	(32 [11–53])	(21 [3–39])
Turiaf (3)	198	40 [33–47]	21 [15–27]	39 [32–46]
Schaefer (4)	271	3 [1–5]	93 [90–96]	4 [2–6]
Gammal (5)	112	35 [26–44]	25 [17–33]	40 [31–49]
Wulfsohn (6)	18	61 [38–84]	6 [0–17]	33 [11–55]
Hiddlestone (7)	83	39 [24–54]	35 [25–45]	26 [17–35]
Williams (8)	210	42 [35–49]	34 [28–40]	24 [18–30]
Sims[a] (9)	27	0	100	0
Gluck (10)	47	14 [4–24]	43 [29–57]	43 [29–57]
Schatz (11)	366	28 [23–33]	33 [28–38]	35 [30–40]
Stenius-Aarniala (12)	198	18 [12–24]	40 [33–47]	42 [35–49]
White (13)	31	69 [53–85]	22 [7–37]	6 [0–14]
Juniper[b] (14)	16	56	44	0
(control)	(13)	(8)	(77)	(15)

All studies, except Sims and Juniper, reported the percentage (number) of patients who experienced a change in asthma severity during pregnancy.

[a]Spirometry

[b]Twofold change in PC_{20}

Major contributors to the discrepancies between study results may have been differences in outcome measures and different definitions of clinically important change in asthma severity.

Table 3 Medication Scores for the 11 Subjects Who Required Medications During Pregnancy

Subject	Preconception	2nd trimester	3rd trimester	Postdelivery
1	3	1	2	4
2	1.5	1.5	3	4
3	3	2	1	4
4	3.5	3.5	1.5	1.5
5	4	2.5	1	2.5
6	3.5	1	3.5	2
7	3	4	2	1
8	4	1	2.5	2.5
9	4	1.5	1.5	3
10	2	3.5	1	3.5
11	3.5	3.5	2	1
Mean	3.18	2.27	1.91	2.64

The effect of pregnancy on medication requirements was significant ($p = 0.0032$)
Scores were obtained by within-subject ranking of the minimum amount of medication required during each time period to keep symptoms controlled: 1, least; and 4, largest amount of medication required.
Source: Ref. 14.

fact, the 1-sec forced expiratory volume (FEV_1) and FEV_1/vital capacity (VC) ratios also tended to improve during pregnancy, but these differences did not reach statistical significance.

Stenius-Aarniala et al. (12) also used medication requirements during pregnancy to estimate clinical severity and carefully defined criteria for increasing medications. However, they do not indicate what criteria were used for reducing them, nor have they reported whether there were any changes in airflow limitation or symptoms during pregnancy, even though these were recorded. Assessments were made at enrollment, during the last month of pregnancy, and more frequently if symptoms were troublesome. This approach may have tended to overestimate deteriorations, since patients who improved or stayed the same would not have had these additional evaluations.

Complete objective data from the other prospective studies could have been most useful. White et al. (13) collected alternate-day peak flow measurements from all their patients and asked them to score the severity of asthma symptoms and bronchodilator use in a diary. They plotted the data, looked for patterns and then, unfortunately, presented only the results from 10 subjects who reported a subjective improve-

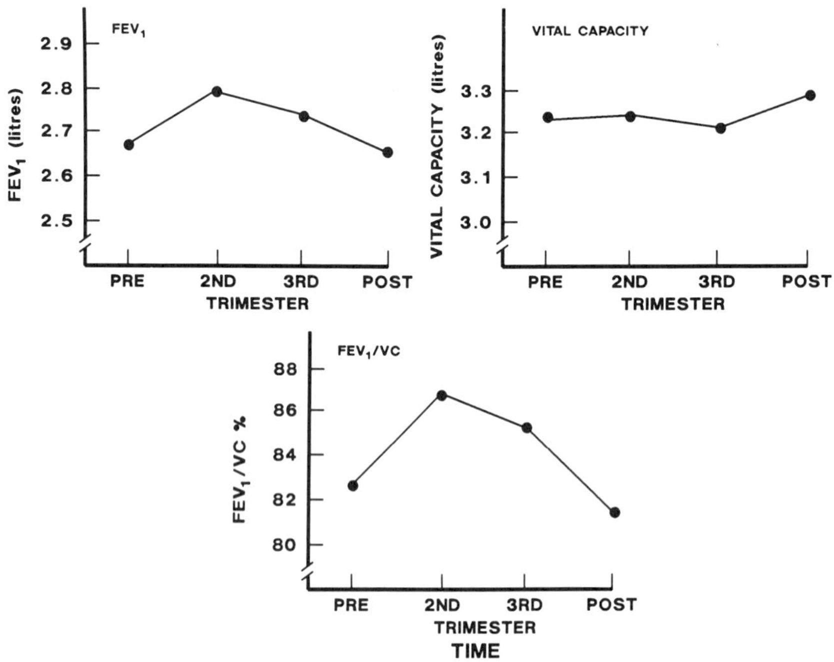

Figure 1 Spirometry measured before, during, and after pregnancy showing that the significant reduction in medication use during pregnancy ($p = 0.032$) was not at the expense of good asthma control. (From Ref. 14.)

ment during the third trimester and 11 patients in whom there was a subjective deterioration postpartum. In both analyses, the objective data in the selected subjects confirmed the subjective impression. The patients of Schatz et al. (11) kept daily symptom and medication diaries, but the results of only 75 of the 330 subjects who entered the study are presented. They were classified on the basis of the patient's own subjective assessment of how their asthma had been during their prenancy and included 25 who reported an improvement, 25 a deterioration, and 25 who remained the same. Based on analysis of physician-interpreted diary cards, the authors concluded that (a) asthma symptoms seemed to improve in the last 4 weeks of pregnancy compared with weeks 17–36 (Figure 2), (b) asthma symptoms in women reporting an improvement in asthma during pregnancy progressively decrease during pregnancy (Figure 3), and (c) asthma symptoms in women reporting a worsening in asthma during pregnancy are particularly increased during

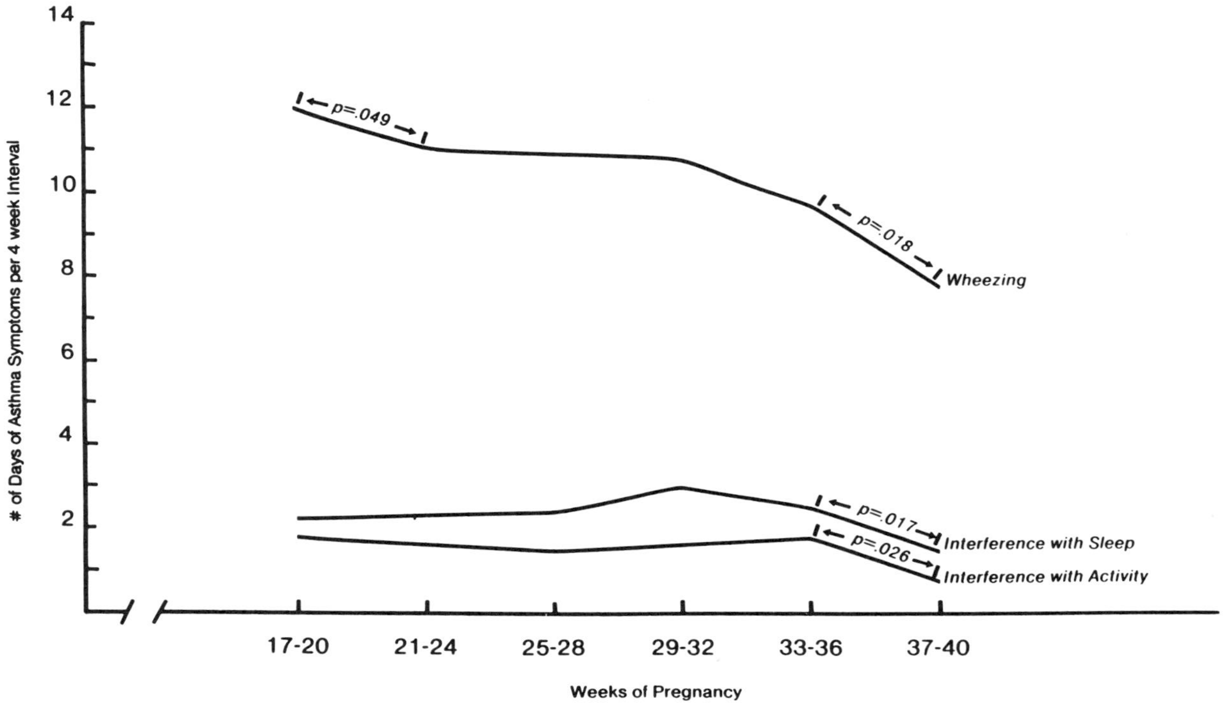

Figure 2 Mean number of symptomatic days (total days of wheezing, days of interference with sleep caused by asthma, days of interference with normal daily activity caused by asthma) versus 4-week gestational intervals in 75 selected women. (From Ref. 11.)

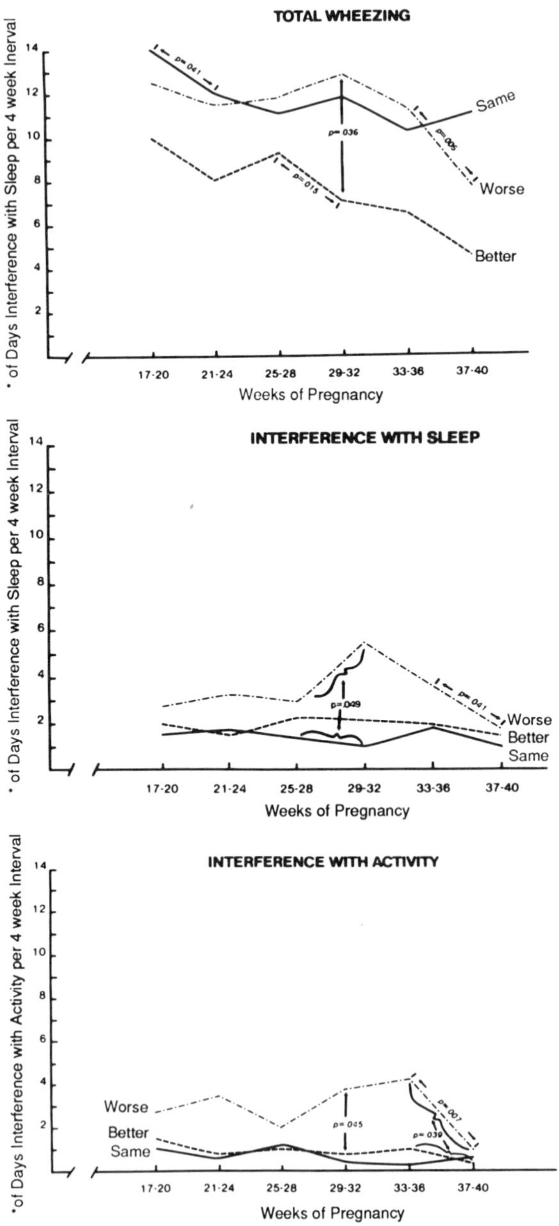

Figure 3 Mean number of symptomatic days versus 4-week intervals from 17 weeks of pregnancy to 12 weeks postpartum in each of 25 women who reported their asthma as getting better, getting worse, or staying the same during pregnancy. (From Ref. 14.)

weeks 29–36 (see Figure 3). However, since these 75 patients were not a random sample and there is no indication of the generalizability of these patients to the remaining 255, these patterns can only be interpreted with caution.

In most of the case series studies (1,4–6) and in two prospective ones (11,13), the patients' own recall of how their asthma behaved during pregnancy has been used as the primary outcome measure. There is no need to belabor the limitations of such assessments. Not only are physicians and asthmatics very unreliable at assessing the severity of asthma by symptoms alone (19,20), but pregnancy itself can alter many factors (e.g., mood, general health state, exercise) that may confound the perception of the asthma. Even back in 1953, Gandevia (2) recognized that ". . . any retrospective investigation based on subjective phenomenon is open to error . . . the patient's opinion regarding the state of her asthma while under treatment may be misleading." This is especially important if there is a delay between the pregnancy and the investigation. For instance, Jensen (1) interviewed patients several years after pregnancy.

In other studies (5,7,8,10), the investigators determined whether asthma had improved, deteriorated, or stayed the same using clinical outcomes such as wheeze, medication change, hospital admissions, exacerbations. These are certainly more objective than the patient's own estimation, but are still uncalibrated. What one investigator may consider a clinically important change another might interpret as natural fluctuation in the disease. This may be one of the reasons why the results from these studies appear very contradictory. For instance, in Hiddlestone's study (7), 5% were reported as staying the same, whereas in the study by Gluck and Gluck (10), 43% fell in this category.

With objective outcome measures, it is easier to define a clinically important change. Let us take an example. Of the 16 subjects who conceived in our study (14), 11 showed a numerical improvement in airway responsiveness during pregnancy and 5 a deterioration. Of the 11 who improved, 9 showed a greater than twofold improvement in PC_{20} (the dose of methacholine needed to provoke a 20% fall in FEV), the change that is usually considered to be of clinical significance. However, in all those who showed a deterioration, the change was less than twofold. Therefore, clinically 9 improved and 7 stayed the same. This example also demonstrates another limitation of the ordinal outcome (better, the same, worse). The magnitude of improvement necessary to be called an improvement may not be equivalent to the magnitude of deterioration interpreted as a deterioration (i.e., the clinical difference between no change and improvement may not be the same as the clinical difference between no change and deterioration). For instance, an exacerbation requiring additional medication may be more blatant and more readily interpreted as a deterioration than an equivalent improvement in which change in medication is less dramatic. Therefore, the bias in ordinal outcomes is likely to be underreporting of improvements. The same care in interpretation should also be applied to the studies by Williams (8) and Gluck and Gluck (10) which reported that women with more severe asthma before pregnancy were more likely to experience worsening of their asthma during pregnancy than women with milder prepregnancy asthma.

Airway Responsiveness

There is a very close association between airway responsiveness to methacholine and clinical asthma severity (21) and, therefore, changes in responsiveness during pregnancy might be expected to reflect the severity of the disease. We measured airway responsiveness to methacholine before, during, and after pregnancy and showed a twofold improvement in the mean PC_{20} between preconception and the second trimester, which deteriorated slightly but not significantly during the third trimester (Figure 4) (14). One month after delivery, the mean PC_{20} was not significantly different from preconception. The overall effect of pregnancy on airway responsiveness was significant ($p=0.033$), and the magnitude of this change was significantly greater than the natural fluctuations observed in the nonpregnant control data. There was a linear relation between preconception PC_{20} and the magnitude of change during pregnancy, showing that the subjects with the most hyperresponsive airways initially showed the greatest improvement during pregnancy (Figure 5). Of the 11 subjects who improved, 9 showed a greater than twofold improvement in responsiveness, whereas in the 5 who deteriorated, the change was less than twofold.

OTHER FACTORS AFFECTING CLINICAL ASTHMA SEVERITY DURING PREGNANCY

Clinical research would be much simpler if the intervention of interest could be the only factor affecting the target disease. Unfortunately, this can rarely be true and, in asthma, we have a condition that is often affected by several external factors. These include allergen exposure, viral respiratory infections, the actual medications used to treat the condition and, particularly during pregnancy, gastroesophageal reflux. Ideally, one would like to hold the effect of all of these constant, but the best that can be done is to minimize the effect, document exposure, and take exposure into account in the analysis. Very few studies have

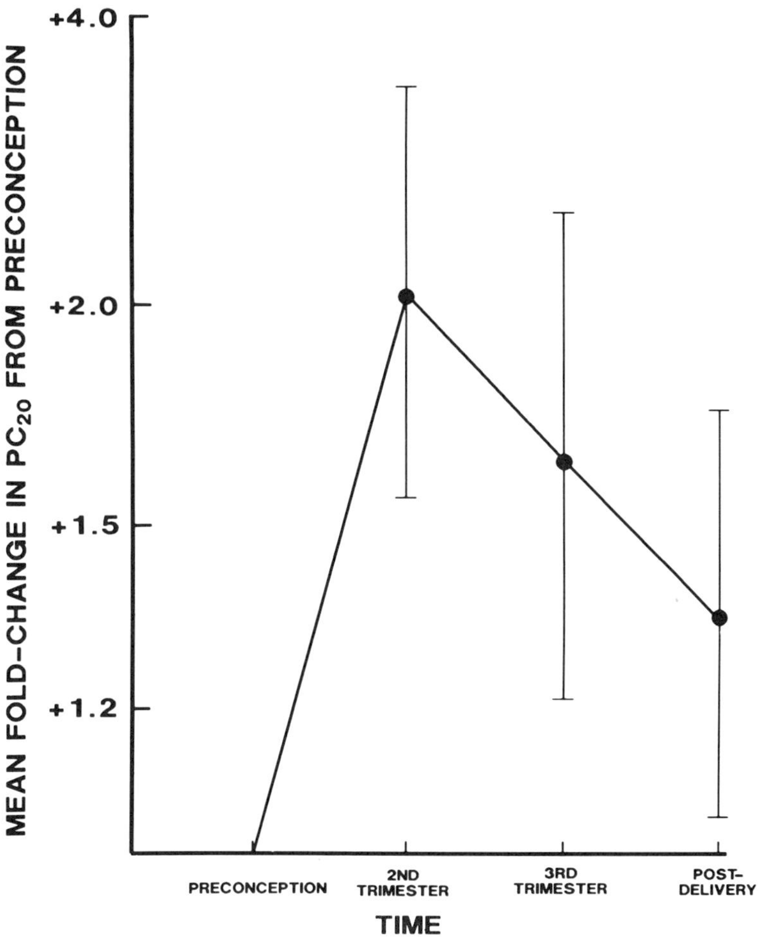

Figure 4 Within-subject mean change in airway responsiveness to methacholine from preconception expressed as a fold change in PC_{20}. The overall effect of pregnancy was significant ($p = 0.033$). The difference between preconception and postdelivery is accounted for by subjects who required regular inhaled steroids throughout the study. (From Ref. 14.)

considered these sources of contamination and cointervention, and this omission may also have contributed to the discrepancies in results (Table 2).

Asthma Medications

Recent studies have shown that the regular use of inhaled steroids can

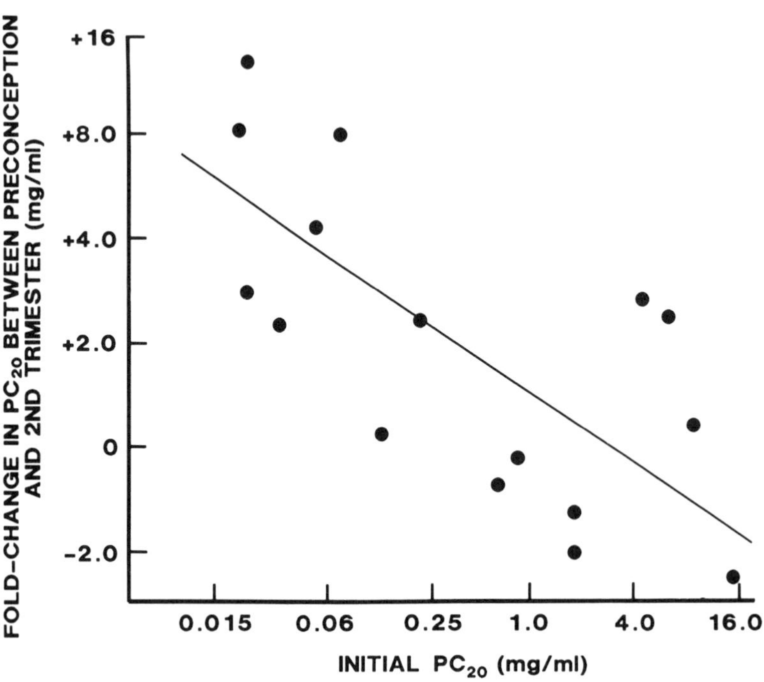

Figure 5 The relation between the initial level of airway responsiveness and change in responsiveness between preconception and the second trimester showing that subjects with the greatest improvements were most hyperresponsive initially ($p = 0.014$). (From Ref. 14.)

improve clinical asthma severity and airway responsiveness (22), whereas the regular use of high-dose inhaled β-agonists may cause a worsening (23). In our study (14), all subjects used β-agonists less than four times per day, but 8 of the 16 who conceived used inhaled steroids regularly throughout the study. In these 8 patients, the mean improvement in airway responsiveness between preconception and postdelivery was greater than a doubling concentration of methacholine, which was significantly different from the very stable airway responsiveness observed in the non–steroid-dependent patients. This inhaled steroid effect accounts fully for the fact that the mean airway responsiveness for the entire group did not return completely to the preconception value after delivery (see Figure 4), and it occurred totally independently of the effect of the pregnancy on asthma. Similar medication effects do not appear to have been considered in other studies. However, systematic changes over time, independent of pregnancy, are difficult to detect unless one has preconception data.

Gastroesophageal Reflux

As serum progesterone rises during pregnancy, there is an associated relaxation of the smooth muscle of the lower esophageal sphincter (24), with the result that one-third of all women experience reflux, heartburn, and indigestion during pregnancy (25,26). In nonpregnant asthmatics, reflux is associated with asthma symptoms (27), and surgical (28) and medical treatment (29) of the reflux has resulted in improvement in asthma symptoms. Although we instituted a conservative treatment regimen for patients who developed reflux, there was a significant worsening of heartburn and burping during pregnancy (14). Both were also significant within-subject covariates for the primary outcomes, but adjusting for them did not affect the overall interpretation of the study. In some studies, in which reflux was not treated during pregnancy, the asthma symptoms associated with the reflux may have been erroneously interpreted as being caused directly by the pregnancy.

Allergens

The inhalation of airborne allergens, such as pollens, animal danders, and house dust, will not only produce immediate bronchoconstriction in sensitized asthmatics, but will often lead to increased airway responsiveness to methacholine and histamine, as well as to a deterioration in clinical asthma severity (30,31). Although it is often impossible to avoid these exposures, documentation of such events allows them to be taken into account in the analysis. Four studies considered the possible importance of allergen exposure and atopy. Williams observed no relation between the season of the year of delivery and the condition of asthma during pregnancy (8). Both Hiddlestone (7) and Stenius-Aarniala et al. (12) found that results in atopic and nonatopic subjects were similar, although Hiddlestone did observe a trend towards greater improvement in extrinsic patients during pregnancy (7). In our study, patients were asked at each clinic assessment whether they were currently or had recently been in contact with an allergen to which they were sensitive (14). Exposures were scored and included as covariates in the statistical analysis. Although the effects of allergens appear to have made little difference in the results of the studies for which they have been taken into consideration, they should not be ignored. For instance, if by chance a large number of pollen-sensitive women were pregnant during the late summer, this might erroneously be interpreted as a deterioration in asthma owing to pregnancy, rather than to the allergen.

Upper Respiratory Tract Infections

Viral respiratory tract infections that produce acute bronchitis often result in an increase in asthma symptoms and a deterioration in airway responsiveness (32). There is some evidence that there is a decrease in cell-mediated immunity during pregnancy (33,34), which could make the patient more susceptible to viral infections, and it has been reported that viral respiratory infections are the most common precipitants of severe asthma during pregnancy (8). We treated infections with antibiotics and, where necessary, increased asthma medications (14). Infections occurring within a month of any clinical assessment were scored similarly to allergen exposure, and these scores were included as covariates in the analysis. In our study, they made no difference to the conclusions (14), but in studies in which infections are treated less vigorously, they might affect the outcome.

MULTIPLE PREGNANCIES

Jensen (1), Gammal and Warraki (5), Williams (8), Schatz et al. (11), and Stenius-Aarniala et al. (12) followed women during two or more pregnancies to evaluate whether the course of asthma during successive pregnancies is consistent. Once again, it is important, when reviewing the results, to take into consideration the biases associated with uncontrolled subjective recall, the method used in most of these studies. Nevertheless, the results are fairly consistent. Schatz et al., looking at two consecutive pregnancies, demonstrated 58.8% concordance ($p = 0.019$) when patients were asked to rank asthma during each pregnancy as being better, the same, or worse than when they were not pregnant (11). Other data support this observation. Gammal and Warraki reported consistency in asthma deterioration in 29 of 33 patients and consistency of improvement in 23 of 28 patients (5). Williams reported consistency in 63% of his subjects, but 21% of the subjects showed marked variation (8). Jensen noted that each multipara stated that she responded in exactly the same manner during all her pregnancies (1). Although Stenius-Aarniala et al. followed 13 women during more than one pregnancy, they report that medication was checked and adjusted at an earlier stage during the second pregnancy and, as a result, asthma may have been better controlled (12).

SYMPTOMS DURING LABOR AND DELIVERY

There have been no controlled studies formally looking at the effect of labor and delivery on asthma severity, but two groups of investigators have reported their observations. Schatz et al. reported the frequency of patient-reported asthma symptoms during labor and delivery (11). Ninety percent of their 366 subjects reported no symptoms of asthma at all during labor and delivery. Of the 37 patients who did have symptoms, 20 patients (54%) required no acute treatment, 15 patients (41%) used inhaled bronchodilators, and 2 patients (5%) received intravenous aminophylline. Similarly, Stenius-Aarniala et al. reported that symptoms were mild during labor and easily controlled with an inhaled β-agonist and that no patients required intensive asthma treatment (12).

MECHANISMS

Our study (14) and the data of Gandevia (2), both of which included control data on nonpregnant women, suggest that the changes in asthma observed during pregnancy are more than just the random fluctuations in the natural course of the disease. This is supported by the observations of most of the uncontrolled during-after prospective cohort studies (10,11,13) and by the case series study by Jensen (1), all of which reported that asthma changes that occurred during pregnancy generally reverted to the prepregnancy state within 3 months postpartum. Although the mechanisms involved in the changes in asthma during pregnancy have not been defined, there are several gestational physiological changes that have the potential to improve or worsen asthma, either directly or indirectly. Some of these have been proposed by Schatz and Zeiger (Table 4). Other possible mechanisms include the direct effect of progesterone and estrogen on airway smooth muscle (14), the suppressed proliferation of interleukin 2-dependent cells (14), and increased atrial natriuretic factor-induced bronchodilation. Quite possibly some of the between-subject variance observed in the studies of the effect of pregnancy on asthma can be attributed to different mechanisms varying in influence among patients.

SUMMARY

Although 14 reported studies have examined the effect of pregnancy on asthma, it is still not possible to draw any definite conclusions. In this review, we have examined the practical difficulties associated with addressing this question and have considered some of the methodo-

Table 4 Physiological Changes During Pregnancy That May Affect the Course of Asthma

Factors that may improve asthma
Progesterone-mediated bronchodilation
Estrogen or progesterone-mediated potentiation of β-adrenergic stimulation
Decreased plasma histamine-mediated bronchoconstriction (owing to increased circulating histaminase)
Pulmonary effects of increased serum free cortisol
Increased glucocorticoid-mediated β-adrenergic responsiveness
Increased prostaglandin E-mediated bronchodilation
Prostaglandin I_2-mediated bronchial stabilization
Increased half-life or decreased protein-binding of endogenous or exogenous bronchodilators
Factors that may worsen asthma
Pulmonary refractoriness to cortisol owing to competitive binding to glucocorticoid receptors by elevated progesterone, aldosterone, or deoxycorticosterone
Increased prostaglandin $F_{2\alpha}$-mediated bronchoconstriction
Decreased functional residual capacity with resultant airway closure during tidal breathing and altered ventilation/perfusion ratios
Increased major basic protein reaching the lung
Increased viral or bacterial respiratory infection-triggered asthma
Increased gastroesophageal reflux
Increased stress

Source: Ref. 35.

logical problems and the pitfalls into which some studies have tumbled. We have looked at the importance of taking into consideration all the other factors that can affect asthma, such as medications, infections, reflux, and allergens. Although some studies have yielded results in which we can place far more confidence than others, there is still a need for further prospective work. Ideally, future studies should enroll consecutive patients, preconception, from a broad population base, and all patients should be accounted for at the end of the study. There should be matched, nonpregnant asthmatic controls. All data should be included in the analysis and reported, and the primary outcomes should be validated objective and subjective measurements of asthma severity. Until we have several methodologically sound studies showing consistent results, there will be uncertainty about the effect of pregnancy on asthma, and the search for possible mechanisms will be frustrated.

ACKNOWLEDGMENT

We wish to thank Dr. Gordon Guyatt for his valuable suggestions for this manuscript.

REFERENCES

1. Jensen K. Pregnancy and allergic disease. Acta Allergol 1953; 6:44–53.
2. Gandevia B. Note on course of bronchial asthma and vasomotor rhinitis during pregnancy. Royal Melbourne Hosp Clin Rep 1953; 23:72–74.
3. Turiaf J. L'asthme et ses rapports avec les secretions hormono-genitales. Donnees statistiques, physio-pathologiques et therpeutiques. J Fr Med Chir Thorac 1958; 12:597–622.
4. Schaefer G, Silverman F. Pregnancy complicated by asthma. Am J Obstet Gynecol 1961; 82:182–191.
5. Gammal MT, Warraki S. Pregnancy and asthma. J Egypt Med Assoc 1963; 46:903–910.
6. Wulfsohn NL, Politzer WM. Bronchial asthma during menses and pregnancy. S Afr Med J 1964; 38:173.
7. Hiddlestone HJH. Bronchial asthma and pregnancy. NZ Med J 1964; 63:521–523.
8. Williams DA. Asthma and pregnancy. Acta Allergol 1967; 22:311–323.
9. Sims CD, Chamberlain GVP, de Swiet M. Lung function tests in bronchial asthma during and after pregnancy. Br J Obstet Gynaecol 1976; 83:434–437.
10. Gluck JC, Gluck PA. The effects of pregnancy on asthma: a prospective study. Ann Allergy 1976; 37:164–168.
11. Schatz M, Harden K, Forsythe A, Chilingar L, Hoffman C, Sperling W, Zeiger RS. The course of asthma during pregnancy, postpartum, and with successive pregnancies: a prospective analysis. J Allergy Clin Immunol 1988; 81:509–517.
12. Stenius-Aarniala B, Piirila P, Teramo K. Asthma and pregnancy: a prospective study of 198 pregnancies. Thorax 1988; 43:12–18.
13. White RJ, Coutts II, Gibbs CJ, MacIntyre C. A prospective study of asthma during pregnancy and the puerperium. Respir Med 1989; 83:103–106.
14. Juniper EF, Daniel EE, Roberts RS, Kline PA, Hargreave FE, Newhouse MT. Improvement in airway responsiveness and asthma severity during pregnancy. Am Rev Respir Dis 1989; 140:924–931.
15. Department of Clinical Epidemiology and Biostatistics, McMaster University Health Sciences Centre. How to read clinical journals: IV. To determine etiology or causation. Can Med Assoc J 1981; 124:985–990.

16. Sackett DL. Bias in analytic research. J Chronic Dis 1979; 32:51–63.
17. Juniper EF. The effect of pregnancy and the menstrual cycle on airway responsiveness and asthma severity [Dissertation]. Hamilton, Ontario: McMaster University, 1988.
18. Yernault JC. Dyspnoea, wheezing and respiratory insufficiency in pregnancy: was it bronchial or cardiac asthma? Eur Respir J 1990; 3:247–248.
19. Adelroth E, Hargreave FE, Ramsdale EH. Do physicians need objective measurements to diagnose asthma? Am Rev Respir Dis 1986; 134:704–707.
20. Burdon JGW, Juniper EF, Killian KJ, Hargreave FE, Campbell EJM. The perception of breathlessness in asthma. Am Rev Respir Dis 1982; 126:825–828.
21. Hargreave FE, Ryan G, Thomson NC, O'Byrne PM, Latimer K, Juniper EF, Dolovich J. Bronchial responsiveness to histamine and methacholine in asthma: measurement and clinical significance. J Allergy Clin Immunol 1981; 68:347–355.
22. Juniper EF, Kline PA, Vanzieleghem MA, Ramsdale EH, O'Byrne PM, Hargreave FE. Effects of long-term treatment with an inhaled corticosteroid (budesonide) on airway hyperresponsiveness and clinical asthma severity in nonsteroid-dependent asthmatics. Am Rev Respir Dis 1990; 142:832–836.
23. Sears MR, Taylor DR, Print CG, Lake DC, Li Q, Flannery EM, Yates DM, Lucas MK, Herbison GP. Regular inhaled beta-agonist treatment in bronchial asthma. Lancet 1990; 336:1391–1396.
24. Bortoff A. Progesterone reduces slow wave propagation velocity and decreases electrical coupling between intestinal muscle cells. In: Weinbeck M, ed. Motility of the digestive tract. New York: Raven Press, 1982; 445–450.
25. Fisher RS, Roberts GS, Grabowski CJ, Cohen S. Altered lower esophageal sphincter function during early pregnancy. Gastroenterology 1978; 74:1233–1237.
26. Ostrick DG, Cowley DJ, Sharp DS, Skinner L, Ganguli PC. A study of gastroesophageal reflux in late pregnancy. In: Vantrappen G, ed. Proceedings of the fifth international symposium of gastrointestinal motility. Belgium: Typoff Press, 1975:358–362.
27. Kjellen G, Brundin A, Tibbling L, Wranne B. Oesophageal function in asthmatics. Eur J Respir Dis 1981; 62:87–94.
28. Perrin-Foyalle M, Bel A, Braillon G, Lombard-Platet R, Kofman J, Harf R, Montagnon B, Pacheco Y, Perpoint B. Asthme et reflux gastro-oesophagien. Resultats de la cure chirurgicale chez 50 malades. Poumon Coeur 1980; 36:231–237.
29. Kjellen G, Tibbling L, Wranne B. Effect of conservative treatment of oesophageal dysfunction on bronchial asthma. Eur J Respir Dis 1981; 62:190–197.

30. Cockcroft DW, Ruffin RE, Dolovich J, Hargreave FE. Allergin-induced increases in non-allergic bronchial reactivity. Clin Allergy 1977; 7:503–513.
31. Boulet L-P, Cartier A, Thomson NC, Roberts RS, Dolovich J, Hargreave FE. Asthma and increases in nonallergic bronchial responsiveness from seasonal pollen exposure. J Allergy Clin Immunol 1983; 71:399–406.
32. Empey DW, Laitinen LA, Jacobs L, Gold WM, Nadel JA. Mechanisms of bronchial hyperreactivity in normal subjects after upper respiratory tract infection. Am Rev Respir Dis 1976; 113:131–139.
33. Finn R, St Hill CA, Govan AJ. Immunological responses in pregnancy and survival of foetal homograft. Br Med J 1972; 3:150–152.
34. Jones E, Curzen P, Gaugas JM. Suppressed activity of pregnancy plasma on mixed lymphocyte reaction. J Obstet Gynaecol 1973; 80:603–607.
35. Schatz M, Zeiger RS. Allergic disease in pregnancy. In: Gleicher N, ed. Principles and practice of medical therapy during pregnancy, 2nd ed. East Norwalk, CT: Appleton–Lange, 1991:437.
36. Merkouris RW, Miller FC, Catanzarite V, Rigg LA, Quirk JG, Vesely DL. Increase in the plasma level of the N-terminal and C-terminal portions of the prohormone of atrial natriuretic factor during normal pregnancy. Am J Ob Gyn 1990; 162:859–864.
37. Chanez P, Mann C, Bousquet J, Chabrier DE, Godard D, Braquet P, Michel FB. Atrial natriuretic factor (ANF) is a potent bronchodilator in asthma. J All Clin Immunol 1990; 86:321–324.

12

Severe Asthma and Pregnancy: The Northwestern University Experience

Paul A. Greenberger and Roy Patterson

Northwestern University Medical School, Chicago, Illinois

Asthma is a disease characterized by smooth-muscle contraction of large or smaller bronchi, or both, with hypersecretion of mucus (1). The smooth-muscle contraction reverses with therapy or spontaneously, and bronchi are hyperresponsive. This definition of asthma is general because asthma itself is considered a complex disease and is not only a condition of abnormal smooth-muscle contraction. In severe asthma, it is recognized increasingly that inflammation of the airways is a major factor in the disease, as presented in detail later. For the purpose of this chapter, *severe asthma* will be defined by asthma of such severity that daily medications are necessary to prevent episodes of wheezing dyspnea, nocturnal wheezing, emergency room visits, hospitalizations, and fatalities.

Recent Advances in Asthma

There has been greater appreciation of mast cell activation products in asthma, such as bronchoconstricting prostaglandins (PG) (e.g., $PGF_{2\alpha}$ and PGD_2), leukotrienes C_4 and D_4, and platelet-activating factor (2), and specific antagonists have been effective in inhibiting agonist-induced bronchoconstriction (3–5). However, currently available leukotriene D4 or 5-lipoxygenase antagonists, platelet-activating factor or cyclooxygenase antagonists have not been clearly demonstrated to inhibit an IgE-mediated allergen bronchial response. At one time, asthma was considered to be a condition of β-adrenergic agonist deficiency and, indeed, it might be appealing to propose that the profound bronchial hyperresponsiveness of asthma is a form of denervation supersensitivity of the bronchi. There are no convincing data to support either hypothesis, and β-adrenergic agonists are valuable pharmacologic agents in management of acute and chronic asthma. New knowledge of a variety of compounds called neuropeptides have been the focus of continued investigation (6,7). Substance P, which is located in sensory nerves near the bronchial epithelium, can activate mast cells, cause increases in capillary permeability and bronchial glandular secretion, and induce bronchoconstriction (2). Asthma is characterized histologically by patchy denudation of bronchial epithelium in addition to mucous obstruction of bronchi and smooth-muscle hypertrophy. Recent evidence suggests that a bronchial epithelium-derived relaxing factor may be lost in asthma, which could contribute to the abnormal function of asthma (8).

Cellular products from eosinophils, such as major basic protein, have been identified at sites of bronchial epithelium denudation in asthma (9). Platelet-activating factor (PAF) is a potent eosinophil chemoattractant, synthesized by eosinophils (10), in addition to being a bronchospastic agonist and aggregator of platelets. The eosinophil not only results in bronchial epithelium injury, but produces PAF, which attracts even more eosinophils. Leukotriene B_4, which is synthesized by mast cells, has neutrophil chemoattractant effects that may be relevant in the late (3–11 hr) bronchial response following allergen challenge. Alveolar macrophages synthesize leukotrienes (LT), primarily LTB_4 (11), PAF (12), and cytokines, which involve lymphocyte proliferation and activation (6). The relative contributory effects of mast cells, eosinophils, macrophages, lymphocytes, and neutrophils remain to be clarified, but emphasize the tremendous complexity of asthma and the challenges involved in understanding the control of bronchial tone.

Asthma has been considered an inflammatory condition, especially in patients with long-term medication requirements when compared with patients who have sporadic asthma promptly managed by avoidance or by temporary bronchodilator use. Following inhalation of an allergen, some patients experience both an immediate bronchial reaction and a late reaction (6). Initially, it was thought that the late bronchial reaction resulted in greater bronchial hyperresponsiveness to other stimuli, such as exercise or cold air. Some evidence suggests that bronchial hyperresponsiveness occurs several hours after the early bronchial response when airway caliber [1-sec forced expiratory volume (FEV_1) and forced vital capacity (FVC)] is normal, but before the late bronchial response (13).

Patients usually are aware of an immediate bronchial response to an allergen, such as a cat, if there is sudden exposure. However, a late bronchoconstrictive response, hours later, may be indolent or severe, but in either event, not considered by the patient to be related to the exposure to cat dander hours earlier. Long-term exposure to an animal in a sensitive patient often results in daily respiratory symptoms poorly controlled with an increasing number of medications. Patients may be unaware of or deny temporal associations between exposure and symptoms. Removal of the animal from the environment can reduce the concentration of airborne allergen such that there is improvement in respiratory status and decreased need for medications. This principle is especially relevant during pregnancy.

The many advances in knowledge about asthma suggest that asthma be considered a chronic condition of unknown etiology and one for which current approaches to management can result in outcomes for the gravida and fetus that are the same or close to what occurs in the general population (14–20).

Pregnancy Outcomes in General

Information concerning the outcomes of pregnancy in the general population has been published (14). *Prematurity*, defined as gestation of fewer than 37 weeks, occurs in about 10% of pregnancies. Birth weights of less than 2500 g are present in approximately 7%, and major malformations occur in 2.5–3.0%. These malformation figures can reach 6–9% if reexamination of the infant occurs in the first 9–12 months of life. The incidence of stillbirths is 8:1000, neonatal deaths (within the first month) 7:1000, and maternal deaths 8:100,000. The mean birth weight from the National Center for Health Statistics is 3370 g (14). Alternative "general population" data have recently been derived from a survey of 4412 pregnancies in medical residents and 4236 pregnancies in wives of medical residents (21). Miscarriages occurred in 12–14%, stillbirths in 2:1000–5:1000, preterm deliveries in 6.0–6.5%, and birthweight less than 2500 g in 3.0–4.3%.

Outcomes of Pregnancies in Gravidas with Asthma

The adverse effects of inadequately controlled asthma during gestation can be devastating in terms of pregnancy outcomes. Maternal fatalities have been reported in women who experienced frequent serious episodes of wheezing (22). Neonatal deaths and stillbirths have occurred in the same setting (23). Some studies have noted increased rates of preterm births and intrauterine growth retardation in the infants of gravidas with asthma (23–25). Pregnancy termination has been performed in an attempt to stop life-threatening episodes of asthma in the gravida (26). Alternatively, several studies have demonstrated pregnancy outcomes similar or close to that of the general population (14–20,25). Effective control of severe asthma during gestation often requires use of oral corticosteroids, such as prednisone and inhaled beclomethasone dipropionate (14,18,19,20,25). The currently available information suggests that the failure to use these drugs in the management of severe asthma during pregnancy is a greater danger than the potential adverse effects from their use (14,18–20,25).

PHYSIOLOGIC CHANGES DURING GESTATION

General (see also Chapters 1 and 2)

Progesterone concentrations increase and cause hyperventilation during gestation. Increases in plasma concentrations of estrone, estradiol, and estriol occur, but it is not established what, if any, effects relating to asthma occur. Similarly, both bound and free cortisol are elevated during gestation. There is a modest decrease in delayed hypersensitivity reactions during gestation, perhaps from increased free cortisol, but the clinical relevance to asthma is doubtful.

Uterine blood flow increases tenfold from about 50 mL/min in the nongravid state to 500 mL/min at term (27,28). Uterine blood flow during gestation can be compromised by hypotension and severe hyperventilation with marked hypocarbia (29). Decreased fetal oxygen tension can result from hypocarbia-associated uterine artery vasoconstriction, reduced maternal venous return from increased intrathoracic pressure during acute asthma, and the leftward shift of the maternal oxyhemoglobin dissociation curve attributable to respiratory alkalosis. Additional complicating factors may include maternal anemia or hemoglobinopathy. In gravidas with normal hemoglobin levels, pregnancy does not change the P_{50}, or oxygen pressure in maternal blood at which hemoglobin is 50% saturated with oxygen (26–28 mm Hg).

Cardiac stroke volume is unchanged, but diastolic pressure falls as peripheral resistance is reduced. The resting heart rate increases 10–20 beats per minute, and cardiac output increases by 30–50% by the second trimester. Total body water expands by 8.5 L. The blood volume increases by as much as 60% and, because the increase is in intravascular fluid, but not red cell mass, the hemoglobin concentration declines. The expected mild anemia of pregnancy can be aggravated in the presence of preexisting iron deficiency in gravidas who have not had prenatal care. The expansion of total body water and intravascular volume have some clinical implications for intravenous fluids. Although dehydration must be corrected, excessive fluid administration in gravidas whose peripheral resistance is low can cause noncardiac pulmonary edema.

Respiratory Changes (see also Chapter 3)

The maternal hyperventilation during gestation alters the usual arterial blood gases such that the PO_2 ranges from 90 to slightly over 100 mmHg, depending on data in different studies (29). The Pco_2 drops to 25–32 mmHg and pH varies from 7.40 to 7.47. A gravida who presents with acute asthma and has a Pco_2 of 35 mmHg is suffering from some degree of alveolar hypoventilation. The diaphragm moves cephalad, and there is a reduction in the generated negative intrathoracic pressure (30). In that an adaptive response during acute asthma is increased negative intrathoracic pressure (to apply more radial bronchodilating traction on bronchi), the gravida may become susceptible to more serious attacks of asthma during gestation. This possibility needs to be confirmed.

The major pulmonary function changes are 15–25% reductions of functional residual capacity (the amount of air remaining in the lung at the end of a normal or tidal breath) and residual volume (trapped gas) (31,32). The vital capacity is unchanged, but the quantity of air moved during resting ventilation (tidal volume) is increased. As the frequency of respiration is unchanged, the increased tidal volume results in greater minute ventilation. Minute ventilation rises by 20–50% over nongravid values. Serial measurements of bronchial responsiveness in women before the onset of pregnancy and during gestation did not reveal any large changes in bronchial tone (33). Thus, primary factors other than bronchial hyperresponsiveness must contribute to worsening of asthma during gestation (see Chapter 11).

CLASSIFICATION OF ASTHMA SEVERITY DURING GESTATION

In evaluating the gravida, it is useful to define the type of asthma present. Some types of asthma are listed in Table 1. In the assessment of the patient with asthma who is pregnant, it is necessary to consider the physiological "dyspnea of pregnancy" that occurs in the first two

Table 1 Classification of Asthma During Gestation

Asthma classification	IgE-triggering factors of asthma
Extrinsic	Yes
Intrinsic	No
Mixed	Yes
Potentially fatal asthma	Some cases
Malignant potentially fatal asthma	Some cases
Aspirin-sensitive asthma	Usually not
Adolescent asthma	Some cases
Asthma and allergic bronchopulmonary aspergillosis	Yes

Table 2 Criteria for the Diagnosis of Potentially Fatal Asthma

1. History of respiratory arrest or intubation from asthma
2. History of respiratory failure without intubation
3. Two or more episodes of status asthmaticus despite oral corticosteroids
4. Two or more episodes of pneumothorax or pneumomediastinum from asthma

trimesters (37). No wheezing or ronchi are present in such patients. Additional information concerning the differential diagnosis of gestational asthma may be found in Chapter 13.

Potentially Fatal Asthma

It is important to identify patients who meet the criteria for the diagnosis of potentially fatal asthma (34) or malignant potentially fatal asthma (35). The cumulative fatality rate in patients with potentially fatal asthma is over 7% despite our very best efforts. This fatality rate is 1000 times higher than the overall fatality rate from asthma (34). Specific criteria for potentially fatal asthma are listed in Table 2. These criteria refer to major asthma events from which patients survive. However, rare patients do exist who suffer a life-threatening or fatal respiratory arrest from asthma without prior warning. Thus, these criteria for identifying the high-risk patient with asthma will not predict all patients who die of asthma. Some patients with potentially fatal asthma are so noncompliant with medications, office visits, and most all physician's advice that they are a threat to themselves in terms of survival. The term *malignant potentially fatal asthma* has been proposed for such patients who are almost impossible to manage (35). Even long-acting injectable corticosteroids (36), which are undesirable because of the risk of adverse effects, especially hyperglycemia, during gestation, become impossible to administer in these patients who are unable or unwilling to keep ambulatory appointments.

Specific questions to determine the severity of the gravida's asthma include (a) current medications for asthma and other medical conditions, with emphasis on whether there is overuse of β-adrenergic agonists; (b) exercise tolerance; (c) presence of nocturnal wheezing and medication use; (d) coughing during inspiration; (e) recent hospitalizations or emergency treatment for respiratory symptoms; and (f) development of symptoms consistent with viral upper respiratory syndromes, purulent rhinitis, bronchitis, or sinusitus.

Peak Expiratory Flow Monitoring

There is increasing interest in personal peak expiratory flow monitoring at home as well as during ambulatory visits (38). However, because certain patients, especially adolescents, may be noncompliant and submit "expected" values to their physicians, the actual benefit in terms of prevention of emergency room visits, hospitalizations, and in identifying subclinical asthma exacerbations remains to be established. For example, if a gravida is stable according to the six parameters of assessment mentioned in the foregoing, is asymptomatic, or has minimal symptoms, and has no wheezing on examination, the benefit of requiring her to record daily peak expiratory flow rates is questionable.

In the gravida with severe asthma, the main emphasis should be on moderate to high doses of inhaled beclomethasone dipropionate and alternate-day prednisone if necessary. This approach has been successful in preventing repeated exacerbations of asthma and in achieving clinical stability (20,25). Some physicians believe that use of personal expiratory flow rate monitoring formalizes the process of medication use and improves care from that perspective. In this context, the recordings represent an index of compliance.

Pregnancy in Adolescents

Pregnancy in adolescents with severe asthma has been associated with a high frequency of hospitalizations and emergency room visits (18). During 28 pregnancies in 21 adolescents with severe asthma, there were 22 hospitalizations and 20 emergency room visits during 56 asthma exacerbations. Most asthma exacerbations were attributable to upper respiratory tract infections or noncompliance with medical advice. No maternal or fetal deaths occurred. One infant was found to have cerebral palsy at the age of 9 months. The mother had numerous episodes of status asthmaticus during gestation and was noncompliant. In an effort to prevent continued hospitalizations from asthma with its associated hypoxemia and respiratory distress, we administered a long-acting corticosteroid, depot methyl prednisolone, to help prevent a fatality in the gravida.

In the absence of asthma, the child born from an adolescent pregnancy has increased likelihood of physical and developmental abnormalities (39). Preterm births and gestational hypertension are more frequent during adolescent pregnancies. From a management perspective, many adolescents desire to be medication-free. Repeated exacerbations of asthma that may be life-threatening can occur when the gravida has asthma of such severity and rejects effective long-term therapy. Emphasis in these patients should include regular administration of inhaled beclomethasone dipropionate in doses up to 16–20 inhalations per day, alternate-day prednisone on a maintenance basis, or short courses of daily oral corticosteroids such as prednisone (18). The latter are effective in preventing emergency room visits in adolescent gravidas whose asthma deteriorates (18).

CHOICE OF THERAPY

General Measures

Asthma therapy requires accurate diagnosis, classification of asthma (see Table 1), consideration of additional major medical diagnoses (cystic fibrosis, allergic bronchopulmonary aspergillosis, or others), avoidance measures, appropriate pharmacotherapy, and in some patients allergen immunotherapy. Communication with the physician managing the obstetrical aspects of the pregnancy is necessary (40). Some important general measures during gestation include smoking cessation, effective prenatal care, avoidance of recreational drugs and alcohol abuse, physician availability, prompt treatment for asthma exacerbations, and a management regimen that is not excessively demanding for the gravida. For example, especially for the adolescent gravida with severe or potentially fatal asthma, pharmacotherapy should include inhaled beclomethasone dipropionate and, if necessary, alternate-day prednisone as the cornerstones of maintenance therapy (18). Some general recommendations, as they apply to management of severe asthma, are listed in Table 3.

Table 3 Some General Recommendations During Management of Severe Asthma

1. Discontinue smoking and recreational drugs
2. Consider IgE-mediated triggers of asthma, such as animals in the home.
3. Exclude allergic bronchopulmonary aspergillosis
4. Appreciate limitations in pharmacotherapy as bronchodilators help mild more than severe asthma
5. After emergency therapy, discharge gravidas on prednisone therapy
6. Start oral steroids promptly for anticipated problem patients whose course deteriorates.
7. Antibiotics can help resolve purulent rhinitis or bronchitis, but oral corticosteroids likely will be required to prevent status asthmaticus
8. After hospitalizations for asthma, alter discharge medications to prevent recurrences of status asthmaticus
9. Choose medications of established efficacy and safety
10. It is better to intensively treat the gravida during an exacerbation, rather than undertreat

Pharmacotherapy

The appropriateness of pharmacotherapy during gestation has been established reasonably well for the management of asthma. Most of the commonly used medications are considered appropriate for use during gestation (14,16,17,19,20,25,41). General aspects of the use of medication during pregnancy are described in detail in Chapter 7, but certain points will be emphasized here.

The best data to support the administration of medication during gestation are derived from experience in human pregnancies in whom therapeutic doses are used at conception or during the first trimester. Information can be gained from a lack of case reports reporting teratogenic effects and from birth-defect registries. The period of organogenesis in human gestations is during days 13–56. The rest of the gestation is a period for growth and development. In humans the fraction of gestation during which organogenesis occurs is short, whereas growth and functional development is long compared with animals, which often are tested for teratogenic effects of drugs. As a generalization, many drugs that are considered appropriate for use in human pregnancies induce teratogenic effects in animals. For example, the administration of high doses of cortisone acetate to pregnant rabbits can induce cleft palate formation. However, systemic or oral corticosteroids in doses necessary for management of asthma do not produce an excessive number of teratogenic effects of any kind (19,25).

Most congenital malformations are not caused by maternal use of medications. However, examples of known human teratogens include lithium, isotretinoin, ethanol (dose-related), thalidomide, diethylstilbesterol, inorganic iodides, carbamazepine, valproic acid, tetracycline, and streptomycin.

Drugs considered appropriate for administration at conception and during gestation are listed in Table 4. Published data and long experience support the use of such medications. For acute exacerbations, either subcutaneous epinephrine or terbutaline may be administered. An alternative approach is use of metered-dose inhalers or nebulized delivery systems (see Appendix). Severely dyspneic gravidas may be unable to inspire deeply enough to permit delivery of inhaled β-adrenergic agonists to lower airways. Terbutaline may be appropriate to administer in early gestation, but specific human data are limited (40). Other β-adrenergic agonists may be suitable alternatives (17), but there are even fewer human data to support their use. Theophylline is an effective bronchodilator on a short- or long-term basis and can be administered during gestation. Some recent studies in nonpregnant patients with asthma have not demonstrated benefit of theophylline

Table 4 Appropriate Therapy for Management of Severe Asthma During Gestation

1. General measures to reduce bronchial hyperresponsiveness
   - Allergen avoidance
   - Cessation of smoking
2. Inhaled beclomethasone dipropionate (8–20 inhalations daily)
3. Inhaled epinephrine or terbutaline
4. Theophylline with caution
5. Prednisone or methylprednisolone
   - Brief courses
   - Alternate-day or rarely daily
6. Depot methylprednisolone for malignant potentially fatal asthma or noncompliant gravidas
7. Cromolyn[a]
8. Antibiotics: penicillins, erythromycin, older cephalosporins
9. Allergen immunotherapy
10. Influenza immunization (after first trimester)

[a]Cromolyn is not routinely used for management of ambulatory patients with severe asthma.

when added to β-adrenergic agonists (42,43). However, it appears premature to discard theophylline from the management of the acutely ill gravida who may not be responding to epinephrine or terbutaline. In this setting, early administration of systemic corticosteroids is essential.

For ambulatory management of many gravidas with severe asthma, beclomethasone dipropionate (8–20 inhalations daily) and inhaled terbutaline or epinephrine provide effective asthma control. Some gravidas will require alternate-day prednisone, daily prednisone, or rarely depot methylprednisolone in cases of malignant potentially fatal asthma. Essentially all patients with severe asthma during pregnancy can be managed with these medications. The gravida must be taught effective inhaler technique whether or not an extender device is used. When the gravida develops severe coughing, wheezing dyspnea, or purulent bronchitis, rhinitis, or sinusitis, an increase in medications in indicated. A short course of prednisone, 30–60 mg daily, for 5–7 days may be advised and an appropriate antibiotic administered. The blood glucose level may be increased during gestation when oral corticosteroids are administered. During an exacerbation of asthma in gravidas who already require daily medications, additional theophylline or β-adrenergic agonists often produce limited to no additional benefit in terms of asthma control. More effective anti-inflammatory therapy, such as from a short course of prednisone, will help prevent emergency room visits and status asthmaticus.

Patient information sheets may be used for the asthmatic gravida, and some examples have been published concerning asthma during pregnancy (Table 5) and corticosteroids during pregnancy (Table 6) (40). Patients should contact their physicians when there has been a significant increase in symptoms so that additional pharmacotherapy can be instituted. Similarly, should the gravida be treated in the emergency room or office for an exacerbation of asthma, a short course of prednisone (44) should be administered to prevent complications from asthma that can result in maternal hypoxemia and stress for the fetus.

At the time of labor, hydrocortisone, 100 mg intravenously, should be administered to gravidas with severe asthma requiring corticosteroids and repeated every 8 hrs. This therapy provides for sufficient corticosteroid coverage should a cesarean section be required. Once the gravida is able to take her oral and inhaled medications, parenteral corticosteroids can be discontinued.

ACKNOWLEDGMENT

Supported by USPHS Grant Al 11403 and the Ernest S. Bazley Grant.

Table 5 Patient Information Sheet: Drug Therapy for the Pregnant Patient with Allergic Rhinitis or Asthma

Definitions: A drug or therapy that we consider appropriate for use in pregnancy is one that normally has been reported or otherwise shown to have no risk for the fetus or mother in human studies. This information is recorded in published medical journals. There are various drugs or therapies that may not be unsafe, but have not been proved to be appropriate; we do not recommend use of such drugs or therapies. The following drugs or therapies have been proved appropriate in human studies:

Antiasthmatic medications
- Theophylline
- Aminophylline
- Epinephrine by inhalation or by injection
- Ephedrine
- Cromolyn
- Prednisone
- Methylprednisolone
- Beclomethasone dipropionate by inhalation

Allergen immunotherapy (allergy shots)

Influenza immunization in second or third trimester

Antibiotics
- Erythromycin
- Penicillin derivatives

Antirhinitis medication
- Chlorpheniramine
- Diphenhydramine
- Tripelennamine
- Beclomethasone dipropionate by nasal spray
- Cromolyn

All allergic and asthmatic patients can be managed by these drugs singly or in combination.

We consider it of great importance to prevent the low oxygen levels that may occur in the mother during asthmatic episodes. Early treatment of asthma episodes is indicated, and you should call your physician for increasing symptoms as well as keep scheduled outpatient visits.

We would be happy to discuss any questions or comments that you may have about this information.

Other medication may be required for pregnancy as evaluated and prescribed by your obstetrician.

Source: Ref. 40.

Table 6 Patient Information Sheet: Use of Cortisone-Type Medications for Asthma During Pregnancy

We believe that cortisone-type medications, such as prednisone or inhaled drugs of this type (e.g., Vanceril, Beclovent), are required to help control your asthma.
Poorly controlled severe asthma (frequent wheezing, coughing, and shortness of breath) is a risk to your health and may be a risk for your baby. A study done at Northwestern University determined that mothers with poorly controlled asthma delivered babies with smaller birth weights than babies born to mothers with well-controlled asthma. Thus, every effort is made to keep your asthma well controlled during pregnancy.
There are a variety of complications from cortisone-type medications that are dose-independent. Cleft palates have been reported in offspring of rabbits exposed to very high doses of cortisone-type compounds in early pregnancy. This had led to a fear that their use in humans might similarly affect the baby. However, the amount of cortisone-type compounds used to produce these abnormalities in rabbits was much greater than that required to control human asthma. Several studies of the use of cortisone-type compounds in human pregnancy, including studies done at Northwestern University, showed no abnormalities that could be associated with the treatment. Thus, we believe that prednisone and beclomethasone dipropionate (Vanceril or Beclovent) should be used during pregnancy to help control severe asthma. The smallest dose of Vanceril or Beclovent and prednisone necessary to prevent severe asthma will be used.
It is most important that your asthma be managed properly at all times and especially now that you are pregnant. No medications should be taken unless your physician prescribes them. If you are prescribed prednisone, you must notify your obstetrician of this because prednisone may increase your blood sugar levels. You may be required to have your blood sugar measured during your pregnancy.

Source: Ref. 40.

REFERENCES

1. American College of Chest Physicians, American Thoracic Society. Pulmonary terms and symbols. Chest 1975; 67:583–593.
2. Friedman MM, Kaliner MA. Human mast cells and asthma. Am Rev Respir Dis 1987; 135:1157–1164.
3. Hsie HK-H. Effects of PAF antagonist, BN 52021, on the PAF-, methacholine-, and allergen-induced bronchoconstriction in asthmatic children. Chest 1991; 99:877–882.
4. Manning PJ, Watson RM, Margolskee DJ, Williams VC, Schwartz JI, O'Byrne PM. Inhibition of exercise-induced bronchoconstriction by MK-571, a po-

tent leukotriene D_4-receptor antagonist. N Engl J Med 1990; 323:1736–1739.

5. Israel E, Juniper EF, Callaghan JT, Mathur PN, Morris MM, Dowell AR, Enas GE, Hargreave FE, Drazen JM. Effect of a leukotriene antagonist, LY 171883, on cold air-induced bronchoconstriction in asthmatics. Am Rev Respir Dis 1989; 140:1348–1353.
6. Woolcock AJ. Asthma-what are the important experiments? Am Rev Respir Dis 1988; 138:730–744.
7. Barnes PJ. Neuropeptides in the lung: localization, function and pathophysiologic implications. J Allergy Clin Immunol 1987; 79:285–295.
8. Barnes PJ, Cuss FM, Palmer JB. The effect of airway epithelium on smooth muscle contractility in bovine trachea. Br J Pharmacol 1985; 86:685–691.
9. Filley WV, Holley KE, Kephart GM, Gleich GJ. Identification by immunofluorescence of eosinophil granule major basic protein in lung tissues of patients with bronchial asthma. Lancet 1982; 2:11–16.
10. Lee TC, Lenihan DJ, Malone B, Roddy LL, Wasserman SI. Increased biosynthesis of platelet-activating factor in activated human eosinophils. J Biol Chem 1984; 259:5526–5530.
11. Martin TR, Altman LC, Albert RK, Henderson WR. Leukotriene B_4 production by human alveolar macrophages: a potential mechanism for amplifying inflammation in the lung. Am Rev Respir Dis 1984; 129:106–111.
12. Arnoux B, Duval D, Beneviste J. Release of platelet activating factor (PAF-acether) from alveolar macrophages by calcium ionophore A23187 and phagocytosis. Eur J Clin Invest 1980; 10:437–441.
13. Durham SR, Craddock CF, Cookson WO, Benson MK. Increases in airway responsiveness to histamine precede allergen-induced late asthmatic responses. J Allergy Clin Immunol 1988; 82:764–770.
14. Greenberger PA, Patterson R. The outcome of pregnancy complicated by severe asthma. Allergy Proc 1988; 9:539–543.
15. Schatz M, Harden K, Forsythe A, Chilingar L, Hoffman C, Sperling W, Zeiger RS. The course of asthma during pregnancy, postpartum, and with successive pregnancies: a prospective analysis. J Allergy Clin Immunol 1988; 81:509–517.
16. Stenius-Aarniala B, Piirila P, Teramo K. Asthma and pregnancy: a prospective study of 198 pregnancies. Thorax 1988; 43:12–18.
17. Schatz M, Zeiger RS, Harden KM, Hoffman CP, Forsythe AB, Chilingar LM, Porreco RP, Benenson AS, Sperling WL, Saunders BS, Kagnoff MC. The safety of inhaled β-agonist bronchodilators during pregnancy. J Allergy Clin Immunol 1988; 82:686–695.
18. Apter AJ, Greenberger PA, Patterson R. Outcomes of pregnancy in adolescents with severe asthma. Arch Intern Med 1989; 149:2571–2575.
19. Schatz M, Patterson R, O'Rourke J, Zeitz S, Melam H. Corticosteroid therapy for the pregnant asthmatic patient. JAMA 1975; 23:804–807.
20. Greenberger PA, Patterson R. Beclomethasone dipropionate for severe asthma during pregnancy. Ann Intern Med 1983; 98:478–480.

21. Klebanoff MA, Shiono PH, Rhoads GG. Outcomes of pregnancy in a national sample of resident physicians. N Engl J Med 1990; 323:1040–1045.
22. Bahna SL, Bjerkedal T. The course and outcome of pregnancy in women with bronchial asthma. Acta Allergol 1972; 27:397–406.
23. Gordon M, Niswander KR, Berendes H, Kantor AG. Fetal morbidity following potentially anoxigenic obstetric conditions. VII. Bronchial asthma. Am J Obstet Gynecol 1970; 106:421–429.
24. Schatz M, Zeiger RS, Hoffman CP. Intrauterine growth is related to gestational pulmonary function in pregnant asthmatic women. Chest 1990; 98:389–392.
25. Fitzsimons R, Greenberger PA, Patterson R. Outcome of pregnancy in women requiring corticosteroids for severe asthma. J Allergy Clin Immunol 1986; 78:349–353.
26. Gelber M, Sidi Y, Gassner S, Ovadia Y, Spitzer S, Weinberger A, Pinkhas J. Uncontrollable life threatening status asthmaticus: an indication for termination of pregnancy by cesarean section. Respiration 1984; 46:320–322.
27. Assali NS, Rauramo L, Peltonen T. Measurement of uterine blood flow and uterine metabolism. VIII. Uterine and fetal blood flow and oxygen consumption in early human pregnancy. Am J Obstet Gynecol 1960; 79:86–98.
28. Quilligan EJ. Maternal physiology. In: Danforth DN, ed. Obstetrics and gynecology. Philadelphia: Harper & Row, 1982:326–341.
29. Greenberger PA, Patterson R. Management of asthma during pregnancy. N Engl J Med 1985; 312:897–902.
30. Prowse CM, Gaensler EA. Respiratory and acid–base changes during pregnancy. Anesthesiology 1965; 26:381–392.
31. Alaily AB, Carrol KB. Pulmonary ventilation in pregnancy. Br J Obset Gynaecol 1978; 85:518–524.
32. Cugell DW, Frank NR, Gaensler EA, Badger TL. Pulmonary function in pregnancy. I. Serial observations in normal women. Am Rev Tuberc 1953; 67:568–597.
33. Juniper EF, Daniel EE, Roberts RS, Kline PA, Hargreave FE, Newhouse MT. Improvement in airway responsiveness and asthma severity during pregnancy. Am Rev Respir Dis 1989; 140:924–931.
34. Walker CL, Greenberger PA, Patterson R. Potentially fatal asthma. Ann Allergy 1990; 64:487–493.
35. Detjen PF, Greenberger PA, Grammer LC, Patterson R. Malignant potentially fatal asthma: a management strategy. Allergy Proc 1992; 13:27–33.
36. Chandler MJ, Grammer LC, Patterson R. Noncompliance and prevarication in life-threatening asthma. NER Allergy Proc 1986; 7:367–370.
37. Tenholder MF, South-Paul JE. Dyspnea in pregnancy. Chest 1989; 96:381–388.
38. Cross D, Nelson HS. The role of the peak flow meter in the diagnosis and management of asthma. J Allergy Clin Immunol 1991; 87:120–128.

39. Martimer EA. Adolescent pregnancy. In: Berhrman RE, Vaugh VC III, eds. Nelson textbook of pediatrics, 12th ed. Philadelphia: WB Saunders, 1983:188.
40. Patterson R, Greenberger PA, Frederiksen MC. Asthma and pregnancy: responsibility of physicians and patients. Ann Allergy 1990; 65:469–472.
41. Wilson J. Utilization du cromoglycate de sodium au cours de la grosse. Acta Ther [Suppl] 1982; 8:45–51.
42. Self JH, Abou-Shala N, Burns R, Stewart CF, Ellis RF, Tsiu SJ, Kellerman AL. Inhaled albuterol and oral prednisone therapy in hospitalized adult asthmatics. Does aminophylline add any benefit? Chest 1990; 98:1317–1321.
43. Fanta CH, Rossing JH, McFadden ER. Treatment of acute asthma: is combination therapy with sympathomimetics and methylxanthines indicated. Am J Med 1986; 80:5–10.
44. Chapman KR, Verbeek PR, White JG, Rebuck AS. Effect of a short course of prednisone in the prevention of early relapse after the emergency room treatment of acute asthma. N Engl J Med 1991; 324:788–794.

13

The Management of Asthma During Pregnancy

Michael Schatz

Kaiser-Permanente Medical Center and University of California, San Diego, School of Medicine, San Diego, California

The management of asthma during pregnancy is important for both quantitative and qualitative reasons. Quantitatively, asthma is one of the most common potentially serious medical problems to complicate pregnancy. Retrospective data suggest that asthma complicates 1% of pregnancies (1), although recent unpublished data from the Kaiser-Permanente Asthma and Pregnancy Study suggest a prevalence of at least 3%. Qualitatively, experiencing and managing asthma during pregnancy is unique for the patient and her physician because the effect of both the illness and the treatment on the developing fetus as well as the patient must be considered. This chapter will review general concepts of asthma pathogenesis and therapy, specific goals of gestational therapy, nonpharmacologic and pharmacologic management of asthma during pregnancy, and the obstetrical management of the asthmatic patient. In addition, management guidelines for pregnant women with severe asthma are presented in Chapter 12 and the recommendations of the National Asthma Education Program Working Group on Asthma and Pregnancy are described in the Appendix.

ASTHMA GENERAL CONCEPTS

Definition

Symptomatic asthma may be defined as fluctuating degrees of chest wheezing, cough, or tightness associated with reversible obstructive airways disease or with bronchial hyperreactivity. Although most patients with asthma report the symptom of wheezing, and most patients who describe chest wheezing can be shown to have asthma, each may occur independently of the other. For example, in some patients, cough or dyspnea without wheezing may represent the sole symptom of asthma (2,3). Conversely, wheezing may occasionally be caused by processes other than asthma (see later discussion).

Etiology and Pathogenesis

The cause of asthma is unknown. However, certain pathophysiological mechanisms are currently considered important. First, there appears to be a genetic predisposition to asthma, although the exact mode of inheritance and the specific inherited defect(s) remain to be defined (4). Second, the airway hyperreactivity of asthma may be related to abnormalities of smooth muscle, abnormalities of bronchoconstricting and bronchodilatory neurogenic reflexes, β-adrenergic hyporesponsiveness, or α-adrenergic hyperresponsiveness (5). Third, eosinophilic airway mucosal inflammation triggered by IgE-mediated reactions, viral infections, and possibly other mechanisms, is currently recognized as being important in both the clinical manifestations and bronchial hyperreactivity of asthma (6). Finally, abnormalities in production of mucus and in mucociliary function are documented in patients with asthma (7).

Triggering Factors

Several types of exposures are known to trigger symptoms in patients with asthma (8). *Allergies* to pollen, mite, mold spores, and animal dander may trigger symptoms in allergic subjects. *Respiratory infections*, particularly viral infections and bacterial sinusitis, are probably the most important triggers of severe asthma and, apparently, may induce long-lasting clinical asthma in previously asymptomatic subjects. *Exercise*, if it is vigorous enough, will trigger asthma in most patients, and some patients wheeze only with exercise. *Aspirin* and other nonsteroidal anti-inflammatory drugs may trigger wheezing in approximately 10% of adult asthmatics, especially steroid-dependent patients and those with nasal polyps. *Irritants, aeropollutants, and meteorologic changes* all may trigger asthma, apparently nonspecifically. Finally, approximately one-third of women report exacerbation of their asthma several days *premenstrually* (9,10). Although premenstrual asthma occurs more frequently in women with more severe asthma, no clear relation has been documented between the occurrence of premenstrual asthma and the subsequent course of asthma during pregnancy.

Diagnosis

Most patients who complain of intermittent wheezing associated with chest tightness or cough can be shown to have asthma. Although the demonstration of auscultatory wheezing is more objective than subjective wheezing alone, the objective diagnosis of asthma depends on the demonstration of reversible obstructive airways disease on pulmonary function tests (11). It may be more difficult to demonstrate airway obstruction in patients with infrequent asthma episodes or in those with cough-variant asthma. In these circumstances, the diagnosis may be confirmed by methacholine testing (12). However, since methacholine testing is not generally recommended during pregnancy (13), pregnant patients whose history is consistent with asthma, but who lack pulmonary function confirmation thereof, should be considered for therapeutic trials of antiasthma medication after other causes of symptoms (see later) are excluded. A positive response to asthma therapy would support the diagnosis of asthma in such patients, which could then be confirmed by methacholine challenge postpartum, if indicated.

Various conditions must be considered in the differential diagnosis of asthma (8) (Table 1). *Mechanical obstruction* of the larynx, trachea, or main bronchi or *laryngeal dysfunction* are suggested by wheezing prominently over the trachea, inspiratory and expiratory obstruction on flow volume loops, and poor responsiveness to bronchodilators; these diagnoses are confirmed endoscopically. *Chronic bronchitis-emphysema* (14) should be considered in a smoker with irreversible airway obstruction, and α_1-antitrypsin deficiency (15) should be considered in a nonsmoking pregnant woman with irreversible obstructive airway disease. *Carcinoid syndrome* is suggested by episodes of flushing, diarrhea, and hypotension associated with wheezing and may be confirmed by finding elevated levels of urinary 5-hydroxyindolacetic acid (5-HIAA). *Hyperventilation* is suggested by the occurrence of dyspnea without wheezing associated with perioral and peripheral paresthesia and normal pulmonary function tests. *Cystic fibrosis* (16) should be considered in patients with persistent airway obstruction, especially when associated with a family history of cystic fibrosis, symptoms of exocrine pancreatic insufficiency, nasal polyps, or sinusitis.

Several conditions are particularly important in the differential diagnosis of asthma during pregnancy. *Dyspnea of pregnancy* generally presents in early or late pregnancy as dyspnea without wheezing or

Table 1 Differential Diagnosis of Asthma

Condition	Distinguishing features		
	History/physical	Pulmonary function	Laboratory
Mechanical obstruction (larynx, trachea, main bronchi)	History of injury, aspiration, hemoptysis Wheezing over the trachea	Inspiratory and expiratory obstruction on flow volume loop No response to bronchodilators Normal maximum midexpiratory flow rate	Endoscopy diagnostic
Laryngeal dysfunction	Wheezing over the trachea	Same as above	Endoscopy reveals adduction of vocal cords during symptomatic episodes
Chronic bronchitis/ emphysema	Smoking Daily productive cough Family history of emphysema	Irreversible airway obstruction	α_1-Antitrypsin deficiency
Pulmonary edema	Nocturnal dyspnea Wheezing may occur Cardiomegaly Gallop rhythm Valvular disease Tocolytic therapy	Decreased forced vital capacity	Chest x-ray: cardiomegaly, pulmonary venous hypertension, interstitial edema Echocardiography: mitral or aortic valve disease, left ventricular dilatation or hypertrophy, hypocontractile left ventricle in peripartum cardiomyopathy
Pulmonary embolism	*Sudden* onset of dyspnea/ wheezing		Arterial hypoxemia Abnormal perfusion on ventilation/perfusion scan Pulmonary angiography diagnostic
Carcinoid syndrome	Episodes of flushing,		Urine 5-hydroxyindole acetic

	diarrhea, hypotension associated with wheezing		acid (5-HIAA) elevated
Dyspnea of pregnancy	No associated wheezing or cough Early or late pregnancy	Normal	
Hyperventilation syndrome	Dyspnea without wheezing Perioral and peripheral paresthesias	Normal	Respiratory alkalosis (blood gases)
Amniotic fluid embolism	Acute respiratory distress during labor or delivery Cyanosis Shock Bleeding Wheezing may occur		Disseminated intravascular coagulation Demonstration of fetal elements in the maternal circulation
Cystic fibrosis	Family history of cystic fibrosis Chronic obstructive pulmonary disease Symptoms of exocrine pancreatic insufficiency Coexisting atopy common	Abnormal in 85–90% of adults Small + large-airway obstruction usual, but restrictive impairment may be seen early in course	Sweat chloride determination by pilocarpine iontophoresis >80 mEq/L chloride in adults (>98%) Abnormal sinus radiographs (>95%) Sputum culture of *Pseuodmonas* sp. (>60%) Chest radiography abnormalities (>98%) include hyperinflation, subsegmental atelectasis, increased bronchial markings, bronchiectasis 72-hr stool fat elevated Glucose intolerance

Source: Ref. 87.

cough and with normal pulmonary function tests. Patients with asthma can usually differentiate this dyspnea from chest symptoms caused by asthma. *Pulmonary embolism* may occur during pregnancy and usually presents with the sudden onset of chest pain, hemoptysis, and dyspnea, sometimes associated with wheezing. *Pulmonary edema* may cause wheezing ("cardiac asthma"), but the presence of cardiomegaly, left ventricular dysfunction, gallop rhythm, valvular disease, and interstitial pulmonary edema on physical examination, chest radiographs, or echocardiograms suggest the correct diagnosis. Two causes of pulmonary edema unique to pregnancy are tocolytic therapy (17) and peripartum cardiomyopathy (18). Finally, *amniotic fluid embolism* usually presents with acute respiratory distress during labor or delivery associated with cyanosis, shock, and bleeding, but the presentation may include bronchospasm (19).

GESTATIONAL ASTHMA MANAGEMENT

Goals of Therapy

Clinical data demonstrating the potential effects of asthma on pregnancy have been reviewed in Chapter 10. The results of two of these studies relate specifically to the goals of asthma therapy during pregnancy. First, data from Greenberger and Patterson (20) suggest that prevention of acute asthmatic episodes will improve perinatal outcome. These authors reported a significantly lower birthweight (2920 g) in the infants of mothers hospitalized for asthma during pregnancy compared with infants of mothers not requiring emergency therapy for gestational asthma (3354 g) (20). Prevention of acute episodes potentially involves (a) avoiding triggering factors (see following discussion), (b) early contact with the physician for increasing symptoms, and (c) avoidance of daily wheezing and optimizing pulmonary function.

Recent data further support optimizing pulmonary function as an important therapeutic goal during pregnancy. The Kaiser-Permanente study has demonstrated a direct relation between individual mean second forced expiratory volume (FEV_1) in asthmatic mothers during pregnancy and subsequent infant birthweight (21). Moreover, an inverse relation between mean FEV_1 and the occurrence of asymmetric intrauterine growth retardation was demonstrated that was independent of the effects of maternal smoking or medication use (21).

Nonpharmacologic Aspects of Management

The identification of potentially avoidable triggering factors is an important aspect of nonpharmacologic asthma management that may improve clinical well-being and decrease the need for pharmacologic intervention. Identification of allergic and nonallergic triggering factors and allergen environmental control measures are discussed in Chapter 5. It is particularly important for the pregnant asthmatic woman to discontinue smoking during pregnancy. First, smoking may predispose to increased asthma, complicating bronchitis or sinusitis, with an increased need for medication. Second, the increased perinatal morbidity attributed to smoking may be additive to that conferred by maternal asthma (21).

Careful follow-up by physicians experienced in managing asthma is an essential aspect of optimal gestational asthma management. Asthmatic patients requiring regular medication should be routinely evaluated at least monthly. In addition to symptomatic and auscultatory assessment, objective measures of respiratory status [optimally spirometry, minimally with peak expiratory flow rates (PEF)] should be obtained on every clinic visit. In addition, patients with more severe or labile asthma should be considered for home PEF monitoring (22). All pregnant patients with asthma should have facilitated access to their asthma physician for increased symptoms (23).

Psychological changes during pregnancy and their implications for medical management are reviewed in Chapter 6. It is particularly important that pregnant patients with asthma are educated about their illness and its interaction with pregnancy. Several examples of educational material for pregnant asthmatic patients have been published (23–25) (see also Appendix). Such education should improve patient compliance and reduce patient anxiety. It is also important that effective three-way communication exists among the physician managing the asthma, the patient, and the obstetrician.

Immunotherapy may be indicated for some asthmatic women of childbearing age. Immunotherapy during pregnancy is discussed in detail in Chapter 5. In general, it may be *continued* in patients who appear to be deriving benefit therefrom and who are not experiencing systemic reactions, but benefit-risk considerations do not favor *beginning* immunotherapy during pregnancy for most women.

Use of Specific Asthma Medications During Pregnancy

Safety data on the use of specific medications during pregnancy are discussed in Chapter 8. This section will highlight certain benefit-risk considerations in the use of specific asthma medications during pregnancy.

Recent data in subjects using inhaled *β-agonist bronchodilators* during pregnancy (26,27) support their gestational use. Their use is also supported by their efficacy with minimal associated side effects (28). Current data are insufficient to determine the safest specific inhaled β-agonist bronchodilator to use during pregnancy. In fact, any of the inhaled bronchodilators may be safe owing to their minimal systemic effects (26). Although recent studies have primarily used albuterol (28) or metaproterenol (26), both of these drugs are teratogenic in animals and possess a Food and Drug Administration (FDA) category C pregnancy rating (29). Terbutaline is currently being evaluted in the Kaiser-Permanente Asthma Pregnancy Study because of its relative β_2-selectivity (30), duration of action (30), reassuring animal studies (29), and lack of adverse effect on uterine blood flow (31). Oral β-agonists are not generally recommended for use during pregnancy because of lack of human data during early pregnancy, potential inhibition of labor during later pregnancy (32), and increased side effects, with little increased benefit in most subjects properly using inhaled β-agonists.

Theophylline has been a time-honored drug for use during pregnancy. However, its "first-line" use during pregnancy is being reevaluated because of (a) frequent gastrointestinal and central nervous system side effects; (b) occurrence of neonatal theophylline toxicity in some infants of mothers requiring theophylline at term (33); (c) the potential association in one study of its regular use with chronic gestational hypertension and prematurity (34); and (d) the availability of inhaled medications (*cromolyn*, *beclomethasone*) that appear to be safe during pregnancy (35,36), cause fewer maternal side effects, and may have advantages over theophylline in their anti-inflammatory–prophylactic effects (37). Actually, the use of inhaled corticosteroids during pregnancy is supported more by their efficacy and apparent lack of systemic effects at recommended doses than by the data that exist on their gestational use (36). Beclomethasone is generally recommended when an inhaled corticosteroid is indicated during pregnancy, since it has been available longer and some reassuring data on its use have been published.

The overall role of *anticholinergics* in the treatment of asthma remains undefined. No human data exist on the use of inhaled atropine or ipratropium for asthma during pregnancy, although animal data for ipratropium are reassuring (30). Several studies do suggest that the effects of inhaled anticholinergics may be additive to the effects of inhaled β-agonists in the treatment of acute asthma (38–40).

Although animal data have suggested adverse effects of the use of *systemic corticosteroids* during pregnancy (41), most of the human data have been reassuring (33). This difference may, in part, relate to the typical use of prednisone or methylprednisolone in humans (versus cortisone in animals), which has relatively poor fetal penetration (42,43). Recent data have associated the regular maternal use of 10 mg daily of prednisone throughout pregnancy with lower infant birth weight in nonasthmatic subjects receiving prednisone for pregnancy maintenance (44). However, regular prednisone administered during only the early first trimester (45) and employing smaller amounts of prednisone (21) have not been shown to lower infant birth weight. Moreover, review of data on the adverse effects of severe asthma on pregnancy (see Chapter 10), as well as the overall published experience concerning the use of oral corticosteroids for asthma during pregnancy (33) suggest that patients who require regular prednisone for control of their asthma would still be at greater risk from their uncontrolled disease than from the lowest effective dose of prednisone.

Pharmacologic Outpatient Management of Chronic Asthma

Medications suggested for the prophylactic management of chronic asthma are shown in Table 2A. The reliance on the use of inhalational therapy seems quite appropriate during pregnancy, but respiratory tract penetration of the drugs must be optimized by appropriate inhalation technique and the use of spacer devices (28). Medications should generally be added one by one until adequate control is achieved. As has been pointed out previously, "interpatient variability in asthma severity, compliance, and medication tolerance will lead to a variety of dosages and combinations of these medications which will ultimately

Table 2 Outpatient Management of Gestational Asthma

A. Prophylactic therapy (medications are generally considered sequentially as indicated)
   1. Regular inhaled cromolyn (2 puffs tid to qid)
   2. Inhaled beclomethasone (2–4 puffs bid to qid)
   3. Regular oral theophylline (generally long-acting preparations bid)
   4. Oral prednisone at lowest effective dose, preferably on alternate days
B. Therapy for increased symptoms
   1. Inhaled terbutaline (up to 3 puffs q3hr)
   2. Oral theophylline
   3. Oral prednisone course
   4. Antibiotics (generally amoxicillin, erythromycin, or cefaclor) for documented or suspected bacterial sinusitis, bronchitis, or pneumonia

be required to achieve acceptable asthma control in the individual patient'' (46).

The management of increased asthma symptoms unassociated with acute respiratory distress is shown in Table 2B. One must maintain a high index of suspicion for complicating bacterial respiratory infections during pregnancy, particularly for bacterial sinusitis, which has been estimated to be six times more common during pregnancy than in non-pregnant patients (47).

Management of Acute Gestational Asthma

Assessment

The management of acute gestational asthma begins with a proper assessment (48–51). A brief history should attempt to ascertain the duration of the attack, the apparent precipitating event, the presence of upper respiratory infection (especially with fever and purulent mucus), current medication (especially theophylline and corticosteroids), and any prior history of respiratory failure or intubation. The physical examination should particularly attempt to identify features suggestive of severe asthma, including use of accessory muscles, diaphoresis, pulsus paradoxus greater than 18, inability to lie down comfortably, pulse rate faster than 120, and respiratory rate faster than 30.

The first objective laboratory measurement to be obtained should be a PEF or an FEV_1. Nowak et al. (52) have shown that patients with an initial FEV_1 higher than 1 L or PEF of over 200 L/min will have a Po_2 higher than 60 and a Pco_2 lower than 42, and initial blood gas analyses may be deferred in such patients. However, blood gas concentrations should be obtained in patients presenting with values less than the foregoing or in those not responding to therapy. In interpreting blood gas values in women with acute asthma during pregnancy, it must be remembered (see Chapter 3) that blood gas analysis in the normal pregnant woman reveals a higher Po_2 (102–116 mmHg) and a lower Pco_2 (28–30 mmHg) than in the nonpregnant state. Thus, a Pco_2 higher than 35 mmHg or a Po_2 lower than 70 mmHg associated with acute asthma will represent more severe respiratory compromises during pregnancy than will similar blood gas values in the nongravid state.

Pulse oximetry may be considered as a noninvasive alternative to blood gas analysis when CO_2 retention appears unlikely. However, studies of the accuracy of oximetry and consideration of the oxyhemoglobin disassociation curve suggest that only an oximetry-determined O_2 saturation of 95 or higher can be considered sufficient evidence of adequate oxygenation (53).

A chest x-ray examination should not be obtained routinely, consistent with the recommended practice in nonpregnant patients presenting with acute asthma (54). However, a chest x-ray film taken with a shielded abdomen is felt to constitute no increased risk during pregnancy (55) and should be obtained in patients in whom pneumonia, pneumothorax, or pneumomediastinum is suggested; in those not responding to therapy; and in those admitted to the hospital (48). A baseline serum potassium level should be obtained, since β-agonists and corticosteroids may lower the serum potassium concentration, and a baseline serum glucose concentration should be obtained to look for hypoglycemia [to which pregnant patients may be unusually susceptible (56), particularly if not eating properly] or hyperglycemia (caused by corticosteroids or pregnancy).

Therapy

Supplemental oxygen (initially 3–4 L/min by nasal cannula) should be administered, adjusting F_{IO_2} to maintain a P_{O_2} of 70 or higher or O_2 saturation by pulse oximetry of 95 or higher (57). Intravenous fluids (containing glucose if the patient is not hyperglycemic) should be administered, initially at a rate of at least 100/mL/hr.

The recommended pharmacologic management of acute gestational asthma is summarized in Table 3. Most authors suggest nebulized β-agonists, rather than epinephrine, as the initial bronchodilator of choice for acute asthma in nonpregnant patients (48,49), and information on the use of inhaled β-agonists during pregnancy (discussed earlier) as well as the apparent equal efficacy of epinephrine and inhaled β-agonists in the treatment of acute asthma (58–60) suggest that this recommendation does not need to be altered during pregnancy.

Parenteral corticosteroids should be administered along with initial therapy to patients taking regular corticosteroids. In addition, McFadden recommends that intravenous corticosteroids be used in subjects with severe initial impairment who do not demonstrate a 30–40% improvement after 1 hr of intensive β-agonist therapy (49). Fitzgerald and Hargreave also support the early use of corticosteroids for acute asthma, pointing out that, "In all reviews of asthma mortality, failure to appreciate the severity of the attack . . . and failure to treat the condition with steroids have been important contributing factors" (48). There are no data on the pharmacokinetics of exogenous corticosteroids administered during pregnancy, and dosages of corticosteroids recommended for pregnancy are generally no different from those recommended for nonpregnant patients. Although there is insufficient data to determine the optimal dose of parenteral corticosteroids to be

Table 3 Pharmacologic Management of Acute Asthma During Pregnancy

1. Nebulized terbutaline (2–4 mg + 2 mL saline)
   May be repeated every 20–30 min, monitoring pulse rate, until respiratory distress corrected, $Po_2 \geq 70$, $Pco_2 < 35$
   Then taper to q4hr maintenance
2. Intravenous methylprednisolone (with initial therapy in patients on regular corticosteroids and for those with poor response during first hour of treatment)
   125 mg q6hr initially
   Taper as patient improves
3. Consider anticholinergics for patients responding poorly—nebulized atropine (0.025–0.050 mg/kg) or metered-dose ipratropium (2–4 puffs with spacer device) every 6 hr
4. Consider intravenous aminophylline. If it is to be used for
   Patient not receiving oral theophylline: 5 mg/kg over 20–30 min, then maintenance dose
   Patients receiving oral theophylline: stat theophylline level (< 5 μg/mL: 2.5 mg/kg over 20–30 min, then maintenance dose; ≥ 5 μg/mL: proceed to maintenance dose)
   Maintenance dose (initially) 0.5 mg/kg per hr following response, side effects and serum theophylline levels
5. Subcutaneous terbutaline 0.25 mg if not responding to the above therapy

used in patients with acute asthma, Haskell et al. (61) showed that three 125-mg doses of methylprednisolone every 6 hr was somewhat superior to 15 or 40 mg every 6 hr.

A recent meta-analysis of studies evaluating the efficacy and therapeutic index of intravenous aminophylline in the management of acute asthma was inconclusive (62). Although intravenous aminophylline may be considered, particularly in patients responding poorly to other therapy, its benefit in general may not outweigh its risks. If intravenous aminophylline is to be used, pharmacokinetic studies during pregnancy (63–65) suggest that the loading dose (mg/kg) recommendation for theophylline requires no modification during pregnancy, but the initial maintenance dose guidelines should be more conservative (see Table 3). In addition, studies have suggested that protein binding of theophylline decreases during pregnancy, such that there is an approximately 15% increase in free drug for any total drug concentration (63,66). This suggests that a lower therapeutic range (5–15 μg/mL) than is often recommended may be appropriate during pregnancy.

Hospitalization

Ten to fifteen percent of nonpregnant patients presenting to the emergency room will require hospital admission (51). The following pulmonary function criteria for admission have been recommended: Posttherapy $FEV_1 < 60\%$ predicted (52), < 2.0 L (67,68) or < 400 mL greater than pretherapy (69), or posttherapy PEF < 300 (68). Other criteria for admission include initial respiratory failure (even with improvement); the presence of complications such as pneumonia, pneumothorax, or cardiac arrhythmias; and repeat emergency room visit within 72 hr (51,57). Certainly, criteria for admission of the pregnant asthmatic should be no less liberal, and the coexistence of uterine contractions or fetal distress with acute asthma would also necessitate admission. When the pregnant asthmatic is hospitalized, both medical and obstetrical supervision is required.

Intubation was required in 2.3% of 811 consecutive hospitalized, nonpregnant patients (70), and two cases during pregnancy have been recently reported (71). The criteria for intubation in nonpregnant patients are as follows (50,51,57): (a) $Po_2 < 60-65$ on maximum supplemental O_2, (b) uncompensated respiratory acidosis ($Pco_2 > 55$, pH < 7.2), and (c) inability to clear secretions and the need to protect the airway owing to altered mental status. Although these criteria may also be applied to pregnant patients, it has been suggested that pregnant patients should be intubated earlier in the stage of respiratory acidosis (lower Pco_2, higher pH) (72).

Because of airway narrowing from hyperemia, nasotracheal intubation should be avoided during pregnancy (50). Sedation with morphine sulfate is recommended (50). Mechanical ventilation of the pregnant patient is the same as in nongravid patients (50) and weaning criteria are also the same, although it is recommended that pregnant patients maintain the lateral decubitus position during weaning near term to minimize the inferior vena caval compression caused by the gravid uterus (50).

Asthma Management During Labor and Delivery

Fortunately, substantial asthma symptoms during labor in women whose asthma has been controlled during pregnancy are unusual. In one study (73), 90% of asthmatic women experienced no asthma symptoms during labor and, of those who did, only half required treatment (4.1% inhaled bronchodilators, 0.5% intravenous aminophylline). Nonetheless, it is suggested that daily prophylactic medication (cromolyn, beclomethasone, or theophylline) be continued during labor. Asthma symptoms during labor requiring therapy should be treated initially with inhaled terbutaline by metered-dose inhaler or mechanical nebulizer (see Table 3). If the patient's asthma responds poorly to inhaled β-agonists, intravenous methylprednisolone should be administered. For persistent symptoms, inhaled anticholinergics and intravenous aminophylline may be considered (see Table 3). For patients receiving regular corticosteroids or who have received frequent courses during pregnancy, supplemental parenteral corticosteroids for the stress of labor and delivery are recommended: 100 mg hydrocortisone intravenously at admission, followed by 100 mg intravenously every 8 hr for 24 hr or until the absence of complications is established.

OBSTETRICAL MANAGEMENT OF ASTHMATIC PATIENTS

The obstetrical management of asthmatic women during pregnancy is generally the same as for nonasthmatic women (see Chapter 2). There are, however, several circumstances in which the presence of asthma may influence obstetrical treatment decisions. Prostaglandins may be used to induce labor for therapeutic abortion or for fetal death during the second trimester. Intravenous prostaglandin $F_{2\alpha}$ has been reported to cause bronchospasm in one patient with a history of asthma (74), and prostaglandin $F_{2\alpha}$ by the intravenous (75) or intraamniotic (76) route has also been reported to cause airway obstruction in nonasthmatic subjects. Although prostaglandin E_2 is generally considered to have bronchodilator properties, clinical bronchospasm has been observed in three patients receiving transcervical or intraamniotic prostaglandin E_2 (77), and intravenous prostaglandin E_2 has also been reported to cause increased lung resistance in seven other nonasthmatic subjects (75). It would appear that intravenous, intraamniotic, and transcervical prostaglandins for induction of labor should be avoided, if at all possible, in asthmatic subjects. If a prostaglandin is required for induction of labor, prostaglandin E_2 suppositories may be considered, with airway function and clinical respiratory status monitored closely, and prophylactic treatment with intravenous methylprednisolone also considered. Alternatively, concentrated oxytocin has been recently reported to be as effective as prostaglandin E_2 vaginal suppositories for mid–second-trimester labor induction (78).

Recently, intracervical or intravaginal application of prostaglandin E_2 gel has been used for cervical ripening before induction of labor during the third trimester. This procedure has not been reported to cause bronchospasm or airway obstruction (79). Specifically, prostaglandin E_2 gel applied by pessary for cervical ripening has been reported in nine asthmatic women without apparent adverse effects (80).

Ergonovine or methylergonovine may be used to stimulate myometrial contractions to reduce uterine blood loss postabortion or postpartum. Three cases of asthma exacerbation in patients receiving ergonovine for this purpose have been reported (81–83), and ergonovine has also been shown to cause contraction of tracheal smooth muscle in vitro (81). Thus, ergonovine derivatives should be avoided, if possible, in asthmatic women. If it must be used, careful monitoring and pretreatment with intravenous methylprednisolone are recommended.

β-Adrenergic antagonists may also exacerbate asthma, and all efforts should be made to avoid their use in the management of gestational hypertension in asthmatic women. When such drugs are essential in asthmatic women for the management of recalcitrant hypertension during pregnancy, a more selective β-adrenergic antagonist, such as atenolol or metoprolol (84), should be used. However, the cardioselectivity of these drugs is relative rather than absolute, and asthmatic women receiving atenolol or metoprolol must be carefully monitored for possible deterioration of their respiratory status.

Obstetrical management during labor and delivery of women with controlled asthma is identical with such management in nonasthmatic women, including the preference for regional versus general anesthesia. When general anesthesia is required for cesarean section, halogenated anesthetic agents to supplement balanced general anesthesia must be used with caution because, although they possess bronchodilator activities (85), their similar relaxing effects on uterine musculature have been associated with increased blood loss at cesarean section (86).

REFERENCES

1. Gordon M, Niswander KR, Berendes H, Kantor AG. Fetal morbidity following potentially anoxigenic obstetric conditions. VII. Bronchial asthma. Am J Obstet Gynecol 1970; 106:421.
2. Corrao WH, Brenner SS, Irwin RS. Chronic cough as the sole presenting manifestation of bronchial asthma. N Engl J Med 1979; 300:633–637.
3. Lusk JA, Winterbauer DF, Dreis DF, et al. Dyspnea of unknown etiology: prospective study of 92 consecutive cases. Am Rev Respir Dis 1986; 133:A56.
4. Gerrard JW. Genetic factors in the development of asthma. In: Weiss ER, Segal MS, Stein M, eds. Bronchial asthma: mechanisms and therapeutics, 2nd ed. Boston: Little, Brown & Co, 1985:24–29.

5. Nadel JL, Sheppard D. Mechanisms of bronchial hyperreactivity in asthma. In: Weiss ER, Segal MS, Stein M, eds. Bronchial asthma: mechanisms and therapeutics, 2nd ed. Boston: Little, Brown & Co, 1985:30–36.
6. Busse WW, Reed CE. Asthma: definition and pathogenesis. In: Middleton E, Reed CE, Ellis EF, et al., eds. Allergy: principles and practices, 3rd ed. St Louis: CV Mosby, 1988:969–998.
7. Wanner A. Airway mucus and the mucociliary system. In: Middleton E, Reed CE, Ellis EF, et al., eds. Allergy: principles and practice, 3rd ed. St Louis: CV Mosby, 1988:541–558.
8. Mathison DA. Asthma in adults: diagnosis and treatment. In: Middleton E, Reed CE, Ellis EF, et al., eds. Allergy: principles and practices, 3rd ed. St Louis: CV Mosby, 1988:1063–1092.
9. Gibbs CJ, Coutts II, Lock R, Finnegan OC, White RJ. Premenstrual exacerbation of asthma. Thorax 1984; 39:833–836.
10. Eliasson O, Scherzer HH, DeGraff AC. Morbidity in asthma in relation to the menstrual cycle. J Allergy Clin Immunol 1986; 77:87–97.
11. Pennock BE, Rogers RM, McCaffree DR. Changes in measured spirometric index. What is significant. Chest 1981; 80:97–99.
12. Chai H, Farr RS, Froehlich LA, et al. Standardization of bronchial inhalation challenge procedures. J Allergy Clin Immunol 1975; 56:323–327.
13. Huff BB, ed. Physicians' desk reference. Oradell, NJ: Medical Economics, 1992:1912.
14. Lalli CM, Raju L. Pregnancy and chronic obstructive pulmonary disease. Chest 1981; 80:759–761.
15. Giesles CF, Buehler JH, Depp R. alpha$_1$-Antitrypsin deficiency. Severe obstructive lung disease and pregnancy. Obstet Gynecol 1977; 49:31–34.
16. Palmer J, Dillon-Baker C, Tecklin JS, et al. Pregnancy in patients with cystic fibrosis. Ann Intern Med 1983; 99:596–600.
17. Howler F. Pulmonary edema associated with beta$_2$ sympathomimetic treatment of premature labor. Anesth Intensive Care 1984; 12:143.
18. Adler AF, Davis MR. Peripartum cardiomyopathy: Two case reports and a review. Obstet Gynecol Surv 1986; 41:675–682.
19. Scoggin CH. Pulmonary disorders. In: Abrams RS, Wexler P, eds. Medical care of the pregnant patient. Boston: Little, Brown & Co. 1983:249.
20. Greenberger PA, Patterson R. The outcome of pregnancy complicated by severe asthma. Allergy Proc 1988; 9:539–543.
21. Schatz M, Zeiger RS, Hoffman CP, et al. Intrauterine growth is related to gestational pulmonary function in pregnant asthmatic women. Chest 1990; 98:389–392.
22. Plaut TF. Peak flow: the key to success in asthma treatment. Am J Asthma Allergy Pediatr 1988; 1:172–177.
23. Patterson R, Greenberger PA, Frederiksen MC. Asthma and pregnancy: responsibility of physicians and patients. Ann Allergy 1990; 65:469–472.
24. Schatz M. Asthma and pregnancy: questions and answers. Asthma Allergy Found Am N Engl Chap Bull 1989; 5, (2).

25. Ziment I. Taking care of asthma when you're pregnant. J Respir Dis 1989; 10:91–92.
26. Schatz M, Zeiger RS, Harden K, et al. The safety of inhaled beta-agonist bronchodilators during pregnancy. J Allergy Clin Immunol 1988; 82:686–695.
27. Stenius-Aarniala R, Piirila P, Teramo K. Asthma and pregnancy: a prospective study of 198 prenancies. Thorax 1988; 43:12–18.
28. Newhouse MT, Dolovich MG. Control of asthma by aerosols. N Engl J Med 1986; 315:870–874.
29. Huff BB, ed. Physicians' desk reference. Oradell, NJ: Medical Economics. 1992:674, 2118.
30. Nelson HS. beta-Adrenergic therapy. In: Middleton EJ, Reed CE, Ellis ER, et al, eds. Allergy: principles and practice, 3rd ed. St Louis: CV Mosby 1988:647–665.
31. Akerlund M, Andersson KE. Effects of terbutaline on human myometrial activity and endometrial blood flow. Obstet Gynecol 1976; 47:529.
32. Schatz M, Hoffman CP, Zeiger RS, Falkoff R, Mellon M. The course and management of asthma and allergic disease during pregnancy. In: Middleton E, Reed CE, Ellis EF, et al, eds. Allergy: principles and practice, 3rd ed. St Louis: CV Mosby, 1988:1093–1155.
33. Labovitz E, Spector S. Placental theophylline transfer in pregnant asthmatics. JAMA 1982; 247:286.
34. Schatz M, Zeiger RS, Hoffman CP, et al. Preterm and low birthweight infants of asthmatic mothers: clinical correlations. J Allergy Clin Immunol (Abst) 1988: 81:275.
35. Wilson J. Utilization de cromoglycate de sodium a cours de la grossessa. Acta Ther 1982; 8 (suppl):45–51.
36. Greenberger PA, Patterson R. Beclomethasone dipropionate for severe asthma during pregnancy. Ann Intern Med 1983; 98:478–480.
37. Du Toit JI, Salome CM, Woolcock AJ. Inhaled corticosteroids reduce the severity of bronchial hyperresponsiveness in asthma but oral theophylline does not. Am Rev Respir Dis 1987; 136:1174.
38. Beck E, Robertson C, Galdes-Sebaldt M, Levison H. Combined salbutamol and ipratropium bromide by inhalation in the treatment of severe asthma. J Pediatr 1985; 107:605.
39. Ward MJ, MacFarlane JT, Davies D. A place for ipratropium bromide in the treatment of severe acute asthma. Br J Dis Chest 1985; 79:374.
40. Rebuck AS, Chapman KR, Abboud R, et al. Nebulized anticholinergic and sympathomimetic treatment of asthma and chronic obstructive airways disease in the emergency room. Am J Med 1987; 82:59.
41. Fainstat T. Cortisone-induced congenital cleft palate in rabbits. Endocrinology 1954; 55:502.
42. Beitins IZ, Bayard F, Ances IG, et al. The transplacental passage of prednisone and prednisolone in pregnancy near term. J Pediatr 1972; 81:936.

43. Levitz M, Jansen V, Dancis J. The transfer and metabolism of corticosteroids in the perfused human placenta. Am J Obstet Gynecol 1978; 132:363.
44. Reinisch JM, Simon NG, Karow WG, Gandelman R. Prenatal exposure to prednisone in humans and animals retards intrauterine growth. Science 1978; 202:436–438.
45. Smith KD, Steinberger E, Rodriguez-Rigan LJ. Prednisone therapy and birth weight. Science 1979; 206:96.
46. Schatz M, Zeiger RS. Allergic diseases. In: Gleicher N, ed. Medical therapy in pregnancy, 2nd ed. East Norwalk, CT: Appleton and Lange, 1992:435.
47. Sorri M, Hartikainen-Sorri AL, Karja J. Rhinitis during pregnancy. Rhinology 1980; 18:83–86.
48. Fitzgerald JM, Hargreave FG. The assessment and management of acute life-threatening asthma. Chest 1989; 95:888–894.
49. McFadden ER. Therapy of acute asthma. J Allergy Clin Immunol 1989; 84:151–158.
50. Hollingsworth HM, Pratter MR, Irwin RS. Acute respiratory failure in pregnancy. J Intensive Care Med 1989; 4:11–34.
51. McDonald AJ. Asthma. Emerg Med Clin North Am 1989; 7:219–235.
52. Nowak RM, Tomlanovich MC, Sarkar DD, et al. Arterial blood gases and pulmonary function testing in acute bronchial asthma: predicting patient outcome. JAMA 1983; 249:2043–2046.
53. Ries AL. Oximetry—know thy limits. Chest 1987; 91:316.
54. Findley LJ, Sahn S. The value of chest roentgenograms in acute asthma in adults. Chest 1988; 80:535–536.
55. Swartz WM, Reichling BA. Hazards of radiation exposure for pregnant women. JAMA 1978; 239:1907.
56. Pritchard JA, MacDonald PC, Gant MF, eds. The placental hormones, and maternal adaptation to pregnancy. In: Williams obstetrics. Norwalk, CT: Appleton-Century-Crofts, 1985.
57. Brenner BE. Bronchial asthma in adults: presentation to the emergency department. Part II. Am J Emerg Med 1983; 3:306–333.
58. Uden DL, Goetz DR, Kohen DP, Fifield GC. Comparison of nebulized terbutaline and subcutaneous epinephrine in the treatment of acute asthma. Ann Emerg Med 1985; 14:229.
59. Pancorbo S, Fifield G, Davies S, et al. Subcutaneous epinephrine versus nebulized terbutaline in the emergency treatment of asthma. Clin Pharm 1983; 2:45.
60. Elenbaas RM, Frost GL, Robinson WA, et al. Subcutaneous epinephrine vs nebulized metaproterenol in acute asthma. Drug Intell Clin Pharm 1985; 19:567.
61. Haskell RJ, Wang BM, Hansen JE. A double blind randomized clinical trial of methylprednisolone in status asthmaticus. Arch Intern Med 1983; 143:1324–1327.
62. Littenberg B. Aminophylline treatment in severe, acute asthma. JAMA 1988; 259:1670–1684.

63. Gardner MJ, Schatz M, Cousins L, et al. Longitudinal effects of pregnancy on the pharmacokinetics of theophylline. Eur J Clin Pharmacol 1987; 32:289.
64. Frederiksen MC, Ruo TI, Chow MG, Atkinson AJ. Theophylline pharmacokinetics in pregnancy. Clin Pharmacol Ther 1986; 40:321.
65. Carter BL, Driscoll CE, Smith GD. Theophylline clearance during pregnancy. Obstet Gynecol 1986; 68:555.
66. Connelly TJ, Rhuo TI, Fredericksen MC, Atkinson AJ. Characterization of theophylline binding to serum proteins in pregnant and nonpregnant women. Clin Pharm Ther 1990; 47:68–72.
67. Verbeek PR, Chapman KR. Asthma; who to send home, when to hospitalize. J Respir Dis 1986; 7:15–31.
68. Nowak RM, Pensler MI, Sorker DD, et al. Comparison of peak expiratory flow and FEV_1 admission criteria for acute bronchial asthma. Ann Emerg Med 1982; 11:64.
69. Kelsen SG, Kelsen DP, Fluge BF, et al. Emergency room assessment and treatment of patients with acute asthma. Adequacy of the conventional approach. Am J Med 1978; 64:622–628.
70. Scoggin CH, Sahn SA, Petty TH. Status asthmaticus: a nine-year experience. JAMA 1977; 238:1158.
71. Schreier L, Cutler RM, Saigel V. Respiratory failure in asthma during the third trimester: report of two cases. Am J Obstet Gynecol 1989; 160:80–81.
72. Stauffer JL. Emergency treatment of pregnant asthmatic patients. J Respir Dis 1983; 4:37–42.
73. Schatz M, Harden K, Forsythe A, et al. The course of asthma during pregnancy, postpartum and with successive pregnancies: a prospective analysis. J Allergy Clin Immunol 1988; 81:509–517.
74. Fishburne JI Jr, Brenner WE, Braaksma JT, Hendricks CH. Bronchospasm complicating intravenous prostaglandin $F_{2\alpha}$ for therapeutic abortion. Obstet Gynecol 1972; 39:892.
75. Smith AP. The effects of intravenous infusion of graded doses of prostaglandin $F_{2\alpha}$ and E_2 on lung resistance in patients undergoing termination of pregnancy. Clin Sci 1973; 44:17.
76. Kreisman H, Van de Wiel W, Mitchel CA. Respiratory function in prostaglandin-induced labor. Am Rev Respir Dis 1975; 11:564.
77. Fraser IS, Brach JH. Comparison of extra- and intra-ammniotic prostaglandins for therapeutic abortion. Obstet Gynecol 1974; 43:97.
78. Winkler CL, Gray SE, Hauth JC, Owen J, Tucker JM. Mid-second trimester labor induction: concentrated oxytocin compared with prostaglandin E_2 vaginal suppositories. Obstet Gynecol 1991; 72:297–300.
79. Rayburn WF. Prostaglandin E_2 gel for cervical ripening and induction of labor: a critical analysis. Am J Obstet Gynecol 1989; 160:529–534.
80. Lao TT, Huengsburg M. Labour and delivery in mothers with asthma. Eur J Obstet Gynecol 1990; 35:183–190.

81. Louie S, Kraznowski JJ, Bukantz SC, Lockey RF. Effect of ergometrine on airway smooth muscle contactile responses. Clin Allergy 1985; 15:173.
82. Sellers WFS, Long DR. Bronchospasm following ergometrine. Anesthesiology 1979; 34:909.
83. Crawford J. Bronchospasm following ergometrine. Anesthesiology 1980; 35:397.
84. Doany W, Brinkman CR. Antihypertensive drugs in pregnancy. Clin Perinatol 1987; 14:783–806.
85. Marx GF. Obstetric anesthesia in the presence of medical complications. Clin Obstet Gynecol 1974; 17:165.
86. Gilstrap LC, Hauth JC, Henkins GDV, Patterson AR. Effect of type of anesthesia on blood loss at cesarean section. Obstet Gynecol 1987; 69:328.
87. Schatz M, Zeiger RS. The management of asthma, rhinitis, and anaphylaxis during pregnancy. In: Lee RV, ed. Current obstetric medicine. 1991:78–79.

14

The Diagnosis and Treatment of Rhinosinusitis During Pregnancy and Lactation

Gary A. Incaudo

University of California, Davis, School of Medicine, Davis, California

Upper airway congestive symptoms during pregnancy have been recognized since the turn of the century (1), yet relatively little has been written concerning this problem, despite its frequency and occasional severity. Among randomly selected pregnancies, as many as 30% of patients will report substantial symptoms of rhinitis, and this figure may be higher among patients with preexisting atopic disease (2,3). Furthermore, the diagnosis of sinusitis in pregnancy may be as high as 1.5%, which represents a sixfold increase over the frequency observed in a nonpregnant population (4). There is understandable reluctance on the part of physicians caring for pregnant patients to employ the modalities commonly used in the diagnosis and management of rhinitis because of fetal risk factors, the time-limited nature of pregnancy, and the litiginous nature of the American public. Nevertheless, the risk of sinusitis and the effect rhinitis may have on the pregnant mother's eating, sleeping, and emotional well-being suggest that rhinitis during pregnancy should be actively evaluated and treated.

OVERVIEW OF NASAL PHYSIOLOGY IN PREGNANCY

In the normal nasal airway, optimal mucosal secretion and nasal patency depend on a fine balance between adrenergic and cholinergic stimuli. α-Adrenergic stimulation causes vasoconstriction and will increase nasal patency. In contrast, cholinergic stimulation induces both hypersecretion and vasodilatation giving rise to stuffiness and rhinorrhea. Factors that affect this autonomic balance include body cooling, exercise, change in body position, emotional disturbance, and atmospheric conditions.

The nose functions principally to air-condition the more delicate lower airway. The nose strives to maintain inspired air at 32°C, at 98% relative humidity, and free of dust and foreign vapors. Most water-soluble gases and particles larger than 10 μm are wholly filtered in the nose. Particles trapped in the mucociliary escalator mechanism are cleared every 10–15 min. This same escalator is one of the essential factors in promoting sterility within paranasal sinuses, despite heavy bacterial colonization within the nasal passages.

The nasal mucosa of the pregnant female differs histologically from the nonpregnant state. As early as 1956, Henderson made the observation that the columnar epithelium of the nose is subject to hormonal influence in a manner similar to the uterine cervical surface (5). In 1982, Toppozada et al., using electron microscopy (EM) and histochemical assays, demonstrated mucous gland hyperactivity, increased mucopolysaccharide in the ground substance, and increase phagocytic activity in the nasal mucosa of asymptomatic pregnant women (6). Excessive autonomic activity was not felt to be present, based on cholinesterase activity measurements in these studies, in contrast with earlier animal-derived data (7).

The rise in endogenous hormones, especially estrogens, has been indirectly incriminated as the source of the respiratory changes seen in pregnancy. Primate studies have linked estrogens to nasal mucosal swelling as well as perivascular edema (8). Similarly, Toppozada found highly comparable histological changes in estrogen–progesterone contraceptive users, strengthening a hormonal role (9). However, Bende could find no differences quantitatively in serum levels of estradiol, progesterone, or vasoactive intestinal polypeptide in pregnant patients with rhinometrically documented nasal congestion and a pregnant, symptom-free control group (10). Nasal vascular pooling from vascular smooth-muscle relaxation induced by progesterone or simply from increased circulating blood volume also has been suggested as sources of turbinate swelling (4).

The increased incidence of nasal mucosal hyperemia, epistaxis, and edema has been suggested as indirect evidence that nasal vascular pooling in pregnancy does, indeed, exist (11). However, in contradiction to such a single unifying physiological concept, Schatz and Zeiger described 348 pregnant asthmatic women with preexisting rhinitis, 15%

of whom experienced improvement in their nasal symptoms during pregnancy, often in association with improvement in their asthma (12). Perhaps, end-organ responsiveness to normally circulating hormones during pregnancy would serve to unify these conflicting studies, but such a hypothesis has yet to be demonstrated (Table 1).

In examining the nasal mucosa of pregnant women complaining of nasal congestion, EM and histochemical changes compatible with allergic disease have been described. Suggestions for the origins of this finding are varied and ill defined. In 1903, Roseman and Anderson demonstrated that guinea pigs could be sensitized to extracts of placental proteins (13). Placental proteins, fetal proteins, or endogenous hapten, all were incriminated as potential antigens in allergic pregnant women by Urbach and Gottaib in 1946 (13). Specific immunological reactions to endogenous hormones also have been incriminated by some authors (14,15), but discounted by others (16). The origin of these histological findings may simply lie in the enhancement of a preexisting atopic state. Both Schatz (17) and Mabry (2) have noted clinically that most women with rhinitis during pregnancy have had preexisting nasal symptoms.

OVERVIEW OF NASAL PATHOPHYSIOLOGY DURING THE CHILDBEARING YEARS

Factors of importance that upset the normal physiologic activity of the nose do so by means of either disrupting airflow or interrupting mucociliary clearance. Common causes of a dysfunctional nose pertinent to pregnancy are viral infections, allergic reactions to inhalant aeroallergens, chronic ambient air pollution, anatomical deformities obstructing air and mucous flow, abuse of topical vasoconstrictive drugs, and bacterial infections of the paranasal sinuses.

Common viral infections induce direct tissue damage to the nasal mucosa, with resultant inflammation and its consequences. Some indirect consequences of viral invasion are nasal mucosal hyperactivity through alteration in receptor responsiveness and impaired nasal mucociliary clearance. Secondary bacterial invasion is enhanced in these circumstances, especially from the heavily colonized nasal cavity to the paranasal sinuses.

Immunoglobulin E has emerged from the 1960s as the mediator of classic allergic reactions. The IgE-producing cells are located in the respiratory and gastrointestinal tracts. With appropriate stimulation in the susceptible host, homocytotropic, antigen-specific IgE antibodies are produced and fixed to mast cells and circulating basophils. The

Table 1 End-Organ Hypothesis of Hormonal Influence on Rhinosinusitis During Pregnancy

Preexisting Rhinitis States	Stress	Depressed Immunity(?)	Hormonal Influences
↘	↓	↙	↙
	"RHINITIS OF PREGNANCY"		
	⇅		
	Sinusitis		

"classic" allergic response has grown increasingly complex with the realization of late and delayed reactions being common accompaniments. Foxen et al. and Capel believed that nasal allergy was exacerbated or initiated by pregnancy (18,19). A more recent study failed to demonstrate any consistent change in serum IgE during pregnancy (20). The precise influence of pregnancy on each of the complex immunological steps involved in the allergic reaction has yet to be adequately described.

Cigarette smoke, formaldehyde, ozone, and sulfur dioxide are important air pollutants capable of provoking rhinitis symptoms, especially in the hyperreactive airway. Although not yet fully verified, it is likely that various environmental pollutants and chemicals are capable of nonspecifically stimulating the sensory nerves and the nerve terminals of the autonomic nervous system as well as the mast cells and epithelial cells to produce nasal hyperactivity. The increasing frequency with which women smoke, the increasing use of synthetic materials, the increasing prevalence of women in the workplace, and the generally deteriorating ambient air quality in our cities, all are relevant issues during the childbearing age.

Anatomical findings, such as septal deflections, polyps, and turbinate hypertrophy, all serve as potential additional sources of nasal obstruction in this aged group. The degree of obstruction induced will vary according to the extent and location of the anatomical blockage. Turbinate hypertrophy and polyps generally represent the end product of more severe nasal disease. A thorough investigation should ensue in light of these physical findings. Boggy, pale turbinates, with clear mucoid discharge, generally represent the eosinophilic forms of rhinitis, of which IgE-mediated disease is the most common example.

The actual extent and responsible mechanisms for the increased prevalence of bacterial respiratory infections during pregnancy remain uncertain. There is clearly a depression of maternal cell-mediated immunity during pregnancy, but this appears to be a selective process and not of a profound degree (see Chapter 4). Most evidence supports normally functioning humoral maternal immunity during gestation (20). There are, as yet, no immunological reasons defined to explain the observed increased frequency of infectious respiratory diseases during pregnancy.

Limited clinical observations have been made concerning bacterial rhinosinusitis in pregnancy. The organisms do not appear to be different from those found in the nonpregnant state. The peak onset was the second trimester in one study (4). This same study revealed that the classic symptoms and signs of sinusitis were absent in nearly half of the women studied with documented purulent sinusitis during pregnancy. Even in the nonpregnant state, sinusitis can be notoriously subtle in its clinical presentation, with very little in the patient history or physical findings to support a firm diagnosis (21). Considering the sixfold increased frequency of sinusitis in pregnancy, a high degree of suspicion must be considered in any pregnancy marked by persistent rhinitis of unknown cause.

Complaints of ear congestion, fullness, or stuffiness are frequently encountered during pregnancy. The responsible disorder is usually limited to the following conditions: (a) acute or subacute otitis media, (b) serious otitis media, (c) eustachian tube obstruction, or (d) patulous eustachian tubes. This latter condition, although not unique to pregnancy, is found most commonly during pregnancy. Clinical clues to this disorder are aggravation of symptoms in the upright position, by exercise, and by nervousness, as well as a sense of disturbed hearing owing to autophony. The frequency of onset of patulous eustachian tubes increases with each trimester and typically resolves postpartum (22). Derkay described 20 pregnant volunteers with symptoms of eustachian tube dysfunction, 80% of whom had demonstrable eustachian tube abnormalities by functional testing. Nineteen percent, or 3 of 16, demonstrated patulous eustachian tubes as evidenced by impedance variation synchronous with respiration (23). Hormonal factors may be significantly correlated with this disorder, as evidenced by its frequency both in pregnancy and in women who take birth control pills, but a direct cause-and-effect relation remains to be established (24,25). The differentiation of patulous eustachian tubes from the other aforementioned disorders of the middle ear space is important in that decongestants aggravate and antibiotics have very little effect on this clinical problem.

DIAGNOSTIC APPROACH

The combination of a carefully obtained history and physical examination commonly suggests the etiology of rhinitis in pregnancy (Table 2). Nasal cytologic examination is generally underused, but extremely helpful in many cases. The presence of eosinophils in the nasal mucosa or secretions is strong circumstantial evidence for an allergic cause and directs ancillary investigative procedures and treatment. If the identification of a potential allergen would be useful for formulating avoidance instructions, in vitro methodology, such as selective radioallergosorbent (RASI) or enzyme-linked immunosorbent assay (ELISA) testing is preferable. Routine skin testing during pregnancy is not recom-

Table 2 Differential Diagnosis of Rhinitis in Pregnancy

Allergic rhinitis
Bacterial rhinosinusitis
Rhinitis medicamentosa
"Vasomotor rhinitis"
Structural nasal obstruction
Eosinophilic nonallergic rhinitis
Nasal polyposis

mended because of the potential risk of anaphylaxis and subsequent adverse fetal effects (26–28).

The presence of purulent nasal discharge, facial pain or discomfort, and nasal cytologic appearance demonstrating neutrophils with phagocytosed bacteria in the nasal mucus strongly suggest purulent rhinosinusitis. However, rhinitis unaccompanied by any of these classic findings may still be based on sinus disease. Hence, the diagnosis of sinusitis would escape detection unless a sinus radiograph or maxillary antral puncture and culture is pursued. Limited sinus radiographs or maxillary antral washings should be considered when necessary for confirmation (29). Although physicians are rightfully cautious about ordering radiographs during pregnancy, the threshold dose of pelvic radiation exposure for induction of a congenital defect is considered to be 10 rad, more than 1000-fold greater than the amount of radiation received from routine diagnostic radiologic studies (30). A-mode ultrasonography has been suggested as a safe and efficacious screening modality for sinus disease (31). Unfortunately, if negative, it is not sufficiently sensitive, compared with radiography, to be used as a substitute for diagnosing sinus disease (32). A therapeutic trial of carefully selected broad-spectrum antibiotics may be pursued as an initial approach to the resistant case of rhinitis in pregnancy in whom there are no other clinical findings to suggest sinusitis. However, prolonged antibiotic therapy is not justifiable without confirmatory studies.

Several published reports suggest that allergic rhinitis, bacterial rhinosinusitis, and rhinitis medicamentosa are the most common causes of rhinitis during pregnancy (see Table 2) (2,3). Rhinitis medicamentosa has been cited as possibly being so common owing to a logical preference pregnant women would have for topical versus systemic medications to relieve their symptoms. Structural abnormalities, eosinophilic nonallergic rhinitis, and nasal polyps are also occasionally seen in pregnant women.

Much less common is the syndrome of *vasomotor rhinitis of pregnancy*. Nasal congestion from vasomotor instability develops most prominently in the second and third trimesters in this disorder and usually disappears within 5 days postpartum (33), although any accompanying eustachian tube dysfunction may persist for 4–10 weeks (23). Schatz and Zeiger have subcategorized gestational rhinitis that is not classifiable to any known disorder into two overlapping, nonallergic, noninfectious, noneosinophilic forms, which they term *nonspecific postnasal drip* and *vasomotor 'rhinitis'*. They feel that the former is a gestational hormonal effect on nasal mucus, whereas the latter more "stuffy" disorder represents the nasal vascular effects described previously (12). It is the knowledge of these prevalent etiologies of rhinitis in pregnancy that allows the physician to dictate a logical, direct, and cost-effective diagnostic scheme.

TREATMENT

In choosing among drug therapy options during pregnancy, efficacy must be considered, along with risk of inducing adverse effects on survival or development (see Chapter 8). In 1979, the Food and Drug Administration (FDA) mandated that all drugs approved after November 1, 1980, must include in the package insert all available information about the teratogenic and nonteratogenic effects of the drug during pregnancy. No rhinitis medication labeled since 1980 meets the requirements for pregnancy category A: "Adequate and well-controlled studies in pregnant women have failed to demonstrate a risk in later trimesters" (34). This, then, represents a major problem for the physician in choosing a drug during pregnancy, in that no rhinitis medication can be considered "safe" on the basis of "adequate and controlled clinical trials" (35), and such trials are likely never to be done. One way to manage pregnant patients with rhinitis in a medicolegal risk-free environment is to refuse to be responsible for their treatment during pregnancy. A more reasonable choice is to emphasize nonpharmacologic approaches, such as humidification, avoidance of irritants or allergens, and applying a judicious amount of tolerance to symptoms. Once medication is deemed necessary, the decision should be discussed with the patient referencing its benefits, risks, and alternatives. The discussion should be carefully documented in the medical record, along with a statement of the patient's consent.

The transfer of maternally ingested medications into breast milk has been extensively reviewed, although not all the medications used in the treatment of rhinitis are mentioned (36,37). Nearly all drugs pass into the breast milk. This fact, however, does not presuppose an adverse effect on the newborn, since many drugs will have already been inactivated, remain unabsorbed, or be destroyed in the infant's gut. The newborn, especially if premature, may be more sensitive to the negative effects of certain therapeutic agents because of a greater blood–brain barrier permeability, poorer enzyme conjugating capacity, diminished protein-binding capability, and decreased glomerular filtration rate. In general, if a drug is released for use in infancy, it can be safely administered to the lactating mother. Because of a lag time before a drug appears in breast milk, it may be best for the nursing mother to try to take short-acting formulations and use them 15 min after nursing and 3–4 hr before the next feeding, to minimize breast milk concentrations of the drug in question (38).

The information available concerning the safety of drugs used in the treatment of rhinitis during pregnancy is derived from two major studies and from sporadic case reports or small series describing the outcome of using a given drug in pregnancy. The first major work, and still the most quoted, was the Collaborative Perinatal Project (CPP), which involved 50,282 women studied at 12 centers during 1959–1965 (39). "Standardized relative risk" values were derived using the ratio of malformation rates in exposed to nonexposed mother–child pairs. A relative risk greater than 1.5 was considered suggestive of a cause-and-effect relation. However, despite the large number of women examined, this study suffered because the number of mothers exposed to any single therapeutic agent was small, creating a problem in defining true toxicity or safety to the satisfaction of all. Furthermore, there are many newer drugs being used for rhinitis, such as nasal cromolyn, topical beclomethasone and flunisolide, and the H_1-selective antihistamines terfenadine and astemizole, for which data are sparse or lacking. Because of the complexities in analyzing the data from the CPP, the authors warn that "none of the associations . . . should be regarded as anything more that hypothesis requiring independent confirmation" (39) and also that "Influences of causality based solely on our data are not appropriate" (40).

A second and more recent investigation analyzed pharmacy records of 6837 pregnant women who delivered between July 1977 and December 1979. Termed, the Group Health Cooperative (GHC) study, it equated prescriptions filled as long as 3 months before conception with drug exposure. This approach has drawn criticism and clouded interpretation of their data (12). The available gestational safety data for individual drugs used in the management of rhinitis is summarized in Chapter 8.

Decongestants

For the occasional episode of nasal congestion that may be interfering with sleep, oxymetazoline HCl drops or spray used as minimally as possible may suffice. The risk of rhinitis medicamentosa with continued use of this agent beyond 3–5 days should be emphasized. Although there may be little or no appreciable absorption of topical oxymetazoline at recommended doses, overdoses of topically applied imidazolines [e.g., oxymetazoline (Afrin), xylometazoline (Neo-Synephrine II)] carry the risk of hypertension followed by rebound hypotension and shock (41). Moreover, a nonreactive stress test and late decelerations (suggestive of uteroplacental insufficiency) occurred in a pregnant patient using four times the recommended dose (42). Should nasal obstruction require further therapy, pseudoephedrine 30–60 mg every 6 hr or 120 mg time-release capsule every 12 hr can be considered. A study of 6837 maternal–infant pairs demonstrated a less-than-expected incidence of malformations with the use of pseudoephedrine in conjunction with brompheniramine (43). All other α-adrenergic agonists studied by the CPP (epinephrine, phenylephrine, phenylpropanolamine) were associated with significantly increased risks of fetal malformation. Furthermore, all these agents can theoretically induce uterine vascular constriction. There are no specific data available concerning the use of decongestants during lactation.

Antihistamines

Patients with known eosinophilic allergic or nonallergic rhinitis accompanied by prominent sneezing and rhinorrhea may benefit from antihistamine therapy. Tripelennamine, 25–50 mg, as needed every 6 hr to a maximum of 200 mg/day can be recommended as the safest antihistamine for use during pregnancy, given available studies and the "antiquity" of this drug. Since antihistamines have little or no effect on nasal congestion, many patients would benefit from the addition of pseudoephedrine to this treatment plan. If intolerance or tachyphylaxis intervened, other antihistamines may be considered, but the risk/benefit ratio must be carefully considered, since the data is particularly unclear. The CPP reported statistically significant associations between brompheniramine and total congenital malformations, whereas chlorpheniramine was associated with an increased risk of ear and eye malformations and inguinal hernia (40). A later study by Jick et al. did not substantiate this finding with brompheniramine (43). An increased risk with diphenhydramine was also noted in the CPP and extended specifically to cleft lip and palate in a Finnish study (44). Animal teratogenicity in several species treated with hydroxyzine (45) prompted particular concern for this drug with additional suggestive risk emerging from the CPP data. However, no unusual congenital malformation prevalence was seen in another study of 74 women given hydroxyzine in the first trimester for gestational nausea and vomiting (46). Reassurance is suggested from data of Nelson and Forfar, who found significantly less antihistamine use in a group of mothers of infants with congenital malformations compared with matched controls (47). However, taken together, these data suggest that, if H_1 antihistamines, other than tripelennamine, are needed during pregnancy, they are best used only after the first 4 lunar months.

The regular maternal use of anithistamines at the time of delivery poses a further set of potential clinical mishaps. Parkin described a 5-day-old infant with tremulousness and diarrhea following the maternal ingestion of 150 mg of diphenhydramine daily throughout pregnancy (48). Another mother was reported who used 400 mg of hydroxyzine daily throughout her pregnancy and gave birth to an infant who demonstrated a transient narcoticlike withdrawal symptom complex (49). Finally, maternal antihistamine use has been associated with retrolental fibroplasia in infants with a birth weight of less than 1750 g (50). These data suggest that the regular maternal ingestion of antihistamines, especially in high doses, should be terminated as soon as possible before delivery in an attempt to minimize neonatal withdrawl risk, or should be avoided altogether in women at risk for delivery of very low birth weight infants.

Some adverse effects might be expected from breast milk containing maternally ingested antihistamines. This has, in fact, rarely proved to be true (51). A report incriminating clemastine as the cause of drowsiness and irritability in a nursing 10-week-old infant has been published (52). Clemastine concentrations in breast milk were 25–30% of the maternal serum values, but none could be detected in the infant's serum. The infant in this report showed resolution of symptoms within 24 hr after drug termination.

The trend in antihistamine research is being directed toward the development of highly selective, nonsedative drugs that reportedly do not cross the blood–brain barrier. Such therapeutic agents currently available in the United States, terfenadine and astemizole, currently carry a class C rating. It may be important to note that cetirizine, a newly developed H_1-selective antihistamine soon to be released, is a metabolic product of hydroxyzine, an antihistamine the safety in pregnancy of which has been a subject of controversy noted earlier.

Cromolyn Sodium

Animal and human data suggest that cromolyn sodium is safe in pregnancy, although there is no pregnancy data specifically on intranasal or ophthalmic use. Several points should be emphasized in considering the use of cromolyn sodium in pregnancy for allergic rhinoconjunctivitis. First, animal studies have not shown any harmful effects on the fetus at nontoxic maternal doses (53). Second, very little systemic absorption of cromolyn is seen with topical application. Finally, Wilson has reported a 1.35% congenital malformation rate among 296 asthmatic women who used cromolyn for asthma throughout their pregnancy, which is well within the expected frequency seen within the general pregnant population (54). For women with allergic rhinoconjunctivitis, we feel that intranasal or ophthalmic cromolyn sodium may be considered a treatment of choice.

Corticosteroids

Animal studies have suggested that corticosteroids may have adverse effects on the developing fetus when taken systemically. Particular attention has been paid to cleft palate, although intrauterine growth retardation, placental insufficiency, fetal resorption, and spontaneous abortion have also been described (55,56). The overall data concerning the use of systematic corticosteroids during human pregnancy are not so ominous. In fact, a large body of information on humans published in the past 25 years has not confirmed the fears generated by animal studies. Even though the controversy persists, the topical use of poorly absorbed or first-pass–metabolized derivatives, such as beclomethasone and flunisolide, respectively, for eosinophilic rhinitis during pregnancy, especially after the first trimester, seems justified. Because of their high topical potency and metabolic characteristics, very little if any of these drugs would be expected to reach the fetus during maternal intranasal use, but no specific information is available. In addition, the apparent safety of inhaled beclomethasone in the management of asthma during pregnancy suggests that the intranasal route of this drug also should be safe (57). For patients with significantly symptomatic nasal polyposis or eosinophilic rhinitis not responsive to antihistamine–decongestants or nasal cromolyn, intranasal beclomethasone can be considered, since human data during pregnancy are available. Occasionally, oral corticosteroids may be necessary for severe nasal polyps or eosinophilic nonallergenic rhinitis not responding to the foregoing modalities. Ideally, the oral forms should be withheld until after the first 4 lunar months.

With the exception of extremely high parenteral doses in status asthmaticus, the use of corticosteroids in the lactating mother poses no substantial threat in the infant. A 50-mg dose of prednisone in the lactating mother would transfer to the neonate less than 20% of its daily physiological corticosteroid requirement (58).

Antibiotics

Antibiotics remain the treatment of choice for bacterial sinusitis complicating rhinitis in pregnancy or lactation. Placental transfer of antibiotics has been documented (59). β-Lactam antibiotics and erythromycin (other than the estolate salt) appear to be safe during pregnancy and lactation (60,61). In contrast, tetracycline has reportedly produced impaired bone growth when administered early in pregnancy and discoloration and hypoplasia of the deciduous teeth when administered late in pregnancy and during lactation. Maternal hepatic injury has also been reported with tetracyclines when used during pregnancy (11,62,63). Although trimethoprim–sulfamethoxazole is an excellent antibiotic choice for sinusitis, especially in the penicillin-allergic patient, sulfonamides may induce bilirubin toxicity by competing for albumin-binding sites if present in the immediate newborn period. Furthermore, the folic acid antagonistic properties of trimethoprim may induce anemia (63).

The drugs of choice for the treatment of bacterial sinusitis in pregnancy and during lactation are ampicillin or amoxicillin. Clavulanic acid, a β-lactamase inhibitor, has been added to amoxicillin and marketed as Augmenten. Clavulanic acid carries a category B FDA rating, with no evidence of teratogenicity in animals; however, virtually no human pregnancy data are available. Although Augmenten may be a superior combination for the treatment of bacterial sinusitis, its use during pregnancy should be reserved for resistant infections with known β-lactamase-producing bacteria.

Erythromycin is commonly mentioned as an alternative drug in the treatment of sinusitis in the penicillin-allergic setting. However, an increased incidence of persistent sinus disease caused erythromycin-resistant strains of *Haemophilus influenzae* B has been reported, limiting its usefulness (64). Nevertheless, in such a clinical circumstance, erythromycin still appears as a reasonable alternative, especially in the last trimester of pregnancy. If it can be documented that the penicillin-allergic patient had used cephalosporins safely subsequent to the penicillin-allergic reaction, cefaclor (Ceclor) or cefuroxime (Ceftin) may be considered. A penicillin-allergic patient in whom cephalosporin tolerance has not been documented and whose sinusitis is not responding to erythromycin should be skin tested to penicillin (see Chapter 17). If the skin test results are negative, an oral challenge under observation with cefaclor or cefuroxime is recommended. If the skin tests are positive, an alternative antibiotic or penicillin desensitization (see Chapter 17) should be considered, depending on the particular clinical circumstances.

Since decreased serum levels of penicillins, cephalosporins, and erythromycin have been observed in pharmacokinetic studies of pregnant women, larger doses of these drugs are recommended (65). Dosages of 500 mg three times each day of amoxicillin, Augmenten, erythromycin and cefaclor are reasonable for gestational bacterial rhinosinusitis.

Humidification, Cleansing, and Avoidance Maneuvers

Nasal irrigation methods deserve mention as a useful nonpharmacologic modality in the treatment of sinusitis during pregnancy. This can take the form of a topically applied nasal saline mist available over-the-counter (OTC) or tepid physiological saline washed through the nose using either a bulb syringe, ear syringe, or more vigorously with a Water Pik and special nasal adapter. Avoidance of airborne allergens or irritants such as smog and smoke by staying indoors on high-risk days or through the purchase and use of an high-efficiency particulate air (HEPA) filter should also be considered, depending on the clinical circumstances.

Immunological Management

For the pregnant patient with known allergic disease, allergen avoidance is particularly important (see Chapter 5). Avoiding known allergens, when possible, will not only improve maternal well-being, but also minimize needs for pharmacologic intervention. If all pertinent allergens have not been identified before the pregnancy, identification of the offending agents may be of benefit. Because skin testing with potent antigens may be associated with systemic reactions, and since abortions and other adverse fetal effects have been associated with maternal anaphylaxis, skin testing should be replaced with in vitro methods, such as RAST tests to identify pertinent allergens (66). Historical information will usually suggest if house dust, mold, animal dander, or pollen are involved. Avoidance instructions can be empirically given in these circumstances. However, in selected patients, especially when dealing with indoor animals, selected RAST testing may be necessary to demonstrate the need for more vigorous avoidance maneuvers.

By similar reasoning, the initiation of immunotherapy during pregnancy should be avoided (67) (see Chapter 5). However, aside from the risk of systemic reactions, most authors recommend that allergen immunotherapy may be continued in patients who have experienced clinical benefit and who have not experienced systemic reactions (68). Consideration should be given to lowering the maintenance dose routinely to minimize the chance of a systemic reaction.

SUMMARY

The symptomatic human respiratory nasal mucosa in pregnancy represents a challenge to the physician both in terms of its diagnosis and therapy. Although there are several unique influences of pregnancy that adversely affect nasal mucosa, there is growing recognition that most symptomatic nasal problems are, in fact, expressions of known diagnostic entities in the nonpregnant state. In approaching gestational rhinitis, emphasis should be placed on making an accurate diagnosis so that specific and, therefore, limited medicinal intervention can be used. At the same time, the physician should remember that there is morbidity associated with ignoring this clinical problem altogether. Particular attention should be placed on the diagnosis and treatment of sinusitis, which may have a unique tendency for occurrence during pregnancy. Subtleties in clinical symptomatology and reluctance to use radiographs make sinusitis a particularly elusive diagnosis. Specialty consultation with otolaryngology or allergy may, at times, be necessary in the extremely symptomatic pregnant woman before an accurate diagnosis and successful therapeutic recommendations can be made.

The medicolegal atmosphere in the United States today unfortunately suggests that absolute safety for the fetus can only be guaranteed by practicing therapeutic nihilism for all women from puberty to menopause (57) (see Chapter 9). For those physicians choosing to take up this therapeutic challenge, emphasis should be placed on making the appropriate diagnosis so that therapy can be directed as accurately, yet as minimally, as necessary to achieve the desired therapeutic outcome. Some guidelines have been presented to assist the physician in choosing the "safest" form of therapy for the rhinological entities that commonly occur during pregnancy (Table 3). In the individual clinical situation, management decisions must be made only after establishing an exact clinical diagnosis and giving full consideration to the therapeutic risks, benefits, and alternatives. Moreover, the physician's interpretation of the benefit/risk ratio and the therapeutic decisions based

Table 3 Safest Treatment Choices of Common Rhinological Problems in Pregnancy

Type	Nonpharmacologic choices	Pharmacologic choices
Allergic rhino-conjunctivitis	Avoidance of antigens; continue successful immunotherapy	Topical cromolyn Na; tripelennamine +/− pseudoephedrine; beclomethasone (topical)
Bacterial rhinosinusitis	Nasal irrigation; sinus irrigation for resistant cases	Topical oxymetazoline for $<$ 6 days; antibiotics $\times$ 3 wk
Rhinitis medicamentosa	Discontinue topical vasoconstrictors	Pseudoephedrine +/− tripelennamine; beclomethasone (topical)
Vasomotor rhinitis	Nasal irrigation	Pseudoephedrine +/− tripelennamine; topical oxymetazoline for $<$ 6 days

thereon must be fully explained to and approved by the pregnant patient and documented in the patient's record.

REFERENCES

1. MacKinzie JN. The physiological and pathological relations between the nose and the sexual appearance of man. Alïenst Neurol 1898; 19:219–239.
2. Mabry RL. Intranasal steroid injection during pregnancy. South Med J 1980; 73:1176–1179.
3. Mabry RL. Rhinitis of pregnancy. South Med J 1986; 79:965–971.
4. Sorri M, Bortikanen-Sorri AL, Karja J. Rhinitis during pregnancy, Rhinology 1980; 18:83–86.
5. Henderson ID. Cyclical changes in female mucous. J Clin Endocrinol 1956; 16:905–909.
6. Toppozada H, Michaels L, Toppazada M, El-Ghazzawi I, Talaat M, Elwany S. The human respiratory nasal mucosa in pregnancy. J Laryngol Otol 1982; 96:613–626.
7. Reynolds SRM, Foster FI. Acetylcholine-equivalent content of the nasal mucosa in rabbits and cats, before and after administration of estrogen. Am J Physiol 1940; 131:422–425.
8. Taylor M. An experimental study of the influence of the endocrine system on the nasal respiratory mucosa. J Laryngol Otol 1961; 75:972–979.

9. Toppozada H, Toppozada M, El-Ghazzawi I, Elwany S. The human respiratory nasal mucosa in females using contraceptive pills. J Laryngol Otol 1984; 98:43–51.
10. Bende M, Hallgarde U, Sjogren C, Uvnas-Moberg K. Nasal congestion during pregnancy. Clin Otolaryngol 1989; 14:385–387.
11. Schatz M, Hoffman CP, Zeiger RS, Falkoff R, Mellon M. The cause and management of asthma and allergic diseases during pregnancy. In: Middleton E Jr, Reed CE, Ellis EF, et al., eds. V Allergy: principles and practice, 3rd ed. St Louis: CV Mosby 1988; 1093–1155.
12. Schatz M, Zeiger RS. Diagnosis and management of rhinitis during pregnancy. Allergy Proc 1988; 9:545–554.
13. Urabach E, Gottiab PM. In: Allergy, 2nd ed. New York: Grune & Stratton 1946; 128, 861.
14. Flarer F, Serri IF, Cotton DWK. Proceedings of the IXV international congress of dermatology. Amsterdam: Excerpta Medica 1974; 853.
15. Zondeck B, Bromberg YM. Endocrine allergy—clinical reactions of allergy to endogenous hormones and their treatment. J Obstet Gynecol Br Emp 1947; 54:1–19.
16. Helmy AM, El-Ghazzawi IF, Mandour MA, Shehata MA. The effect of oestrogen on the nasal respiratory mucosa. J Laryngol Otol 1975; 39:1229–1241.
17. Schatz M. Asthma and rhinitis of pregnancy: who's at risk? J Respir Dis 1986; 7:14–15.
18. Foxen EH, Preston TD, Lack JA. The assessment of nasal airflow: a review of past and present methods. J Laryngol Otol 1971; 85:811–825.
19. Capel LH. Recent advances in otolaryngology. London: Churchill-Livingstone 1973; 235.
20. Falkoff R. Maternal immunologic changes during pregnancy: a critical appraisal. Clin Rev Allergy 1987; 5:287–300.
21. Incaudo GA, Gershwin ME, Nagy SM. The pathophysiology and treatment of sinusitis. Allergol Immunopathol 1986; 14:423–434.
22. Bluestone CD. Assessment of eustachian tube function. In: Jerger J, ed. Manual of impedance audiometry. Dobbs Ferry: American Electromedics, 1975.
23. Derkay CS. Eustachian tube and nasal function during pregnancy: a prospective study. Otolaryn Head Neck Surg 1988; 99:558–566.
24. Plate S, Johnsen NJ, Pedersen SN, Thomsen KA. The frequency of patulous eustachian tubes in pregnancy. Clin Otolaryngol 1979; 4:393–400.
25. Pulec JL. Diseases of the eustachian tube. In: Paparella MM, Shumrick DA, eds. Otolaryngology, 2nd ed. Philadelphia: WB Saunders 1983; 1410–1411.
26. Entman SS, Moise KJ. Anaphylaxis in pregnancy. South Med J 1984; 77:402.
27. Erasmus C, Blackwood W, Wilson J. Infantile multicystic encephalomalacia after maternal bee sting anaphylaxis during pregnancy. Arch Dis Child 1982; 57:785–787.

28. Klein VR, Harris AP, Abraham RA, Neibyl JR. Fetal distress during a maternal systemic allergic reaction. Obstet Gynecol 1984; 64(suppl):15s–17s.
29. Swartz HM, Reichling BA. Hazards of radiation exposure for pregnant women. JAMA 1978; 239:1907–1908.
30. Jones KL, Chernoff GF. Environmental influences on fetal development: effects of chemical and environmental agents. In: Creasy RK, ed. Maternal and fetal medicine. Philadelphia: WB Saunders, 1984.
31. Landman MD. Ultrasound screening for sinus disease. Otolaryngol Head Neck Surg 1986; 94:157–154.
32. Shapiro G, Furukawa C, Pierson W, Gilbertson E, Bierman CW. Blinded comparison of maxillary sinus radiography and ultrasound for diagnosis of sinusitis. J Allergy Clin Immunol 1986; 77:59–64.
33. Mohun M. Incidence of vasomotor rhinitis during pregnancy. Arch Otolaryngol 1943; 37:699–709.
34. Specific requirements on content and format of labelling for human prescription drugs. Fed Reg 1979; 44:37462.
35. Briggs GG, Freeman RK, Yaffe SJ. Drugs in pregnancy and lactation. Baltimore: Williams & Wilkins, 1986; xxi.
36. Gardner DK, Rayburn WF. Drugs in breast milk. In: Rayburn WF, Zuspan FP, eds. Drug therapy in obstetrics and gynecology. Norwalk, CT: Appleton-Century-Crofts. 1982.
37. Lawrence RA. Drugs and breast feeding. Semin Perinatol 1979; 3:271–279.
38. Catz CS, Giacoia GP. Drugs and breast milk. Pediatr Clin N Am 1972; 19:151–162.
39. Heinonen OP, Slone D, Shapiro S. Birth defects and drugs in pregnancy. Littleton, MA: PSG Publishing, 1977.
40. Slone D, Shapiro S. Drugs and pregnancy [letter]. Ann Intern Med 1979; 90:275.
41. Ballen JC, ed. American Medical Association drug evaluation. Chicago: American Medical Association, 1980.
42. Baxi LV, Gindoff PR, Pregenzer GJ, Parras MK. Fetal heart rate changes following maternal administration of a nasal decongestant. Am J Obstet Gynecol 1985; 153:799–800.
43. Jick H, Holmes LB, Hunter JR et al. First trimester drug use and congenital disorders. JAMA 1981; 246:343–346.
44. Saxin I. Cleft palate and maternal diphenhydramine intake [letter]. Lancet 1974; 1:407.
45. King CTG, Howell J. Teratogenic effects of buclizine and hydroxyzine in the rat and chlorcylizine in the mouse. Am J Obstet Gynecol 1966; 95:109.
46. Erez S, Schifrin BS, Dirim O. Double-blind evaluation of hydroxyzine as an antiemetic in pregnancy. J Reprod Med 1971; 7:57–61.
47. Nelson MM, Forfar JO. Association between drugs administered during pregnancy and congenital abnormalities of the fetus. Br Med J 1971; 1:523–527.

48. Parkin DE. Probable Benedryl withdrawal manifestation in a newborn infant. J Pediatr 1974; 85:580.
49. Prenner BM. Neonatal withdrawal syndrome associated with hydroxyzine hydrochloride. Am J Dis Child 1977; 131:529.
50. Zierler S, Purohit D. Prenatal antihistamine exposure and retrolental fibroplasia. Am J Epidemiol 1986; 123:192–196.
51. White GT, White MK. Breast feeding and drugs in human milk. Vet Hum Toxicol 1980; 22(suppl):1–11.
52. Kok THHG, Taitz LS, Bennett MJ, Holt DW. Drowsiness due to clemastine transmitted in breast milk [letter]. Lancet 1982; 1:914.
53. Dykes MHM. Evaluation of an anti-asthmatic agent cromolyn sodium (Aarane, Intal). JAMA 1974; 227:1061–1072.
54. Wilson J. Utilisation du cromoglycate de sodium au cours de la grossesse. Acta Therap 1982; 8(suppl):45.
55. Blackburn WR, Kaplan HS, McKay DG. Morphologic changes in the developing rat placenta following prednisolone administration. Am J Obstet Gynecol 1965; 92:234–236.
56. Fraser FC, Watter BE, Fainstat JD. The experimental production of cleft palate with cortisone and other hormones. J Cell Comp Physiol 1954; 43(suppl 1):237–245.
57. Greenberger PA, Patterson R. Beclomethasone dipropionate for severe asthma during pregnancy. Ann Intern Med 1983; 98:478–481.
58. Hill RM, Tennyson LM. The lactating allergic patient: which drugs cause concern for the infant? Immunol Allergy Prac 1984; 6:221–227.
59. Charles D. Placental transmission of antibiotics. Obstet Gynecol Annu 1979; 8:19–25.
60. Hill RM, Tennyson LM. The effect of maternal allergy medications on the fetus. Immunol Allergy Prac 1985; 7:80–91.
61. Greenberg F. The potential teratogenicity of allergy and asthma treatment in pregnancy. Immunol Allergy Prac 1985; 7:4–9.
62. Holt GR, Mabry RL. ENT medications in pregnancy. Otolaryngol Head Neck Surg 1983; 91:338–341.
63. Schwerz RH. Considerations of antibiotic therapy during pregnancy. Obstet Gynecol 1981; 58(suppl):955–956.
64. Helin I, Andreasson L, Jannert M, Petterson H. Acute sinusitis in children—results of different therapeutic regimens. Heli Pediat Acta 1982; 37:83–90.
65. Philipson A. Pharmacokinetics of antibiotics in pregnancy and labour. Clin Pharmacokinet 1979; 4:297–309.
66. Francis N. Abortion after grass pollen injection. J Allergy 1941; 12:559.
67. Greenberger PA. Pregnancy and asthma. Ches 1985; 87(suppl):85s–87s.
68. Metzger WJ, Turner E, Patterson R. The safety of immunotherapy during pregnancy. J Allergy Clin Immunol 1978; 61:268–271.

15

Anaphylaxis in Pregnancy

Stephen I. Wasserman

University of California, San Diego, San Diego, California

Anaphylaxis is a true allergic emergency that can prove fatal. Fatalities from anaphylaxis have been demonstrated to occur within minutes, and it is the obligation of the physician to be prepared to recognize and treat this allergic emergency. Obviously, in pregnancy there is a twofold risk, in that the patient, the fetus, or both, may be harmed during an anaphylactic reaction. The purpose of this chapter is to review our understanding of this important clinical entity, to define some of the unique pathophysiological mechanisms in pregnant patients undergoing anaphylaxis, and to identify the best modalities for treatment.

DEFINITION AND ETIOLOGY

Anaphylaxis is the most critical of allergic emergencies. It may reach its peak within minutes and can prove fatal despite rapid treatment (1). Although the term *anaphylaxis* has been defined by some to indicate only IgE-mediated reactions with other similar non-IgE reactions termed *anaphylactoid*, it is preferable to use the term anaphylaxis to describe the clinical syndrome regardless of immune mechanism, as during such an episode its immunochemistry cannot be immediately ascertained. Manifestations of anaphylaxis include the nonspecific findings of flushing, pruritus, a metallic taste in the mouth, and a sense of impending doom. These symptoms may then be rapidly followed by one or more subsequent events, including urticaria and angioedema; upper (laryngeal edema) or lower airway obstruction; gastrointestinal manifestations of nausea, vomiting, abdominal cramping, and diarrhea; and the cardiac manifestations of dysrhythmia, hypoperfusion, third-space vascular loss, hypotension, and cardiovascular collapse. In addition, uterine cramping has been reported. These signs and symptoms may occur together or singly. Differing mechanisms may be responsible for the events triggering anaphylaxis as noted in Table 1.

EPIDEMIOLOGY

Anaphylaxis does not favor any particular time of year, occupation, sex, race, or geographic predisposition, except as these might expose individuals to particular anaphylactic-eliciting agents. Very little is known about the risk of anaphylaxis to any particular stimulus, and the risk of fatal anaphylaxis is even less well-defined. Fractions of a percent of patients receiving penicillin, or stung by Hymenoptera experience anaphylaxis, whereas fatal anaphylaxis to penicillin has been reported at a rate of 0.002% (2). It is thought that the risk of anaphylaxis increases directly with the number of encounters with medications or specific antigens, and that the parenteral route of administration of an antigen appears to be more likely to cause anaphylaxis than are other

Table 1 Mechanisms of Anaphylaxis

A. IgE mediated agents
   1. Antibiotics
   2. Foreign proteins
   3. Other therapeutic agents (eg. allergen extracts, vaccines, muscle relaxants, thiopental)
   4. Foods
B. Immune complexes/complement mediated events
   1. Blood or blood products
C. Modulators of arachidonic acid metabolism
   1. Non-steroidal anti-inflammatory drugs
D. Agents which directly degranulate mast cells and basophils
   1. Opiates
   2. Radiocontrast media
   3. Dextran
   4. Highly charged compounds
E. Exercise
F. Idiopathic

routes of administration. It remains controversial whether the atopic state predisposes persons to an increased risk of anaphylaxis. Although it is common practice to limit medications to which the pregnant patient is exposed, one must remember that even the most innocuous of drugs can be implicated in anaphylactic reactions. In addition, several important medications used to control pain or to assist in labor and delivery, such as oxytocin (3), have been implicated in anaphylactic reactions.

MECHANISMS

Immunoglobulin E-Mediated Anaphylaxis

For many agents, the participation of IgE has been proved or appears highly likely. This can be identified through the use of appropriate skin or blood (radioallergosorbent technique; RAST) testing, both of which identify antigen-specific IgE. Of particular importance are the antibiotics, including penicillin and other β-lactam antibiotics, with sulfanilamide derivatives also being an important cause of anaphylactic reactions. Foreign proteins, either as therapeutic agents (such as horse serum), or hymenoptera venom, have also been identified to be important causes of IgE-mediated anaphylaxis. A wide variety of foods have been identified to cause anaphylaxis, with peanuts, eggs, shellfish, and nuts being most important. Several therapeutic and diagnostic agents, including general anesthetics (4); muscle-relaxing agents (5); synthetic hormones, such as oxytocin (3) and progesterone (6); and, most recently, latex gloves (7) have been shown to cause IgE-mediated anaphylactic episodes in pregnant patients.

Immune Complex-Mediated Anaphylaxis

The administration of blood and blood products, particularly those that contain immunoglobulin A (IgA), have been known to induce immune complex-mediated anaphylactic episodes, presumably through the release of mast cell-activiting anaphylatoxins during the consumption of complement (8). Immune complexes are formed in patients who lack IgA or who have generated IgG antibodies to IgA for uncertain reasons. Similarly, aggregated proteins, particularly aggregated immunoglobulins, can also induce this syndrome.

Agents that Alter Arachidonic Acid Metabolism

Urticaria, angioedema, and anaphylactic responses to nonsteroidal anti-inflammatory drugs may be noted in as many as 0.5–1% of the general population (9). Intolerance to these compounds is often unrecognized, and their use may precipitate severe and profound reactions, particularly severe asthmatic episodes, accompanied by profound watery rhinorrhea or urticaria. As this reaction generally precedes more slowly than anaphylaxis and is much less often associated with hypotension, it can usually be distinguished from anaphylaxis. Nonetheless, nonsteroidal anti-inflammatory compounds can cause events that are impossible to distinguish from anaphylaxis.

Agents that Directly Degranulate Mast Cells and Basophils

Anaphylactic reactions to a whole host of therapeutic agents have been shown to be due to the ability of these compounds to directly release histamine (and presumably other important mediators) from peripheral blood basophils or mast cells. Agents known to cause such reactions include opiates (10), neuropeptides, highly charged compounds, plasma expanders, and radiocontrast media (11). Although these reactions are not due to antibody and, therefore, can be unpredicable on reexposure, individuals having had a reaction to one of these compounds run a much higher risk than the normal population of subsequently reacting to the same compound on reexposure. With radiocontrast media, risk is highest with intravenous use, and diminishes with exposure through the arterial or intravesicular route and with nonionic agents.

Exercise Anaphylaxis

In some persons, profound exercise, including the physical stress of labor and delivery (12), may precipitate anaphylaxis directly. This anaphylactic reaction may occur only after eating and, occasionally, only after eating a specific food. In some patients with food-associated exercise anaphylaxis, IgE-mediated food allergy has been demonstrated (13).

Idiopathic Anaphylaxis

In some patients who experience recurrent episodes of anaphylaxis, no inciting cause can be identified, despite rigorous and thorough analysis. Such persons are said to suffer from idiopathic anaphylaxis (14).

Clinical and Pathophysiologic Findings

The course of anaphylaxis, its onset, duration, and manifestations vary immensely among patients. As noted earlier, the integument, airway, cardiovascular system, gastrointestinal tract, and reproductive system may be affected singly, or in combination. Involvement of the airway and cardiovascular systems is of primary importance to mortality, with most fatal cases being due to respiratory complications and a significant minority being due to cardiovascular collapse. Symptoms usually occur within minutes of introduction of the causative agent, and it is rare for anaphylaxis to occur more than 1 hr after exposure to the eliciting stimulus.

Initial signs and symptoms often include flushing and pruritus, which may be accompanied by a sense of unease and light-headedness. Urticaria and angioedema, if they occur, may progress rapidly, but rarely persist for more than 24 hr.

Upper airway obstruction from laryngeal edema may progress, with associated swallowing difficulties, hoarseness, and eventually airway obstruction, which may lead to death from asphyxia. Lower airway obstruction (asthma) occurs more commonly in individuals who have underlying asthma, but may appear in the absence of a past history of asthma, and certainly may occur in the absence of upper airway obstruction.

Nausea, vomiting, diarrhea, and cramping abdominal pain are felt to be more common in individuals who are reacting to an ingested anaphylactic agent; however, they may accompany anaphylaxis induced by any route.

Reproductive system reactions, including uterine cramping, may be of special importance in the pregnant individual. However, miscarriage has only rarely been reported from uterine activation as a consequence of anaphylaxis (15).

Cardiovascular collapse is of obvious great importance, and may be due to cardiac arrhythmia, hypoxia, or vascular volume loss. This manifestation of anaphylaxis is of particular importance because of the known consequences of diminished uterine blood flow to fetal well-being. Myocardial infarction, as well as diminished myocardial performance, also occurs in anaphylaxis.

In rare instances, the first manifestation of anaphylaxis may be loss of consciousness. Death may occur within minutes or may be delayed for days to weeks. However, these late deaths are due to the consequences of early events, such as hypoxia and hypotension. It is commonly stated that the later the onset of the reaction, the less severe. Although logical, this is unproved. Recently, biphasic anaphylactic reactions, with severe early manifestation, followed by spontaneous recovery, and then a second recrudescence have been described (15). Not all observers agree that such late anaphylactic reactions occur or are important clinicial manifestations of anaphylaxis. However, some observers feel this is an important area requiring further research and may prove of clinical relevance.

PATHOLOGIC AND LABORATORY MANIFESTATIONS

The pathological and laboratory diagnosis of acute anaphylaxis is of very little clinical use. Pathological studies of patients dying of anaphylaxis have demonstrated acute airway hyperinflation, laryngeal edema, increased bronchial secretions, peribronchial vascular congestion, and eosinophilic infiltration (17). The upper airway edema associated with laryngeal edema is not inflammatory. No pathological markers exist for acute cardiovascular collapse; however, occasionally myocardial infarction may be identified. Electrocardiographic abnormalities may occur as a consequence of direct effects on the heart of anaphylactic mediators or may ensue following severe hypoxia, and include a T-wave flattening and inversion, conduction defects, bundle-branch block, superventricular arrhythmias, and currents of injury. Congestion of visceral organs, including the spleen and liver, have been described, as have edema or hemorrhage of various organs, such as the gut.

The laboratory analysis in anaphylaxis is likewise of relatively little clinical use in the acute setting. Hemocentration may occur when shock is present, owing to third-space fluid losses. Enzyme markers of myocardial ischemia or injury can occasionally be identified. Elevations in mast cell mediators, including histamine and, more recently, tryptase, have also been reported (18,19).

The diagnosis of anaphylaxis is often obvious, with its abrupt onset and characteristic constellation of findings. Of great importance is the complaint of pruritus by the patient, and the identification of flushing, urticaria, and tachycardia. In the absence of these findings, the differential diagnosis of anaphylaxis is more difficult. One of the most difficult differential diagnostic syndromes is that of vasovagal syncope. This often occurs following an injection or other painful or stressful stimulus, which may be particularly pertinent in the pregnant state. In vasovagal collapse, flushing is uncommon, and bradycardia is the rule. Patients experiencing vasovagal collapse often complain of nausea, but rarely of pruritus. Airway (upper or lower) obstruction does not complicate this syndrome. Instead, profuse diaphoresis often ensues. The pulse is slow, although profound hypotension, and even seizure activity may complicate vasovagal collapse.

In the case of upper airway edema, particularly laryngeal edema, the diagnosis of hereditary angioedema must be considered (20). Airway obstruction secondary to this disorder usually is slow in onset and prolonged, and it is *not* accompanied by urticaria, pruritus, or hypotension. Often a family history of similar reactions can be elicited. Hereditary angioedema is due to an absence of the functional inhibitor of the first component of complement. This disorder responds slowly to androgens, but not to antihistaminics, epinephrine, or glucocorticoids.

Causes of acute collapse must also be considered in the differential diagnosis, including such disorders as myocardial infarction, cardiac arrhythmia, pulmonary embolism, seizure, or stroke. All should be easily differentiable from anaphylaxis. A disorder known as laryngopathia gravidarum has been described during pregnancy in which progressive upper airway obstruction can occur (21). This is a slowly developing condition that should be easily distinguishable from anaphylaxis (see Chapter 16).

PATHOGENESIS

Anaphylaxis is thought to be due to mediators generated from activated mast cells and basophils (22). Activation of these cells can occur by IgE-mediated mechanisms or through a variety of other immune or nonimmune triggers. Such triggers include histamine-releasing factors produced by monocyte–macrophages and lymphocytes (23); complement fragments (3a and C5a), generated during complement activation; and direct membrane activation, especially by highly charged or membrane-active agents, such as neuropeptides and opiates.

Histamine is felt to be the central effector molecule of anaphylaxis. This amine is known to be responsible for many of the clinical manifestations of anaphylaxis, including urticaria secondary to endothelial disconnections and edema formation, as well as pruritus and flushing. Histamine also has a direct constrictor effect on the coronary circulation, and it may mediate bronchoconstriction. Thus, histamine may participate in many of the cardiovascular and respiratory changes associated with anaphylaxis. Leukotrienes (C_4,D_4), prostaglandin D_2, platelet-activating factor, and adenosine also have the ability to induce wheal-and-flare reactions, cause bronchoconstriction, and mediate cardiac depression and hypotension and, thereby, may be important contributing mediators in anaphylaxis or some of its manifestations.

The neutral proteases, tryptase and chymase, may not only prove useful as markers of mast cell participation in asthma, but may also mediate several of the respiratory changes seen in anaphylaxis. Finally, cytokines, especially tumor necrosis factor (24), are known to participate in septic shock, and their production by mast cells suggests they may play a role in the hypotension of anaphylaxis as well.

PREVENTION

It is clear that the most important aspect of anaphylaxis treatment is its prevention. Simple rules can be extremely helpful here. Patients should receive no medications that are not required, and those with known anaphylactic sensitivity should either avoid the stimulus or have appropriate treatment kits, which include injectable epinephrine, available. If patients are to receive medications, this should be done in an office setting where the effect of the medication may be observed, particularly if the parenteral route is to be used, as this appears to increase the risk of anaphylaxis. Clearly, taking a complete medical history, and educating the patient on unexpected exposures and cross-reacting medications are very important rules of thumb. If these simple rules are followed, many anaphylactic episodes may be avoided.

The physician also must be aware of uniquely important causes of anaphylaxis in pregnancy. For example, certain professions may predispose anaphylactic sensitization to unique antigens. For example, those in the medical and nursing professions are at risk for latex sensitization, and the role of latex gloves in inducing puerperal anaphylaxis has recently been demonstrated (7). The physician should also be aware that oxytocin (3) has been implicated as a direct mast cell degranulating agent and, in addition, some patients may develop anaphylaxis during labor and delivery as a manifestation of exercise anaphylaxis (12). A recent report indicates that progesterone also may cause IgE-mediated anaphylaxis (6).

If a patient must be exposed to a required therapy known to induce anaphylaxis, then desensitization must be undertaken. Since effective substitutes for nearly all antibiotics in almost all situations are available, the appropriate first step is to use an effective, non–cross-reacting antibiotic to treat anaphylactically sensitive patients. However, in special circumstances, such as subacute bacterial endocarditis caused by a penicillin-sensitive organism, or syphilis in the penicillin-allergic pregnant patient, it may be necessary to use an antibiotic to which the patient is allergic. If so, the technique of desensitization must be undertaken. This technique, although dangerous in itself, does through its successful performance enable individuals to receive medications to which they are anaphylactically sensitive. It is best done through the oral route, and it has been demonstrated successful for such drugs as penicillin and aspirin (25,26). The mechanism by which such oral desensitization is effective is uncertain. It does not confer lifetime safety, but rather, permits the use of the drug for a single course only.

When one is required to use an agent often associated with anaphylaxis (i.e., heterologous sera), but that has not done so in the patient previously, an attempt to address the presence of host sensitivity should be undertaken. This can be done by a prick–puncture skin test or an in vitro test, searching for antigen-specific IgE antibodies. Skin testing can be dangerous and care should be undertaken if it is to be performed (27). Prick–puncture skin testing appears to be the safest route and is available for the testing of various antibiotics, foods, hormones, proteinaceous drugs, and hymenoptera venom. If anaphylactic sensitivity is determined, then patients should avoid these drugs or compounds, be desensitized if their use is necessary, or receive true immunotherapy, as with venom anaphylaxis. In this latter example, it appears that the cost/benefit ratio favors the continuation of venom immunotherapy, even during pregnancy if anaphylactic sensitivity is known to be present (28).* The use of drugs that are known to cause direct histamine release, such as radiocontrast media, may best be undertaken in prior reactors by premedicating individuals with H_1 antihistamines, ephedrine, and glucocorticoids to prevent the effects of such mast cell activation (29).

TREATMENT

A detailed protocol for the medical management of anaphylaxis is described in Table 2. Effective treatment is immensely assisted by the rapid recognition of anaphylaxis symptomatology. Delay in therapy is associated with increased mortality (30). The patient should be placed in the left lateral decubitus position. A blood pressure of at least 90 mmHg should be maintained. The treatment of choice in anaphylaxis is epinephrine (Adrenalin). Although as an α-adrenergic agonist epinephrine may decrease uterine blood flow, its unique benefits in anaphylaxis outweigh its potential risks. It must be remembered that fetal distress may accompany anaphylaxis, which may lead to central nervous system abnormalities and even neonatal death if inadequately treated (32,33). Thus, aqueous epinephrine at a 1:1000 concentration, 0.3–0.5 mL should be immediately administered through the intramuscular or subcutaneous route. This can be repeated every 10–30 min as tolerated and required. Although some physicians advocate the use of intravenous epinephrine, its use has been

* However, it would appear that venom immunotherapy should be initiated during pregnancy only in patients with unusually high exposure risks.

Table 2 Kaiser-Permanente Severe Anaphylaxis Protocol*

Modify as desired, cross off nonapplicable orders

1. Call physician STAT.
2. P,R, BP every 5 min or every 2 min if BP < 90 mm Hg.
3. Patient wt. ________ kg.
4. O_2 at 6L/min by nasal cannula.
5. If systolic BP < 90 mm Hg, use Trandelenburg's position, place patient on left side and ECG monitor.
6. Continue ice and tourniquets if reaction secondary to injection, skin test, or sting.
7. Continue epinephrine (1:1000), 0.3 mL IM in deltoid, repeat every 10 min if reaction persists. In addition, give either half or equivalent dose into site of skin test injection or sting.
8. Start IV with 18 or 19 gauge needle or intercath, infuse Ringer's lactate; start wide open then check with physician for rate or volume (may require 3 to 10 L).

CONSIDER:

9. Benadryl (diphenhydramine hydrochloride; 50 mg/mL): 1 mL IV piggyback in 50 mL over 5 min.
10. Methylprednisolone (125 mg/2 mL) 2 mL in 50 mL IV piggyback over 5 min. Don't mix with Benadryl.
11. If wheezing, use terbutaline (2 mg/mL), 2.0 mL added to 2 mL saline and nebulize.
12. If symptoms persist, ranitidine (50 mg/2mL) 2 mL in 50 mL IV piggyback infused in 5 min.
13. If systolic BP less than 90 mm Hg and pulse less than 60/min, give atropine (1 mg/10 mL) 5 mL IV push, may repeat 10 mL if necessary in 5 to 10 min.
14. If still hypotensive, or hypotension recurs, use maintenance epinephrine: 1 mL epinephrine (1:1000) to 10 mL saline and infuse over 10 min. Consider repeating if still hypotensive, perfusing immediately after previous dose.
15. If still hypotensive, or hypotension recurs, use maintenance epinephrine: 1 mL epinephrine (1:1000) in 250 mL D_5 W (4 μg/mL) and infuse at 15 mL/hr (1 μg/min). Titrate every 5 min to maintain systolic BP ≥ 90 mm Hg. Maximum dose 60 mL/hr = 4 μg/min.
16. If still hypotensive, discontinue maintenance epinephrine and infuse dopamine (400 mg/5 mL): mix 5 mL with 250 mL IV solution (1.6 mg/mL) and start infusion at 0.15 × ________ kg (4 μg/kg/min) = ________ mL/hr to maintain systolic BP ≥ 90 mm Hg. Titrate every 5 min to maintain systolic BP ≥ 90 mm Hg (usual maximum dose 5 × infusion rate = 20 μg/kg min).
17. If ventricular dysrhythmia occurs, use lidocaine (100 mg/5 mL) acutely: 0.05 × ________ kg = ________ mL IV bolus which may be repeated in 5 min. Consider twice the dose in 15 min if necessary.
18. If dysrhythmia persists, lidocaine (2 g/50 mL) maintenance dosage: add 50 mL to 500 mL, D_5 W, and start infusion at 30 mL/hr (2 mg/min).
19. Consider glucagon if patient on β-blocker and anaphylaxis persists. Add 1 mL glucagon diluting solution to glucagon vial and infuse 0.5 mL IV push. May repeat if necessary.
20. If wheezing persists and patient is on no previous theophylline for past 24 hours, give bolus of aminophylline (500 mg/20 mL) 0.2 × ________ kg = ________ mL IV in 50 mL IV solution over 20 min.

*From Schatz M, Zeiger RS: Allergic diseases, in Gleicher N (ed): *Medical Therapy In Pregnancy*, ed 2. East Norwalk, Conn. Appleton-Lange, 1992, p. 435. Used by permission.

associated with myocardial infarction and death, and it should be reserved for those individuals who are in extremis, even after the use of subcutaneous epinephrine. When used intravenously the 1:1000 concentration of epinephrine should be diluted a further 10- to 100-fold, and administered slowly. If the cause of anaphylaxis has been an injected drug or venom, a portion of the epinephrine should be injected directly into the local site in an attempt to delay absorption of the inciting agent.

Some obstetricians favor the use of ephedrine as a first line of treatment to reduce the α-adrenergic effects of epinephrine on uterine blood flow (31,33). This may be tried initially, but has been reported to be less effective than epinephrine in the treatment of anaphylaxis in pregnancy (33,34).

Parenteral diphenhydremine (50 mg intramuscularly or intravenously) should generally be administered for persistent symptoms. Should airway obstruction persist, maintenance of the airway, either through mechanical intubation, or tracheostomy, if necessary, must be undertaken. Oxygen administration and the use of theophylline or inhaled β-adrenergic agonists may be useful should lower airway obstruction (i.e., bronchospasm) be identified.

Vascular collapse from third-space loss or fall of effective peripheral resistance should be treated not only with epinephrine, but also by intravenous fluids. Other modalities that have been demonstrated to be useful in some instances of anaphylaxis include antihistamines, which may be beneficial in the treatment of prolonged or severe hypotension. Repeated large doses of glucocorticoids, such as 125 mg of methylprednisolone (Solu-Medrol) intravenously, may be of benefit, although this has never been conclusively demonstrated. A recent issue has been the recognition of anaphylaxis in patients receiving β-adrenergic blocking agents. Such drugs limit the effectiveness of β-adrenergic agonists and may make the treatment of anaphylaxis quite difficult. Patients who are receiving β-adrenergic blocking drugs should be counselled regarding the difficulty of treating anaphylaxis, and their physician should be aware of the use of such drugs before administering any agent, particularly those with a high incidence of inducing anaphylaxis. Some advocate the use of glucagon to reverse β-adrenergic blockade in the anaphylactic setting, although the utility of this maneuver has not been proven.

PROGNOSIS

In general, anaphylaxis is rapidly responsive to the administration of adrenaline and fluids, and both mother and fetus do well (31). In the case of severe prolonged hypotension, maternal and fetal death can occur. In addition, severe prolonged hypotension may lead to severe abnormalities in the fetus, despite the recovery of the mother (32,33). For these reasons, the recognition and prompt treatment of anaphylaxis is essential. The rapid institution of treatment is an essential cornerstone of the therapy, but despite recognition and intervention, death has been reported even in well-staffed and prepared hospital facilities.

REFERENCES

1. James LP, Austen KF. Fatal systemic anaphylaxis in man. N Engl J Med 1964; 270:597–603.
2. Idsoe O, Gruthe T, Wilcox RR, et al. Nature and extent of penicillin side reactions with particular references to fatalities from anaphylactic shock. Bulletin, World Health Org 1968; 38:159–188.
3. Kawarabyashi T, Narisawa Y, Nakimura K, et al. Anaphylactoid reaction to oxytocin during cesarian section. Gyn and Obst Inv 1988; 25:277–279.
4. Baldo BA, Fisher M, Harle D. Allergy to Thiopentone. Clin Rev of Allergy 1991; 9:295–307.
5. Vervloet D. Allergy to muscle relaxants and related compounds. Clin Aller 1985; 5:501–508.
6. Meggs W, Peskovitz O, Metcalfe D, et al. Progesterone sensitivity as a cause of recurrent anaphylaxis. N Engl J Med 1984; 311:1236–1238.
7. Lavent J, Malat R, Smiejan JM, et al. Latex hypersensitivity after natural delivery. J Aller Clin Immunol 1992; 89:779–780.
8. Vyas GN. Perkins HA, Feudenberg HH. Anaphylactoid transfusion reactions associated with anti-IgA. Lancet 2:1968; 312–315.
9. Chafee FH, Settipane G. Aspirin intolerance: I. Frequency in an allergic population. J Aller Clin Immun 1974; 53:193–199.
10. Flacke JW, Flacke WE, Bloom B, et al. Histamine release by four narcotics: a double blind study in humans. Anest and Analgesia 1987; 66:723–730.
11. Brash RC, Rockoff SD, Kuhn C, et al. Contrast media as histamine liberators: II. Histamine release into venous plasma during intravenous pyelography in man. Invest Rad 1970; 5:510–513.
12. Smith HS, Hare M, Hoggarth C, et al. Delivery as a cause of exercise-induced anaphylactoid reaction: Case report. Brit J Obst & Gynecol 1985; 92:1196–1198.
13. Kidd JM, Cohen SH, Sosman HA, et al. Food-dependent exercise-induced anaphylaxis. J Aller Clin Immunol 1983; 71:407–411.

14. Wiggins CA, Dykewicz MS, Patterson R. Idiopathic anaphylaxis: classification, evaluation and treatment of 123 patients. J Allergy Clin Immunol 1988; 83:849–855.
15. Francis N. Abortion after grass pollen injection. J All 1941; 12:559–563.
16. Stark BJ, Sullivan TJ. Biphasic and protracted anaphylaxis. J Aller Clin Immunol 1986; 78:76–83.
17. Delage C, Irey NS. Anaphylactic deaths: A clinicopathologic study of 43 cases. J Forensic Sci 1972; 17:525–540.
18. Smith PL, Kagey-Sobotka A, Bleeker ER, et al. Physiologic manifestation of human anaphylaxis. J Clin Invest 1980; 66:1072–1080.
19. Schwartz LB, Louis RA, Austen KF. Tryptase from human pulmonary mast cells, purification and characterization. J Biol Chem 1981; 256:119–39.
20. Chappatte O, Deswite M. Hereditary angioneurotic edema and pregnancy: case reports and review of the literature. Brit J Obst Gyne 1988; 95:938.–942.
21. Bhatia PL, Singh MS, Jha BK. Layrngopathia gravidarum. Ear Nose Throat J 1981; 60:408–412.
22. Sheffer AL. Anaphylaxis. J Aller Clin Imm 1985; 75:227–233.
23. Grant JA, Alam R, Alam R, Letbrown MA. Histamine releasing factors and inhibitors: historical perspectives and possible implications in human illness. J Aller Clin Imm 1991; 88:683–693.
24. Walsh LJ, Trinchieri G, Waldorf HA, et al. Human dermal mast cells contain a released tumor necrosis factor α, which induces endothelial leukocyte adhesion molecule 1. Proc Natl Acad Sci 1991; 88:4220–4224.
25. Pleskow W, Stevenson D, Mathison DA, et al. Aspirin desensitization and aspirin sensitive asthmatic patients: clinical manifestations and characterization of the refractory period. J Allergy Clin Immunol 1981; 69:11–19.
26. Sullivan TC, Yecies LD, Shatz GS, et al. Desensitization of patients allergic to penicillin using orally administered beta lactam antibiotics. J Allergy Clin Immunol 1982; 69:275–282.
27. Blanton WB, Sutphin AK. Death during skin testing. Am J Med 1949; 217:169–173.
28. Schwartz HJ, Golden DBK, Lockie RF. Venom immunotherapy in the hymenoptera-allergic pregnant patient. J Aller Clin Imm 1990; 85:709–712.
29. Kelly JF, Patterson R, Leiberman P, et al. Radiographic contrast media studies in high risk patients. J Allergy Clin Immunol 1978; 62:181–184.
30. Barnard JH. Studies of 400 hymenoptera sting deaths in the United States. J Allergy Clin Immunol 1973; 52:259–264.
31. Klein VR, Harris AD, Abraham RA, Niebyl JR. Fetal distress during a maternal systemic allergic reaction. Obstet Gynecol 1984; 64 (suppl):155–175.

32. Erasmus C, Blackwood W, Wilson J. Infantile multicystic encephalomalacia after maternal bee sting anaphylaxis during pregnancy. Archives of Disease of Child 1982; 57:785–787.
33. Entman SS, Maise KJ. Anaphylaxis in pregnancy. South Med J 1984; 77:402.
34. Gallagher JS. Anaphylaxis in pregnancy. Obstet Gynecol 1988; 71:491–493.

16

Cutaneous Diseases During Pregnancy

Joseph Alcalay

Tel-Aviv University, Tel-Aviv, Israel

Robert S. Zeiger

University of California, San Diego, School of Medicine, and Kaiser-Permanente Medical Center, San Diego, California

I will greatly increase the pangs of your childbearing; in pain shall you bring forth children.—Genesis 3:16

Cutaneous disorders during pregnancy represent common afflictions that cause moderate concern and frequent pruritus to the parous woman. A systematic approach to the diagnosis of the allergic and immunological skin diseases during pregnancy should help institute appropriate therapy to alleviate suffering. This chapter will emphasize the specific dermatoses of pregnancy (Table 1), as well as the two more common atopic cutaneous diseases, urticaria–angioedema and atopic dermatitis. An understanding of these conditions will aid the concerned clinician in the care of the pregnant woman.

AUTOIMMUNE DISEASES

Herpes Gestationis (Pemphigoid Gestations)

Herpes gestationis is a specific skin disease of pregnancy and the puerperium. There is no relation between herpes gestationis and the herpes virus. *Herpes* comes from the Green word *to creep*, and Galen was the first to use this term to describe any dermatosis characterized by the formation of small vesicles, occasionally in clusters. Herpes gestationis is an intensely pruritic, yet exceedingly uncommon eruption. Early reports estimated the incidence to be from 1:3000 to 1:10,000 pregnancies (1,2). Kolodny in 1969 (2) counted the numbers of patients between

Table 1 Comparative Characteristics of the Pruritic Dermatoses of Pregnancy

	Herpes gestationis	Pruritic folliculitis of pregnancy	Prurigo gestationis	PUPPP[a]	Impetigo herpetiformis[b]	Pruritus gravidarum
Onset and incidence	Second trimester; rare	4th to 9th mo; rare	25th to 30th wk; 0.3–2%	Last trimester; 0.5%	Second half of pregnancy; rare	Last trimester; common (0.02–2.4%)
Gravidity preference	Multigravidas	None	None	Primigravidas	None	None
Distribution	Generalized: buttocks, abdomen, extremities, mucous membranes	Shoulders, back, buttocks, abdomen, thigh, "acne of pregnancy"	Trunk and extremities (extensor surfaces)	Abdomen with spread to extremities; striae involved: face spared	Intertriginous zones and thighs	Abdomen, trunk, extremities
Clinical lesions	Erythematous papules, vesicles bullae Constitutional symptoms	Follicular erythematous papules	Excoriated erythematous papules	Erythematous papules and urticarial plaques; excoriations rare	Small, sometimes coalescent pustules; constitutional symptoms	No primary lesions; excoriations
Pruritus	Moderate to severe	Moderate	Moderate	Severe	Mild to none	Mild to severe
Histology	Subepidermal bullae often containing eosinophils	Acute sterile folliculitis, dermal edema, and perivascular infiltrates	Parakeratosis, acanthosis, with dermal perivesicular infiltration of lymphocytes	Spongiotic dermatitis with superficial mixed perivascular inflammation	Spongioform and intraepidermal pustule	Nonspecific cholestasis of liver; no skin biopsy data
Immunofluorescence	C_3 deposition at basement membranes in lesional skin	Negative	Negative	Negative	ND	ND

Laboratory abnormalities	Peripheral blood eosinophilia; ↑ HLA-B8 and DR3; circulating HG factor (autoantibody)	None	None, but associated with atopy?	None	↓ Ca^{2+}, ↑ ESR, ↑ WBC	↑ Bile acid; abnormal liver functions (variable)
Treatment	Systemic steroids as topical steroids usually inadequate	10% benzoyl peroxide and 1% hydrocortisone	Topical antipruritics, oral antihistamines	Topical steroids; systemic steroids if necessary	Ca^{2+}, vitamin D, systemic steroids	Topical antipruritics, cholestyramine
Complications	Maternal: ↑ infection; fetal: prematurity and stillbirth; blisters in neonate	None	None	None	Maternal: prostration, renal failure, cardiac failure, death; Fetal: abortion, stillbirth, neonatal death	Maternal: none; fetal: prematurity
Prognosis	May flare postpartum Recurrences common in subsequent pregnancies	Clears postpartum Recurs in one third of patients	Clears postpartum Recurrences uncommon	Clears postpartum Recurrence rare	Clears postpartum, recurs earlier in subsequent pregnancies	Clears postpartum Recurrences common in subsequent pregnancies

[a]Pruritic urticarial papules and plaques of pregnancy.
[b]Possibly pustular psoriasis exacerbated by pregnancy.
ND, No data; *ESR*, erythrocyte sedimentation rate; *WBC*, white blood cell count.
Source: Ref. 5.

1945 and 1967 in two university hospitals in St. Louis. Although his estimation was 1:10,000, he was able to find only two patients with the disease among 113,000 deliveries. Holmes et al. found two cases of herpes gestationis during 21 years at St. Thomas Hospital in London (3). During that time there were approximately 84,000 deliveries; this brings the incidence to 1:42,000. An incidence of 1:50,000 was reported by Shornick et al. from the Dallas–Fort Worth area (4).

Clinical Presentation

Herpes gestationis is a vesiculobullous disease. It may begin between the second trimester and 1 week postpartum, with an average onset of 21 weeks (3). Severe chronic pruritus is found in all patients suffering from herpes gestationis, with the pruritus sometimes preceding the eruption. In more than 90% of patients, the eruption begins in the umbilical area (Figure 1), with subsequent symmetric involvement extending to the trunk and extremities. Its onset consists of urticarial papules, erythematous plaques (Figure 2), small vesicles, and bullae (Figure 3). The average interval between the onset of the papules and the bullous lesions can be 4 weeks (3). The morphology may show

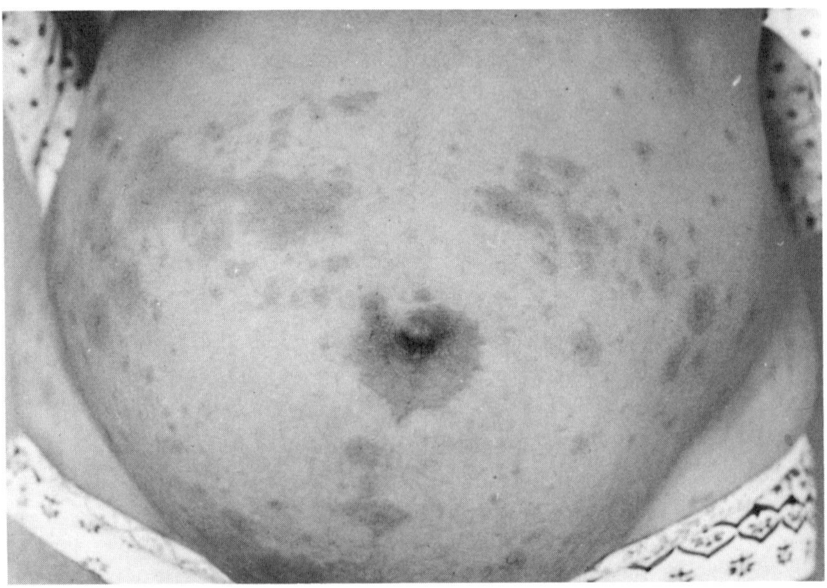

Figure 1 Herpes gestationis: involvement of the umbilical area with typical urticarial plaques.

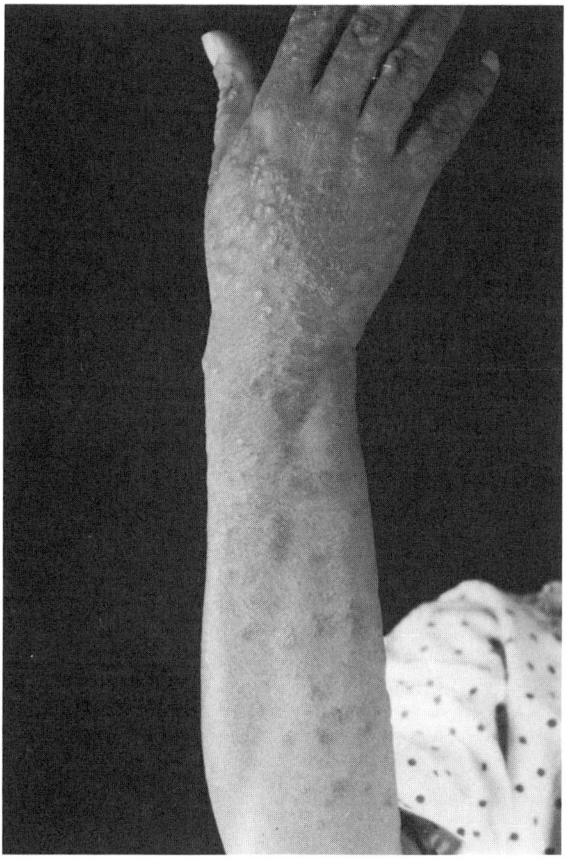

Figure 2 Herpes gestationis: edematous papules and plaques.

target lesions, annular lesions, and polycyclic lesions. The vesicles and bullae can be seen in the periphery of the plaques. Involvement of the face and oral and genital mucosa is uncommon. Blisters may develop on uninvolved skin. When the blisters rupture, they leave denuded areas covered with brown-yellow or hemorrhagic crusts. Pustules without vesicles or bullae have also been reported (5). Because of a few similarities to bullous pemphigoid, an autoimmune blistering disease of the elderly, Holmes and Black suggested the name pemphigoid gestationis (6,7). The disease manifests with exacerbations and remissions and with a tendency toward spontaneous clearing at the end of the last trimester. Marked exacerbation after delivery is the rule (3). The lesions

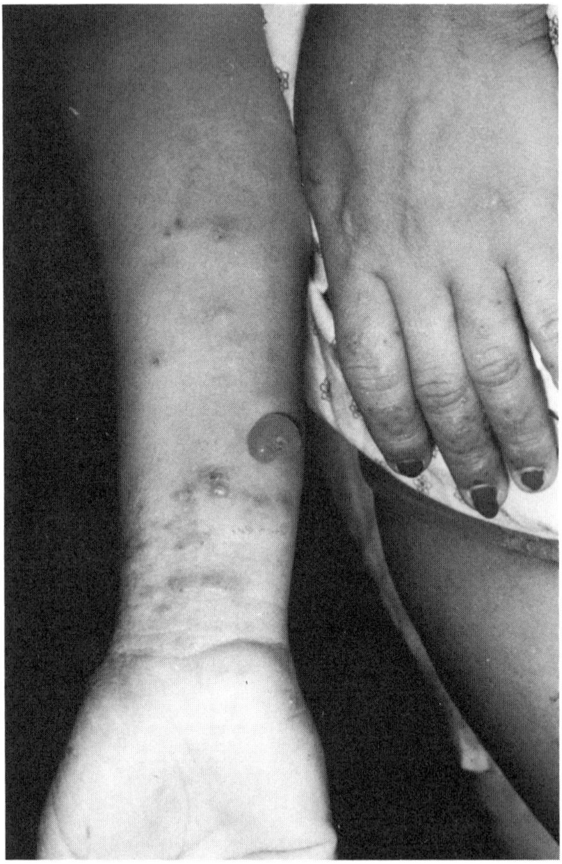

Figure 3 Herpes gestationis: tens bulla on normal appearing skin.

heal without scarring, but postinflammatory hyperpigmentation is common. The first episode of herpes gestationis occurs mainly in a multigravid patient, and it tends to recur in subsequent pregnancies (8). Moreover, in each subsequent pregnancy, it tends to appear earlier and to be more severe. In some patients, the disease continues after the puerperium. Minor exacerbations may occur postpartum after menstruation for several months (9) and also after use of oral contraceptives.

Fetal Morbidity

Fetal morbidity is one of the controversial subjects surrounding herpes gestationis. In 1978, Lawley et al. reported that the rate of stillbirths among these patients was 7.7%, compared with 1.3% in the general population (10). They did not find a higher incidence of spontaneous abortions in herpes gestationis patients. They also found a higher incidence of premature babies, 23% compared with 5–10% in the general population. Holmes and Black also found an impaired fetal prognosis in herpes gestationis (11). They found a significant increase in the frequency of small-for-dates babies and concluded that patients with herpes gestationis should deliver in maternity units with facilities for intensive care of the newborn. In contrast, Shornick et al. found no increased risk of fetal morbidity or mortality (4).

Cutaneous involvement of the newborn of mothers with herpes gestationis occurs in up to 10% of cases (12). A recent study reported pustular herpes gestationis in a newborn who experienced a favorable outcome (13).

Etiology and Pathogenesis. For many years the etiology of herpes gestationis remained obscure, but, with the advent of immunoflourescent techniques, it has become clear that herpes gestationis is an autoimmune disease. In 1973, Provost and Tomasi reported the deposition of complement in the skin of herpes gestationis patients (14). The authors described a "herpes gestationis factor" that activated complement through the alternative pathway and later was identified as an IgG (15,16). A recent study demonstrated that herpes gestationis factor is an IgG1 antibody, with inferred complement-binding activity (17). There seems to be no correlation between the titer of antibodies and disease activity.

The association of herpes gestationis with pregnancy and some trophoblastic tumors suggests that a placental antigen cross-reacting with the skin may trigger the autoimmune response. In 1987, Ortonne et al. demonstrated for the first time, by using both complement-fixing immunofluorescence and immunoelectronmicroscopy, that herpes gestationis factor was bound to the basement membrane zone of the amnion (18). This finding demonstrates the antigenic similarity between the basement membrane of the amnion and the skin. With sera from patients with herpes gestationis, Morrison et al. demonstrated that 89% of the sera that had herpes gestationis factor activity recognized a 180-kd epidermal protein by immunoblotting (19). This 180-kd protein was not recognized by sera from other pregnant women. Kelly et al. also demonstrated that sera of herpes gestationis patients mainly recognized a 180-kd epidermal protein (20), although a few patients showed antibodies against a 220-kd protein that is known as the bullous pemphigoid antigen.

We know today that the initiation of the immune response in some autoimmune diseases is associated with aberrant expression of major histocompatibility complex (MHC) class II antigens in the target tissues (21). Aberrant expression of MHC class II molecules occurs in herpes gestationis (22,23).

There is now convincing evidence that the activation of complement in herpes gestationis is through the classic pathway (16,24). Recently, Scheman et al. demonstrated evidence for eosinophil degranulation in the pathogenesis of herpes gestationis (25). By using indirect immunofluorescence with antibody to human eosinophilic granule major basic protein, they showed the existence of this protein within tissue eosinophils and exterior to eosinophils in the involved dermis.

Associated Diseases. Isolated reports about the association of herpes gestationis with other diseases are found in the literature. Holmes et al. reported that 43 of herpes gestationis patients had thyroid autoantibodies and 21% had Graves' disease (3). Other coincidental diseases include atopy, alopecia areata, alopecia totalis, and ulcerative colitis (12). It has been reported in association with hydatidiform mole (26) and choriocarcinoma (27,28). The association of herpes gestationis and a human chorionic gonadotropin-producing germ cell tumor has also been reported (29).

Laboratory Findings

Routine laboratory findings are usually normal. Several studies showed mild eosinophilia and leukocytosis (10,30). Immunofluorescent studies show that all patients with herpes gestationis have linear deposition of C3 at the basement membrane zone. Indirect immunofluorescence is positive for C3 in 91% of the patients (31). In 21% of the patients, deposition of IgG is seen in direct immunofluorescence at the dermoepidermal junction. Levels of hormones, such as plasma and urinary estriol or human chorionic gonadotropin, are also normal. A significant and strong genetic predisposition occurs in herpes gestationis patients. HLA-DR3 is found in 61–85% of the patients, and the combination of HLA-DR3 and HLA-DR4 is found in 43–45% of the patients (9,32).

Treatment

The treatment of choice is systemic steroids. The dosage varies between 40 and 60 mg/day. This dose is usually sufficient to control the activity of the disease. The dose can be tapered within 2 weeks after clinical improvement. According to Shornick (12) many patients can control their disease with a modest dose such as 10–20 mg daily. Topical corticosteroids may be beneficial, but usually do not eliminate the blisters. Other treatment modalities, such as dapsone, pyridoxine, gold, and methotrexate, have been reported without much success.

Linear Immunoglobulin M Dermatosis of Pregnancy

In 1988, we reported a case we believed was a unique new dermatosis of pregnancy (33). A 39-year-old woman presented in her 37th week of gestation with an intensely pruritic eruption on the trunk and extremities. The eruption was composed of red follicular papules with few pustules (Figure 4). Direct immunofluorescence test revealed a dense linear deposition of IgM along the dermoepidermal junction (Figure 5). The eruption and the immunofluorescence findings disappeared 6 weeks after delivery. Since the first description of this disease there have been no other reported cases. It is possible that linear IgM der-

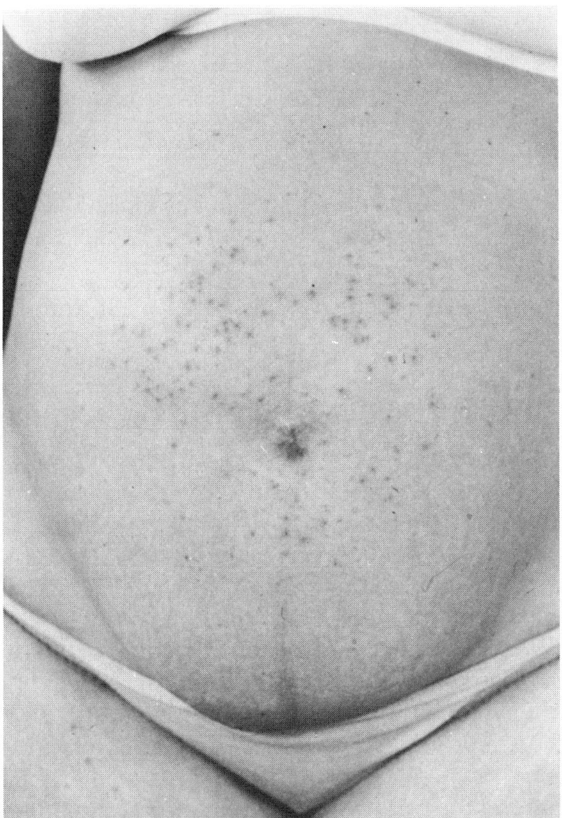

Figure 4 Follicular papules on abdomen in linear IgM dermatosis of pregnancy.

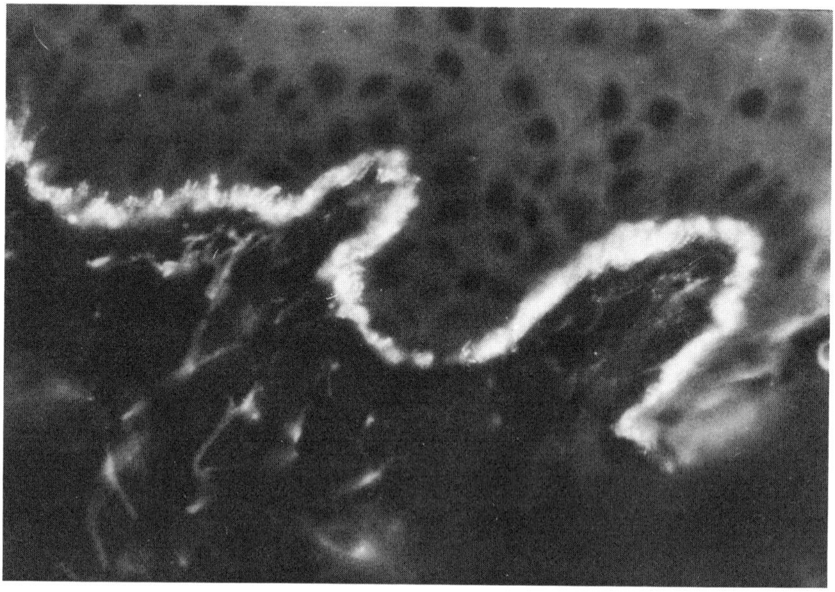

Figure 5 Linear deposition of IgM along the dermoepidermal junction.

matosis is a rare disease and only careful search will lead to the detection of other cases.

Autoimmune Progesterone Dermatitis of Pregnancy

Autoimmune progesterone dermatitis is a well-recognized entity of recurrent episodes of urticaria and erythema multiforme that occurs in the luteal phase of each menstrual cycle (34). This clinical entity is attributed to a hypersensitivity to endogenous progesterone. Autoimmune progesterone dermatitis of pregnancy (APDP) is distinct from autoimmune progesterone dermatitis. It was described once in 1973 by Bierman (35) who described a patient who in two successive pregnancies had an acneiform eruption on the buttocks and extremities. In both pregnancies the eruption developed during the first 2 weeks, and both terminated in spontaneous abortion. There was a unique papulopustular eruption together with transient arthritis and peripheral and tissue eosinophilia. Administration of an oral contraceptive mixture resulted in severe exacerbation of the clinical and laboratory features of the disease. Intradermal test with aqueous extracts of progesterone resulted in an hypersensitivity reaction. The author summarized that "APDP appears to be a disease sui generis." To my knowledge no other cases have been reported, indicating that it is a very rare disease.

PRURITIC URTICARIAL PAPULES AND PLAQUES OF PREGNANCY

Several eruptions of pregnancy with similar clinical features have been described under different names. The clinical features include erythematous papules and plaques, as well as urticarial plaques accompanied by severe itching. In 1941, Costello reviewed erythema multiforme gestationis, which was characterized by erythematous patches with urticarial-like lesions (36). Toxemic rash of pregnancy was described by Bourne as an intense pruritus followed by red wheals with central papules (37). An eruption that falls within this spectrum of disease consists of extremely pruritic macules, papules, and urticarial plaques (38). In 1979, Lawley et al. described an intensely pruritic cutaneous eruption characterized by urticarial papules and plaques under the name pruritic urticarial papules and plaques of pregnancy (PUPPP) (39). This terminology is widely used today to describe the most common eruption of the pregnant woman. Holmes and Black suggested lumping all these eruptions under the name "polymorphic eruption of pregnancy" (7). One should appreciate the spectrum of disease when evaluating these disorders (40). The incidence of PUPPP is estimated to be between 1:120 and 1:240 pregnancies (3,37).

Clinical Features

In 90% of the cases the eruption starts in the abdomen (41). It is symmetric, mostly involves the flexor areas of the upper extremities, the abdomen, thighs, legs, it is occasionally noted on the buttocks (Figure 6), and is rarely found on the face (42). The lesions consist of erythematous, urticarial plaques and erythematous small papules. Severe pruritus accompanies the eruption. Targetlike lesions and blisters are sometimes seen (3,43). The periumbilical area is spared in PUPPP and, in many cases, lesions can be seen within the striae atrophicae (distansae) (44) (Figure 7). Seventy-six to ninety-three percent of the patients are primigravid at the onset of the eruption (43,44). The PUPPP usually starts in the third trimester or occasionally shortly after delivery (41,43). The rash clears up spontaneously shortly after delivery or in the early period of the puerperium (42,45) and does not recur in subsequent pregnancies. Excoriated lesions are infrequently seen in PUPPP (39).

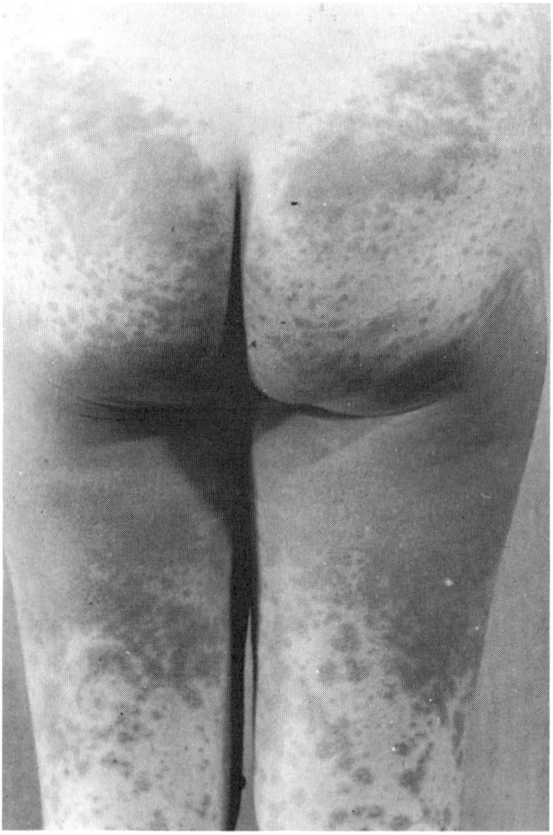

Figure 6 Pruritic urticarial papules and plaques of pregnancy: typical lesions on buttocks and thighs.

Fetal Outcome

Since the report by Lawley et al. (39), it has been understood that, in contrast to herpes gestationis, there is no increased fetal morbidity or mortality associated with PUPPP (39). Callen and Hanno reported normal delivery and normal fetal outcome in 15 patients with PUPPP (43). Several other reports confirmed a normal fetal outcome (42,46,47). To date, there has been one report of cutaneous involvement of the infant (48), which may actually have been toxic erythema of the newborn. An increased prevalence of twin delivery has been reported in PUPPP,

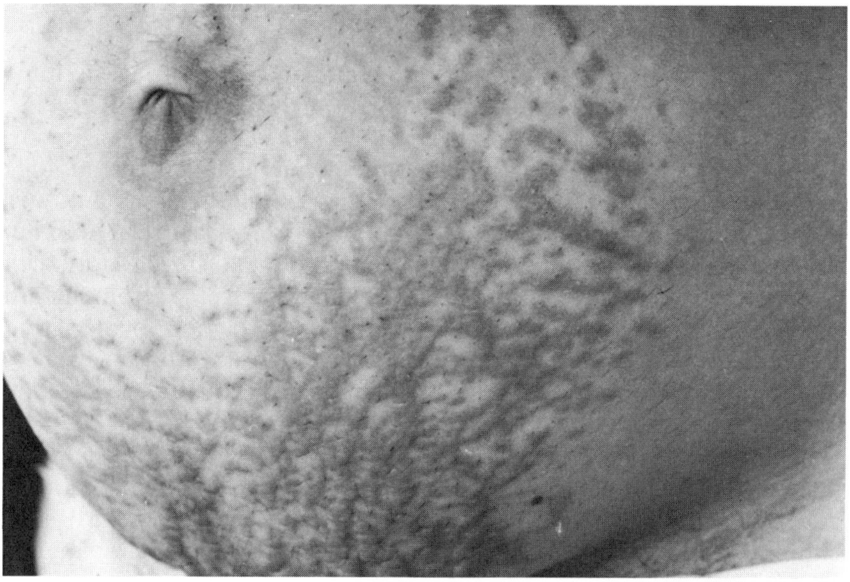

Figure 7 Erythematous urticarial plaques involving the striae atrophicae (distansae) in pruritic urticarial papules and plaques of pregnancy.

varying from 16 to 33% (39,44,49). Recently, Bunker et al. reported severely symptomatic polymorphic eruption of pregnancy in three pregnant women with twins (50). A higher neonatal birth weight has also been found in neonates of mothers with PUPPP than in those of controls (51).

Laboratory Findings

Routine laboratory workup reveals changes usually seen in women in the third trimester of pregnancy (44). Direct immunofluorescence assay from lesional or perilesional skin reveals only granular deposition of C3 at the dermoepidermal junction (41) or in the dermal blood vessel walls (44). Histopathological examination reveals a superficial middermal perivascular lymphohistiocytic infiltrate. Eosinophils are seen together with mild papillary edema. There is a correlation between the intensity of the inflammatory response and the presence of epidermal involvement (52). Subepidermal blisters occur occasionally (53), and increased dermal fibroblasts have been reported in several patients (54).

Etiology

The etiology of PUPPP is unknown. In contrast with herpes gestationis there is no increased prevalence of any HLA class II antigens in PUPPP. None of the PUPPP patients demonstrated HLA-DR3 or HLA-DR4 antigens (44). A role for circulating immune complexes in the etiology has been suggested. By using C1q solid-phase binding assay and polyethylene glycol precipitation of IgG, Kasp-Grochowska et al. could not find any circulating immune complexes in polymorphic eruption of pregnancy (55). However, by using a solid-phase polyclonal rheumatoid factor-binding assay, they found a significant reduction in the circulating immune complexes in the acute stage of the eruption. They speculated that leakage of small immune complexes through dermal blood vessels plays a role in the etiology of the disease.

We have investigated the possibility of an autoimmune mechanism (47). Serum autoantibodies such as antinuclear, antismooth muscle, antithyroid, antimitochondrial, and antigastric parietal cell antibodies were not found. Results of hormonal evaluation of these patients, which included a subunit of human chorionic gonadotropin, estradiol, cortisol, and urinary estriol, were normal and could not point toward a hormonal etiology (47).

Cohen et al. found a significantly increased maternal weight gain in patients with PUPPP (51). They suggested that the increased abdominal distention and trauma to the overlying skin triggers the inflammatory response of PUPPP.

Treatment

This is a self-limiting disease. Symptomatic treatment is needed to control the itching and includes calamine lotion, topical corticosteroids, and antihistamines.

PAPULAR ERUPTIONS OF PREGNANCY

Papular eruptions of pregnancy are a group of dermatoses characterized by the appearance of pruritic papules on the trunk and extremities. The dermatoses included in this section lack precise clinical descriptions.

Prurigo Gestationis

A pruritic eruption characterized by closely excoriated grouped papules was described in 1904 by Besnier (56). The eruption was located on the extensor surfaces of the arms, forearms, dorsum of the hands, thighs, legs, and feet. It started at the last trimester and persisted until delivery. Mild postinflammatory hyperpigmentation remained after the eruption cleared. Histological and laboratory data were not available. Cases of prurigo gestationis have not been reported in the last few decades. No fetal complications were reported.

Papular Dermatitis of Pregnancy

In 1962 Spangler et al. described 12 patients with an intensely pruritic generalized eruption that consisted of erythematous papules (57). In many cases hemorrhagic crusts covered the papules. The lesions did not appear in crops. The time of onset varied from the first to the last month of pregnancy. This disease recurs in subsequent pregnancies and appears associated with high fetal mortality. Abnormalities noted in the 12 patients included (a) elevated urinary human chorionic gonadotropin during the last trimester, (b) lowered plasma hydrocortisone level, and (c) shortened hydrocortisone half-life. Subsequently, Spangler and Emerson (58) extended the hormonal evaluation in patients with papular dermatitis of pregnancy and found lower estrogen levels. Resolution of the disease was achieved with stilbestrol therapy without the occurrence of fetal loss. Since these reports no other cases of the disease have been reported. Holmes and Black believe that papular dermatitis of pregnancy is the same as prurigo gestationis and that the high fetal mortality was overestimated (31).

Pruritic Folliculitis of Pregnancy

A pruritic papular eruption with a pattern of folliculitis was described by Zoberman and Farmer in 1981 (59). Six women developed pruritic folliculitis between the fourth and ninth month of gestation. In five patients the eruption was widespread and the sixth patient had an eruption limited to the arms and abdomen. In one patient, the eruption cleared spontaneously in 1 week. There was no increase in fetal morbidity or mortality. The lesions cleared spontaneously at delivery or during the postpartum period. Histopathological features of folliculitis were seen in five patients. Direct immunofluorescence test of the lesions did not show deposition of immunoglobulin or complement. Holmes and Black reported two additional cases with similar clinical features (31). They suggested that pruritic folliculitis of pregnancy is a form of hormonally induced acne and not a specific dermatosis of pregnancy (31).

Pruritic Papules of Pregnancy

Although the main clinical presentation of this dermatosis is a papular eruption, it can also be classified in the spectrum of PUPPP. Rahbary described 16 women in whom a pruritic papular eruption developed in the first, second, and mostly in the third trimester (60). The papules were sometimes accompanied by erythematous or urticarial background. The lesions were generalized in distribution and histopathological examination showed toxic dermatitis. Follow-up of 8 cases showed that 62% resolved completely after delivery.

PUSTULAR ERUPTIONS OF PREGNANCY

Impetigo Herpetiformis

Impetigo herpetiformis is a pustular eruption that appears during pregnancy. Controversy exists whether impetigo herpetiformis is a specific dermatosis of pregnancy or whether it is a variant of psoriasis (61,62). The disease was described in five pregnant women by von Hebra in 1872 (63), who noted that the disease presented during the last 3 months of pregnancy and occasionally as early as the first trimester. Ross et al. reported a case of impetigo herpetiformis that presented during the puerperium (64). The eruption consists of erythematous patches occurring in intertriginous areas, with small pustules in the periphery. In contrast to all of the other dermatoses of pregnancy, pruritus is uncommon. The pustules rupture, leaving denuded areas, and the erythema spreads centrifugally. The eruption is accompanied by high fever, chills, diarrhea, and vomiting. Among the specific dermatoses of pregnancy, impetigo herpetiformis is associated with the highest fetal mortality (65–67). Several cases of impetigo herpetiformis have been associated with hypocalcemia (68–70). The etiology of impetigo herpetiformis is still an enigma. The treatment of choice is the administration of systemic steroids.

URTICARIA AND ANGIOEDEMA

Urticaria represents a common dermatological response to diverse physical, allergic, chemical, infectious, and emotional triggers, which manifests as circumscribed elevated pruritic and erythematous lesions. Edema of the superficial dermis characterizes the lesion. *Angioedema* results from extension of this edema to deeper areas of the dermis, subcutaneous tissue, or submucosa (71). For both urticaria and angioedema, convention defines acute disease as persistence of symptoms for less than 6 weeks, and chronic as those persisting longer.

Incidence, Etiology, and Pathophysiology

Although at least one episode of urticaria is common in individuals (up to 20%), chronic or recurrent symptoms are uncommon, occurring with a cumulative prevalence of less than 2% (71). For chronic urticaria/angioedema, causation remains unknown in over 90% of cases, leading to the principal classification of idiopathic urticaria/angioedema. During pregnancy, urticaria/angioedema can occur from any of the causes, agents, and mechanisms responsible during the nonpregnant state (Table 2). On the other hand, urticaria/angioedema may be limited to pregnancy and recur with subsequent pregnancies. This chronic urticaria/angioedema syndrome of pregnancy which occurred in 3 of 438 (0.5%

Table 2 Common Causes of Urticaria/Angioedema

IgE-mediated mechanisms
Antibiotics (particularly penicillins and cephalosporins)
Foreign proteins, including heterologous serum, ACTH, hormones, enzymes, venom, and protamine
Other therapeutic materials, such as allergen extracts, vaccines, muscle relaxants, ethylene oxide, and thiopental
Foods (especially egg, shellfish, nuts, seeds, fish, celery, milk, and legumes)
Immune complex or complement-mediated mechanisms
Whole blood
Cryoprecipitate
Immunoglobulin
Plasma
Methotrexate
Arachidonic acid metabolism-modulating agents
Aspirin
Other nonsteroidal anti-inflammatory drugs
Direct mediator-releasing agents
Opiates
Curare
Radiocontrast medium
Dextran
Mannitol
Pentamidine
Polymyxin B
Thiamine

Source: Ref. 88.

incidence) consecutive pregnancies, possibly may be caused by allergic sensitization to endogenous hormones, particularly progesterone (72). As described earlier, sensitivity to progesterone during pregnancy has been termed *autoimmune progesterone dermatitis of pregnancy* since 1971, appearing as a papulopustular eruption associated with transient arthritis, peripheral and tissue eosinophilia, miscarriage, and delayed intradermal sensitivity to aqueous progesterone (73). A similar syndrome also has been described 7–10 days premenstrually (74). Moreover, administration of progesterone intramuscularly in affected patients reproduces symptoms within 1 hr; in contrast, cyclically administered conjugated estrogens control the urticaria (73,74). As noted earlier, progesterone injection has also been implicated in anaphylaxis during pregnancy (73).

Hereditary angioedema (HANE) is an uncommon, generally autosomal dominant systemic disorder in which a deficiency or malfunction of C1-esterase inhibitor leads to a failure to adequately modulate the activated complement cascade. Recent data suggest that the resulting formation of kininlike fragments and other pharmacologically active mediators trigger the myriad of clinical signs and symptoms of HANE. These include attacks of nonpruritic and nonurticarial angioedema of the subcutaneous tissue and submucosa of the extremities, abdomen, lips, face, and larynx, the frequency of which ranges from every few days to once a year (75). Severe abdominal colic, vomiting, and guarding without fever, leukocytosis, elevated sedimentation rate, or rigidity typically occur owing to edematous involvement of the bowel wall. Differentiation of HANE-induced abdominal crises from a surgical or obstetrical abdominal emergency is crucial to prevent needless exploratory surgery. HANE-induced laryngeal edema causes hoarseness, dysphagia, and occasionally life-threatening upper airway obstruction. Although episodes are often sporadic, they often may be triggered by trauma (minor or major dental, surgical, and accidental), stress, infections, and wide fluctuations in temperature. A familial pattern is typical, but not invariable. During pregnancy, 23 of 25 pregnant women with HANE reportedly markedly fewer, or an absence of, attacks from the fourth to ninth months. Moreover, 10 women with a total of 25 pregnancies did not experience angioedema during vaginal delivery, despite its traumatic potential (75). Generally, pregnancy exerts a profound amelioration of HANE, although recurrent worsening during multiple pregnancies (75,76) and postpartum exacerbations may occur (76). In addition, tragically HANE has triggered localized perineal swelling after delivery, resulting in secondary irreversible shock and death (77). Moreover, a primary attack of HANE on the third postpartum day, precipitated by a spontaneous vaginal delivery, has recently been described, illustrating the importance of maintaining a high level of suspicion for emergence of this condition when evaluating labial swelling in the puerperium (78).

Diagnosis

The cause of urticaria/angioedema, if one is to be found, can be elicited by a thorough history and careful physical examination. Should a cause not be readily identified, laboratory evaluation of chronic urticaria/angioedema should be limited to screening with a complete blood count, urinary analysis, and erythrocyte sedimentation rate. Diagnostic tests reserved for confirmation of diagnostic suspicions are noted in Table 3.

One must differentiate gestational urticaria/angioedema from such dermatological entities as autoimmune progesterone dermatitis of pregnancy, polymorphic eruption of pregnancy, other pruritic dermatoses of pregnancy, and laryngopathia gravidarum. The first three disorders are discussed in the foregoing and are summarized in Table 1.

Laryngopathia gravidarum appears as an acute or chronic, noninfectious, somewhat inflammatory disorder of laryngeal tissue seen in the multigravida (79). Although the acute form presents before parturition, the chronic entity occurs throughout pregnancy, recurring with subsequent pregnancies. Spontaneous resolution occurs postpartum with both forms. Typical symptoms of laryngopathia gravidarum include (a) progressive dyspnea, sporadically requiring artificial ventilation, (b) hoarseness, (c) nonfebrile sore throat and odynophagia, (d) malaise, (e) lymphadenopathy, (f) cough, and (g) elevated erythrocyte sedimentation rate (40–60 mm/hr) and normal white blood count. Patchy localized edema and congestion are noted in the larynx and frequently the epiglottis, but not the aryepiglottic folds, arytenoids, vestibular region, or true vocal cords. Microscopic abnormalities are limited to the submucosa, which appears edematous because of infiltration with lymphocytes and plasma cells. Owing to its resolution postpartum, pregnancy hormones have been implicated in its causation (79).

Prevention and Treatment

Identification and avoidance of triggering agents or causes (see Table 2) remain the hallmark of treatment to prevent symptoms and obviate pharmacological intervention. During pregnancy, tripelennamine (25–50 mg every 6 hr or 100 mg sustained-release bid) continues as the recommended initial H_1-antihistamine for symptomatic control of urticaria/angioedema. Ephedrine (25–50 mg every 6 hr) or substitution

Table 3 Diagnostic Tests for Urticaria/Angioedema During Pregnancy

Suspected disorder	Procedure
Food, drug, or inhalant allergy	Diary and trial avoidance of causal agent RAST
Physical	
Dermatographism	Stroke skin with tongue blade
Cold	Ice cube on forearm for 5 min Cryoglobulins, cryofibrinogen
Cholinergic	Methacholine skin test (postpartum)
Solar	Expose skin to light wave lengths Protoporphyrin/coproporphyrins
Vibratory	Vortex skin for 4 min
Pressure	Weights to extremity for 10 min
Aquagenic	Expose hand to tap-water at varying temperatures
Exercise	History
Infectious	Appropriate cultures/titers Stool for ova/parasites
Cutaneous or systemic vasculitis	Skin or tissue biopsy with immunofluorescence Immunoglobulin analysis Antinuclear antibody Thyroid antimicrosomal antibody Complement profile
Hereditary angioedema (HANE)	C4, C2, CH_{50} C1-esterase inhibitor by functional and protein analysis
Malignancy	CH_{50}, C1, C1-esterase inhibitor
Idiopathic	History with negative tests

Source: Ref. 88.

with hydroxyzine (10–25 mg every 6 hr) may be necessary for refractory cases. Systemic corticosteroids occasionally are required for severe recalcitrant urticaria or angioedema. Acute, severe urticaria/angioedema requires aggressive therapy modeled after that used for anaphylaxis (see Chapter 15).

Attenuated androgen prophylaxis generally is not required, nor warranted, for the treatment of HANE during pregnancy, since the potential for drug-related fetal damage (80) includes female masculination and pseudohermaphroditism and spontaneous abortion (81). Effective contraception during androgen therapy should be maintained by women of childbearing potential with HANE to prevent these adverse fetal effects from occurring during early pregnancy before confirmation of pregnancy.

Vaginal deliveries appear safe for HANE patients (75). Cesarian sections, on the other hand, require preoperative transfusion of two units of fresh-frozen plasma to prevent episodes (79). Regional is preferred to general anesthesia to avoid endotracheal intubation, which could trigger laryngeal edema. HANE-induced life threatening laryngeal edema during pregnancy requires rapid and aggressive therapy including (a) androgenic therapy (stanozolol 4 mg qid), (b) standard emergency measures for reversing airway obstruction (endotracheal intubation and, if necessary, tracheostomy), and (c) intravenous fluid replacement if hypovolemia develops (79). The usual therapeutic modalities for angioedema (epinephrine, antihistamines, and corticosteroids) typically are ineffective in most patients during acute HANE attacks (75). Postpartum episodes of HANE must be recognized rapidly and aggressive therapy instituted, including large-volume fluid replacement of third-space losses and reinstitution of androgenic therapy (75).

ATOPIC DERMATITIS

Definition, Etiology, and Pathogenesis

The characteristic features of atopic dermatitis, an eczematous disorder that occurs in about 1–2% of adults, include (a) pruritis, (b) chronicity, (c) typical morphology and distribution, and (d) a genetic predisposition to develop allergic rhinitis, asthma, and food allergy. The spectrum of symptoms may extend from a mild isolated small circumscribed patch (nummular eczema) to severe generalized exfoliative erythroderma. The acute condition evidences erythema, dermal edema, excoriations, and weeping; whereas the chronic stage reveals scaling, thickening, hyperpigmentation, and fissuring. The antecubital and popliteal fossae, neck, upper trunk, perioral and periorbital areas, and hands represent areas of proclivity in adults (82).

Up to 70–80% of subjects with atopic dermatitis evidence elevated serum IgE levels, peripheral eosinophilia, and often specific IgE to foods (most during infancy) and inhalants, which historically may trigger the cutaneous symptoms. Alterations in cell-mediated immunity, reduced T lymphocytes, loss of circulating suppressor–cytotoxic T cells, increased numbers of circulating Fcε RII mononuclear cells, depressed neutrophilic and mononuclear cell chemotactic activity, and elevated mononuclear cell phosphodiesterase activity have been observed to varying degrees in patients with atopic dermatitis (82–84). Abnormal cutaneous findings frequently include white dermographism (a white line, rather than a wheal, in response to skin stroking), a greater dermal constrictor response to cold, reduced whealing to histamine, reduced delayed hypersensitivity reactions on patch testing, exaggerated response to methacholine, pallor instead of erythema to nicotinic acid, diminished reactions to β-adrenergic stimulation, and increased dermal mast cells. These findings may also be observed, although less frequently, in patients with other chronic dermatoses. The pathogenesis of atopic dermatitis is thought to involve an abnormal immunological mechanism in atopics that leads to the cutaneous release from mast cells of such mediators as histamine, eosinophilic chemotactic factors, leukotrienes, and others (83). Eczematous lesions evidence depending on the severity of involvement, varying degrees of irregular parakeratosis and hyperkeratosis, with irregular acanthosis and spongiosis. Recently, increased numbers of dendritic Langerhans' cells were found in chronic lesions; an elevated proportion of T-helper to T-suppressor lymphocytes was seen in dermal infiltrates; greater numbers of mast cells, but not basophils, were observed in lesions; and large quantities of eosinophil basic protein, a potentially toxic product of eosinophil leukocytes, were observed to permeate abnormal skin (83,85).

Diagnosis

To aid in the diagnosis of atopic dermatitis, specific diagnostic criteria have been formulated and are summarized in Table 4 (84). Typical-appearing atopic dermatitis is easily differentiated from such cutaneous disorders as (a) seborrheic dermatitis, which appears as greasy scaling areas on a yellow-red base over the scalp, forehead, and flexor areas; (b) allergic contact dermatitis, which evidences acute, patchy, and streaky lesions, correlating with exposure to contactants; (c) other immunological disorders, including the hyper-IgE syndrome, which demonstrates recurrent cold abscesses, severe local and systemic infections to *Candida* and *Staphylococcus*, coarse facies and skeletal abnormalities, and markedly elevated serum IgE levels; dermatitis herpetiformis, which has severe refractory pruritus, blistering, and excoriations frequently associated with sprue and wheat sensitivity; Wiskott–Aldrich syndrome, which presents with purpura from thrombocytopenia and systemic infections from immunological abnormalities; chronic granulomatous disease, which manifests recurrent skin abscesses, fistulas, pneumonia, hepatosplenomegaly, and abnormal nitroblue tetrazolium test and generation of oxygen radicals; and (d) cutaneous lymphomas,

Table 4 Diagnostic Criteria for Atopic Dermatitis

A. Absolute features
   1. Pruritus
   2. Flexural lichenification in adults
   3. Chronic or recurrent tendency
      plus

B. Two or more of the following features:
   1. Personal or family atopic history (asthma, allergic rhinitis, or atopic dermatitis)
   2. Specific IgE (skin test or RAST)
   3. White dermographism (a white line rather than a wheal in response to skin stroking) or delayed blanch to methacholine
   4. Anterior subcapsular cataracts
      or

C. Four or more of the following features:
   1. Xerosis/ichthyosis/hyperlinear palms
   2. Pityriasis alba
   3. Keratosis pilaris
   4. Facial pallor/infraorbital darkening
   5. Dennie-Morgan infraorbital fold
   6. Elevated serum IgE
   7. Keratoconus
   8. Tendency toward nonspecific hand dermatitis
   9. Tendency toward recurrent dermal infections

Source: Ref. 88.

such as mycosis fungoides, Sezary's syndrome, and Hodgkin's disease, which may present early with pruritic dermal lesions involving linear thickening of flexural surfaces (82).

Interrelations Between Pregnancy and Atopic Dermatitis

Of 117 women with mild to severe atopic dermatitis, pregnancy was associated with clearing or definite improvement in 3% and definite exacerbation in 1% (86). In contrast, in a recent questionnaire-based study, atopic dermatitis was reported to worsen in 52%, improve in 24%, and remain unchanged in 24% of 50 women during 88 full-term pregnancies. Moreover, worsening of atopic dermatitis occurred by 20 weeks in 80% of those women reporting worsening of atopic dermatitis during pregnancy (87). Prospective follow-up studies with clinical scoring are necessary to confirm these findings.

Prevention and Treatment

During pregnancy the treatment of atopic dermatitis must focus on avoidance of triggering factors, such as known food and inhalant allergens; irritating agents, such as wools and chemicals; excessive perspiration and heat; unwarranted stress; occlusive clothing; and other known exacerbants. Topical therapy that has proved efficacious for atopic dermatitis includes (a) moisturizes and lubricants to alleviate dryness (Neutrogena hand cream, Aveeno lotion, Eucerin cream), and (b) cleansers such as Cetophil lotion instead of soaps, and aluminum acetate (Burow's solution) or baking soda soaks to reduce inflammation, weeping, and pruritis. When clinically indicated, oral antihistamines should be administered at the lowest effective dose, initiating therapy with tripelennamine in doses similar to those given for urticaria/angioedema. Hydroxyzine may be necessary for recalcitrant pruritus. A similar conservative approach should be followed for topical corticosteroid use. Corticosteroid treatment should be initiated, when clinically indicated, with the least potentially adrenal suppressive preparations such as hydrocortisone (0.5–2.5%). Use of the more potent topical corticosteroid preparations should be reserved for the more recalcitrant areas or patients. Administration of corticosteroids by intralesional or systemic injections should be avoided. Infectious exacerbations, generally secondary to *Staphylococcus aureus* colonization, should be treated with penicillinase-resistant synthetic penicillins or erythromycin in those allergic to penicillin (see Chapter 17) (88).

REFERENCES

1. Russel B, Thorne NA. Herpes gestationis. Br J Dermatol 1957; 69:339–357.
2. Kolodny RC. Herpes gestationis: a new assessment of incidence, diagnosis, and fetal prognosis. Am J Obstet Gynecol 1969; 104:39–45.
3. Holmes RC, Black MM, Dann J, James DCO, Bhogal B. A comparative study of toxic erythema of pregnancy and herpes gestationis. Br J Dermatol 1982; 106:499–510.
4. Shornick JR, Bangert JL, Freeman RG, Gilliam JN. Herpes gestationis: clinical and histologic features of twenty-eight cases. J Am Acad Dermatol 1983; 8:214–224.
5. Bercovitch L, Bogaars HA, Murray DO. Pustular herpes gestationis. Arch Dermatol 1983; 119:91–93.
6. Holmes R, Black MM, Williamson PM, Scutt RWB. Herpes gestationis and bullous pemphigoid: a disease spectrum. Br J Dermatol 1980; 103:535–541.
7. Holmes RC, Black MM. The specific dermatoses of pregnancy: a reappraisal with special emphasis on a proposed simplified clinical classification. Clin Exp Dermatol 1982; 7:65–73.

8. Holmes RC, Jurecka W, Black MM. A comparative histopathological study of polymorphic eruption of pregnancy and herpes gestationis. Clin Exp Dermatol 1983; 8:523–529.
9. Holmes RC, Black MM, Jurecka W, Dann J, James DCO, Timlin D, Bhogal B. Clues to the etiology and pathogenesis of herpes gestationis. Br J Dermatol 1983; 109:131–139.
10. Lawley TJ, Stingl G, Katz SI. Fetal and maternal risk factors in herpes gestationis. Arch Dermatol 1978; 114:552–555.
11. Holmes RC, Black MM. The fetal prognosis in pemphigoid gestationis (herpes gestationis). Br J Dermatol 1984; 110:67–72.
12. Shornick JR. Herpes gestationis. J Am Acad Dermatol 1987; 17:539–556.
13. Guillet G, Nougue J, Oksman F. Herpes gestationis in mother and erythemato-pustulous rash in the newborn with positive direct immunofluorescence. A transfer of the disease *Dermatologica*. 1988; 176:143–147.
14. Provost TT, Tomasi TB. Evidence for complement activation via the alternate pathway in skin diseases. I. Herpes gestationis, systemic lupus erythematosus and bullous pemphigoid. J Clin Invest 1973; 52:1779–1787.
15. Katz, SI, Hertz KC, Yaoita H. Herpes gestationis: immunopathology and characterization of the HG factor. J Clin Invest 1976; 57:1434–1441.
16. Jordon RE, Heine KG, Tappeiner G, Bushkell LL, Provost TT. The immunopathology of herpes gestationis: immunoflourescence studies and characterization of HG factor. J Clin Invest 1976; 57:1426–1433.
17. Kelly SE, Cerio R, Bhogal BS, Black MM. The distribution of IgG subclasses in pemphigoid gestationis: PG is an IgG1 autoantibody. J Invest Dermatol 1989; 92:695–698.
18. Ortonne JP, Hsi BL, Verrando P, Bernerd F, Pautrat G, Pisani A, Yeh CJG. Herpes gestationis factor reacts with amniotic epithelial basement membrane. Br J Dermatol 1987; 117:147–154.
19. Morrison LH, Labib RS, Zone JJ, Diaz LA, Anhalt GJ. Herpes gestationis autoantibodies recognize a 180-kD human epidermal antigen. J Clin Invest 1988; 81:2023–2026.
20. Kelly SE, Bhogal BS, Wojnarowska F, Whitehead P, Leigh IM, Black MM. Western blot analysis of the antigen in pemphigoid gestationis. Br J Dermatol 1990; 122:445–449.
21. Bottazo GF, Pujol-Borrel R, Hanafusa T, Feldman M. Hypothesis: role of aberrant HLA-DR expression and antigen presentation in induction of endocrine autoimmunity. Lancet 1983; 2:1115–1118.
22. Kelly SE, Fleming S, Bhogal BS, Wojnarowska F, Black MM. Immunopathology of the placenta in pemphigoid gestationis and linear IgA disease. Br J Dermatol 1989; 120:735–743.
23. Borthwick GM, Holmes RC, Stirrat GM. Abnormal expression of class II MHC antigens in placenta from patients with pemphigoid gestationis. Placenta 1988; 9:81–94.
24. Carruthers JA, Ewins AR. Herpes gestationis: studies on the binding characteristics, activity and pathogenic significance of the complement-fixing factor. Clin Exp Immunol 1978; 31:38–44.

25. Scheman AJ, Hordinsky MD, Groth DW, Vercellotti GM, Leiferman KM. Evidence for eosinophil degranulation in the pathogenesis of herpes gestationis. Arch Dermatol 1989; 125:1079–1083.
26. Tindall JG, Rea TH, Schulman I, Quismorio P. Herpes gestationis in association with a hydatidiform mole. Arch Dermatol 1981; 117:510–512.
27. Slazinski L, Degefu S. Herpes gestationis associated with choriocarcinoma. Arch Dermatol 1982; 118:425–428.
28. Tillman WG. Herpes gestationis with hydatidiform mole and chorioepithelioma. Br Med J 1950; 1:1471.
29. Sorensen LH, Beck HI, Sogaard H. Herpes gestationis in association with neoplasma malignum generalisata. A case report. Acta Derm Venerol (Stockh) 1985; 120:96–100.
30. Starks GC. Herpes gestationis. A report of two cases. J Reprod Med 1984; 29:493–495.
31. Holmes RC, Black MM. The specific dermatoses of pregnancy. J Am Acad Dermatol 1983; 8:405–412.
32. Shornick JK, Stastny P, Gilliam JN. High frequency of histocompatibility antigens HLA-DR3 and DR4 in herpes gestationis. J Clin Invest 1981; 68:553–555.
33. Alcalay J, Ingber A, Hazaz B, David M, Sandbank M. Linear IgM dermatosis of pregnancy. J Am Acad Dermatol 1988; 18:412–415.
34. Hart R. Autoimmune progesterone dermatitis. Arch Dermatol 1977; 113:426–430.
35. Bierman SM. Autoimmune progesterone dermatitis of pregnancy. Arch Dermatol 1973; 107:896–901.
36. Costello MJ. Eruptions of pregnancy. NY State J Med 1941; 41:849–855.
37. Bourne G. Toxemic rash of pregnancy. Proc R Soc Med 1962; 55:462–464.
38. Nurse PS. Prurigo of pregnancy. Australas J Dermatol 1968; 9:258–267.
39. Lawley TJ, Hertz KC, Wade RD, Ackerman AB, Katz SI. Pruritic urticarial papules and plaques of pregnancy. JAMA 1979; 241:1696–1699.
40. Alcalay J, Wolf JE. Pruritic urticarial papules and plaques of pregnancy: the enigma and the confusion. J Am Acad Dermatol 1988; 19:1115–1116.
41. Alcalay J, Ingber A, David M, Hazaz B, Sandbank M. Pruritic urticarial papules and plaques of pregnancy: a review of 21 cases. J Reprod Med 1987; 32:315–316.
42. Alcalay J, David M, Sandbank M. Facial involvement of pruritic urticarial papules of pregnancy [letter]. J Am Acad Dermatol 1986; 15:1048.
43. Callen JP, Hanno R. Pruritic urticarial papules and plaques of pregnancy (PUPPP). A clinicopathologic study. J Am Acad Dermatol 1981; 5:401–405.
44. Yancey KB, Hall RP, Lawley TJ. Pruritic urticarial papules and plaques of pregnancy. Clinical experience in twenty-five patients. J Am Acad Dermatol 1984; 10:473–480.
45. Noguera J, Moreno A, Moragas JM. Pruritic urticarial papules and plaques of pregnancy. Acta Derm Venerol (Stockh) 1983; 63:35–38.

46. Ahmed AR, Kaplan R. Pruritic urticarial papules and plaques of pregnancy. J Am Acad Dermatol 1981; 4:679–681.
47. Alcalay J, Ingber A, Kafri B, Segal J, Kaufman H, Hazaz B, Sandbank M. Hormonal evaluation and autoimmune background in pruritic urticarial papules and plaques of pregnancy. Am J Obstet Gynecol 1988; 158:416–420.
48. Uhlin SR. Pruritic urticarial papules and plaques of pregnancy. Involvement in mother and infant. Arch Dermatol 1981; 117:238–239.
49. Stoller HE. Pruritic urticarial papules and plaques of pregnancy. JAMA (Letter) 1980; 243:2156.
50. Bunker CB, Erskine K, Rustin MH, Gilkes JJ. Severe polymorphic eruption of pregnancy occurring in twin pregnancies. Clin Exp Dermatol 1990; 15:228–231.
51. Cohen LM, Capeless EL, Krusinski PA, Maloney ME. Pruritic urticarial papules and plaques of pregnancy and its relationship to maternal–fetal weight gain and twin pregnancy. Arch Dermatol 1989; 125:1534–1536.
52. Moreno A, Noguera J, Moragas JM. Polymorphic eruption of pregnancy: histopathologic study. Acta Derm Venerol (Stockh) 1985; 65:313–318.
53. Holmes RC, McGibbon DH, Black MM. Polymorphic eruption of pregnancy with subepidermal vesicles. J R Soc Med 1984; 77(suppl):22–23.
54. Ingber A, Alcalay J, Sandbank M. Multiple dermal fibroblasts in patients with pruritic urticarial papules and plaques of pregnancy. A clue to the etiology. Med Hypoth 1988; 26:11–12.
55. Kasp-Grochowska E, Beck J, Holmes RC, Black MM, Timlin D. The role of circulating immune complexes in the etiology of polymorphic eruption of pregnancy. Arch Dermatol Res 1984; 276:71–73.
56. Besnier E, Brock L, Jacquet L. La pratique dermatologique, 1. Paris. Masson et Cie, 1904, Tone IV, p 74–75.
57. Spangler AS, Reddy W, Bardawil WA, Roby CC, Emerson K. Papular dermatitis of pregnancy. A new clinical entity? JAMA 1962; 181:577–581.
58. Spangler AS, Emerson K. Estrogen levels and estrogen therapy in papular dermatitis of pregnancy. Am J Obstet Gynecol 1971; 110:534–537.
59. Zoberman E, Farmer ER. Pruritic folliculitis of pregnancy. Arch Dermatol 1981; 117:20–22.
60. Rahbari H. Pruritic papules of pregnancy. J Cutan Pathol 1978; 5:347–352.
61. Katzenellenbogen I, Feuerman EJ. Psoriasis pustolosa and impetigo herpetiformis. Single or dual entity. Acta Derm Venerol (Stockh) 1966; 46:86–94.
62. Oosterling RJ, Nobrega RE, Du Boeuff JA, Van der Meer JB. Impetigo herpetiformis or generalized pustular psoriasis? Arch Dermatol 1978; 114:1527–1529.
63. von Hebra F. Ueber einzlne wahrend swangerschaft, dens wachenbette unde bei uterinal krankheiten der frauen zu beobachtende haut-krankheiten. Wein Med Wochenschr 1872; 48:1197–1202.

64. Ross MG, Tucker DC, Hayashi RH. Impetigo herpetiformis as a cause of postpartum fever. Obstet Gynecol 1984; 64:49s–51s.
65. Beveridge GW, Harkness RA, Livingstone JRB. Impetigo herpetiformis in two successive pregnancies. Br J Dermatol 1966; 78:106–112.
66. Oumeish OY, Farraj SE. Some aspects of impetigo herpetiformis. Arch Dermatol 1982; 118:103–105.
67. Lotem M, Katzenelson V, Rotem A, Hod M, Sandbank M. Impetigo herpetiformis—a variant of pustular psoriasis or a separate entity? J Am Acad Dermatol 1988; 20:338–341.
68. Gentele H, Lodin A, Odqvist-Niordson AM. Impetigo herpetiformis in conjunction with parathyroprival tetany. Acta Derm Venerol (Stockh) 1957; 37:387–393.
69. Bajaj AK, Swarup V, Gupta OP, Gupta SC. Impetigo herpetiformis. Dermatologica 1977; 155:292–295.
70. Moynihan GD, Ruppe JP. Impetigo herpetiformis and hypoparathyroidism. Arch Dermatol 1985; 121:1330–1331.
71. Soter NA, Wasserman SI. Clinical manifestations pathogenesis and therapeutic approaches in urticaria/angioedema. Dermatol Dig 1979; 18:17–32.
72. Champion RH, Roberts SOB, Carpenter RG, Roger JH. Urticaria and angioedema. Br J Dermatol 1969; 81:588–597.
73. Meggs WJ, Pescouitz OH, Metcalfe D, et al. Progesterone sensitivity as a cause of recurrent anaphylaxis. N Engl J Med 1984; 19:1236–1238.
74. Farah F, Shtaklu A. Autoimmune progesterone urticaria. J Allergy Clin Immunol 1971; 48:257–261.
75. Frank MM, Gelfand JA, Atkinson JP. Hereditary angioedema: the clinical syndrome and its management. Ann Intern Med 1976; 4:580–593.
76. Warin RD, Cunliffer WT, Greaves MW, Wallingtion TB. Recurrent angioedema: familial and estrogen induced. Br J Dermatol 1986; 115:731–734.
77. Postnikoff IM, Pritzker KP. Hereditary angioneurotic edema: an unusual case of maternal mortality. J Forensic Sci 1979; 24:473–478.
78. Cunningham DS, Jensen JT. Hereditary angioneurotic edema in the puerperium. A case report. J Reprod Med 1991; 36:312–313.
79. Bhatia PL, Singh MS, Jha BK. Laryngopathia gravidarum. Ear Nose Throat J 1980; 60:408–412.
80. Stiller RJ, Kaplan BM, Andreoli JW. Hereditary angioedema and pregnancy. Obstet Gynecol 1984; 64:133–135.
81. Adverse effects of danazol in pregnancy [editorial]. Ann Intern Med 1982; 96:672–673.
82. Zeiger RS. Atopic dermatitis of childhood: current concepts and management. Immunol Allergy Pract 1981; 3:198–210.
83. Hanifin JM. Atopic dermatitis. In: Middleton E, Reed EC, Ellis EF, et al, eds. Allergy: principles and practice, 3rd ed. St Louis: CV Mosby, 1988:1403–1428.

84. Hanifin JM, Lobitz WC. Newer concepts of atopic dermatitis. Arch Dermatol 1977; 113:663–670.
85. Sampson H. Pathogenesis of eczema. Clin Exp Allergy 1990; 20:459–467.
86. Roth HL, Kierland RR. The natural history of atopic dermatitis. Arch Dermatol 1964; 89:209–214.
88. Schatz M, Hoffman CP, Zeiger RS, et al. The course and management of asthma and allergic disease during pregnancy. In: Middleton E, Reed CE, Ellis EF, et al, eds. Allergy: principles and practices, 3rd ed. St Louis: CV Mosby 1988:1093–1155.
87. Kemmett D, Tidman MJ. The influence of the menstrual cycle and pregnancy on atopic dermatitis. Br J Dermatol 1991; 125:59–61.
88. Schatz M, Zeiger RS. Allergic disease in pregnancy. In: Gleicher N, ed. Principles and Practice of Medical Therapy in Pregnancy, 2nd ed. East Norwalk, CT: Appleton–Lange 1992:435–454.

17

Immunologically Mediated Adverse Drug Reactions in Pregnancy

Eric Macy

Kaiser-Permanente Medical Center and University of California, San Diego, School of Medicine, San Diego, California

BACKGROUND

Pregnant women appear to be no more likely to have allergic reactions to medications than nonpregnant women, but actual data on rates of adverse drug reactions and drug allergies have not been prospectively collected (1). Given the general avoidance of all but essential medications in pregnancy, actual episodes of allergic reactions are fairly uncommon. Recent reviews on drug allergy by DeSwarte (2) and Anderson and Adkinson (3) and a treatment summary compiled by Patterson et al. (4) are good sources for further reading on the general principles of drug allergy. A summary of these general principles relative to pregnant women and a review of drugs likely to be given in pregnancy that have been reported to induce adverse or immunologically mediated reactions are the subjects of this chapter.

Frequency

In general surgical patients, immunologically mediated drug reactions have been estimated to account for fewer than 10% of the 1:10,000 rate of fatal drug reactions (2). The remainder of serious adverse drug reactions proceed by direct toxic, metabolic, or idiosyncratic mechanisms. A similar rate of fatal drug reactions has been quoted for the general medical population, although a slightly higher fraction, 10–

25%, may proceed by an immunological mechanism (5). Obstetrical patients can be expected to have this same theoretical 1:100,000 rate of life-threatening immunologically mediated adverse drug reactions. Immunologically mediated adverse reactions of less severity occur more frequently. A given reaction may have additional morbidity in the obstetrical population, with the potential for an adverse effect on the fetus, either from the reaction itself or the treatment of the reaction. Mild immunologically mediated reactions occur in up to 5% of individuals (3). These are almost exclusively cutaneous reactions with very little morbidity.

As part of the preparation of this chapter, a retrospective survey of adverse drug reaction reports generated on the obstetrical service at the San Diego Kaiser Foundation Hospital was performed to provide actual data on the occurrence of severe, acute potentially immunologically mediated drug reactions during labor and delivery. From January 1988 to June 1990, over which time about 12,500 live births occurred, no episodes of fatal anaphylaxis were reported. There was one reported reaction to phenytoin, two episodes associated with antibiotics (penicillin and metronidazole), and three reactions to agents used in epidural anesthesia. Although this form of reporting invariably underreports both mild and delayed-onset reactions, it does support the prevailing opinion that severe acute drug reactions and specifically immunologically mediated reactions in pregnant women are rare during labor and delivery.

Types of Reactions

The term *allergic* loosely refers to a subgroup of adverse drug reactions mediated by specific antibody or T-cell recognition of the drug, generally functioning as a hapten. This review will be restricted to known Gell and Coombs type I–IV reactions and only indirectly consider toxic, idiosyncratic, and other types of reactions (6). It will concentrate on true allergic, IgE-mediated or type I reactions, as these have the most dramatic presentation and, although rare, are potentially life-threatening to both the mother and baby.

If the term allergic was restricted to adverse reactions secondary to preformed IgE, much of the confusion with the term would be removed. The term *immunological drug reaction* could be used for type II, III, and IV reactions and the term *adverse drug reaction* would encompass all other mechanisms.

The obstetrical literature, like much of the general medical literature, has unfortunately perpetuated a sloppy use of the word allergic in the characterization of adverse drug reactions. A good example of this is a report by Bruner et al. about intolerance of antithyroid medications in a pregnant woman (7). Although they state that thioamide toxicity, a syndrome of uncertain pathogenisis, but consisting of a delayed onset purpuric papular rash, with occasional associated arthralgias, parathesias, headaches, nausea, and alopecia, was the mechanism for drug intolerance, the word *allergy* appears in the title and throughout the discussion. There was no documentation of an immunological mechanism responsible for the reaction in the report. Mechanisms of adverse reactions need to be characterized at least as mediated through a specific immune mechanism, preferably IgE, before they are labeled *allergic*.

IMMUNOLOGICAL MECHANISMS AND CLINICAL SYMPTOMS

Gell and Coombs Classification

The Gell and Coombs classification system provides a useful starting point to characterize clinically relevant immunological reactions (5). Potential adverse responses to drugs fall into all four Gell and Coombs types (6).

Type I reactions are mediated by preformed IgE bound to mast cells. The cross-linking of IgE by relevant therapeutic agents, either serving as haptens on autologous proteins or as complete antigens, releases preformed and newly synthesized mediators. This clinically results in urticaria, angioedema, and anaphylaxis.

Type II reactions involve antibodies, generally IgG, that either cross-react with native cell surface antigens or react with haptenated self. The result is cellular destruction, such as the hemolytic anemia seen with penicillin or methyldopa.

Type III reactions involve antibodies that, instead of directly binding to cells, form poorly soluble immune complexes with relevant antigens and activate complement. Complement activation is then responsible for the pathological changes seen. The serum sickness reactions seen with phenytoin or heterologous sera are clincal examples.

Type IV reactions are T–cell-mediated, the classic example being contact dermatitis. A similar mechanism is responsible for the nephritis seen with nonsteroidal anti-inflammatory medications.

The hallmarks of immunological reactions are specificity and memory. In general, unless there is a cross-reaction, an individual must be exposed to the drug and develop a specific immune response to it before experiencing an immunologically mediated adverse reaction. If the drug persists in the body or is continually given, a reaction could occur during the first course of treatment or because of a single treatment. It would be much more common for a reaction to occur with subsequent treatments. The IgE antibody, in particular, seems to develop more readily in individuals given intermittent dosing with the sensitizing agent. Bee-sting allergy represents a good example of this. Cutaneous and intramuscular are the most sensitizing routes of exposure for the development of IgE because the antigen tends to persist and continuously stimulate the immune system. Oral exposure is intermediate, and intravenous administration is the least immunogenic. In contrast, once the individual is sensitized, oral exposure has the lowest likelihood of inducing anaphylaxis, and intravenous has the highest because it can degranulate a large number of sensitized mast cells quickly.

Type I or Immunoglobulin E-Mediated Allergic Reactions

Immunoglobulin E-mediated reactions in their most extreme form, anaphylaxis, with its immediate life-threatening sequelae, is what justly inhibits physicians from administering medications to individuals who are "allergic" to them. Other immunologically mediated adverse reactions proceed much more slowly, are less likely to be fatal, and generally improve with discontinuation of the medication. Delayed-onset skin rash, rarely IgE mediated and not predicted by immediate-type hypersensitivity skin testing, probably represents the most common clinical symptom associated with immunologically mediated reactions.

The IgE-mediated reactions comprise

1. Cutaneous urticarial eruptions
2. Angioedema of the skin, respiratory and digestive system mucosa
3. Asthma
4. Hypotension, shock, and death.

The pathogenisis of these reactions is the result of preformed IgE bound to mast cells and basophils combining with antigen, which results in the release of preformed and late-phase or newly synthesized mediators. The effect of these mediators both on vascular permeability and on vascular, respiratory, and digestive system smooth muscle results in most of the changes seen.

Direct mast cell release bypassing IgE occurs in anaphylactoid reactions, such as those seen with intravenous contrast medium or opiates. The acute clinical scenario and treatment of anaphylactoid reactions are similar to true anaphylaxis. The important difference is that skin testing is not predictive. Premedication with corticosteroids and antihistamines helps prevent anaphylactoid reactions in those with a history of contrast medium reactions.

DIAGNOSIS

History

The history is the key to prevention. As with politics, so with medicine, those who ignore the past are bound to repeat it.

Given an initial allergic drug reaction, there appear to be persons who are at higher risk for repeating both allergic and nonallergic drug reactions. Sullivan at the 1990 American Academy of Allergy and Immunology annual meeting presented unpublished data showing a markedly increased rate of adverse reactions to a variety of unrelated antibiotics in a group of general medical patients selected for an initial systemic reaction to penicillin. Of 312 patients with a previous systemic reaction to penicillin, 20% also had an adverse reaction to an unrelated drug, and 7% had two or more reactions to different unrelated drugs. The serious associated secondary reactions included eight patients with anaphylaxis, seven with drug fever, five with Stevens–Johnson syndrome, and four with serum sickness.

An important element in the history is the time between drug exposure and onset of reaction. As a general rule, the reaction of preformed IgE bound to mast cells in anaphylaxis starts in seconds to minutes; that of preformed IgG mediating a reaction through complement begins in hours; boosted T cells infiltrate skin containing a foreign antigen in 1–2 days; new IgM and IgG can be produced and mediate a serum sickness reaction within 1–2 weeks; and newly sensitized cells can mediate contact dermatitis within 1–2 weeks.

The route of exposure in both the historical reaction and anticipated drug administration is important, with parenteral exposures more immediately life-threatening than oral or cutaneous administration. Clinical symptoms, such as systemic angioedema, urticaria, wheezing, and hypotension after drug exposure, all indicate a potential IgE-mediated anaphylactic or direct mast–cell-release anaphylactoid reaction.

Uneventful rechallange with a drug that has previously evoked a reaction, whether anticipated and controlled or inadvertent, can progress to very different conclusions depending on the timing of the exposures and the exact nature of the adverse reactions. Consider the following two patients, using penicillin as an example.

Patient A previously had a rash after penicillin had been given during an Epstein–Barr virus infection; then, subsequently, tolerated a 10-day course of oral dicloxicillin, without any adverse effect. There is a high probability that this patient does not have any IgE to penicillin.

Patient B had life-threatening anaphylaxis 10 min after intramuscular penicillin 20 years ago and just recently tolerated a course of oral penicillin. This second patient may have just stimulated new high levels of IgE and may have anaphylaxis with the next parenteral exposure to penicillin.

Antigen specific IgE levels tend to fade in the absence of exposure, and reboosting theoretically can occur from occult sources such as traces of antibiotics in foodstuffs. Legal considerations bias recommendations relative to anaphylaxis and, thus, my recommendations are very conservative: **All pregnant patients with a history of prior adverse reaction to penicillin should be penicillin skin tested within 48 hr of any anticipated use of penicillin.** Penicillin skin testing is very safe (10).

The recommendation stands even though only some of these patients (such as Patient B above) are likely to be penicillin skin test-positive. If skin tested and negative, both patients have about a 1–3% chance of having a delayed onset skin rash with penicillin, often a mild type III reaction, about the same rate as the general population. Even if negative, given the good positive history of anaphylaxis in the second patient, there would be approximately a 0.1% chance of subsequent anaphylaxis. This is about 100 times higher than the first patient, who would have the same risk as any random person in the population, between 1:100,000 and 1:1 million (8).

Despite what has been previously stated, in pediatric populations, prophylactic penicillin skin testing of "penicillin allergic" children far in advance of anticipated use of penicillins has been quite safe and useful (9). There are several important differences to consider. Most patients told that they were allergic to penicillin had only rashes and not true anaphylaxis. Most children are given only oral penicillins. Although several hundred children have been tested and followed by Mendelson et al. (9), the true frequency of anaphylaxis to oral penicillin is very rare. Parenteral penicillins are needed in most circumstances that may be anticipated in the sick obstetrical patient and, therefore, much higher rates of anaphylaxis could be anticipated.

Skin Testing

Skin testing is still the most useful and quickest way to safely identify the presence of medication-specific IgE, but unfortunately, it is restricted by the drugs available for use. Drugs are generally small molecules that function as haptens, and appropriate skin test reagents require knowledge of the exact drug metabolite that is the causative hapten. There are alternative chemically reactive forms for a number of drugs, well illustrated by penicillin, which has at least four significant determinants (10). Sulfa drugs, aminoglycosides, cephalosporins, and monobactams, all are antibiotics that potentially can be used in skin testing. Unfortunately, skin testing is unsatisfactory for these drugs because adequate reagents—specifically reactive forms or minor determinants—are not commercially available, and the native drugs as solitary reagents possess neither high specificity nor sensitivity. Protein medications, such as vaccines, insulin, and heterollogous sera, do not have this problem, because the drug is an intact antigen in its own right and capable of cross-linking IgE without functioning as a hapten.

Skin testing cannot be reliably performed with drugs that induce direct mast cell release, such as quaternary ammonium neuromuscular blockers, intravenous contrast material, dextran, polygelatin, or opiates. It also will not work with drugs that do not haptenate readily, such as erythromycin. When skin testing with untested reagents, adequate negative controls need to be done on nonsensitive subjects to ensure the material used for skin testing is not a direct cutaneous irritant.

In Vitro Testing

In vitro testing for antigen-specific IgE to drugs by enzyme-linked immunosorbent assay (ELISA) or radioallergosorbent technique (RAST) are now available only in research settings, but this is a very exciting area of potential advance. Specific tests have been developed for β-lactams, sulfonamides, quaternary ammonium neuromuscular blockers, and many proteins, including vaccines and serum proteins. Commercial availability of these reagents is anticipated. Drugs, such as sulfonamides, which in vivo require hepatic metabolism to be transformed to a reactive form that is able to haptenate to carrier proteins before interaction with IgE, could be provided in the relevant form directly in an in vitro test. Identification of metabolites is a complex and time-consuming process. Given the variation in immune responses among individuals, often a panel of haptens must be used to identify all truely allergic individuals.

TREATMENT

Acute Immunoglobulin E-Mediated Reactions

Epinephrine is the mainstay of immediate treatment for systemic IgE-mediated reactions. The rapid intramuscular or subcutaneous administration of 0.3 mL of 1:1000 epinephrine is essential as soon as a systemic allergic reaction is suspected. (See Chapter 15 for further discussion of treatment of drug-induced anaphylaxis.)

Delayed Onset Immunologically Mediated Reactions

Discontinuation of the offending drug is the mainstay of treating type II, III, and IV reactions. The current recommendation for the treatment of Stevens–Johnson syndrome with significant skin sloughing is supportive and relies on the principles of burn management. In pediatric studies, systemic steroids have yet to be shown effective (11). This is a very controversial area, with impassioned but anecdotal arguments both for and against use. In the adult literature the current prevailing opinion supports the use of systemic steroids for the treatment of this syndrome (12). Milder skin reactions may just be treated supportively.

The use of topical steroids to suppress an ongoing contact dermatitis is preferred to systemic administration. As discussed in Chapter 8, systemic steroids appear to be safe in pregnancy and, occasionally, are necessary in the treatment of severe drug eruptions. Mild skin itching or urticaria can usually be safely controlled with tripelennamine, 50 mg every 4–6 hr.

Desensitization

Desensitization can be achieved in individuals with high levels of preformed IgE to a particular medication by the controlled administration of increasing amounts of the agent. Clinically, systemic effects will be seen within minutes to 1 hr after parenteral exposure to a drug for which an individual has drug-specific IgE. Life-threatening reactions virtually always begin well within the first hour of exposure. Fifteen to 20 min has been selected as the time between doses in desensitization protocols for IgE-mediated reactions, because adverse reactions generally become evident in this interval. The patient may complain of a flushed or hot feeling, itchy skin, hives, throat tightness, shortness of breath, wheezing, stomach upset, or proceed rapidly to shock. Oral exposure causes less acute and generally less severe symptoms, as opposed to an equivalent dose administered intravenously. The oral route is therefore preferred and has been exploited in penicillin desensitization protocols, since oral forms are available (see later). Five to seven orders of magnitude less drug than the final therapeutic dose is generally selected as the starting dose for desensitization, and stepwise increases of between two- and tenfold are generally used.

Contrast Medium Anaphylactoid Reaction Prophylaxis

Pregnant women with a history of an anaphylactoid reaction to intravenous contrast medium who require subsequent exposure should be treated with a slight modification of the protocol of Anderson and Adkinson (3). Nonionic material should be employed, if possible. Prednisone 50 mg is given every 6 hr for three doses, beginning 13 hr before the procedure. Tripelennamine, 50 mg, is given orally 1 hr before the procedure. Test doses are not helpful and should not be given.

SPECIFIC MEDICATIONS

It is generally considered prudent to avoid medications in pregnant women. However, there are situations in pregnancy when medications are needed. These occur when the assumed benefit from administration outweighs potential adverse effects. Following are specific medications, which pregnant women may receive for indicated disorders, that at the same time may lead to immunologically mediated and other adverse reactions (Table 1).

Penicillins

Syphilis (both primary and secondary disease) in adults and congenital syphilis reached their highest overall rate in 40 years in the United States in 1988. Prolonged courses of parenteral penicillins remain the best treatment for central nervous system syphilis. Inadequately treated syphilis has significant documented fetal morbidity. Thus, the need for exposure to penicillins in pregnant women who are penicillin-allergic is probably at an all time high. β-Lactam antibiotics may also be required during pregnancy in women with histories of penicillin allergy whose respiratory infections are not responding to erythromycin, with or without sulfonamides.

Penicillin Skin Testing

A history of previous anaphylaxis or systemic reaction to penicillin mandates skin testing to penicillin before subsequent use. Appropriate reagents include the major determinants, benzylpenicillin and benzylpenicilloyl polylysine (Pre-Pen, Taylor Pharmacal Co. Decatur, Illinois) and the minor determinants, benzylpenicilloic acid and benzylpenilloic acid (Table 2). Previous delayed-onset rash associated with penicillin, whether erythematous, fixed drug eruption, or even urticarial, is generally not indicative of high risk for subsequent anaphylaxis, but

Table 1 Adverse Drug Reactions in Pregnancy with Emphasis on Immunological and Allergic Mechanisms

Medication	Primary Known Mechanisms	Ref.
Angiotensin-converting enzyme inhibitors	Other	13, 14
Aldomet (methyldopa)	Type II	15
β-Blockers	Other	16
Barbiturates	Type I	17–19
Dextran	Other	20, 21
Heparin	Type II, I	22, 23
Heterologous sera	Type III, I	4, 24
Human serum albumin	Type I	25
Hydralazine	Type III	15
Insulin	Type I	26–28
Latex gloves	Type I, IV	30
Local anesthetics	Other, type I	18, 19, 31
$MgSO_4$	Other	32
Nonsteroidal anti-inflammatory drugs	Other, type IV	4
Opiates	Other	18, 19, 33
Other antibiotics (sulfonamide, aminoglycosides, macrolides)	Type I, other	2
Oxytocin	Type I, other	17, 34–36
Penicillins/cepholasporins/monobactams	Types I, II, III	10, 37–40
Phenytoin	Type III, other	41
Polygelatin	Other	42
Propylthiouracil	Other	7
Quaternary ammonium muscle relaxants	Other, type I	15, 43
Radiographic contrast medium	Other	29
RhoGAM (Rh_oD immune globulin)	Type III, other	44, 45
Vitamin K	Other	46

prudence should mandate skin testing and, if positive, penicillin avoidance, or administration by a desensitizing protocol. Skin testing, however, does not predict delayed onset rashes. Skin testing is empirically considered valid for a 48-hr period, as it may potentially, albeit rarely, cause de novo production or boosting of IgE.

Table 2 Penicillin Skin Testing

I. Reagents	
Benzylpenicilloyl-polylysine	(6×10^{-5} M)
Benzylpenicillin	(6000 U/mL or 10^{-2} M)
(Not commercially available):	
Benzylpenicilloic acid[a]	(10^{-2} M)
Benzylpenilloic acid[a]	(10^{-2} M)
Histamine (positive control)	(1.0 mg/mL)
Buffered saline (negative control)	

II. Procedure
1. Scratch or prick test is done first.
2. Negative tests are followed by intradermal tests using 0.02 mL of each reagent administered with a 27-guage needle.
3. The tests are read at 20-min, with larger than 4 mm of wheal in the presence of erythema being interpreted as a positive test.
4. Both the positive and negative controls must work as expected.

[a]Benzylpenicilloic acid and benzylpenilloic acid are more stable in solution when stored at −70°C, but may be kept at −20°C. In the anhydrous form they can be stored at 4°C. They can be prepared by the method of Levine and Redmond (47).

Immunological Cross-Reactions Between β-Lactams

Antibiotics that cross-react to a high degree with penicillins include all of the modified or semisynthetic penicillins and imipenim (Table 3). Cephalosporins cross-react less frequently and less predictably, but skin testing for cephalosporin allergy outside of a research setting is not feasible because of the difficulty in obtaining or producing appropriate minor determinants and the low predictive yield of skin testing with the native drugs. The increasing size of the side chains in second- and third-generation cephelosporins tend to dominate the immunological reactivity. Monobactams, in general, and aztreonam, in particular, tend not to cross-react with penicillin and can be safely given in most penicillin-allergic individuals, although rare individuals with dual sensitivities have been reported. The primary side chain of aztreonam is identical with that of ceftazidime, and these two drugs do share immunological cross-reactivity.

Jarish–Herxheimer Reactions

All systemic reactions in pregnant women with syphilis treated with penicillins are not allergic in origin, as Jarish–Herxheimer reactions also occur and can result in preterm labor, preterm delivery, or fetal death (40). These delayed reactions occur 4–8 hr after penicillin ther-

Table 3 β-Lactam Immunological Cross-Reactivity Relative to Penicillin

High
Penicillin
Penicillinase resistant penicillins
All semisynthetic penicillins
Imipenim (core structure dominates)
Low
First-generation cephalosporins
Second-generation cephalosporins (fewer cross-reactions with large side chains)
Very low
Monobactams
Third-generation cephalosporins (side chains dominate)

apy and are still of uncertain pathogenesis, although they have been shown not to be the result of systemic endotoxin release. Similar reactions have been seen in the treatment of Lyme disease.

Penicillin Desensitization

Penicillin, as well as other medications causing IgE-mediated reactions, can be administered under strict guidelines in a sensitized individual using the general method outlined by Sullivan, and reported in a series of 15 pregnant women by Wendel et al. (37). Sullivan has summarized the rational for the preference of oral desensitization (38).

1. Deaths from oral penicillin are extremely rare.
2. Drug polymers and contaminating penicillin mold will not be absorbed orally.
3. Blood levels rise gradually after oral dosing, allowing more univalent haptenation to occur that will be unable to cross-link IgE.
4. No life-threatening reactions have occurred in more than 90 reported cases of oral desensitization.
5. Parenteral desensitization regimens have been described, but have a higher incidence of untoward effects (39).

The following procedure and protocol for oral penicillin desensitization has been adapted by most institutions and was first described by Wendel et al. (37). Patients are selected if

1. They have positive reactions to penicillin skin test reagents.
2. They are infected with an organism sensitive to β-lactam antibiotics.

3. No alternative antibiotics are available.
4. The infection is life-threatening.
5. The risk of a fatal allergic reaction is considered to be of less risk than the potentially fatal outcome from the infection if β-lactam antibiotics are not used.

Written consent is ideally obtained from the patient, patient's family, patient's physicians, and infectious disease consultant. The procedure is done under continuous monitoring by a physician, with life-support equipment available. The procedure is initiated in the morning if possible. An intravenous line is established. Epinephrine, other emergency medications, and resuscitation equipment are at the bedside. No premedication is given. No lapses in therapy are allowed after desensitization is achieved, and nurses are alerted to the possibility of a severe late-onset reaction.

Oral desensitization is begun using penicillin G, 100 units (U) in 50 mL of water, and doubling the dose of penicillin every 15 min until 400,000 U in 50 mL of water has been given. Commercial oral suspensions of penicillin G are made up to the appropriate dilutions in water, or carbenicillin tablets are crushed, weighed, and given with 50 mL of water (Table 4). The procedure continues with 200,000 U, 400,000 U, and 800,000 U, given subcutaneously at 15-min intervals. Finally 1 million U is given intramuscularly, and intravenous therapy is started within 15 min. No lapses in therapy are permitted. The patient is continually monitored for at least 1 hr after the first intravenous dose is completed. If a severe reaction occurs, it is treated as necessary and, when the patient is stabilized, the dose given before the reaction is repeated and the protocol proceeds. About 30% of patients can be expected to develop an urticarial eruption 6–48 hr after IV treatment is started. The rashes are treated with an antihistamine (tripelennamine, 50 mg), if needed, and the penicillin is continued.

This procedure does not cure penicillin allergy. It merely allows the safe administration of penicillin to an individual with IgE directed against penicillin. If therapy is allowed to lapse, there is a potential for a booster effect on IgE production and a high probability of subsequent anaphylaxis when penicillin is next administered. Carbenicillin may then be given twice a day to maintain desensitization in an individual who may need repetitive courses of penicillins, such as a patient with cystic fibrosis.

Insulin

Anaphylaxis to insulin is rare, but the setting of gestational diabetes is one of the instances for which intermittent use of insulin (which pre-

Table 4 Protocol for Oral Penicillin Densensitization

Dose	Units (if using penicillin G)	Micrograms (if using carbenicillin)	Route
1	100	60	PO
2	200	120	PO
3	400	240	PO
4	800	480	PO
5	1,600	960	PO
6	3,200	2,000	PO
7	6,400	4,000	PO
8	12,800	8,000	PO
9	25,000	16,000	PO
10	50,000	32,000	PO
11	100,000	64,000	PO
12	200,000	125,000	PO
13	400,000	250,000	PO
14	200,000	125,000	SC
15	400,000	250,000	SC
16	800,000	500,000	SC
17	1 million	500,000	IM
18	First intravenous dose		IV

Notes: Doses 1–18 are given at 15-min intervals. No longer than 12 hr between intravenous doses is permitted without repeating the procedure. A total of 5 hr and 15 min are required if no adverse reactions occur. Should a reaction occur, treat the reaction and, when stabilized, resume the protocol, repeating the dose before the one that caused the reaction.

disposes to insulin allergy) may be undertaken. Human insulin is currently the preferred product for primary administration in the new-onset diabetic patient who is pregnant, since human insulin is less immunogenic than animal insulins. Apparent IgE-mediated reactions can occur even to human products in individuals previously sensitized to animal insulins, as reported by Gossain et al. (26) and Bodendorfer et al. (27).

In patients exhibiting systemic insulin allergy during pregnancy, desensitization can be achieved by administration of subcutaneous regular insulin starting at 1/10,000 U and increasing the dosage by tenfold increments every 15 min until the desired dose is achieved, under constant observation as described in the foregoing for penicillin desensitization (4). It is then preferable to maintain the individual on a regimen of at least twice-daily regular insulin to maintain the desensitization. If there is an interruption in the therapy, repeat desensitization is recommended.

Local cutaneous reactions to insulin are much more common and usually disappear with continued therapy. The associated itching generally responds to antihistamines such as tripelennamine. Increasingly large local reactions may precede systemic reactions.

Heparin

Heparin may be responsible for rare IgE-mediated reactions, in addition to mediating a thrombocytopenia of type II immunological origin, resulting in enhanced platelet sequestration without platelet lysis (6). Heparin and antiheparin IgG form complexes and then bind to platelets through the IgG Fc to glycoprotein 1b, independently of the von Willebrand factor site. De Boer et al. have reported the successful treatment of a pregnant woman, with deep venous thrombosis, with the low-molecular-weight heparin preparation Fragmin, who had a previous adverse reaction to native heparin (22).

Oxytocin

Rare case reports of apparent IgE-mediated reactions to oxytocin have been published, and in several of the cases, the preservative chlorobutanol or possibly associated anesthetic agents, such as thiopental, were implicated (17,34–36). Anaphylaxis to oxytocin is so rare that there is no practical way to screen for its occurrence other than history.

Oxytocin desensitization could theoretically be achieved in a fashion similar to insulin desensitization: start with 0.02 mU (20 μU) of oxytocin intramuscularly and double the dose every 15 min. The target intramuscular dose to be tolerated would be 450 mU or greater, equivalent to the cumulative dose that would be given intravenously over 15 min at 30 mU/min. This procedure has yet to be tested and should be done only with resuscitation equipment available, as with any desensitization procedure. Intravenous oxytocin could theoretically be started 15 min after the 450 mU or greater intramuscular dose was tolerated.

Magnesium Sulfate

A report of two anecdotal cases of urticarial eruptions apparently secondary to magnesium sulfate ($MgSO_4$) has been published (32). However, the patients refused rechallange, and no immunological studies were performed. It seems extremely doubtful that an IgE-mediated or any immunologically mediated mechanism was involved.

Anesthetic Agents

Anesthesia provides the greatest potential risk of severe adverse drug reactions to women during labor and delivery. With the cesarean section rate unfortunately, and probably unnecessarily, as high as 20–50% in some hospitals, many women are exposed to this morbidity. Often the exact cause of what appears to be an anaphylactoid reaction is difficult to determine (48–50).

Local Anesthetics

True IgE-mediated reactions to local anesthetic agents are extremely rare, but have been identified. The vast majority of local or systemic reactions are pharmacologic reactions, inadvertent intravenous administration, or toxic effects. Thus, using the smallest amount possible and avoiding intravenous administration minimizes these occurrences. Skin testing and provocative challenges for local anesthetics have been outlined elsewhere (4). Preservatives have not been shown to be a significant problem in local anesthetics, and the use of preservative-free material is not routinely recommended.

Opiates and Fentanyl

Opiates as a class are direct mast cell releasing agents. Codeine has been classically used as a positive control for immediate hypersensitivity skin testing, although histamine itself is now is more widely used. Morphine has been widely reported to cause direct mast cell release and urticarial eruptions.

Fentanyl administered epidurally has been reported to cause an anaphylactoid reaction (33). Fentanyl is in general a poor direct mast cell histamine releaser, but it is still probably functioning in this capacity, as the data for specific IgE directed against it is weak.

Thiopental

Thiopental, a barbiturate, may rarely be the cause of an IgE-mediated reaction (17). There is no good data on frequency, nor on rates of cross-reaction with other barbiturates.

Neuromuscular Blockers

Quaternary ammonium neuromuscular blockers are all capable of direct mast cell mediator release, but the newer agents are orders of magnitude less efficient at this, as opposed to curare (51). There may be rare individuals able to make IgE to these agents, and this antibody may cross-react throughout this class of agents through the quaternary ammonium group. As optimal neuromuscular blocking agents contain two quaternary nitrogens separated by 12–20 A, these agents are theoretically capable of serving as bivalent reagents, directly cross-linking IgE and bypassing the need for haptenation.

SUMMARY

Outside of penicillins and insulin, there is very little useful specific information published concerning drug allergy in pregnancy. Most reports are just anecdotes and do not provide data on risks of reactions or benefits for particular interventions. A rational approach can still be undertaken by using the general medical literature on drug allergy. Avoidance thus should be the mainstay of treatment of drug allergy in pregnancy, and history is the key to avoidance. Desensitization, if needed, can be safely achieved in pregnant women. The IgE-mediated anaphylactic reactions and anaphylactoid reactions need to be treated aggressively.

REFERENCES

1. Schatz M, Hoffman CP, Zeiger RS, Falkoff R, Mellon M. The course and management of asthma and allergic disease in pregnancy. In: Middleton E, Reed EE, Ellis EF, et al, eds. Allergy: principles and practice, 3rd ed. St Louis: CV Mosby, 1988:1093–1155.
2. DeSwarte RD. Drug allergy: an overview. Clin Rev Allergy 1988; 4:143–169.
3. Anderson JA, Adkinson NF. Allergic reactions to drugs and biologic agents. JAMA 1987; 258:2891–2899.
4. Patterson R, DeSwarte RD, Greenberger PA, Grammer LC. Drug allergy and protocols for management of drug allergies. N Engl Regional Allergy Proc 1986; 7:325–342.
5. Coombs RRA, Gell PGH. Classification of allergic reactions responsible for clinical hypersensitivity and disease. In: Gell PGH, Coombs RRA, Lachmann PJ, eds. Clinical aspects of immunology, 3rd ed. Oxford: Blackwell Scientific Publications, 1975:761–781.
6. Coleman JW. Allergic reactions to drugs: current concepts and problems. Clin Exp Allergy 1990; 20:79–85.
7. Bruner JP, Landon MB, Grabbe SG. Diabetes mellitus and Graves' disease in pregnancy complicated by maternal allergies to antithyroid medication. Obstet Gynecol 1988; 72:443–445.

8. Sullivan TJ. Drug allergy. In: Middleton E, Reed EE, Ellis EF, et al, eds. Allergy: principles and practice, 3rd ed. St Louis: CV Mosby, 1988:1523–1536.
9. Mendelson LM, Ressler C, Rosen JP, Selcow JE. Routine elective penicillin allergy skin testing in children and adolescents: study of sensitization. J Allergy Clin Immunol 1984; 73:76–81.
10. Saxon A, Beall GB, Rohr AS, Adelman DC. Immediate hypersensitivity reactions to beta-lactam antibiotics. Ann Intern Med 1987; 107:204–215.
11. Prendiville JS, Hebert AA, Greenwald MJ, Esterly NB. Management of Stevens–Johnson syndrome and toxic epidermal necrolysis in children. J Pediatr 1989; 115:881–887.
12. Patterson R, Dykewicz MS, Gonzalzles A, Grammer LC, Green D, Greenburger PA, McGrath KG, Walker CL. Erythema multiforme and Stevens–Johnson syndrome. Descriptive and therapeutic controversy. Chest 1990; 98:331–336.
13. Kreft-Jais C, Plouin PF, Tchobroutsky, Boutry MJ. Angiotension converting enzyme inhibitors during pregnancy. Br J Obstet Gynaecol 1988; 95:420–423.
14. Raia JJ Jr, Barone JA, Byerly WG, Lacy CR. Angiotensin-converting enzyme inhibitors: a comparative review. Drug Intell Clin Pharm Ann Pharmacother 1990; 24:506–525.
15. Mitchell JA, Gillam EMJ, Stanley LA, Sim E. Immunotoxic side-effects of drug therapy. Drug Safety 1990; 5:169–178.
16. Toogood JH. beta-Blocker therapy and the risk of anaphylaxis. Can Med Assoc J 1987; 136:929–933.
17. Giuffrida JG, Singh S, Bizzarri DV. Anaphylaxis to thiopental or oxytocin. Anesthesiol Rev 1981; 8:30–33.
18. Parnass SM, Schmidt KJ. Adverse effects of spinal and epidural anaesthesia. Drug Safety 1990; 5:179–194.
19. Stoelting RK. Allergic reactions during anesthesia. Anesth Analg 1983; 62:341–356.
20. Paull J. A prospective study of dextran-induced anaphylactoid reactions in 5745 patients. Anaesth Intensive Care 1987; 15:163–167.
21. Fanous LH, Gray A, Felmingham J. Severe anaphylactoid reactions to dextran 70. Br Med J 1977; 2:1189–1190.
22. de Boer K, Heyboer H, ten Cate JW, Borm JJJ, van Ginkel CJW. Low molecular weight heparin treatment in a pregnant woman with allergy to standard heparins and heparinoid. Thromb Haemost 1989; 61:148.
23. Mayou SC, Kelly SE, McGibbon DH. Local cutaneous sensitivity to subcutaneous heparin. Br J Dermatol 1987; 117:664–665.
24. Macy E, Bulpitt K, Champlin RE, Saxon A. Anaphylaxis to infusion of autologous bone marrow: an apparent reaction to self mediated by IgE antibody to bovine serum albumin. J Allergy Clin Immunol 1989; 83:871–875.

25. Stafford CT, Lobel SA, Fruge BC, Moffitt JE, Hoff RG, Fadel HE. Anaphylaxis to human serum albumin. Ann Allergy 1988; 61:85–88.
26. Gossain VV, Rovner DR, Mohan K. Systemic allergy to human (recombinant DNA) insulin. Ann Allergy 1985; 55:116–118.
27. Bodendorfer TW, Brown MB, Frankel EH, Palay BH, Fulp SR. Desensitization with human (recombinant DNA) insulin. Drug Intell Clin Pharm 1985; 19:827–829.
28. Yap PK. Primary allergy to monocomponent porcine insulin. Postgrad Med J 1985; 61:629–630.
29. Greenberger PA, Patterson R. Adverse reactions to radiocontrast media. Prog Cardiovasc Dis 1988; 31:239–248.
30. Turjanmaa K, Reunala T, Tuimala R, Karkkainen T. Allergy to latex gloves: unusual complication during delivery. Br Med J 1988; 297:1029.
31. Erkkola R, Kanto J, Maenpaa J, Kero P, Hovi-Viander M, Viander M. Allergic reaction to an amide local anesthetic in segmental epidural analgesia. Acta Obstet Gynecol Scand 1988; 67:181–184.
32. Thorp JM Jr, Katz VL, Campphell D, Ceefalo RC. Hypersensitivity to magnesium sulfate. Am J Obstet Gynecol 1989; 161:889–890.
33. Zucker-Pinchoff B, Ramanathan S. Anaphylactic reaction to epidural fentanyl. Anesthesiology 1989; 71:599–601.
34. Kawarabayashi T, Narisawa Y, Nakamura K, Sugimori H, Oda M, Taniguchi Y. Anaphylactoid reaction to oxytocin during cesarean section. Gynecol Obstet Invest 1988; 225:277–279.
35. Hofmann H, Goerz G, Plewig G. Anaphylactic shock from chlorobutanol-preserved oxytocin. Contact Derm 1986; 15:241–260.
36. Slater RM, Bowles BJM, Pumphrey RSH. Anaphylactoid reaction to oxytocin in pregnancy. Anaesthesia 1985; 40:655–656.
37. Wendel GD Jr, Stark BJ, Jamison RB, Molina RD, Sullivan TJ. Penicillin allergy and desensitization in serious infections during pregnancy. N Engl J Med 1985; 312:1229–1232.
38. Stark BJ, Wendel GD, Sullivan TJ. Oral desensitization for penicillin sensitivity. JAMA 1987; 257:1474.
39. Ziaya PR, Hankins GDV, Gilstrap LC III, Halsey AB. Intravenous penicillin desensitization and treatment during pregnancy. JAMA 1986; 256:2561–2562.
40. Klein VJ, Cox SM, Mitchell MD, Wendel GD Jr. The Jarisch–Herxheimer reaction complicating syphilotherapy in pregnancy. Obstet Gynecol 1990; 75:375–379.
41. Silverman AK, Fairley J, Wong RC. Cutaneous and immunologic reactions to phenytoin. J Am Acad Dermatol 1988; 18:721–741.
42. Lund N. Anaphylactoid reaction to infusion of polygelatin (Haemaccel). Anaesthesia 1980; 35:655–659.
43. Matthews MD, Ceglarski JZ, Pabari M. Anaphylaxis to suxamethonium—a case report. Anaesth Intensive Care 1977; 5:235–238.

44. Ring J, Thomas P. Anaphylactoid reaction after injection of anti-rhesus-D-hyperimmunoglobulin. Clin Allergy 1988; 18:510–512.
45. Jones BF, Trevillian PR, Nanra RS. Serum sickness due to Rh (anti-D) immunoglobulin. Aust NZ J Obstet Gynaecol 1984; 24:49–50.
46. Andersen TB, Hindsholm KB, Fallingborg J. Severe complication to phytomenadione after intramuscular injection in woman in labor. Acta Obstet Gynecol Scand 1989; 68:381–382.
47. Levine BB, Redmond AP. Minor haptenic determinant-specific reagins of penicillin hypersensitivity in man. Int Arch Allergy 1969; 35:445–455.
48. Jackson IJB, Bryson MR, McPhail S, Bhala BB. Recurrent anaphylactoid reaction during cesarean section. Anaesthesia, 1989; 44:585–587.
49. Emmott RS. Recurrent anaphylactoid reaction during caesarean section. Anaesthesia, 1990; 45:62.
50. Moscicki RA, Sockin SM, Corsello BF, Ostro MG, Bloch KJ. Anaphylaxis during induction of general anesthesia: subsequent evaluation and management. J Allergy Clin Immunol 1990; 86:325–332.
51. Vervloet D. Allergy to muscle relaxants and related compounds. Clin Allergy 1985; 15:501–508.

18

Genetic Factors in the Development of Allergy

N-I M Kjellman and Lennart Nilsson

University Hospital, Linköping, Sweden

CHARACTERIZATION OF ALLERGIC/ATOPIC DISEASES

Is the Increase in Allergy Genetically Determined?

Allergic diseases, such as allergic rhinoconjunctivitis (hay fever and perennial allergic rhinitis), bronchial asthma, atopic eczema (dermatitis), certain forms of urticaria, and some gastrointestinal allergies, are often called *atopic* (≈ strange or mysterious) (1,2). They share a common genetic background, as demonstrated in pedigree and twin studies (3–6). Edfors-Lubs gave support also for the importance of nongenetic (i.e., environmental) factors (6). Immunoglobulin E-mediated allergy and other forms of hyperreactivity are predominant causes of symptoms and signs of the allergic diseases. Highly predisposed children may show all types of allergic symptoms. In addition, they may show a variety of pharmacologic abnormalities, some of which may be primary and, therefore, genetically predetermined (7,8). The "hyperreactivity" of part of their immune system involving regulation of IgE-mast cells–eosinophils may have given survival advantage (e.g., through a superior protection against parasites) (9–11). This would explain a slow increase in allergic diseases over thousands of years, but hardly the rapid rise in hay fever, for example, over the last decades (12–14). Changing habits and environment must be sought to explain the increase in incidence and prevalence rates of allergic diseases as well as the increase in asthma deaths experienced in many countries during the past 20 years (15,16).

Immunoglobulin E Antibodies and the Definition of Atopy

It is a normal phenomenon to produce low amounts of IgE antibodies (e.g., to egg) at first contact, but subjects with no genetic propensity for allergy soon turn off the production of these antibodies, and most of them never show symptoms when ingesting the allergen in question (17–19). On the other hand, subjects with a genetic propensity for allergy and allergic disease produce higher amounts of IgE antibodies to the foods eaten during infancy, and some of the infants develop symptoms when ingesting these foods. The symptoms may occur from various organs (e.g., from the gastrointestinal tract or skin).

Atopy is defined as a genetic propensity to produce large amounts of IgE antibodies to normal environmental antigens at normal contact and to have difficulties in turning off the production of these antibodies, eventually giving rise to symptoms at renewed contact with the allergen in question (20). When a baby has demonstrated its genetic predisposition for atopy, a whole range of symptoms may have to be expected in the future in response to environmental exposure, cnanges in barrier function, and changes in immune balance (21–23).

Once Atopic, Always Atopic

The *multifactorial* etiology of allergic diseases was already recognized by Salter in 1864 (24). The presence of IgE antibodies to a particular allergen indicates that the person is sensitized to the allergen. It is important to stress, however, that the presence of even large amounts of IgE specific for food or other environmental allergens does not prove current allergy to the particular allergen, but it does suggest a genetic predisposition for allergic disease (25–27). Sensitized subjects who remain asymptomatic when exposed to appropriate doses of the proper allergen are said to have *latent* allergy (27–29). There are also other reasons why sensitization is not always accompanied by symptoms at exposure to the allergen in question. For instance, symptoms may fail to appear unless other factors (adjuvants) are present concomitantly. Adjuvants may temporarily change barrier functions or produce an immune imbalance that may be necessary for the occurrence of symptoms in response to allergen exposure. Allergens relevant for symptoms and type of symptoms may vary considerably during infancy, childhood, and adolescence, but the child who has once demonstrated an atopic constitution remains at high risk for new allergies throughout life (21,30,31).

Which Factors Are Genetic?

Production of IgE antibodies and elevated serum IgE concentrations are hallmarks of immediate-type allergy, with symptoms such as bronchial asthma. When an allergen simultaneously binds to two specific antibodies that are positioned on the surface of a mast cell, a cascade of events occur that together initiate local inflammation and also may produce generalized symptoms. Development of a clinically relevant allergic response depends on the type and amount of environmental allergen exposure, on concomitant exposure to adjuvant factors, and on a variety of host factors. Some of these may be passively acquired through the placenta or through breast milk, but many of them are hereditary (32). Responses to environmental allergens are also influenced by the previous immunological experience of the subject and by age factors (e.g., the maturation of the gut barrier and immune system during infancy) (33–35).

There are possible interindividual differences in antigen uptake and handling, antigen presentation and subsequent immune responses, number of IgE antibodies on mast cells, release of a variety of inflammatory mediators from various cell types, and sensitivity of target cells or target organs to the effects of these mediators. The inflammation initiates swelling caused by edema and infiltration with cells, and eventually it produces tissue damage. The inflamed tissue shows an increased nonspecific responsiveness to various physical and chemical irritants. A state of tissue hyperreactivity of great clinical importance is established and may persist for weeks and even months or years. Genetic factors may be involved in some, if not all, of these steps (36,37).

Toward the Detection of the Basic Defect

Great efforts have been devoted to the investigation of clinical and laboratory aspects of allergic diseases. However, the basic genetic factor or factors remain to be revealed. Several components involved in the pathophysiology of allergic diseases may be major determinants. Among the immunological abnormalities in atopic subjects is a high serum IgE concentration, and the genetic regulation of IgE production is probably most important for the phenotypic expression (38). Several other mechanisms have also been implicated (39–44).

This presentation aims at bringing together information on the interaction between various genetic and environmental factors. The identification of genetically predisposed subjects at high risk for development of allergic diseases will be briefly addressed.

BASIC DEFECT

Immunoglobulin E Production

One of the hallmarks of allergic diseases is the *hyperproduction of IgE* and of allergen-specific IgE antibodies. Elevated serum IgE concentrations are found more often in newborn infants of families with allergic diseases, when compared with neonates from nonatopic families (43). Only rarely have allergen-specific IgE antibodies been demonstrated in newborn infants, supporting the notion that IgE produced antenatally probably is nonspecific (45). High neonatal IgE concentrations are found significantly more often in children who later develop allergic diseases than in children who remain healthy (46,47). Furthermore, IgE antibodies to egg white or cow's milk are found in almost one-third of healthy infants at a time when these foods are introduced into the diet (17). The levels of IgE antibodies are, however, higher in infants who later develop allergic manifestations. Hyperproduction of IgE in humans, spontaneously and especially at allergen exposure, may therefore represent a primary abnormality. This is similar to the situation in high (as compared with low) IgE responder strains among experimental animals (48,49).

Bone Marrow Cells Carry the Primary Defect

Atopic eczema and allergic sensitization may be transferred to a previously nonallergic subject through bone marrow transplanted from an atopic donor (50). The IgE hyperresponsiveness, positive skin tests, and asthma can be transmitted by allogenic bone marrow transplants from asthmatic donors to nonatopic recipients (51,52). The effects were still found 12 months after the transplantation, indicating the possibility of a permanent change in the phenotypic expression. Eczema in subjects with Wiskott–Aldrichs syndrome has been cured together with other manifestations of disease by successful bone marrow transplants (53). These findings strongly suggest that allergic diseases are highly dependent on a particular bone marrow cell line or the balance between cell lines.

An increased ratio between CD4 and CD8-positive T cells, roughly corresponding to an increased helper/suppressor cell ratio, has been demonstrated in subjects with atopic eczema in some, but not all, studies (54,55). The same defect has also been described in infants before the development of symptoms and signs of allergic disease (56), whereas a reduced number of E-rosetting cells were found in infants with a family history of allergic diseases by others (57–59). Taken together, these studies lend support to the hypothesis of a primary defect in a subset of bone marrow cells, probably T cells controlling IgE production by B cells. Whether this functional abnormality also acts on the initial interaction between T cells and antigen-presenting cells, with subsequent imbalance of, for example, interleukin-4/interferon gamma (IL4/IFN-γ) (or other messenger substances), or is solely due to imbalance in the regulation of IgE production by IgE-binding factors, is not yet known. An imbalance between T-cell subsets may also affect the production of mucus through their regulatory effect on the appearance of goblet cells at mucosal sites. Nevertheless, even if it is very important for the clinical manifestations, an excessive IgE synthesis in genetically predisposed subjects may be only one of several consequences of an underlying abnormality.

Receptor Abnormalities

There is some evidence that the genetic defect associated with asthma is inherited as an autosomally dominant trait, at least in some families (60,61). A defect in chromosome 11q was associated with atopy in 85%, with wheeze in 60%, and with a previous diagnosis of asthma in 20% of the patients. The findings are interesting and, if confirmed, they could lead to improved understanding of asthma and other allergic diseases. The nature of the defect is unclear, but surface receptors have been suggested to play a role, as some of them are under control of chromosome 11q (62). Abnormalities in T-cell receptors may be responsible for the IgE hyperresponsiveness after allergen exposure in a subset of infants who are genetically predetermined high IgE responders. Animal experiments (63,64) indicate that high IgE responder strains of mice and rats need considerably higher levels of exposure to potential allergens to induce tolerance (turn off IgE production), compared with low IgE responders. Abnormal handling of antigen or dysregulation of IgE synthesis may be the cause. Atopic T cells have been shown to express and also to release increased amounts of a soluble IgE-binding factor (Fcε RII, CD23) (65,66). This IgE-binding factor augments in vitro synthesis of IgE by atopic B cells. Certainly, these findings could represent a primary defect (67), but they may also be secondary to intracellular defects in T cells of atopic subjects. To assess their importance, a prospective study in high-allergy-risk families is in progress.

Immune Deficiencies Connected With Atopy

It has been suggested that there is a genetic *immune deficiency* underlying the development of allergy (68–72). Besides the imbalance in the function of various T-cell subsets, mentioned earlier, there is very little proof of any primary immunological abnormality. Transient deficiency in the production of IgA in genetic high-allergy-risk babies during early infancy has been suggested, but in two studies this could not be confirmed (70,73,74). The increased occurrence of skin infections with *Staphylococcus aureus* and several viral strains (e.g., molluscum contagiosum) in subjects with atopic eczema is probably due to changes in barrier function and other effects of local allergic inflammation in conjunction with the itching behavior of the subjects (28). Defective phagocytosis has been demonstrated only in subjects with severe dermatitis or inflammation of the skin, but not during remission of the dermatitis. Otitis media, especially otitis media with effusion, is overrepresented among subjects with allergic diseases (75); however, there are other severe generalized infections that are not overrepresented.

Bronchial Hyperreactivity

Another hallmark of bronchial asthma, *bronchial hyperreactivity*, has attracted a great deal of interest in genetic studies. A substantial part of asymptomatic family members of asthmatic subjects showed increased responsiveness to methacholine (76), in contrast to the case in relatives of healthy control subjects. Several studies have demonstrated a better concordance for bronchial responsiveness to exercise or histamine–methacholine in monozygotic, compared with dizygotic, twins (4,77). Animal studies have suggested a recessive manner of genetic transmission of a high bronchial reactivity (78). In humans, bronchial hyperreactivity has been demonstrated in subjects with atopic eczema and hay fever before the development of bronchial asthma, indicating that it is a primary trait characterizing at least some children with a genetic propensity for allergic disease (79,80). There is another study indicating that hyperreactivity is present in all infants, probably from birth on, but most children outgrow their hyperreactivity, whereas, for some reason, others do not (81). It has been suggested that infections or early exposure to allergens and adjuvants may affect this normal maturation of the state of bronchial reactivity.

The mechanisms underlying bronchial hyperresponsiveness may be many. Besides a varying sensitivity on the level of the bronchial smooth muscle, there may be differences in neural transmission or in the balance of transmitter substances, imbalance in the effect of hormones or mediators of inflammation, and differences in mucosal barrier function or endothelial hormone production (82). In humans, there is evidence of separate control of bronchoconstriction by methacholine or histamine and by adenosine or neurokinin A (83,84). The level of hyperreactivity is also influenced by inflammation following upper respiratory tract infections and by exposure to pollutants or allergens (85). Mast cell reactivity and airway inflammation may well be under genetic control similar to smooth-muscle responsiveness, local axon reflexes, and possibly vagal reflexes. Evidently, IgE-associated mechanisms may also be involved in the bronchial hyperresponsiveness. Consequently, it is impossible to point out a single basic factor that could explain hyperreactivity, unless we go down to the cellular level. A genetically determined abnormality in many cells of the body would conceivably explain the diversity of clinical manifestations of the predisposition for atopy.

Intracellular Abnormalities

Phosphodiesterase (PDE; an enzyme reducing the intracellular level of cyclic 3-5-AMP) is increased in mononuclear blood cells of subjects with atopic eczema, but not in contact dermatitis patients (8,39,86,87). Also, in subjects with hay fever a similar increase in PDE has been demonstrated (39). A higher level of PDE was already found in neonates if there was a family history of atopic disease (89,90). The mean PDE concentration was higher in infants with two, compared with one, atopic parent. In consequence, the increase was suggested to be primary and of genetic origin. There is also experimental evidence that a normalization of intracellular PDE concentrations may normalize IgE responsiveness (91). A prospective study evaluating the predictive capacity of analysis of PDE in mononuclear blood cells of newborn infants with varying genetic background is currently in progress (Odelram et al., in preparation). Preliminary data, although confirming a small difference in PDE concentration between neonates with and without a family history of atopic disease, seem disappointing when it comes to the predictive capacity of the neonatal PDE level. This casts some doubt on the origin of the increase in PDE concentrations (primary or secondary). A recent study from Hanifin's group has demonstrated increased protein kinase A and decreased protein kinase C activity in leukocytes from atopic dermatitis patients, which could account for the previously demonstrated increase in PDE activity (92).

Many other possibly primary intracellular abnormalities have yet to be explored, among them a reduced steroid sensitivity of T cells when measured as release of arachidonic acid with phytohemagglutinin (PHA) stimulation (93). The mononuclear cells from atopic subjects also had abnormalities in arachidonic acid metabolism and showed an increased releasability of arachidonic acid (93).

Another abnormality in subjects suffering from allergic disease is an abnormal fatty acid composition of serum lecithin (42). An increase in linoleic acid and a decrease in its metabolites has suggested a reduction in enzymatic activity of Δ^6-desaturase. This may represent a primary abnormality, as similar high linoleic acid contents were found in cord blood lecithin, especially in subjects with a high cord blood IgE concentration (42).

WHAT IS INHERITED?

First, a *general predisposition* to develop allergy and hypersensitivity is inherited, together with a general propensity to develop any atopic disease (62). Thus, allergic diseases are not inherited as specific diseases. If there are ancestors with asthma, hay fever, and urticaria, an infant may start to show his or her atopic constitution by vomiting when fed a cow's milk formula, and the baby may also develop atopic eczema later during infancy. A decade later, hay fever may develop in the child. The particular clinical manifestations are determined by environmental factors, but also genetic and other host factors may have some influence. During the last decades a polygenic heritability has been suggested (94–96).

Second, genetic factors do have an influence on the symptomatology, as there appears to be a genetically based *end-organ sensitivity* (97,98). This is especially seen if both parents have shown the same disease (e.g., bronchial asthma), when the risk for their child to have any atopic disease is seven times higher than with no family history of allergy (98). Similarly, the risk for expressing bronchial asthma is tenfold higher in a child of two asthmatic parents than in a child with no family history of asthma. The manner of genetic transmission of the end-organ sensitivity is still under debate, but a recent study indicates autosomal dominant inheritance (60,99).

Third, the *age at which symptoms begin* seems to be under genetic control. Symptoms tend to start earlier with increasing number of close relatives suffering from allergy (98,100–103). Children of two atopic parents tend to begin having symptoms during early infancy, whereas children with no parental history of allergy are a few years older when symptoms begin. This may merely have to do with the doses needed for sensitization or to the degree of sensitivity to adjuvant factors. It could also depend on differences in maturation of the immune system or of barrier functions.

Fourth, the level of *serum IgE concentrations* is subject to genetic control. The regulation of IgE production is not linked to the human major histocompatibility complex (HLA) (103–105). Children of parents with high serum IgE concentrations tend to show higher serum IgE concentrations than children of parents with low serum IgE concentrations (106). Newborn infants of parent with high IgE concentrations show elevated cord blood IgE concentrations significantly more often than neonates of parents with normal IgE levels (107). The genetic influence is most marked during infancy, but later during childhood environmental factors play a more important role (47). At 11 years of age, no significant difference was seen between serum IgE concentrations of children with a high, compared with a low, neonatal IgE concentration (21). Subjects who show high serum IgE concentrations (from the neonatal period and onward) seem to be more easily sensitized to allergens than those with low IgE concentrations. A low serum IgE concentration does not, however, preclude specific sensitization nor clinically relevant allergy at the time of sampling or during subsequent years. In some subjects with unexpectedly low serum IgE concentrations, IgE complexed with anti-IgE antibodies has been demonstrated (108). The production of such autoantibodies and the transfer of antibodies from the mother to her fetus or infant may also be under genetic control.

Fifth, the predisposition for *specific sensitization* (e.g., to cow's milk protein or to the major allergen of ragweed pollen) seems to be inherited as an HLA-linked trait (109). It appears, however, easier to express the genes in a child who separately (not associated with HLA) also inherited the trait for high IgE production (4). In contrast, the control of IgE antibody production to specific antigens (allergens) seems to be determined by HLA-linked Immune response (*Ir*) genes in cooperation with HLA-linked Immune suppressor (*Is*) genes. A significant association between inheritance of a propensity for allergy to certain components of, for instance, ragweed or rye grass allergens and certain HLA haplotypes, especially Dw2/DR, has been demonstrated in some families, but the association is not consistent in all subjects with IgE antibodies to the allergen in question. Neither is allergy to the particular allergen found in all subjects with identical haplotype, indicating a considerable influence of environmental factors for the phenotypic expression (110).

Sixth, *organ hyperreactivity* (e.g., bronchial hyperreactivity) shows a genetic background (111). The threshold for significant bronchial obstruction by histamine or methacholine is considerably lower in healthy relatives of asthmatics than in those of nonasthmatic subjects. Similarly, healthy relatives of children with atopic eczema often present a history of skin hyperreactivity to wool and certain synthetic fibers.

Seventh, also on a *cellular* level there may be *hyperreactivity* (e.g., for histamine releasability; 21).

The identity of most of the genes involved is as yet unknown. There is some knowledge from animal experiments, especially in the mouse and rat (112). The importance of recent findings in humans is not yet known, as the definition for atopic disease in that particular study was arbitrary (113). The findings remain to be confirmed. Currently, there is no simple explanation for the apparent complexity of the genetic control of allergic disease.

INFLUENCE OF THE FAMILY HISTORY ON THE RELATIVE RISK FOR DEVELOPMENT OF ALLERGIC DISEASE

From a clinical point of view, relative risk indices for allergic disease have been calculated for various ages and in relation to the number of close relatives suffering from atopic disease (114; Table 1). Generally speaking, the relative risk for allergic disease is, at most, doubled by a family history of any allergic disease (the relative risk being 2.0 at 18 months and decreasing to 1.7 at 11 years of age). For instance, atopic diseases had developed in 8.1% of 1701 infants followed from birth to 18 months of age, among them in 5.3% of children with no family history, in 7.5% of those with remote family history, in 11.8% of infants with one atopic parent, in 13.8% of infants with an atopic sibling, and in 23.1% of infants of two atopic parents (115).

The relative risk for a child to develop allergic disease increases accordingly with the number of affected family members (Figure 1). If both parents have the same disease, the relative risk increases by a factor of 7 (98). In a child with a single parental history of allergic

Table 1 Relative Risk (RR) for Development of Any Allergic Disease in Relation to Age and Number of Parents Suffering from Atopic Disease

Number of parents with atopic disease	Age	
	Up to 18 mo	Up to 7 yr
0	1	1
1	1.9	1.6
2	4.4	3.4

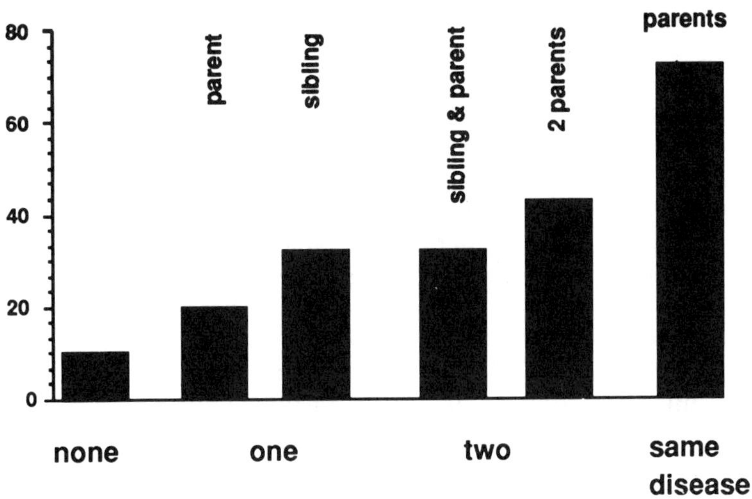

Figure 1 Development of atopic disease in children before 7 years of age (%) in relation to number of atopic family members. (Modified from Ref. 98.)

disease, the cumulative prevalence of such disease is considerably higher if the parent has more than one allergic disease. In a subgroup of infants with no parental history of allergic disease, there is a sibling who currently suffers or previously has suffered from allergic disease. The relative risk for a newborn infant in such a family to develop any allergic disease before school age is about 3 (i.e., three times higher than when there is no immediate family history of allergy) (98). However, a considerable proportion of children with manifestations of allergic disease before 11 years of age (approximately 50% of them) have no immediate family history of allergic disease (21). Approximately half of the rest have a remote family history, which leaves about one-fourth of all children with allergic diseases with no family history of disease whatsoever (21). This, to some extent, may be explained by the fact that allergic diseases may be misdiagnosed, or transient during early years of life and forgotten (21).

EFFECT OF GENETIC AND ENVIRONMENTAL FACTORS ON SENSITIZATION AND ALLERGIC DISEASE

Prevalence of Allergic Disease

The atopic diseases are common conditions, and their prevalence (i.e., frequency of diseases giving symptoms during the past 12 months) seems to be increasing (14). The prevalence of any atopic disease in adolescence is today about 15–20%. The cumulative prevalence (i.e., frequency of diseases now or previously), which is an indicator of the population at high risk for new allergic manifestations, is between 25 and 35% (21). In Sweden and Finland, there is evidence for an increasing asthma prevalence during the last decades from nationwide examinations of conscripts (13,116). Interestingly, the highest increase in Sweden was seen in the northern parts where pollen allergens are sparse. In the United Kingdom, there is good evidence for an increase not only in the consultation rate owing to atopic diseases, but also in the prevalence of, for example, atopic eczema and bronchial asthma (117–119). In the United States, it has been estimated that 35 million Americans suffer from allergic disease, and asthma prevalence rates up to 9–11% have been reported among children (120).

Differences Between Countries

There are great differences in the worldwide prevalence of atopic and allergic diseases. This may partly be explained by differences in genetic predisposition and, in fact, the prevalence of asthma is very high on certain islands with a high rate of inbreeding (121). A more likely explanation for differences in asthma prevalence between regions and over time are differences in exposure to environmental factors, including infections, toxic or irritating chemicals, and allergens. Generally, the prevalence of asthma is higher in industrialized countries than in developing areas, but westernization of the Third World during the last decades is followed by an increase in asthma prevalence. This is particularly seen in urban, as compared with rural areas. This certainly cannot be explained by changes in the human genetic code. However, there is now some evidence that pollutants may affect plants and trees to increase the expression of allergen and to make allergens more readily accessible (e.g., on a pollen grain) (122). This may, to some extent, explain the increase in pollen allergy in urbanized areas (13,123). As environmental factors play a crucial role in the development of allergic diseases, there must be room for a discussion concerning environmental control aimed at preventing the development and severity of symptoms of allergic diseases.

How Common Is a Family History of Allergic Diseases?

The trend for asthma to run in families has been recognized for 300 years (cited in 124). However, the first serious investigation of the genetic influence of atopic diseases was done 75 years ago by Cooke and van der Veer (125). Their conclusion was that dominant heredity determined the development of asthma and hay fever, but later studies have tried to explain heredity in various other ways, including a recessive disease with decreased penetrance and, lately, as a dominant or polygenic disease (113,126). A family history of allergic diseases is reported by a high proportion of subjects with these diseases. The frequency of such a family history varies with the origin of the material, from less than one-half in nonselected materials up to three-quarters in subjects referred to a specialist for severe symptoms of allergy (21,125).

Varying Levels of Exposure Elicit Symptoms

Environmental factors may affect genetically predisposed subjects at considerably lower levels of exposure than are needed for a reaction in a subject without a family history of allergic disease. The difference in concentration of a particular allergen needed for eliciting symptoms may be more than 1 million times between a subject at high and low sensitivity (127). For factors acting as adjuvants, differences in concentrations needed to elicit symptoms may vary between 10 and 1000.

Age Factors, Period of Birth, and Early Feeding

Age factors are important. Sensitization occurs early in genetically predisposed subjects, often as early as during the period of breast-feeding (19). The fact that allergic disease tends to begin at an earlier age with increasing number of allergic relatives was recognized early on by Cooke and van der Veer (125). About 80% of childhood asthma and perhaps more than 90% of childhood atopic eczema begin before school age (128). The natural history of a disease in relation to the family history and the expected exposure, all have to be taken into account when calculation is made of the risk for development of allergic disease. A newborn infant of a family at high risk for allergy is especially prone for pollen allergy and bronchial asthma before school age if born during or immediately before the pollen season (129,130). Breast-feeding appears to delay the onset of allergic symptoms, but only in genetically predisposed infants (74,131). Atopic dermatitis develops more often in infants at high risk for allergy if their breast-feeding mothers are on a normal food intake, when compared with high-allergy-risk babies of mothers who are on an elimination diet (eliminating all milk, egg, and fish, and products thereof) during the first 3 months of lactation (132,133).

Molds, Mites, and Asthma

Bronchial asthma develops more often in genetically predisposed children if they are exposed to an indoor climate favoring growth of molds and mites (134–136). The risk for asthma in a similar environment is only marginally increased in children with no family history of allergic diseases.

CONCLUSIONS AND PRACTICAL CONSEQUENCES

There is ample evidence that environmental factors and age factors play an important role for the phenotypic expression of allergy, bronchial hyperreactivity, and allergic diseases in infancy and childhood. The importance of environmental factors is most evident in subjects with a genetic predisposition for allergy. In some countries, such as Sweden, most neonates now have a family history of allergic diseases, and one out of three newborn infants have an immediate family history of allergic diseases. Therefore, neonates at risk for development of significant allergic manifestations during the next couple of years should be identified by questioning mothers-to-be and fathers-to-be well before the birth of the high-risk baby. There is no doubt about the importance of protecting these babies from tobacco smoke during pregnancy, throughout infancy, and early childhood.

Other recommendations aiming at reducing the effect of allergic predisposition may be valid for only selected newborns at especially high risk for development of allergy—the "high-risk babies." These include babies of two allergic parents (approximately 3% of newborn

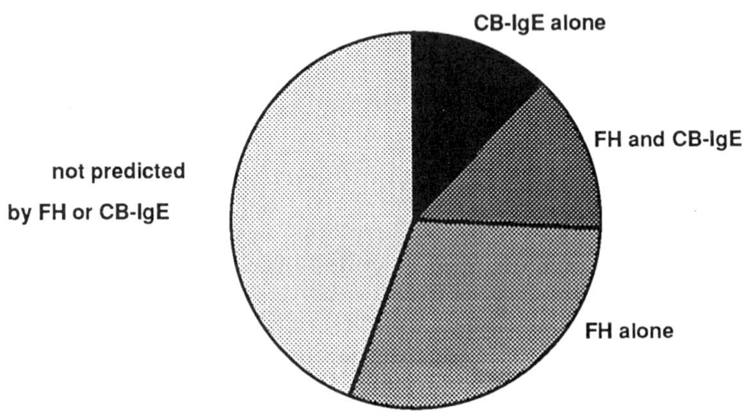

Figure 2 Sensitivity of cord blood IgE determination and family history (FH) for predicting cases of atopic disease in 1654 11 year-old children. (Adapted from Ref. 21.)

infants) and neonates with one of the parents and a sibling suffering from allergic diseases (approximately 8% of neonates). If a baby has a parent who has suffered from especially severe or multiple allergic diseases, then the risk for subsequent allergic disease in the baby is also high enough (above 30% will develop allergic disease before 7 years of age) to motivate prophylactic measures during infancy (see Chapter 23).

It is important to collect relevant information concerning possible allergic symptoms from both parents-to-be. It may sometimes be necessary to make deeper inquiries and to consult previous medical records before recommendations are given. There is not yet an ideal test or a battery of tests to identify *all* subjects at genetic risk for the development of allergic disease. However, a high neonatal IgE concentration is helpful, to some extent, but the sensitivity of neonatal IgE determination is unfortunately too low to warrant a general screening procedure (Figure 2).

REFERENCES

1. Coca AF, Cooke RA. On the classification of the phenomena of hypersensitiveness. J Immunol 1923; 8:163–182.
2. Nelson HS. The atopic diseases. Ann Allergy 1985; 55:441–447.
3. Bazaral M, Orgel H, Hamburger R. Genetics of IgE and allergy: serum IgE levels in twins. J Allergy Clin Immunol 1974; 54:288–304.
4. Hopp RJ, Bewtra AK, Watt GD, Nair NM, Townley RG. Genetic analysis of allergic disease in twins. J Allergy Clin Immunol 1984; 73:265–270.
5. Svartengren M, Ericsson CH, Mossberg B, Camner P. Bronchial reactivity and atopy in asthma discordant monozygotic twins. Ann Allergy 1990; 64:124–128.
6. Edfors-Lubs ML. Allergy in 7000 twin pairs. Acta Allergol 1971; 26:249–285.
7. Blumenthal MN, Amos DB. Genetic and immunologic basis of atopic responses. Chest 1987; 91:176–184.
8. Hanifin JM. Pharmacological abnormalities in atopic dermatitis. Allergy 1989; 44 (suppl 9):41–46.
9. Parks T, Felix K, Subbarao PV, Masrimuthu KM, Rao DC. A genetic study of immunoglobulin E and atopic disease based on families ascertained through asthmatic children. Hum Hered 1990; 40:69–76.
10. IgE, parasites, and allergy [editorial]. Lancet 1976; 1:894–896.
11. Venge P, Shaw M. Parasites and allergy. Allergol Kongressausgabe 1989; 12:96–99.
12. Fleming DM, Crombie DL. Prevalence of asthma and hay fever in England and Wales. Br Med J 1987; 294:279–283.

13. Åberg N. Asthma and allergic rhinitis in Swedish conscripts. Clin Allergy 1989; 19:59–63.
14. Wütrich B. Epidemiology of the allergic diseases: are they really on the increase? Int Arch Appl Immunol 1989; 90:3–10.
15. Woolcock AJ. Beta-agonists and asthma mortality. What have we learned, what questions remain? Drugs 1990; 40:653–656.
16. Burney P. Asthma deaths in England and Wales 1931–85: evidence for a true increase in asthma mortality. J Epidemiol Commun Health 1988; 42:316–320.
17. Hattevig G, Kjellman B, Johansson SGO, Björkstén B. Clinical symptoms and IgE responses to common food proteins in atopic and healthy children. Clin Allergy 1984; 14:551–559.
18. Polmar SH, Lawrence DR, Minnefor AB. Immunoglobulin E in bronchiolitis. Pediatrics 1972; 50:279–284.
19. van Asperen PP, Kemp AS. The natural history of IgE sensitization and atopic disease in early childhood. Acta Paediatr Scand 1989; 78:239–245.
20. Pepys J, Davies RJ. Allergy. In: Clark TJH, Godfrey S, eds. Asthma. London: Chapman and Hall, 1986:126–161.
21. Croner S, Kjellman N-IM. Development of atopic disease in relation to family history and cord blood IgE levels. Pediatr Allergy Immunol 1990; 1:14–20.
22. Charpin D, Vervloet D, Charpin J. Epidemiology of asthma in western Europe. Allergy 1988; 43:481–492.
23. Gerritsen J, Koëter GH, deMonchy JGR, Knol K. Allergy in subjects with asthma from childhood to adulthood. J Allergy Clin Immunol 1990; 85:116–125.
24. Salter HH. On asthma: its pathology and treatment. Philadelphia: Blanchard and Lea, 1864.
25. Hattevig G, Kjellman B, Björkstén B. Clinical symptoms and IgE responses to common food proteins and inhalants in the first 7 years of life. Clin Allergy 1987; 17:571–578.
26. Johansson SGO. The clinical significance of IgE. In: Franklin EC, ed. Clinical immunology update. New York: 1981:123–145.
27. Juhlin-Dannfeldt C. About the occurrence of various forms of pollen allergy in Sweden. Acta Med Scand 1948; 26:563–577.
28. Sampson HA. Pathogenesis of eczema. Clin Exp Allergy 1990; 20:459–467.
29. Horak F. Manifestation of allergic rhinitis in latent-sensitized patients. Arch Otorhinolaryngol 1985; 242:239–245.
30. Blair H. Natural history of childhood asthma. 20-year follow-up. Arch Dis Child 1977; 52:613–619.
31. Kelly WCM, Hudson I, Phelan PD, Pain MCF, Olinsky A. Atopy in subjects with asthma followed to the age of 28 years. J Allergy Clin Immunol 1990; 85:548–557.

32. Kjellman N-IM, Björkstén B. Maternal interaction with her fetus/infant and childhood allergy. Allergologie 1989; 12(S):180–185.
33. Heird WC, Hansen IH. Effect of colostrum on growth of intestinal mucosa. Pediatr Res 1977; 11:406.
34. Axelsson I, Jakobsson I, Lindberg T, Polberger S, Benediktsson B, Räihä N. Macromolecular absorption in preterm and term infants. Acta Paediatr Scand 1989; 78:532–537.
35. Beach RC, Menzies IS, Clayden GS, Scopes JW. Gastrointestinal permeability changes in the preterm neonate. Arch Dis Child 1982; 57:141–145.
36. Chung KF. Mediators of bronchial hyperresponsiveness. Clin Exp Allergy 1990; 20:453–458.
37. Frew AJ, Kay AB. Interactions between lymphoid cells, mast cells and granulocytes in allergic inflammation. Allergol Kongressausgabe 1989; 12:81–84.
38. Holt PG, McMenamin C, Nelson D. Primary sensitisation to inhalant allergens during infancy. Pediatr Allergy Immunol 1990; 1:3–13.
39. Grewe SR, Chan SC, Hanifin JM. Elevated leucocyte cyclic AMP-phosphodiesterase in atopic disease: a possible mechanism for cAMP-agonist hyporesponsiveness. J Allergy Clin Immunol 1982; 70:452–457.
40. Holden CA. Atopic dermatitis: a defect of intracellular secondary messenger systems? Clin Exp Allergy 1990; 20:131–136.
41. Reed CE. Abnormal autonomic mechanisms in asthma. J Allergy Clin Immunol 1974; 53:34–41.
42. Strannegård I-L, Svennerholm L, Strannegård Ö. Essential fatty acids in serum lecithin of children with atopic dermatitis and in umbilical cord serum of infants with high or low IgE levels. Int Arch Allergy Appl Immunol 1987; 82:422–423.
43. Michel FB, Bousquet J, Greillier P, Robinet-Lévy M, Coulomb Y. Comparison of cord blood immunoglobulin E concentrations and maternal allergy for the prediction of atopic diseases in infancy. J Allergy Clin Immunol 1980; 65:422–430.
44. Halonen M, Stern D, Lyle S, Wright A, Taussig L, Martinez FD. Relationship of total serum IgE levels in cord and 9-month sera of infants. Clin Exp Allergy 1991; 21:235–241.
45. Björkstén B, Kjellman N-IM. Perinatal factors influencing the development of allergy. Clin Rev Allergy 1987; 5:339–347.
46. Orgel HA, Hamburger RN, Bazaral M, Gorrin H, Groshong T, Lenoir M, Miller JR, Wallace W. Development of IgE and allergy in infancy. J Allergy Clin Immunol 1975; 56:296–307.
47. Kjellman N-IM, Croner S. Cord blood IgE determination for allergy prediction: a follow-up to seven years of age in 1651 children. Ann Allergy 1984; 53:167–171.

48. Levine BB, Vaz NM. Effects of combination of inbred strain, antigen and antigen dose on immune responsiveness and reagin production in the mouse. Int Arch Allergy Appl Immunol 1970; 39:156–171.
49. Watanabe N, Kojima S, Ovary Z. Suppression of IgE antibody production in SJL mice. I. Nonspecific suppressor T cells. J Exp Med 1976; 143:833–845.
50. Saarinen UM. Transfer of latent atopy by bone marrow transplantation: a case report. J Allergy Clin Immunol 1984; 74:196–200.
51. Agosti JM, Sprenger JD, Lum LG, Witherspoon P, Fisher LD, Storb R, Henderson WR. Transfer of allergen specific IgE-mediated hypersensitivity with allogenic bone marrow transplantation. N Engl J Med 1988; 319:1623–1628.
52. Higenbottam T, Varma N. Asthma: an inherited dysfunction of bone marrow cells? Eur Respir J 1989; 2:921–922.
53. Saurat JH. Eczema in primary immune-deficiencies. Acta Derm Venereol (Stockh) 1985; 114:125–128.
54. Leung DYM, Bhan AK, Schneeberg EE, Geha RS. Characterization of the mononuclear cell infiltrate in atopic dermatitis using monoclonal antibodies. J Allergy Clin Immunol 1983; 71:47–56.
55. Strannegård I-L, Strannegård Ö. The T cell deficiency in atopic disease and its relation to hyperproduction of IgE. Acta Derm Venereol [Suppl] (Stockh) 1981; 95:20–24.
56. Chandra RK, Baker M. Numerical and functional deficiency of suppressor T cells precedes development of atopic eczema. Lancet 1983; 2:1393–1394.
57. Strannegård I-L, Lindholm L, Strannegård Ö. Studies of T lymphocytes in atopic children. Int Arch Allergy Appl Immunol 1976; 50:684–691.
58. Björkstén B, Juto P. Allergy and cell-mediated immunity in infants. In: Businco L, ed. Advances in pediatric allergy. Amsterdam: Excerpta Medica, 1983:19–33.
59. Juto P, Strannegård Ö. T lymphocytes and blood eosinophils in early infancy in relation to heredity for allergy and type of feeding. J Allergy Clin Immunol 1979; 64:38–42.
60. Cookson WOCM, Hopkin JM. Dominant inheritance of atopic immunoglobulin E responsiveness. Lancet 1988; 1:86–87.
61. Hopkin JM. Genetics of atopy. Clin Exp Allergy 1989; 19:263–265.
62. Cookson WOCM, Faux JA, Sharp PA, Hopkin JM. Linkage between immunoglobulin E responses underlying asthma and rhinitis and chromosome 11q. Lancet 1989; 1:1292–1294.
63. Sedgwick JD, Holt PG. Suppression of IgE responses in inbred rats by repeated respiratory tract exposure to antigen: responder phenotype influences isotype specificity in induced tolerance. Eur J Immunol 1984; 14:893–897.

64. Holt PG, Britten D, Sedgwick JD. Suppression of IgE responses by antigen inhalation: studies on the role of genetic and environmental factors. Immunology 1985; 62:586–594.
65. Matsumoto T, Miike T, Takahashi H, Hosoda M, Kawabe T, Yodoi J, Hirashima M. Fc-epsilon RII on T cells and IgE binding factors in children with atopic asthma. Pediatr Allergy Immunol 1990; 1:21–25.
66. Yanagihara Y, Sarfati M, Marsh D, Nutman T, Delespesse G. Serum levels of IgE-binding factor (soluble CD23) in diseases associated with elevated IgE. Clin Exp Allergy 1990; 20:395–401.
67. Kim K-M, Mayumi M, Iwai Y, Tanaka M, Ito S, Mikawa H, Shinomya K. IgE-receptor bearing lymphocytes in allergic and non-allergic children. Pediatr Res 1988; 24:254–257.
68. Kaufman HS, Hobbs JR. Immunoglobulin deficiencies in an atopic population. Lancet 1970; 2:1061–1063.
69. Brasher GW, Bourland PD. The role of IgA in the pathogenesis of atopy. Ann Allergy 1975; 34:137–140.
70. Taylor B, Norman AP, Orgel HA, Stokes CR, Turner MW, Soothill JF. Transient IgA deficiency and pathogenesis of infantile atopy. Lancet 1973; 2:111–113.
71. Björkstén B, Kjellman N-IM. Immunological abnormalities in atopic infants. Allergologie 1989; 12(S):176–179.
72. Richardson VF, Larcher VF, Price JF. A common congenital immunodeficiency predisposing to infection and atopy in infancy. Arch Dis Child 1983; 58:799–802.
73. Kjellman N-IM, Johansson SGO. Soy versus cow's milk in infants with a biparental history of atopic disease: development of atopic disease and immunoglobulins from birth to 4 years of age. Clin Allergy 1979; 9:347–358.
74. Matthew DJ, Taylor B, Norman AP, Turner MW, Soothill JF. Prevention of eczema. Lancet 1977; 1:321–324.
75. Kjellman N-IM, Synnerstad B, Hansson LO. Atopic allergy and immunoglobulins in children with adenoids and recurrent otitis media. Acta Paediatr Scand 1976; 65:593–600.
76. Hopp RJ, Bewtra RK, Nair NM, Watt GD, Townley RG. Methacholine inhalation challenge studies in a selected pediatric population. Am Rev Resp Dis 1986; 134:994–998.
77. König P, Godfrey S. Exercise-induced bronchial lability in monozygotic (identical) and dizygotic (non-identical) twins. J Allergy Clin Immunol 1974; 54:280–287.
78. Pauwels R, van der Straeten M, Weyne J, Bazin H. Genetic factors in non-specific bronchial reactivity in rats. Eur J Respir Dis 1985; 66:98–104.
79. Ford LB, Bewtra AK, Coleman RL, Herbers L, Townley RG. Methacholine challenge as a predictor for asthma [abstr]. J Allergy Clin Immunol 1984; 73:125.

80. van Asperen PP, Kemp AS, Mukhi A. Atopy in infancy predicts the severity of bronchial hyperresponsiveness in later childhood. J Allergy Clin Immunol 1990; 85:790–795.
81. Lesouëf PN, Geelhoed GC, Turner DJ, Morgan SEG, Landau LI. Response of normal infants to inhaled histamine. Am Rev Respir Dis 1989; 139:62–66.
82. Reid LM, Gleich GJ, Hogg J, Kleinerman J, Laitinen LA. Pathology. In: Holgate ST, ed. The role of inflammatory processes in airway hyperresponsiveness. Australia: Blackwell Scientific Publications, 1989:36–79.
83. Joos GF, Pauwels RA, van der Straeten ME. The role of neuropeptides as neurotransmitters of non-adrenergic, non-cholinergic nerves in bronchial asthma. Bull Eur Physiopathol Respir 1988; 23:619–637.
84. Mann JS, Holgate ST, Renwick AG, Cushley MJ. Airway effects of purine nucleosides and nucleotides and release with bronchial provocation in asthma. J Appl Physiol 1986; 61:1667–1676.
85. Charpin D, Kleisbauer JP, Fondarai J, Graland B, Viala A, Govezo F. Respiratory symptoms and air pollution changes in children; the Gardanne Coal-Basin study. Arch Environ Health 1988; 43:22–27.
86. Butler JM, Chan SC, Stevens S, Hanifin JM. Increased leukocyte histamine release with elevated cyclic AMP-phosphodiesterase activity in atopic dermatitis. J Allergy Clin Immunol 1983; 71:490–497.
87. Chan SC, Grewe SC, Stevens SR, Hanifin JM. Functional desensitization due to stimulation of cyclic AMP-phosphodiesterase in human mononuclear leukocytes. J Cyclic Nucleotide Res 1982; 8:211–224.
88. Leung DYM, Geha RS. Immunoregulatory abnormalities in atopic dermatitis. Clin Rev Allergy 1986; 4:67–86.
89. McMillan JC, Heskel NS, Hanifin JM. Cyclic AMP-phosphodiesterase activity and histamine release in cord blood leukocyte preparations. Acta Derm Venereol [Suppl] (Stockh) 1985; 114:24–32.
90. Heskel NS, Chan SC, Thiel ML, Stevens SR, Casperson LS, Hanifin JM. Elevated umbilical cord blood leucocyte cyclic adenosine monophosphate-phosphodiesterase activity in children with atopic parents. J Am Acad Dermatol 1984; 11:422–426.
91. Cooper KD, Kang K, Chan SC, Hanifin JM. Phosphodiesterase inhibition by Ro20-1724 reduces hyper-IgE synthesis by atopic dermatitis cell in vitro. J Invest Dermatol 1985; 84:477–482.
92. Trask DM, Chan SC, Sherman SE, Hanifin JM. Altered leukocyte activity in atopic dermatitis. J Invest Dermatol 1988; 90:526–531.
93. Lans DM, Rocklin RE. Dysregulation of arachidonic acid release and metabolism by atopic mononuclear cells. Clin Exp Allergy 1989; 19:37–44.
94. van Arsdel PP, Motulsky AG. Frequency and heritability of asthma and allergic rhinitis in college students. Acta Genet 1959; 9:101–114.
95. Hasstedt SJ, Meyers DA, Marsh DG. Inheritance of immunoglobulin E: genetic model fitting. Am J Med Genet 1983; 14:61–66.

96. Marsh DG, Meyers DA, Bias WB. The epidemiology and genetics of atopic allergy. N Engl J Med 1981; 305:1551–1559.
97. Gerrard JW, Vickers P, Gerrard CD. The familial incidence of allergic disease. Ann Allergy 1976; 36:10–15.
98. Kjellman N-IM. Atopic disease in seven-year-old children. Incidence in relation to family history. Acta Paediatr Scand 1977; 66:465–471.
99. Hopkin JM. Genetics of atopy. Clin Exp Allergy 1989; 19:263–265.
100. Spain WC, Cooke RA. Studies in specific hypersensitiveness. J Immunol 1924; 9:521–534.
101. Kjellman N-IM. Development and prediction of atopic allergy in childhood. In: Theoretical and clinical aspects of allergic diseases. Stockholm: Almqvist & Wiksell International, 1983:52–73.
102. Wittig HJ, McLaughlin ET, Leifer KL, Belloit JD. Risk factors for the development of allergic disease: analysis of 2,190 patient records. Ann Allergy 1978; 41:84–88.
103. de Weck A, Blumenthal M, Yunis E, Jeannet M. HLA and allergy. In: Dausset J, Svejgaard A, eds. HLA and disease. Baltimore: Williams & Wilkins, 1977:196–211.
104. Marsh DG, Hsu SH, Hussain R, Meyers DA, Freidhoff LR, Bias WB. Genetics of human immune response to allergens. J Allergy Clin Immunol 1980; 65:322–332.
105. Blumenthal M, Mendell N, Yunis E. Immunogenetics of atopic diseases. J Allergy Clin Immunol 1980; 65:403–405.
106. Gerrard JW, Horne S, Vickers P, MacKenzie JWA, Goluboff N, Garson JZ, Maningas C. Serum IgE levels in parents and children. J Pediatr 1974; 85:660–663.
107. Bazaral M, Orgel HA, Hamburger RN. IgE levels in normal infants and mothers and an inheritance hypothesis. J Immunol 1971; 107:794–801.
108. Vassella CV, de Weck AL, Stadler BM. Natural anti-IgE auto-antibodies interfere with diagnostic IgE determination. Clin Exp Allergy 1990; 20:295–303.
109. Blumenthal MN, Yunis E, Mendell N, Elston RC. Preventive allergy: genetics of IgE-mediated diseases. J Allergy Clin Immunol 1988; 78(part 2):962–967.
110. Marsh DG, Hsu SH, Roebber M, Ehrlich-Kautzky E, Freidhoff LR, Meyers DA, Pollard KM, Bias WB. HLA-Dw2: a genetic marker for human immune response to short ragweed pollen allergen Ra5. I. Response resulting primarily from natural antigenic exposure. J Exp Med 1982; 155:1439–1451.
111. Townley RG, Hopp RJ, Bewtra AK, Nair NM. Predictive value of airway reactivity. J Allergy Clin Immunol 1990; 86:650–652.
112. Prouvost-Danon A, Mouton D, Abadie A, Mevel J-C, Biozzi G. Genetic regulation of IgE and agglutinating antibody synthesis in lines of mice selected for high and low immune responsiveness. Eur J Immunol 1977; 7:342–348.

113. Corrigan CJ. News and commentary. Report on a meeting on the advances in the understanding and treatment of asthma, London, England, 1–3 Oct 1990. Clin Exp Allergy 1991; 21:243–248.
114. Kjellman N-IM, Andrae S, Croner S, Hattevig G, Fälth-Magnusson K, Björkstén B. Epidemiology and prevention of allergy. Immunol Allergy Prac 1988; 10:393–400.
115. Croner S, Kjellman N-IM, Eriksson B, Roth A. IgE screening in 1701 newborn infants and the development of atopic disease during infancy. Arch Dis Child 1982; 57:364–368.
116. Haahtela T, Lindholm H, Björkstén F, Koskenvuo K, Laitinen LA. Prevalence of asthma in Finnish young men. Br Med J 1990; 301:266–268.
117. Burr ML. Is asthma increasing? J Epidemiol Community Health 1987; 41:185–189.
118. Taylor B, Wadsworth M, Wadsworth J, Peckham C. Changes in the reported prevalence of childhood eczema since the 1939–45 war. Lancet 1984; 2:1255–1257.
119. Businco L, Cantani A. Epidemiology of childhood atopy. Allergol Kongressausgabe 1989; 12:171–175.
120. Midwinter RE, Morris AF, Colley JRT. Infant feeding and atopy. Arch Dis Child 1987; 62:965–7.
121. Crane J, O'Donnell TV, Prior IA, Waite DA. The relationship between atopy, bronchial hyperresponsiveness, and a family history of asthma: a cross-sectional study of migrant Tokelauan children in New Zealand. J Allergy Clin Immunol 1989; 84:768–772.
122. Kainka-Stänicke E, Behrendt H, Friedrichs KH, Tomingas R. Morphological alterations of pollen and spores induced by airborne pollutants: observations from two different polluted areas in West Germany. Allergy 1988; 43(suppl 7):7.
123. Weeke ER. Epidemiology of hay fever and perennial allergic rhinitis. In: Schlumberger HD, ed. Epidemiology of allergic diseases. Basel: S Karger, 1987:1–20.
124. Wiener AS, Zieve I, Fries JH. The inheritance of allergic disease. Ann Eugen 1936; 7:141–162.
125. Cooke RA, van der Veer A. Human sensitization. J Immunol 1916; 1:201–305.
126. Sibbald B, Turner-Warwick M. Factors influencing the prevalence of asthma among first degree relatives of extrinsic and intrinsic asthmatics. Thorax 1979; 34:332–337.
127. Dreborg S, Björkstén B, Kjellman N-IM, Rimås M. Diagnosis of rhinoconjunctivitis (RC) by history (CH), skin prick test (SPT) and conjunctival provocation tests. Discussion on definition of disease. J Allergy Clin Immunol 1989; 83:265.
128. Åberg N, Engström I. Natural history of allergic diseases in children. Acta Paediatr Scand 1990; 79:206–211.

129. Björkstén F, Suoniemi I, Koski V. Neonatal birch-pollen contact and subsequent allergy to birch pollen. Clin Allergy 1980; 10:585–591.
130. Businco L, Cantani A, Farinella F, Businco E. Month of birth and grass pollen or mite sensitization in children with respiratory allergy: a significant relationship. Clin Allergy 1988; 18:269–274.
131. Saarinen UM, Björkstén F, Knekt B, Siimes MA. Serum IgE in healthy infants fed breast milk or cow's milk-based formulas. Clin Allergy 1979; 9:339–345.
132. Chandra RK, Puri S, Hamed A. Influence of maternal diet during lactation and use of formula feeds on development of atopic eczema in high risk infants. Br Med J 1989; 299:228–230.
133. Hattevig G, Kjellman B, Sigurs N, Björkstén B, Kjellman N-IM. Effect of maternal avoidance of eggs, cow's milk and fish during lactation upon allergic manifestations in infants. Clin Exp Allergy 1989; 19:27–32.
134. Lau S, Falkenhorst G, Weber A, Werthmann I, Lind P, Beuttner-Goetz P, Wahn U. High mite-allergen exposure increases the risk of sensitization in atopic children and young adults. J Allergy Clin Immunol 1989; 84:718–725.
135. Andrae S, Axelson O, Björkstén B, Fredriksson M, Kjellman N-IM. Symptoms of bronchial hyperreactivity and asthma in relation to environmental factors. Arch Dis Child 1988; 63:473–478.
136. Sporik R, Holgate ST, Platts-Mills TAE, Cogswell JJ. Exposure to house-dust mite allergen (Der p I) and the development of asthma in childhood. N Engl J Med 1990; 323:502–507.

19

Environmental Factors in the Development of Allergy

Gunnar Hattevig

Kärnsjukhuset, Skövde, Sweden

Bengt Björkstén

University Hospital, Linköping, Sweden

There are several studies strongly indicating that the prevalence of allergic diseases is increasing in many parts of the world (1–3). As the human genotype has not changed appreciably over the past few generations, it is reasonable to assume that the increase is caused by environmental influences.

Sensitization, as proved by the demonstration of low levels of IgE antibodies directed against environmental allergens, appears to be part of the normal immune response. In most instances, at least in children, these antibodies are only temporary, as the continuing IgE antibody formation is rapidly suppressed. But when genetically predisposed individuals are exposed to an allergen at a time when the regulation of the immune system is impaired, then higher levels of IgE antibodies, lasting for a long time may appear. The more susceptible the person is to sensitization generally, the lower is the allergen dose needed for this to occur. The presence of sensitization does not, by itself, mean that clinical symptoms (i.e., allergic disease) will develop.

There have been several studies attempting to evaluate the effect of various allergy preventive measures (4–15). Even though the results of the studies are not always easily interpreted, they do support the conclusion that some preventive measures may be beneficial. In this chapter various environmental factors known to influence sensitization and the development of allergic disease in children will be discussed as a basis for future allergy prevention recommendations.

PRENATAL FACTORS

Maternal Immunity

The fetus is protected from various external influences by the placental barrier. This barrier is selective, since maternal IgG antibodies as well as various antigens are allowed passage, but maternal IgE, IgA, and IgM are restricted (16). Immunity to various infectious agents is thereby transferred to the fetus.

Less is known about the role of transplacental transfer of maternal immunity. Immunoglobulin IgG antibodies to food antigens are present in cord blood at a higher concentration than in corresponding maternal blood (15). By increasing maternal intake of milk and egg during pregnancy, it is possible to increase maternal antibody concentrations to these foods, and by decreasing the intake, there is a corresponding decrease in antibody concentration (15). Although early reports suggested that maternal IgG antibodies against various foods protected the infant from food sensitization (18,19), more recent and larger studies failed to demonstrate any protection from maternal IgG antibodies (4,12).

Transplacentally transferred immunity by maternal IgG antibodies may protect the baby by reducing the risk for intestinal and respiratory tract infections, similar to that noted with breast-feeding (17). Such infections could possibly change mucosal barrier function and influence immune responses to antigens, including enhanced allergic sensitization.

In contrast to IgG, maternal IgE apparently does not pass through the human placenta (16). However, the human fetus is immunocompetent to produce IgE antibodies, as such antibodies have been demonstrated in in vitro studies of fetal lung and liver tissues, and they have also been isolated in amniotic fluid (20–22). Under normal circumstances, this production is limited; the IgE levels in cord blood are usually very low, often even below the detection level. But elevated levels of cord blood IgE (i.e., $\geq$ 0.6 kU/L) do occur in about 10% of newborns. They are associated with an increased risk for development of allergic disease during infancy and childhood (8,23–25). These IgE antibodies are generally not an indication of intrauterine sensitization, since specific IgE antibodies against known defined allergens are rare, except in the situation of maternal helminth infection (21). The most likely explanation for the presence of elevated levels of IgE in cord serum of allergy-prone babies is a low-grade spontaneous synthesis of polyclonal IgE, secondary to a defective suppression of IgE synthesis (26). This is similar to observations in inbred strains of rats with a high propensity to IgE synthesis (27).

Another explanation is that fetal IgE production may possibly be a consequence of allergens passing through the placenta, thereby inducing an immunological response in the fetus. This possibility is indicated by the observation that proteins eaten by pregnant rats can be isolated both in the serum of their pups and in the amniotic fluid (28). In humans, food allergens are often present in the serum of adults after ingestion of milk and egg (29), but so far there is no documentation of food allergens in the fetal circulation. There are occasional reports of low levels of IgE antibodies against cow's milk in some samples of cord blood (30–32). Furthermore, positive skin prick tests have been elicited in newborns to penicillin, helminths, cow's milk, and grass pollen (32–34). However, in other larger studies, prenatal sensitization could not be confirmed (4,7,15,24,35). It is reasonable to conclude that, although the fetus is not completely protected from allergenic material, it is rarely sensitized in utero.

Transplacental transfer of maternal anti-idiotypic antibodies is another possible explanation for the occasional finding of IgE antibodies in cord blood. Such maternal IgG antibodies directed against the antigen-specific parts of other antibodies have a structure similar to the antigen and can replace it as an immunological stimulus. As a consequence, anti-idiotypic antibodies would have the capacity to stimulate fetal antibody formation. This has been demonstrated as a possible mechanism for transfer of immunity to poliovirus and certain strains of *Escherichia coli* from mother to baby (36). It has been suggested that the IgE synthesis in a newborn baby may be stimulated by a similar mechanism, but there is now no convincing evidence of such a mechanism.

Maternal Diet During Pregnancy

The fact that foods are the dominating allergens in infants, as well as the possibility of prenatal induction of IgE antibody formation, has prompted studies of maternal dietary restrictions during pregnancy as a means to prevent the development of the IgE antibodies and allergy in the babies. Some of these studies are difficult to evaluate, since the maternal diet was not limited to pregnancy, but continued into the lactation period (7,9,10). (Table 1).

Two prospective studies that were mainly limited to studying the effects of dietary manipulation during pregnancy both failed to reveal

Table 1 Prospective Studies Including Control Groups of Dietary Intervention in Infants with a Family History of Allergy

Study	Number	Diet during		Follow-up (yr)	Effect of diet	
		Pregnancy	Lactation		Sens[a]	Disease[b]
Fälth-Magnusson et al., 1987 (5)	181	Yes	Partly	1.5	0	0
Lilja et al., 1991 (14)	163	Yes	Partly	1.5	0	0
Chandra et al., 1986 (9)	71	Yes	Yes	1	–	Less AD
Zeiger et al., 1989 (8)	288	Yes	Yes	2	Less	Less FA
Chandra et al., 1989 (10)	97	No	Yes	1.5		Less AD at 12 mo
Hattevig et al., 1990 (11,12)	115	No	Yes	1.5	Less	Less AD at 3 and 6 mo

[a]Sens, sensitization to food allergy; –, data not presented.
[b]AD, atopic dermatitis; FA, food allergy.

any protective effect. In one of the studies, pregnant women with a family history of allergy were randomly assigned to an unrestricted diet, or to an elimination diet, during the last trimester of pregnancy (4,5). Allergenic foods, such as cow's milk, egg, fish, and peanuts, were excluded in the intervention group. In another prospective study of similarly selected mothers, the participants either ingested a diet low in these foods or a diet with increased amounts of milk and eggs (i.e., at least 1L of milk and one egg daily) (13,14). In contrast to the effect of dietary manipulation of breast-feeding mothers (see later discussion), none of the diets during pregnancy were associated with a reduced risk for food allergy nor of other symptoms of atopic disease in their babies. Thus, neither avoidance of certain allergenic foods nor increased amounts of them to stimulate IgG antibody formation had any appreciable effects on clinical symptoms.

The studies summarized in Table 1 indicate that dietary manipulation of the mothers during pregnancy is not associated with less allergy in their babies unless continued into the lactation period. Consequently, no dietary restrictions should be imposed on pregnant women for allergy prevention purposes.

Other Prenatal Factors

It has been reported that smoking, as compared with nonsmoking, mothers more often give birth to infants with a high neonatal IgE concentration (37,38) (Table 2), although a recent study failed to confirm this finding (39). These earlier studies were not conclusive, however, as they were associated with some methodological shortcomings. In contrast to the role of exposure to tobacco smoke after birth, its role prenatally is still not conclusively proved.

There are also indications that medication administered to pregnant women may affect the rate of allergy in their children. Observations include a possible increase in neonatal IgE concentration in babies of mothers treated with the β-blocking agent, metoprolol [8/19 (42.1%)] vs placebo [2/14 (14.3%; $p = 0.18$)] (40). Intrauterine exposure to metoprolol also tended to be associated with more atopic disease during the first years of life [10/26 (38.5%)], compared with children of placebo-treated mothers [3/20 (15.5%; $p = 0.09$)] (40). Additional studies are needed to evaluate more thoroughly the effect of maternal β-adrenergic blocking agents upon the development of atopy.

The influence of the mothers' disease during late pregnancy on the rate of allergic disease in their children has not been adequately assessed in prospective studies, although it has been postulated that

Table 2 Environmental Factors Encountered During Fetal Life and Early Infancy That May Influence the Development of Allergy

Prenatally
Placental barrier function
Maternal immunity
Maternal smoking
Maternal medication
Maternal health
In infancy
Early introduction of formula
Amount and quality of breast milk
Exposure to tobacco smoke
Early exposure to inhalant allergens
Infections
Neonatal complications

the well-being of pregnant asthmatic women may add to the genetic risk for development of atopic disease in their babies (41).

In conclusion, although much remains to be studied, it is reasonable to assume that maternal immunity, health, and medication, at least during the final part of pregnancy, may have consequences on the incidence of allergy in their babies during early childhood. Whether prenatal factors may also affect the development of allergy later in life remains to be studied.

INFANT FEEDING

Breast-feeding

Early weaning to cow's milk formulas has been associated with an increased rate of allergic disease (42–49), and a protective effect of prolonged breast-feeding was reported in a clinical study of over 10,000 infants as early as 1936 (42). But there are also many studies in which prolonged breast-feeding was not associated with the development of less allergic disease than early administration of cow's milk formulas (50–54). The explanation for these apparently conflicting results may lie in the selection of patients for the studies and that such studies were not truly randomized. Studies showing a protective effect of exclusive breast-feeding have included infants with a genetic propensity to allergy, rather than an unselected group of infants. Also, in successful studies, breast-feeding apparently was associated with an avoidance of other foods (e.g., juices and solid foods). In a Finnish study, 135 babies of atopic families were all breast-fed for 6 months without any cow's milk-based supplements (55). Of these infants, 70 received no other nourishment, and 65 were started on solid foods at the age of 3 months. In the exclusive breast milk group, atopic eczema and food allergy were less frequent than in the solid food group at 1 year of age. Supportive of these findings, it appears that infants exposed directly to many diverse solid food allergens early in infancy tend to develop eczema at a higher rate, but exhibit similar incidences of asthma by 2 years of age (56).

Breast-feeding has many other important advantages over formula feeding, including optimal nutrition, less infection, and psychological factors. Critical reviews indicate, however, that even under the best circumstances, the effect of breast-feeding on the development of atopy or allergy is limited to high-risk individuals and that it appears to merely delay, rather than prevent, the onset of allergy (57). Since a shorter duration of breast-feeding is associated with early introduction of formula and solid foods, it is not fully understood to what extent development of allergy is a consequence of exposure to foreign allergenic foods and to what extent it is a consequence of not receiving breast milk, which contains many immunologically active components (58).

There are several possible explanations for the protective role of breast milk against allergy, including (a) low content of allergens, (b) protection against intestinal and respiratory infections, (c) passive transfer of immunity from the mother by secretory IgA antibodies, and (d) transfer of components that stimulate the maturation of the infantile immune system (Table 3). However, it is well established that human milk may contain food antigens, such as cow's milk proteins and egg, if these

Table 3 Breast-Feeding and Protection Against Allergic Disease

Appears to delay the onset of allergy in genetically predisposed persons.
The allergy-preventive quality of milk may vary, for example,
Maternal diet
Maternal immunity
Several possible protective mechanisms, for example,
Low allergen content
Passive transfer of immunity
Stimulates maturation of immune system
Protects against infections

items are ingested by the mother (59,60). These maternally consumed food allergens reaching the maternal breast milk may sensitize the genetically predisposed breast-fed baby, although such sensitization has not yet been conclusively documented. Breast milk containing specific food allergens, on the other hand, conclusively evoked allergic symptoms during lactation in sensitized infants (35,61).

Hypoallergenic Maternal Lactation Diet

The effects of maternal hypoallergenic diet during lactation have been evaluated in four studies. In two of these studies, however, the maternal antigen avoidance diet had already been started during pregnancy (8,9). One of the studies could document an effect upon atopic dermatitis at 12 months of age. In the second study, Zeiger et al. showed reduced atopic dermatitis, urticaria, or gastrointestinal disease, but no differences in the frequency of asthma and rhinoconjunctivitis (8).

The effect of maternal hypoallergenic diet during the lactation period has been addressed in only two studies. One of them included two randomized groups with and without dietary restrictions for 6 months of lactation (10). After weaning, the infants were given a hydrolysate formula. At 18 months of age, the infants in the maternal diet group had fewer and milder cases of eczema.

In the other study, two matched groups were studied (11,12). Maternal antigen avoidance was adhered to for 3 months after delivery in one group, whereas the other group had no maternal dietary restrictions during the lactation period. Both groups of infants were given a casein hydrolysate formula up to 6 months of age if they were not fully breast-fed. The incidence of atopic dermatitis was significantly lower during the first 6 months of age in infants of mothers adhering to the hypoallergenic diet, when compared with the nondiet group. Furthermore, the maternal diet restrictions resulted in a significantly lower rate of sensitization in the diet infants during the time of restrictions. The follow-up at 4 years of age showed a significant difference in the incidence of atopic dermatitis in the diet children compared with the nondiet children (61A). However, in both studies there were no differences in the frequency of other atopic manifestations.

The results of even a strict maternal hypoallergenic diet are so modest that it is doubtful whether the efforts required for the family are justified. However, parents who have experienced severe atopic disease in themselves and in previous children are sometimes very eager to try preventive measures, even if these have only a temporary effect. Consequently, for such families, individually adapted advice to the mother concerning dietary restrictions during lactation appears worthy.

Immune Effects of Human Milk

As indicated previously, there are several possible explanations for an allergy-preventing role of human milk (see Table 3). It may be secondary to a reduction in the number of intestinal and respiratory infections in the breast-fed baby, as certain infections appear to trigger allergy (discussed later). Passive transfer of immunity is another possibility by which human milk is protective, as in one study it was reported that high levels in breast milk of IgA antibodies against cow's milk protein were associated with fewer allergic symptoms in the babies (62). This observation could not be confirmed, however, in a larger, prospectively done study (6).

Several recent studies indicate that human milk may exert a regulatory role on infant immunity. Observations include an early stimulation of IgA antibody synthesis in breast-fed infants (63,64) and transfer of cell-mediated immunity (65,66) and cytokines (67,69). The precise relation between breast-feeding and infant allergy is thus not fully understood. It is reasonable to assume that any allergy-protective effects of breast-feeding may vary with the individual mothers, as both their diet and their immune status appear to play a role. Also, an allergy-preventing effect of human milk seems to be limited to babies with a genetically determined increased risk for allergic disease (56). This lends further support to the notion that environmental factors associated with an increased rate of allergic disease in children are mainly operative in individuals with a genetic propensity for allergic sensitization and disease.

Conclusions Concerning Breast-feeding and Lactation Diet

Since sensitization may occur during breast-feeding, one may suggest that high-risk infants should not be breast-fed at all, but rather, should be given hypoallergenic formula immediately after birth. However, in the light of all the other advantages of breast-feeding, including both biological and psychological advantages, such advice should not be given at present. Nevertheless, a careful prospective evaluation of such a preventive measure is justifiable.

Even though the results in the literature do not form the basis for any general preventive measures, they increase the insight into the process of sensitization and, thereby, help to increase our understanding of seemingly contradictory case histories described by parents. The mother who, after weaning, reports that the child's eczema has improved is probably just as right as the mother claiming that the eczema in her infant worsened when he or she received an infant formula. In the first case, sensitization to eggs, for example, may have occurred, and the amount of allergen in the breast milk was sufficient to provoke symptoms during lactation. An improvement then took place after weaning when the child was given ordinary food, which for children of that age usually contains no egg protein. Similarly, in the second case, sensitization to, for instance cow's milk, may have occurred, but not to such a degree that the small amounts of cow's milk transferred by breast milk provoked symptoms, whereas such symptoms were provoked when a cow's milk-based formula was introduced.

In conclusion, the prospective studies in which the effect of avoidance of highly allergenic foods by lactating mothers was evaluated indicate that such manipulation of the maternal diet in exclusively breast-fed infants may delay the onset of allergic sensitization and disease in their babies and also result in less severe disease in those who develop allergic symptoms (7–12,49) (see Table 1). Thus, manipulation of the maternal diet may be worthwhile during the lactation period (but not during pregnancy) in families with a genetic predisposition for allergic disease. Maternal diet should, however, be employed only in selected cases, and it should not be recommended indiscriminately, as it imposes a substantial emotional and social stress on the family, as well as a risk for suboptimal nutrition of the mother and infant.

ENVIRONMENTAL FACTORS

Early Exposure to Inhalant Allergens

Several clinical studies indicate that there is a period in early infancy during which exposure to inhalant allergens may enhance development of allergy several years later. Thus, a significantly increased risk for subsequent development of allergy to birch was reported in Finnish children born in the spring (70). Similar results have been reported for grass allergy in the United Kingdom (71) and for ragweed allergy in American children born in the late summer (72). The seasonal influence of allergy appears to be limited to allergy-prone babies, rather than being apparent in the general population (73).

These observations are not limited to pollens, since early exposure to cats (74–76) and house dust mites (76,77) may also result in a higher incidence of sensitization and clinical allergy. Specifically, prospective follow-up from infancy to age 11 of British children from atopic families observed that 16/17 11-year-old children with active asthma were atopic, all sensitized to house dust mites. A significant relation was found between dust mite exposure at age 1 (> 10 μg of mite per gram of dust) and the degree of mite sensitization at age 11 (78). The relation between early exposure to inhalant allergens and allergic disease seems to be limited to children with a congenital propensity for allergy, rather than being present in all children (26). Reasons for the association between early exposure and disease are poorly understood, as clinical symptoms to inhalant allergens usually appear only several years after infancy.

Nonspecific Factors

In addition to allergens, there are several environmental factors that facilitate sensitization to almost any allergen to which the individual is exposed (Table 4). Among these "adjuvant" factors, particularly exposures to tobacco smoke and certain infections appear to play a role in early infancy. The role of tobacco smoke has been substantiated in several studies (39,79). Therefore, it is reasonable to strongly discourage parents from smoking near a young infant, particularly in families with allergic disease. Other nonspecific factors that appear to play a role include industrial air pollution and living in modern tight, poorly ventilated houses (79). Much more research is needed to define the relative role of these and other environmental factors.

The role of infections as a trigger of allergic disease is not fully understood. There are now several studies suggesting an association between respiratory infections and appearance of allergic disease (80–82). Possible explanations for these observations include that infectious agents may (a) facilitate inflammatory reactions and sensitization, (b) alter an immune defense, or (c) act as adjuvants or allergens. It is also well known from animal studies that pertussis bacteria are adjuvants for the induction of IgE antibody formation against various antigens (83). In humans, whooping cough is associated with a prolonged period of bronchial hyperreactivity and IgE antibodies against pertussis toxin,

Table 4 Nonspecific, Adjuvant Factors Enhancing Sensitization to Allergens

Exposure to tobacco smoke
Exposure to outdoor air pollutants
Living in tight, poorly ventilated buildings
Infections

findings commonly demonstrated in children with whooping cough and after pertussis immunization (84).

These specific nonallergen environmental influences seem to play a major role only in individuals with a genetically determined tendency to allergic disease. From extensive experimental work in rodents and analysis of epidemiological data on the appearance of IgE antibodies in infants and children, Holt (27) has proposed that the capacity to produce IgE antibody in response to environmental allergens is genetically controlled through the T-cell system, but the ultimate expression of a genetic potential for high IgE production requires the intervention of additional environmental risk factors (e.g., air pollution). Many of these environmental risk factors appear to function at the level of enhancing contact between allergen and the immune system, particularly by increasing net flux of inhalant allergen across respiratory mucous membranes. At the time of initial contact with an allergen not previously encountered, the immune system responds vigorously. Transient IgE production is part of this normal response. In nonatopic individuals, the initial IgE response is self-limiting and is replaced by a life-long tolerance to the allergen. However, if the individual is simultaneously exposed to appropriate risk factors at the time of initial exposure (e.g., in early infancy), then the immune response may instead steadily increase, giving rise to an expanding pool of memory T cells that effectively prime the immune system, laying the foundation for a state of hypersensitivity to the allergen. Once an allergic inflammatory response to an allergen occurs, this process in turn enhances sensitization to new allergens encountered during the reaction.

CONCLUSIONS

Several environmental factors may increase the risk for sensitization and subsequent development of allergic disease. The first months of life appear to be a period during which babies are particularly susceptible. Sensitization during this period may have long-term consequences. Infants with a genetic propensity to develop allergy and atopic disease seem particularly susceptible to the various environmental influences. As a consequence, a reasonable strategy to employ in the prevention of allergy would be to identify infants at risk early and then to support their families and encourage them to take allergy preventive measures, including exclusive breast-feeding for at least 4–6 months, avoidance of exposure to tobacco smoke and, if possible, avoidance of potent allergens such as house dust mites and furred pets.

REFERENCES

1. Eaton KK. The incidence of allergy—has it changed? Clin Allergy 1982; 12:107–110.
2. Taylor B, Wadsworth J, Wadsworth M, Peckham C. Changes in the reported prevalence of childhood eczema since the 1939–45 war. Lancet 1985; 1:1255–1257.
3. Dowse GK, Turner KJ, Stewat GA, Alphers MD, Woolcock AJ. The association between *Dermatophagoides* mites and the increasing prevalence of asthma in the village communities within the Papua New Guinea Highlands. J Allergy Clin Immunol 1985; 75:75–83.
4. Fälth-Magnusson K, Öman H, Kjellman N-IM. Maternal abstention from cow's milk and egg in allergy risk pregnancy. Allergy 1987; 47:64–73.
5. Fälth-Magnusson K, Kjellman, N-IM. Development of atopic disease in babies whose mothers were receiving exclusion diet during pregnancy. A randomized study. J Allergy Clin Immunol 1987; 80:868–875.
6. Fälth-Magnusson K, Kjellman, N-IM, Magnusson KE. Antibodies IgG, IgA and IgM to food antigens during the first 18 months of life in relation to feeding and atopic disease. J Allergy Clin Immunol 1988; 81:743–749.
7. Zeiger RS, Heller S, Mellon MH, O'Connor R, Hamburger RN. Effectiveness of dietary manipulation in the prevention of food allergy in infants. J Allergy Clin Immunol 1986; 78:224–238.
8. Zeiger RS, Heller S, Mellon MH, Forsythe AB, O'Connor RD, Hamburger RN, Schatz M. Effect of combined maternal and infant food-allergen avoidance on development of atopy in early infancy: a randomized study. J Allergy Clin Immunol 1989; 84:72–89.
9. Chandra RK, Puri S, Suraiya C, Cheema PS. Influence of maternal food antigen avoidance during pregnancy and lactation on incidence of atopic eczema in infants. Clin Allergy 1986; 16:563–569.
10. Chandra RK. Influence of maternal diet during lactation and use of formula feeds on development of atopic eczema in high risk infants. Br Med J 1989; 299:228–230.
11. Hattevig G, Kjellman B, Sigurs N, Björkstén B, Kjellman N-IM. Effect of maternal avoidance of eggs, cow's milk and fish during lactation upon allergic manifestations in infants. Clin Exp Allergy 1989; 19:27–32.
12. Hattevig G, Kjellman B, Sigurs N, Grodzinsky E, Hed J, Björkstén B. The effect of maternal avoidance of eggs, cow's milk and fish during lactation on the development of IgE, IgG and IgA antibodies in infants. J Allergy Clin Immunol 1990; 85:108–115.
13. Lilja G, Dannaeus A, Foucard T, Graff-Lonnevig V, Johansson SGO, Öman H. Effects of maternal diet during late pregnancy and lactation on the development of atopic disease in infants up to 18 months of age—in vivo results. Clin Exp Allergy 1989; 19:473–479.
14. Lilja G, Dannaeus A, Foucard T, Graff-Lonnevig V, Johansson SGO, Öman H. Effects of maternal diet during pregnancy and lactation on the devel-

opment of IgE and egg- and milk-specific IgE and IgG antibodies in infants. Clin Exp Allergy 21 (1991) 2, 195–202.

15. Lilja G, Dannaeus A, Fälth-Magnusson K, Graff-Lonnevig V, Johansson SGO, Kjellman N-IM, Öman H. Immune response of the atopic woman and foetus; effects of high- and low-dose food allergen intake during late pregnancy. Clin Allergy 1988; 18:131–142.
16. Brambell FWR. The transmission of antibodies. In: Brambell FWR, ed. The transmission of immunity from the mother to young. Amsterdam: North-Holland, 1970:242–250.
17. Fallot ME, Boyd J, Oski FA. Breast-feeding reduces incidence of hospital admissions for infection in infants. Pediatrics 1980; 65:1121–1124.
18. Dannaeus A, Johansson SGO, Foucard T. Clinical and immunological aspects of food allergy in childhood. II. Development of allergic symptoms and humoral immune response to foods in infants of atopic mothers during the first 24 months of life. Acta Paediatr Scand 1978; 67:497–504.
19. Casimir G, Gossart B, Vis HL, Duchateau J. Antibody against betalactoglobulin (IgG) and cow's milk allergy [abstr]. J Allergy Clin Immunol 1985; 75:206.
20. Miller DL, Hirvonen T, Gitlin D. Synthesis of IgE by human conceptus. J Allergy Clin Immunol 1973; 52:182–188.
21. Singer AD, Hobel CJ, Heiner DC. Evidence for secretory IgA and IgE in utero [abstr]. J Allergy Clin Immunol 1974; 53:94.
22. Cramer DV, Kunz HW, Gill TJ. III. Immunological sensitization prior to birth. Am J Obstet Gynecol 1974; 120:431–439.
23. Michel PB, Bousquet J, Greillier P, Robinet-Levy M, Coulomb Y. Comparison of cord blood immunoglobulin E concentration and maternal allergy for the prediction of atopic disease in infancy. J Allergy Clin Immunol 1980; 66:422–430.
24. Croner S, Kjellman N-IM, Eriksson B, Roth A. IgE screening in 1701 newborn infants and the development of atopic disease during infancy. Arch Dis Child 1982; 57:364–368.
25. Croner S, Kjellman N-IM. Development of atopic disease in relation to family history and cord blood IgE levels—eleven years follow-up in 1654 children. Pediatr Allergy Immunol 1990; 1:14–20.
26. Björkstén B, Kjellman N-IM. Immunological abnormalities in atopic infants. Allergologie 1989; 12S:176–179.
27. Holt PG, McMenamin C, Nelson D. Primary sensitization to inhalant allergen during infancy. Pediatr Allergy Immunol 1990; 1:3–13.
28. Dahl GMK, Telemo E, Wesström BR, Jacobsson I, Lindberg T, Karlsson BW. The passage of orally fed protein from mother to foetus in the rat. Comp Biochem Physiol 1984; 774:199–201.
29. Huseby S, Jensenius JC, Svehag S-E. Passage of undergraded dietary antigen into the blood of healthy adults. Scand J Immunol 1985; 22:88–92.
30. Businco L, Machetti F, Pellegrini G, Perlini P. Predictive value of cord blood IgE levels in "at risk" newborn babies and influence of type of feeding. Clin Allergy 1989; 13:503–508.

31. Delespesse G, Sarfati M, Lang G, Sehon AH. Prenatal and neonatal synthesis of IgE. Monogr Allergy 1983; 18:83–95.
32. Kimpen J, Callaert H, Embrechts P, Bossmans E. Influence of sex and gestational age on cord blood IgE. Acta Paediatr Scand 1989; 78:233–238.
33. Levin S, Altman Y, Sela M. Penicillin and dinitrophenyl antibodies in newborn and mothers detected with chemically modified bacteriophage. Pediatr Res 1971; 5:87–88.
34. Weil GJ, Hussain R, Kumaraswami V, Tripathy SP, Phillips KS, Oliesen EA. Prenatal allergic sensitization to helminth antigen in offspring of parasite-infected mothers. J Clin Invest 1983; 71:1124–1129.
35. Hattevig G, Kjellman B, Johansson SGO, Björkstén B. Clinical symptoms and IgE responses to common food proteins in atopic and healthy children. Clin Allergy 1984; 14:551–559.
36. Mellander L, Carlsson B, Hanson L-Å. Secretory IgA and IgM antibodies to *E. coli* and poliovirus type I antigens occur in amniotic fluid, meconium and saliva from newborns. A neonatal immune response without antigenic exposure: a result of anti-idiotypic induction? Clin Exp Immunol 1986; 63:555–561.
37. Magnusson CGM. Maternal smoking influences cord serum IgE and IgD levels and increases the risk for subsequent infant allergy. J Allergy Clin Immunol 1986; 78:898–904.
38. Rantakallio P. Relationship of maternal smoking to morbidity and mortality of the child up to age five. Acta Paediatr Scand 1978; 67:621–631.
39. Ownby DR, Johnson CC, Petersen EL. Maternal smoking does not influence cord servor IgE or IgD concentrations. J Allergy Clin Immunol 1991; 88:555–560.
40. Björkstén B, Finnström O, Wichmann K. Intrauterine exposure to beta-adrenergic receptor-blocking agent metroprolol and allergy. Int Arch Allergy Appl Immunol 1988; 87:59–62.
41. Nelson HS. Pregnancy and allergic diseases. In: Bierman CW, Pearlman DS, eds. Allergic diseases of infancy, childhood and adolescence. Philadelphia: WB Saunders, 1980:675–680.
42. Grulee CG, Sanford HN. The influence of breast- and artificial feeding on infantile eczema. J Pediatr 1936; 9:223–225.
43. Kaufman HS. Diet and heredity in infantile atopic dermatitis. Acta Dermatol 1972; 105:400–404.
44. Kaufman HS, Frick OL. The development of allergy in infants of allergic parents. Ann Allergy 1976; 37:410–415.
45. Saarinen UM, Kajosaari M, Backman A, Siimes M. Prolonged breast-feeding as prophylaxis for atopic disease. Lancet 1979; 2:163–166.
46. Chandra RK. Prospective studies of the effect of breast feeding on incidence of infection and allergy. Acta Paediatr Scand 1979; 68:691–696.
47. Juto P, Björkstén B. Serum IgE in infants and influence of type of feeding. Clin Allergy 1980; 10:593–600.

48. Gruskay FL. Comparison of breast, cow and soy feeding in the prevention onset of allergic disease: a 15 year prospective study. Clin Pediatr 1982; 21:486–491.
49. Businco L, Cantani A, Meglio P, Bruno G. Prevention of atopy: results of a long-term (7 months–8 years) follow-up. Ann Allergy 1987; 59:183–186.
50. Halpern SR, Sellars WA, Johnson RB, Anderson DW, Saperstein S, Reisch JS. Development of childhood allergy in infants fed breast, soy or cow's milk. J Allergy Clin Immunol 1973; 51:139–151.
51. Burr ML. Does breast-feeding affect the risk of allergy? Arch Dis Child 1983; 58:561–556.
52. Gordon RR, Ward AM, Nobie DA, Allen R. Immunoglobulin E and eczema–asthma syndrome in early childhood. Lancet 1982; 1:72–74.
53. Hide DW, Guyer BM. Clinical manifestation of allergy related to breast and cow's milk feeding. Arch Dis Child 1981; 56:172–175.
54. Van Asperen PP, Kemp AS, Mellis CM. Relationship of diet in the development of atopy in infancy. Clin Allergy 1984; 14:525–532.
55. Kajosaari M, Saarinen UM. Prophylaxis of atopic disease by six months' total solid food elimination. Acta Paediatr Scand 1983; 72:411–414.
56. Fergusson DM, Harwood LJ, Beautrias AL, et al. Eczema and infant diet. Clin Allergy 1981; 11:325–331.
57. Björkstén B. Does breast-feeding prevent development of allergy? Immunol Today 1983; 4:215–217.
58. Hansson, L-Å, Ahlstedt S, Andersson B, Carlsson B, Fällström S-P, Mellander L, Porras O, Söderström T, Svanborg-Edén C. Protective factors in milk and the development of the immune system. Pediatrics 1985; 75:172–176.
59. Jacobsson I, Lindberg T, Benediktsson B, Hansson B-G. Dietary bovine beta-lactoglobulin is transferred in human milk. Acta Paediatr Scand 1985; 74:342–345.
60. Harmatz PR, Bloch KJ. Transfer of dietary protein in breast milk. Ann Allergy 1988; 61:21–24.
61. Gerrard JW. Allergy in breast-fed babies to ingredients in breast milk. Ann Allergy 1979; 42:69–71.
61A. Sigurs N, Hattevig G, Kjellman B, Kjellman N-IM, Nilsson L, Björkstén B. Appearance of IgE antibodies in relation to atopic disease. A Longitudinal Study. Clin Exp Allergy, in manuscript.
62. Machtinger S, Moss R. Cow's milk allergy in breast fed infants: the role of allergen and maternal secretory IgA antibody. J Allergy Clin Immunol 1986; 77:341–347.
63. Prentice A. Breast feeding increases concentration of IgA in infants urine. Arch Dis Child 1987; 62:792–795.
64. Stephens S. Development of secretory immunity in breast fed and bottle fed infants. Arch Dis Child 1986; 61:263–269.
65. Pittard WB, Bill K. Immunoregulation by breast milk cells. Cell Immunol 1979; 42:437–441.
66. Schlesinger JJ, Covelli HD. Evidence for transmission of lymphocyte responses to tuberculin by breast-feeding. Lancet 1977; 2:529–532.

67. Delespesse G. Presence of IgE suppressor factors in human colostrum. Eur J Immunol 1986; 16:1005–1008.
68. Söder O. Isolation of interleukin-1 from human milk. Int Arch Allergy Appl Immunol 1987; 83:19–23.
69. Shiba Y, Minagawa T, Mito K, Nakane A, Suga K, Honjo T, Nakao T. Effect of breast feeding on responses of systemic interferon and virus-specific lymphocyte transformation in infants with respiratory syncytial virus infection. J Med Virol 1987; 21:7–14.
70. Björkstén F, Suoniemi I, Koski V. Neonatal birch-pollen contact and subsequent allergy to birch-pollen. Clin Allergy 1980; 10:581.
71. Morrison-Smith J, Springett VH. Atopic disease and month of birth. Clin Allergy 1979; 9:153–157.
72. Settipane RJ, Hagy GW. Effect of atmospheric pollen on the newborn. RI Med J 1979; 62:477–482.
73. Croner S, Kjellman N-IM. Predictors of atopic disease: cord blood IgE and months of birth. Allergy 1986; 41:68–70.
74. Suoniemi I, Björkstén F, Haahtela T. Dependence of immediate hypersensitivity in the adolescent period on factors encountered in infancy. Allergy 1981; 36:263–268.
75. Rugtveit J. Environmental factors in the first months of life and the possible relationship to later development of hypersensitivity. Allergy 1990; 45:154–156.
76. Warner JA, Little SA, Pollock I, Longbottom JL, Warner JO. The influence of exposure to house dust mite, cat, pollen and fungal allergens in the home on primary sensitization in asthma. Pediatr Allergy Immunol 1990; 1:79–86.
77. Rowntree S, Cogswell JJ, Platts-Mills TAE, Mitchell EB. Development of IgE and IgG antibodies to food and inhalant allergens in children at risk of allergic disease. Arch Dis Child 1985; 61:727–732.
78. Sporik R, Holgate ST, Platts-Mills TAE, Cogswell JJ. Exposure to house dust mite allergen and the development of asthma in childhood. A prospective study. N Engl J Med 1990; 323:502–507.
79. Andrae S, Axelson O, Björkstén B, Fredriksson M, Kjellman N-IM. Symptoms of bronchial hyperreactivity and asthma in relation to environmental factors. Arch Dis Child 1988; 63:473–478.
80. Frick OL, German DF, Mills J. Development of allergy in children. I. Association with virus infection. J Allergy Clin Immunol 1979; 63:228–241.
81. Welliver RC, Ogra L. The role of IgE in pathogenesis of mucosal viral infections. Ann NY Acad Sci 1983; 21:332.
82. Strannegård I-L, Strannegård Ö. Epstein–Barr virus antibody in children with atopic disease. Int Arch Allergy Appl Immunol 1981; 64:314–319.
83. Pauwels R, Van der Straeten M, Platteu B, Bazin H. The non-specific enhancement of allergy. I. In vivo effects of *Bordetella pertussis* vaccine on IgE synthesis. Allergy 1983; 38:239–246.
84. Hedenskog S, Björkstén B, Blennow M, Granström G, Grandström M. Immunoglobulin E response to pertussis toxin in whooping cough after immunization with a whole cell and an acellular pertussis vaccine. Int Arch Allergy Appl Immunol 1989; 89:156–161.

20

The Natural History of Allergic Disease and Asthma in Childhood

Steven Rubinstein

Stanford University Medical Center, Stanford, California

The duration of any illness or condition is paramount to both the physician and the patient. Knowledge of any precautionary measures that can be taken to ameliorate the severity or shorten the duration of the condition are instrumental in patient care. Longitudinal data can enable physicians, regardless of specialty, to responsibly counsel individuals and parents of those with allergic and asthmatic conditions. This counseling can outline reasonable expectations for the duration of the condition, as well as any interventions that can be taken to minimize its severity. Numerous long-term studies have been undertaken, both retrospectively and prospectively, evaluating the duration of atopic conditions, particularly asthma, and the risk factors for their persistence.

Unfortunately, most studies assessing the natural history of allergic disease are wrought with inherent methodological difficulties. Comparing these studies is even more arduous. Nevertheless, analysis of these studies reveals surprisingly consistent findings. This chapter should help the practitioner more confidently and honestly convey predictions of disease outcome to their patients.

This review assesses both the outcomes and the risk factors determining these outcomes for the most common allergic conditions of childhood. Some epidemiological factors, such as the prevalence or incidence of these conditions, are discussed only in terms of early childhood. Other epidemiological patterns, particularly in later childhood and adulthood, are beyond the scope of this chapter and are reviewed elsewhere (1).

METHODOLOGICAL DIFFICULTIES

Attempting to follow an individual's clinical status over the course of years and decades in a mobile society is fraught with difficulty. Hence, many of the more prolonged prospective studies have occurred in geographic locations where mobility is less likely to take place, such as Australia, Sweden, and Great Britain. Definitions of what constitutes a specific allergic condition, or even an allergic symptom, can vary markedly among researchers. This is particularly apparent for asthma and wheezing. For example, most general cohort studies (those in which a total population group is studied for the presence or persistence of an allergic condition) use patient or parental reporting of any wheezing, or even frequent cough, as criteria for inclusion in an index group. These studies are more likely to have higher incidence rates than those studies that require audible wheezing to be recorded by an examining physician. In addition, these cohort studies tend to underestimate the persistence of the condition (asthma), since many individuals who have experienced only a single symptomatic episode (wheezing) are initially included in the study.

Studies using questionnaires, particularly retrospective studies, are plagued with problems of recall bias. A person's recollection of the frequency or severity of symptoms often does not correlate with findings of practitioners. In addition, certain retrospective studies investigate only those patients with active symptoms, thereby overlooking those who may have "outgrown" the condition. These studies tend to overestimate the persistence of a condition. This is the primary flaw in many of the earlier studies identifying the presence of childhood respiratory conditions as a precursor of subsequent adult respiratory disease (2).

Each researcher uses different criteria to assess the severity of a condition. In general, frequency of a symptom is used as an index of severity. Hence, the severity of those who have frequent, but mild, symptoms will be overestimated in a study, whereas those who ignore their symptoms may be categorized as less severe.

The final concern, and the most difficult, is in comparing study results. In addition to the different criteria used for defining diseases and their severity, follow-up intervals for patients and the methods used to assess their illnesses vary markedly. Although this makes direct comparison of studies impractical, the epidemiological trends found are intriguing and, as noted, remarkably consistent.

THE NATURAL HISTORY OF ATOPY AND ASTHMA IN EARLY CHILDHOOD

The incidence of atopic conditions in infancy and early childhood appears to be influenced by numerous factors. The most significant of these is a familial tendency toward atopy (3–6). There is increasing evidence, however, that environmental exposures in infancy may affect an individual's symptomatic expression of atopy, not only through childhood, but well into adulthood (7–9). Similarly, infectious episodes of the lower respiratory tract in infancy may result in lifelong bronchial hyperreactivity (2,5,10,11).

There are two general types of studies that have evaluated the epidemiology of atopy: longitudinal studies of atopic subjects or those at higher risk for atopy (i.e., infants of atopic parents), and general population cohort studies in which all subjects are evaluated for the presence and persistence of atopic conditions. Many of these studies are reviewed later in this chapter when the specific atopic condition is discussed.

Prospective studies by Van Asperen and Kemp (12) in Australia, Cogswell et al. (13) in Great Britain, and Zeiger, et al. (14) in the United States delineate the early natural history of atopy and skin test reactivity from infancy through early childhood. Their findings are consistent with similar earlier studies (15). Van Asperen and Kemp prospectively studied 79 infants with a family history of atopy every 4 months from birth to 20 months, and again at age 5 (12). Each infant was evaluated clinically and by skin testing to milk, egg, wheat, and dust mite. Cogswell and his group followed 73 children who had one atopic parent prospectively from birth to age 5 (13). Each study patient had a physical examination with skin testing every 3 months from birth through 12 months, and then yearly through age 5. Skin testing was performed for reactions to egg, milk, rye grass, dust mite, dog, and cat. Zeiger et al. prospectively followed 288 infants from atopic parents (~50% bilaterally atopic) from birth with evaluations at 4, 12, 24 (14) and then 36 and 48 months of age (16) which included physical examinations, skin testing, food challenges, and IgE determinations. The results of these studies are discussed later.

Atopic Dermatitis

The cumulative prevalence of atopic dermatitis (AD) in the first 12 months of life in these prospective studies ranged from a low of 11% (14) to a high approaching almost 50% (12) of those children with one or two atopic parents. Most cases start by 4–8 months of age, with few new cases developing after 1–2 years. Van Asperen found that the cumulative prevalence of AD by age 5 increased only to 58% (12). Most children improve significantly or remit by age 5. In fact, Cogswell et al. found that 90% had symptomatically resolved by 1 year of age (13). Zeiger et al. noticed only a 6% period and 20% cumulative prevalence at 4 years of age (16).

The presence of adverse reactions to foods, as well as positive skin tests to foods, is much higher in infants with AD than with other atopic conditions. Cogswell et al. (13) found that 58% of subjects under age 2 with AD had skin test positivity (13); 86% of those with positive tests reacted to foods. Zeiger et al. noted that 67% of infants with atopic dermatitis evidenced positive food skin tests (14). Those with AD had statistically higher serum IgE levels, and egg was the only antigen statistically correlated with the presence of AD (13). Those who had skin test positivity were significantly more likely to have persistence of their skin symptoms through age 5 and to have other associated atopic conditions. By age 5, however, the nature of the skin test reactivity in those with persistent AD appears to change. As the frequency of positive reactions to foods declines, positive reactivity to inhalants increases.

Rhinitis

Very few studies have investigated the incidence of persistent, noninfectious rhinitis in the first several years of life. About 50% of children of atopic parent(s) in Van Asperen's study had prolonged (over 4 weeks) continuous rhinitis by 1 year of age. Two-thirds developed rhinitis by age 5 (12). Most children with rhinitis had episodic symptoms, although about 14% were observed to have continuous symptoms from infancy through age 5. This rhinitis started by 4 months of age in most children. In contrast, Zeiger et al. employing symptoms, nasal eosinophilia, and positive skin tests to diagnose allergic rhinitis, could not identify allergic rhinitis in any of their 4-month-old infants, but found that the frequency of allergic rhinitis increases steadily from a cumulative prevalence of 4% at 1 year to 28% by 4 years (14,16). At each time interval, the periods and cumulative prevalences for allergic rhinitis were similar, indicating that by 4 years of age allergic rhinitis tends to persist, rather than remit as in the case of atopic dermatitis (14,16).

Wheezing, Asthma

Children experiencing a single episode of wheezing (unrelated to bronchiolitis) appear to be at no higher risk for developing asthma than a child never having a wheezing episode (12,13,17). Children of atopic parents, however, are about twice as likely to wheeze by age 5, with about 1-2 of children of atopic parents experiencing at least one episode of wheezing by that age. Approximately 20% of these children will wheeze at least once by 12 months of age. Two or more episodes of wheezing occur by 4 years in about 25% of children of atopic parents (16).

Cohort studies of general population groups have found that about 20% of children by age 7, and 25% by age 16, will have at least one episode of wheezing (4,5). Ultimately between 10 and 15% can be classified as asthmatic (recurrent wheezing episodes) (5,8). In contrast, asthma occurs in about a third of children of atopic parents by age 5 (12,13). Anderson found the prevalence of asthma symptoms in the prior year to be 8% at age 7, 5% at age 11, and 3% at age 16 in a parental questionnaire in 8806 British children (18).

About a half of those with recurrent wheezing at age 5 started wheezing before 1 year of age (12). Recurrent wheezing was rarely found, however, before 4 months of age (15). In those with multiple atopic conditions, asthma generally follows the appearance of atopic dermatitis and persistent rhinitis. Children with atopic parents who develop recurrent wheezing in childhood concurrently experience other atopic conditions (13). These children from atopic parents also have an increased likelihood of having positive skin tests. Cogswell et al. found 89% of asthmatics at age 5 had at least one positive skin test to a battery of six antigens (13).

Those children younger than 2 years of age with skin test positivity and elevated serum IgE levels, who have atopic parents, are more likely to develop asthma (recurrent wheezing) (9,13). Similarly, those with earlier symptoms of recurrent wheezing are significantly more likely to have positive skin tests (at any age) (8,9,13). Persistence of wheezing in early childhood is also related to the degree of bronchial hyperreactivity (17). Other risk factors for the development of asthma are listed in Table 1 and are discussed in detail later.

Skin Test Reactivity and Radioallergosorbent Testing

Infants and children with elevated serum IgE levels and positive skin tests or positive radioallergosorbent tests (RASTs) in early childhood are more likely to have positive skin tests when prospectively studied into adulthood (8,19). This positivity, however, does not necessarily predict persistent clinical symptomatology (discussed later).

Positive skin tests to inhalants in infancy tend to persist and are significantly associated with the early onset of respiratory symptoms

Table 1 Risk Factors for Presence of Asthma in Childhood

Definite[a]
Family history of atopy/asthma
Early lung disease/bronchiolitis
Elevated IgE
Positive skin tests/RAST
Early lung disease/bronchiolitis
Maternal smoking
Concurrent allergic rhinitis
Concurrent atopic dermatitis
Male sex
House dust allergy
High dust mite levels in home (with positive family history)
Probable[b]
House dampness
Immediate food reactivity
Presence of furred animal in home with positive family history of atopy
Eosinophilia (more adults than children)
Maternal smoking while pregnant
Possible[c]
Air pollution exposure
Not breast-fed as infant
Season of birth
Paternal smoking
Unlikely[d]
History of urticaria
Delayed food reactions
Lower respiratory infection after infancy
Social class
No association
IgA, IgG levels
Presence of gas stove in home

[a]Multiple studies show strong statistical significance.
[b]Multiple studies show statistical significance; occasional studies do not.
[c]Some studies show statistical significance and a similar number do not, or a single study showed statistical significance and not evaluated in other studies.
[d]Most studies do not show statistical significance.

(9,12,14). Positive skin test to inhalants develop later than to foods (Figure 1) (12–14). Those to foods tend to develop in infancy and are associated with the presence of atopic dermatitis (12–14) and food allergy (14), but not generally with recurrent wheezing. These positive tests to foods often remit (see Chapter 21), whereas inhalant sensitivity tends to persist in childhood (12–14).

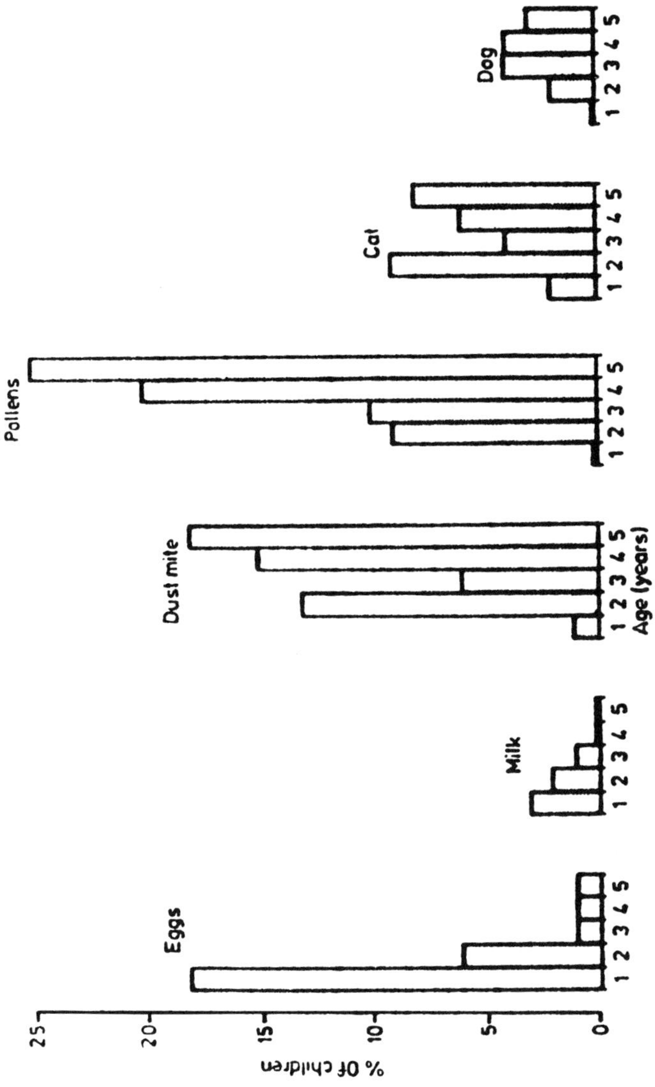

Figure 1 Percentage of children with positive results to skin tests for the six common allergens. (From Ref. 13).

The number of infants with positive skin tests or RAST tests under 1 year of age varies greatly among studies. Soothill et al. found a 48% prevalence of specific IgE reactivity in infants of atopic parent(s) (20), whereas Rowntree et al. showed that less than 10% had specific reactivity (16). The likelihood of skin test or RAST positivity is statistically higher under age 1 (versus nonatopic controls) in children with atopic dermatitis, recurrent wheezing, and immediate food reactions (12,14,21). In infancy there is no correlation between positive skin tests and persistent rhinitis, a single episode of wheezing, gastrointestinal symptoms, or delayed food reactions. In older children, skin test positivity occurs primarily to inhalants and is significantly associated with asthma and allergic rhinitis, but not other atopic conditions (5).

Infants and young children who have specific IgE reactivity to foods only, and not to inhalant allergens, are statistically more likely to develop atopic dermatitis by age 5 (12,13,16). In addition, they are more likely to outgrow their skin reactivity by age 5, although their clinical symptoms are likely to persist. Those who react to inhalants with or without food reactivity are significantly more likely to develop ongoing or recurrent respiratory symptoms by age 5. They are also much less likely to lose their skin test reactivity by this age.

In terms of reactivity to specific allergens, prospective studies of infants of atopic parent(s) have noted about a 15% cumulative prevalence of positive skin tests to egg at 1 year of age (12,14). Conversely, between 2 and 5% reacted to dust mites (12–14). Reactivity to animal proteins and pollens has been reported at this age, but is quite rare (22). By age 4–5, between 50 and 70% of infants who had been skin test-positive to foods become negative (12,13; Zeiger RS, personal communication). On the other hand, once a positive test develops to an inhalant, it is likely to persist for years, frequently into adulthood (8).

Specific reactivity to dust mites increases dramatically by age 2 and continues to rise through age 5 (see Figure 1). Between 15 and 20% of children with atopic parent(s) are skin test positive to dust mite by age 4 (13; Zeiger RS, personal communication). Animal reactivity, as manifested by positive skin tests to cat or dog, reaches a cumulative prevalence of 10% by age 4 in infants of atopic parents (Zeiger RS, personal communication). Pollen reactivity begins later, generally by age 3, probably owing to the more intermittent exposure to pollen than to other aeroallergens. By age 5, however, 25% of Cogswell's subjects reacted to grass, more than any other antigen tested (13). In the prospective study by Zeiger et al. (personal communication), 4-year cumulative prevalences for skin test reactivity to grass was 12% and to mold (*Alternaria* or *Cladosporium*) was 21%.

As childhood progresses into adulthood, the number of positive skin tests increases in individuals with atopic respiratory conditions, with some studies showing up to 88% skin reactivity to at least one inhalant (8,19). In older children and younger adults with clinically apparent allergic conditions and negative skin tests, skin test reactivity nearly always develops over the next few years if the condition persists (19). As in younger children, skin test positivity to inhalants, once present, tends to persist. At 8 years follow-up, Gerritsen found 94% of children initially studied at age 9 to have persistence of skin test reactivity to grass pollen, with 74% persistence of animal dander reactivity (8). All patients maintained reactivity to house dust mite at follow-up. This persisting reactivity to dust mites was also found in a study by Sporik et al. (9).

Risk Factors for the Development of Allergic Disease

The primary risk factors for the development of atopy in childhood are detailed in Chapters 18 and 19. The risk factors for the persistence of asthma, once present, are discussed at length later in this chapter. A summation of the risk factors for the development of asthma itself are shown in Table 1. The risk factors most related to the *development* of an atopic condition, as opposed to its ongoing *persistence* over time are the presence of an elevated IgE level, positive skin tests, or both. Although these are definite risk factors for the presence of asthma and other atopic conditions, they cannot predict the likelihood of their persistence in an individual patient.

Bronchial Hyperreactivity

A genetic predisposition toward allergy and airway hyperreactivity is the most important determinant for atopic asthma. This has been shown in numerous general population cohort studies (3,6), and is beyond the scope of this chapter. Prospective studies of newborn infants also show that an inherent bronchial hyperreactivity predisposes to subsequent lower respiratory infections with wheezing, as well as asthma. Martinez et al. studied pulmonary function (respiratory conductance measured by force oscillometry) in newborn infants and found that those who developed lower respiratory tract infections with wheezing had significantly lower pulmonary function shortly after birth (23). Those infants who measured in the lowest third for certain pulmonary function parameters were 10–16 times more likely to have a wheezing illness. Those with recurrent wheezing episodes in the first year of life had a sixfold risk of a low respiratory conductance value (23).

This risk may not persist, however, into later childhood unless certain environmental circumstances exist. Van Asperen found that the presence of wheezing in infancy was itself not a risk for the presence of bronchial hyperreactivity at age 7 (17). Only those with other atopic conditions or positive skin tests were at risk for later bronchial hyperreactivity. Once bronchial hyperreactivity is present in later childhood, however, the risk for its persistence into adulthood is high (24,25). Further work by Burrows et al. in a prospective evaluation of general population groups, confirmed that atopically predisposed individuals (as measured by serum IgE and skin-testing) are much more likely to manifest asthma in childhood and adulthood (26,27). In addition, only persons with elevated serum IgE had or went on to develop asthma (26,27). These studies, as well as numerous studies cited later, suggest that environmental factors play a critical role in allowing the atopic gene(s) to be expressed.

Inhalant Reactivity

Inhalant exposures, both allergic and nonallergic, in early childhood are definite risk factors for the development of asthma. Nonallergic inhalant exposures (i.e., cigarette smoke) are more likely to be a causative factor in children with or without a genetic tendency toward atopy, whereas allergenic factors, such as dust mite and other inhalant allergens, generally play a role primarily in those with an allergic family history.

Skin test positivity to house dust mites and high levels of exposure to these mites are definite risk factors for the development of asthma and allergic rhinitis in both children and adults (9,28–30). A negative atopic family history reduces, but does not eliminate, this risk.

Van Asperen et al. found six children in his prospective study to be skin test-positive to dust mites at 12 months of age (12). All of these children went on to develop asthma. Every child (119 between ages 6 and 14) with asthma referred to a university allergy clinic in the Netherlands was skin test-positive to dust mite (8).

Sporik et al., in a follow-up of Cogswell's original study group, found that those wheezing in the prior year or actively taking asthma medications at age 11 were significantly more likely to be skin test-positive to dust mites (9). Most of those taking regular bronchodilators were reactive to mites as early as age 2. Those who had wheezing before age 5, but not at age 11, were significantly less likely to be mite-sensitive. The relative risk of having asthma at age 11 if one was skin test-positive to mites approximated 20.

Similarly, Van Asperen et al. found that bronchial hyperreactivity (as measured by responsiveness to methacholine or histamine) was significantly higher in 5 and 7 year olds who were skin test-positive to dust mites and cats, but not to grass or selected foods (17).

Studies from France and China have correlated the degree of mite exposure with the presence of asthma and skin test reactivity to mite (28,29). When mite-infested blankets were introduced into a "mite-free area" in New Guinea, the incidence of adult asthma increased from 0.15 to 7.3% (30). All of those who developed asthma were skin test-positive to mites. General population cohort studies have shown a significantly increased likelihood of wheezing in children living in damp houses, an environment where mites (and molds) thrive (7,31).

Several studies have estimated the actual level of dust mite exposure needed to develop clinical sensitivity. Korsgaard (32) and Lau et al. (33) found that the critical level of exposure for the development of mite sensitization was above 2 μg of the major mite antigen (Der p I) per gram of house dust (about 100 mites per gram). There was a statistically significant correlation between exposures above this level and RAST values to mite, as well as the presence of clinical symptomatology. Eighty-six percent of those exposed to more than 10 μg/g showed positive histamine release from leukocytes, as opposed to 17% of those exposed to less than 0.4 μg/g (33).

Correlating the level of mite exposure in infancy (mite levels determined at 1–2 years of age in bedding and carpet) to the presence of asthma at age 11, Sporik et al. noted that all but 1 of the 17 children with persistent wheezing at age 11 were exposed to levels of more than 10 μg/g of mite (9). In addition, there was a significant relation between the level of exposure at age 1 and the first episode of wheezing. No child exposed to less than 2 μg/g Der p I of dust had symptoms of asthma, and none were skin test or RAST test-positive to mites at age 11.

Although not studied in such detail, early exposure to high levels of any inhalant antigen is likely to be a risk factor for the development of atopic respiratory conditions. This has been shown in retrospective studies of exposure to furry mammals, particularly cats, and to house dampness (molds) in early childhood (7,12,31,34,35). The month of an individual's birth, implying increased pollen or other aeroallergen exposure, in conjunction with a familial tendency, also appears to be a risk factor for the development of allergic disease (36,37). Prospective studies now in progress similarly suggest that exposure to cats and cockroaches increases the likelihood of allergic rhinitis or asthma (38). All of this data signify the importance of early environmental intervention, particularly in those with allergic family histories, in the ultimate prevention or minimization of allergic disease.

Irritants

In addition to the risk of early exposure to aeroallergens, early exposure to aerosolized irritants is a risk factor for the development of ongoing respiratory conditions. These irritants could (a) damage mucosal surfaces or lung tissue itself, or (b) facilitate penetration of foreign substances, predisposing an individual to allergic sensitization. Children exposed to high levels of air pollution are more likely to have allergic rhinitis and asthma (7,39,40). Andrae et al. found an increased prevalence of both conditions in children living in close proximity to a pulp plant in Sweden (7). More specifically, high levels of early exposure to air pollutants (sulfur dioxide, ozone) has been shown to enhance allergic sensitization through respiratory mucosal tissue (41–43).

Passive Smoke

Parental smoking is an obvious factor resulting in both upper and lower airway disease in children. Although some initial retrospective studies showed only a marginal relation between parental smoking and childhood wheezing or asthma (44–47), later well-controlled, prospective studies have undeniably shown a causative relation (40,48–51). This risk is higher when the mother smokes, indicating a probable dose-related risk of smoke, since children usually spend more time with their mothers than with their fathers (52–54). Weitzman et al., in studying data from the Child Health Supplement to the 1981 National Health Survey, found an odds ratio of 2.6 for the presence of asthma (recurrent wheezing episodes) in the first year of life if a mother smoked over one-half pack of cigarettes a day (55). The odds ratio was 2.1 for acquiring asthma by age 5 and 4.7 for the use of chronic asthma medications at age 5 if the mother smoked. Similarly, Cogswell et al. found that the cumulative prevalence of wheezing by age 5 (independent of serum IgE levels) reached 62% with smoking versus 37% with nonsmoking parents (13). Neuspiel et al. further demonstrated that this statistical association persisted to at least age 10 in a prospective national cohort study in England (31). Britten et al., in a multidecade general population cohort study in Great Britain, suggested that this risk persists at least into the mid-30s age range (39).

Studies examining pulmonary function in children (independent of respiratory symptoms) have also shown a detrimental effect of parental smoking, which potentially may impinge on later respiratory function (47,48,51,52,57,58).

Some studies have demonstrated that this increased risk of asthma from passive parental smoke may not be restricted to postnatal exposure. Collins et al. found that fetal rats showed lung hypoplasia with decreased number of alveoli when exposed to tobacco smoke (59). Infants of smoking mothers with no personal or family history of atopy have shown elevated levels of cord IgE and increased development of asthma and other atopic conditions (60). Confirming studies are needed before these findings can be accepted.

Multiple Risk Factors

Many of the risk factors listed in Table 1 are cumulative. Peat et al. found a sixfold risk of moderate or severe bronchial hyperreactivity if a subject had a history of respiratory infection in infancy, a parent with asthma, and positive skin tests (5). There was a twofold risk if the skin test positivity occurred with either early respiratory infection or positive family history. Smoking also appears to be synergistic with other factors in increasing the risk for the development of asthma (44,61). The most notable of these appears to be concurrent atopy, particularly atopic dermatitis (62).

ASTHMA

Retrospective Studies

Numerous retrospective studies have examined the outcome of childhood asthma over various time periods (1). Those studies published since 1960 with a minimum of 10-year follow-up are listed in Table 2 (63–69). These studies cannot be directly compared because of their differing definitions of asthma, its severity, and length of follow-up. Nevertheless, examinations of these studies generally reveal consistent patterns. Roughly one-half of those children with asthma had some degree of respiratory symptoms at follow-up, even after three decades. Approximately one-half of these patients had periodic, mild symptoms; the other half had more severe and persistent symptoms. Jonsson et al. studied a more severe population of hospitalized asthmatics at onset (69). Nevertheless, the outcome was similar, with 45% evidencing persistence (13% severe) 22–32 years later. At 20-years follow-up, Buffum and Settipane found a 5% persistence of severe symptoms in those presenting in childhood with "severe, debilitating" asthma (67). Hence, most of those patients with symptoms at follow-up did experience an overall improvement in their condition, as will be demonstrated again when the prospective studies are discussed.

Two of these retrospective studies have examined asthmatic children at 10- and 20-year intervals, with contradictory findings. Buffum found that the percentage of those with ongoing symptoms decreased from 57% at 10 years to 37% at 20 years (67). Blair looked at the same

Table 2 The Natural History of Asthma: Retrospective Studies

Author (Ref)	N	Age at onset (yr)	Follow-up (yr)	No symptoms at follow-up (%)	Ongoing symptoms at follow-up (%)				Recur (%)
					Mild	Persistent	Severe	Total	
Ryssing and Flensbong (63)	442	Under 15	NS	37	9	54		63	
Buffum (64)	51	NS	10–16	55				45	
Barr and Logan (65)	336	Under 14	17–27	50				48	
Whatley and Guerrant (66)	115	Under 16	15 (median)	53	25	21		46	
Buffum and Settipane (67)	518	"Child"	10	41			6	57	
	136	"Child"	20	55			5	37	
Blair (68)	244	Under 12	10	35	25	37		65	3
	244	Under 12	20	28	24	21		72	27
Jonsson et al. (69)	123	Under 15	22–32	55[a]	27	5	13	45	

NS, not stated

[a]These patients had been symptom-free for a mean of 17 years.

individuals at 10 years and then again at 20 years after the onset of asthma and found more patients symptomatic at 20 years than at 10 years, indicating a marked number (27%) with recurrence of asthma after prolonged symptom-free intervals (68). The mean age of "remission" was 10 years, with the average age of recurrence being 19. This finding of symptomatic recurrence has been demonstrated not only in the prospective studies of asthma, but also in long-term observations of most other atopic conditions.

Prospective studies

The prospective studies examining the long-term course of asthma have shorter follow-up periods than do the retrospective ones. On initial inspection, the results of the prospective studies appear to vary greatly (Table 3) (4,8,21,70–75). Once again, however, the populations studied, methods of evaluation, and definitions of asthma vary markedly among studies. For example, some studies (4,73,74) included any individual who ever wheezed, whereas Johnstone's study included only children with ongoing symptoms at the study onset (75). Consequently, the former studies had fewer patients with persistent symptoms at follow-up than did Johnstone's (75).

Various methods of population selection were used by different authors. Some followed selected symptomatic patients (21,75), others followed randomized cohorts (71,72), and others followed entire population cohorts (4,74). Johnstone followed 63 asthmatic children under age 16 with over three-fourths symptomatic at follow-up (4–14 years) (75). These patients were followed by an allergy specialist, and symptoms were frequent or severe enough to warrant immunotherapy. This preselection bias for increased disease severity as well as the shorter length of follow-up probably explains the higher percentage of patients with persistence compared with other studies.

Foucard and Sjoberg, on the other hand, studied a much younger population (mean age of onset 10 months) 12 years after presentation with wheezy bronchitis (21). Because of the young age, many of these patients were presenting for the first time when studied and likely had an infectious cause for their respiratory symptoms. The low percentage of persistent wheezing at follow-up probably reflects the likelihood that many of these individuals may not have had associated atopy and that their presentations may have been isolated infections.

Giles et al. prospectively followed a birth cohort of children born in a single year in Tasmania in 1961 (74). Questionnaire surveys directed toward respiratory symptoms of wheezing and cough were ini-

Table 3 The Natural History of Asthma: Prospective Studies

Author (Ref)	N	Age 1st studied (yr)	Age at follow-up (yr)	Follow-up (yr)	No symptoms at follow-up (%)	Ongoing symptoms at follow-up (%)	Wheeze (%) Rare	Wheeze (%) Occasional	Wheeze (%) Frequent	Symptoms recur (%)
Gerritsen et al. (8)	119	6–14	22–31	14–20	57	43				
Friberg et al. (70)	20	10.6 (median)	24.9 (median)	14	0	100		75	25	
Anderson et al. (18)										
Severe symptoms at age 7	1608	7[a]	11	4	36	64 (17% severe)				
		7[a]	16	9	64	36 (4% severe)				
All patients		7[a]	11	4	72	28				
		7[a]	16	9	84	16				
Strachan et al.[b] (73)		7[a]	23	11	80	20				
Martin et al. (71)	331	7[a]	14,21	7,14	34	66	21	27	23	45[d]
Kelly et al.[c] (72)	293	7[a]	28	21	32	68[f]	20	22	26	27[e]
Foucard and Sjoborg (21)	81	10 mo (median)	12–17	12	72	28[g]				
Giles et al. (74)	218	7	13,20	6,13	78	22				
Johnstone (75)	63	NS	16	4–14	22	78	8	51	19	

NS, not stated.
[a]These patients had a history of wheezing at or before age 7.
[b]Continued study of Anderson's population.
[c]Continued study of Martin's population.
[d]Symptoms recurred between ages 14–21.
[e]Symptoms recurred between ages 21–28.
[f]Of these, 24% improved, 26% worsened, 50% did not change their condition between ages 21 and 28.
[g]All but one patient with ongoing symptoms improved clinically.

tially sent to all families at age 7, with follow-up of stratified random samples at ages 13 and 20. Only 22% of those wheezing at age 7 experienced wheezing at age 20. Any child with a history of "wheezy breathing" was included at age 7. Hence, numerous patients with single episodes of vague symptomatology and etiology were included. These subjects would be expected to be less likely to wheeze at follow-up, which probably explains the low number of patients with persistent symptoms at age 20.

Anderson and Strachan similarly followed a randomized cohort of 10,557 individuals born in a single week in Britain in 1958 (4,73). Families were sent questionnaires asking if their child "ever had attacks of breathing with wheezing." Follow-up at ages 11, 16, and 23 was performed by questionnaire or interview, with numerous other health and social items also included in the survey. The low prevalence of symptoms at follow-up again probably reflects the liberal inclusiveness of the original survey. When children in this study with more frequent wheezing were evaluated, nearly two-thirds had wheezing at age 11, and approximately one-third had wheezing at age 16. Nevertheless, as most other studies show, nearly all patients demonstrated improvement in their condition, as gauged by frequency of symptoms. This was particularly apparent by age 23, when only 10% of those who had wheezed at or before age 7 had clinical symptoms in the prior year (73).

As noted, all prospective studies show that, even when asthma symptoms persist, they usually improve after prolonged follow-up intervals. This holds true even for those with more severe asthma. Friberg et al. studied 20 males in early adolescence and then again in their mid-20s (70). When initially studied, all had been persistently symptomatic from under 5 years of age, and 60% had been on a long-term systemic corticosteroid regimen. That this was a markedly more severe group than the other studies probably explains the 100% persistence after the 14-year follow-up interval. Despite this persistence, however, only 20% continued to use bronchodilators regularly, and no individual required regular systemic corticosteroids after the age of 12.

The most thorough and well-performed of the prospective studies took place through Royal Children's Hospital in Melbourne (71,72). Randomly selected asthmatics from single-aged cohorts and controls were studied at age 7, 14, 21, and 28. Follow-up included questionnaires, interviews, physical examinations, and pulmonary function testing. At follow-up, the patients were classified into four general categories: (1) no episode of wheezing within the prior 3 years of review; (2) no episodes within 3 months, but within 3 years; (3) an episode within 3 months, but neither very frequent nor persistent symptoms;

(4) very frequent or persistent symptoms over the prior year. The myriad of statistics at the three follow-up periods can be summarized numerous ways. Overall, approximately two-thirds of all patients who had wheezed at or before age 7 had some history of wheezing within 3 years of follow-up at ages 21 and 28. Twenty percent of these individuals with persistent symptoms fell into category 2, and approximately one-quarter fit into category 3. In other words, although these patients had persistent symptoms, they were either infrequent or generally mild. Another quarter of the patients had frequent symptoms (more than once per week). Further categorization of prognosis based on severity (frequency) of wheezing is discussed later under the risk factors.

Of particular note in the Martin and Kelly group (71,72) is the high frequency of recurrence after prolonged symptom-free intervals, similar to the findings of Blair (68). Of those wheezing at age 7, but not at 14 or 21, 27% recurred by age 28. For those wheezing at 7 and 14, but not at 21, 31% recurred by age 28 (71,72).

Gerritsen et al., in a study of 119 children referred to a university allergy department in the Netherlands, found similar percentages of symptomatic persistence (8). After an average of 16 years follow-up, 43% of those clinically similar to Martin and Kelly's foregoing categories 3 and 4 had symptomatic asthma. An interesting side finding was that the average age of symptomatic disappearance occurred at age 15, somewhat later than age 10 found by Blair (68).

The only abnormal physical finding at any age in Martin's and Kelly's studies was an increased prevalence of barrel chest noted at age 14 in the most severe group (71,72). This was not seen at age 21 or 28. There was no alteration of growth in any group at any age. Friberg and associate's more severe, smaller population sample also had several individuals with barrel chest (and reduced height) when initially studied, but this had resolved by follow-up in their mid-20s (70).

Selected patients and controls in Martin and Kelly's study received full pulmonary function testing at age 21 and spirometry at age 28 (72,76). Decrements in pulmonary function were proportional to the severity class at both ages. At age 21, those in categories 3 and 4, and at age 28, those in categories 2 through 4 showed significant abnormalities in most pulmonary function values compared with control groups. Those in category 2 showed evidence of small-airway obstruction with significantly diminished (forced expiratory flow, midexpiratory phase) FEF_{25-75}. Although those in category 1 statistically had normal results of their pulmonary function tests, more than 10% still showed evidence of small-airway obstruction. Fifty-nine percent of this group (no wheezing for at least 3 years) still showed abnormal reactivity to histamine challenge, indicating exaggerated bronchial reactivity, despite the absence of symptoms. This suggests that the potential for symptom recurrence is high, particularly under the proper environmental circumstances. Other retrospective studies in asymptomatic young and middle-aged adults with a prior history of asthma similarly reveal mild abnormalities of pulmonary function (2,77,78). The clinical significance of these abnormalities and their possible relation is unknown.

Giles et al. also prospectively examined pulmonary function tests (74), and, similar to Martin and Kelly, found lower pulmonary function in those with persistent wheezing. In addition, nonwheezers with abnormal pulmonary function tests at age 7 were significantly more likely to wheeze at age 13. Although Friberg's small group evidenced marked symptomatic improvement, significant reductions in all expiratory flow rates persisted compared with healthy adults ($p < 0.001$) (70).

Risk Factors

Severity and Frequency

All studies examining the natural history of asthma have found persistence to correlate directly with the severity of the asthma. Most studies used frequency of symptoms as the indicator of severity, since it is an easy parameter to follow by questionnaire or interview in large studies. Severity based on morbidity, as represented by frequency of asthma hospitalizations, is a risk factor (69,70). In addition, prospective studies that followed asthmatics referred to allergy–asthma centers (where asthma severity is more likely to be greater) showed higher frequencies of asthma persistence than did general population cohort studies. The risk of asthma persistence from childhood and adolescence into early adulthood is best summarized by collation of Martin and Kelly's data (Table 4) (71,72). In individuals with occasional wheezing at age 14, one-fourth will actually have more frequent symptoms at age 21 and one-third at age 28. In individuals with frequent or persistent symptoms at age 14, two-thirds will still have frequent symptoms at age 28, and only 2% will be symptom-free. These numbers can give the clinician a good idea of the likelihood of asthma persistence in a patient, based on the current severity (frequency) of wheezing.

Other Atopy

With the exception of urticaria, the presence of other atopic disease, particularly if persistent, has been shown by numerous authors to increase the likelihood of asthma persistence (Table 5) (4,21,63,65–68,69,72,74,75,79). Giles et al. estimated a fourfold risk of asthma persistence at age 20 if atopic dermatitis or allergic rhinitis was present

Table 4 The Risk of Future Wheezing in All Patients Studied (A) and Based on Asthma Severity (B)

	Age 21(%)	Age 28(%)
A. If wheezing is present before age 14, will it be at 21? at 28?		
None	34	32
Rare	21	20
Occasional	27	22
Frequent	23	26
B. If wheezing is not or rarely present at age 14, will it be at 21? at 28?		
None	55	54
Rare	25	19
Occasional	16	20
Frequent	3	7
If occasional wheezing is present at 14, will it be at 21? at 28?		
None	20	16
Rare	20	22
Occasional	35	30
Frequent	25	32
If frequent or persistent wheezing is present at 14, will it be at 21? at 28?		
None	4	2
Rare	14	19
Occasional	7	11
Frequent	55	68

Source: Collated from Refs. 71 and 72.

(74). In the prospective cohort studies of Anderson et al., several statistical correlations predicting the risk of asthma from ages 7 to 16 were found (4,18). Most notable was the 15-fold greater likelihood of wheezing at age 16 in children with both allergic rhinitis and atopic dermatitis at age 7, compared with those without these disorders (4). Johnstone found that all the asthmatics with concurrent allergic rhinitis had persistent asthma at follow-up (75).

The presence of atopic dermatitis with wheezing appears to be one of the most predictive of all risk factors for persistent asthma (75). Two studies (62,69) found a profound risk of asthma persistence when an individual presented with asthma and atopic dermatitis, but not with other atopic conditions. In contrast with this data and the results of many additional studies (4,21,63,65–68,72,74,75,79,80), the presence of other atopic conditions was not related to asthma persistence in 119 asthmatic children originally aged 6–14 when skin tested in a

Table 5 Persistent Asthma: Association with Other Atopic Disease

Author (Ref)	Allergic rhinitis (AR)	Atopic dermatitis (AD)	AR and AD	Food allergy	Eosinophilia	Elevated IgE	Positive skin test
Anderson et al. (4)	+[a](5–7×)	+[a]	+[a](15×)				
Barr and Logan (65)		+	+				
Blair (68)	+		+[a]				–
Buffum and Settipaine (67)		+		+			Egg +, other –
Foucard and Sjoberg (21)	+	+				–[b]	Cat, pollen +, other –
Geller-Bernstein et al. (79)						–[b]	
Gerritsen et al. (8)	–	–			–	–[b]	–[b]
Giles et al. (74)	+ (4×)	+ (4×)					
Johnstone (75)	+[d]	–					Grass +, other –
Jonsson et al. (69)	–	+					
Kelly et al. (72,80)	+	+[e]			+	+[c]	
Kjellman and Dalen (20)						–[a]	–[a]
Murray and Morrison (62)	+	+					
Ryssing and Flemsborg (63)	+						Mold +, other –
Sporik et al. (9)							Dust mite +
Whatley and Guerrant (66)							–

+ Indicates statistically significant association of this condition or test with persistent asthma.
– Indicates no statistically significant association of this condition or test with persistent asthma.
[a]Significant only if condition present at follow-up.
[b]Indicates predictive of the presence of asthma, but not of asthma persistence.
[c]These associations were made in young adult asthmatics followed into later adulthood.
[d]All subjects with asthma before or concurrent with AR had persistence.
[e]Only the most severe asthmatics had associated AD.

university asthma clinic who evidenced a 57% remission rate of re-evaluation 14–20 years later (8).

Clinical Markers of Atopy

An elevated IgE and multiple positive skin tests are definite predictors of general allergic disease or the risk of developing asthma itself, but numerous studies in asthmatics and other atopic conditions have consistently shown that these laboratory measurements are not statistically predictive of persistence in any person (8,17,21,68,79). However, a recent study showed that the number of positive skin tests, the degree of IgE elevation, and the degree of eosinophilia in adolescence were predictive of asthma severity into adulthood (80). These disparate findings may indicate that at ages beyond early childhood, these specific and nonspecific markers of allergic disease may be better at predicting outcome than in younger-aged groups.

On the other hand, specific skin test reactivity to dust mite does appear to be a risk factor for the persistence of asthma into later childhood, but the risk into adulthood is unclear. Specifically, infants and children under age 5 with wheezing were more likely to have persistent asthma at follow-up in later childhood if they were skin test reactive to dust or dust mite (17). In addition, children demonstrating skin test reactivity to mite after an episode of bronchiolitis evidenced a greater incidence of asthma symptoms at follow-up (81). However, Gerritsen et al. found that, although skin test reactivity to dust mite almost invariably persisted up to 30 years of age, most patients at that time no longer experienced asthma symptoms (8).

Skin test reactivity to other antigens may also be predictive of future wheezing. As shown in Table 5, however, skin reactivity as a predictor of asthma persistence is generally inconsistent. Retrospectively, although several studies have shown that those adults showing skin test positivity to inhalants were more likely to have had asthma as a child (8,80), others could not confirm these findings (26).

In Gerritsen's study of childhood asthmatics followed after 10 years, numerous statistical trends were found in relation to the presence of asthma and persistence of skin test positivity, but none of the clinical variables studied initially proved to be predictive of asthma prognosis (8). Those who had asthma symptoms at follow-up showed no significant differences in the number of positive skin tests, skin test reactivity to specific antigens (animal dander, dust, pollen, mold), total IgE, or eosinophilia from those who were symptom-free. Kjellman, following 58 children admitted for asthma (average age 9) over 8 subsequent years

(19), similarly found skin test reactivity increased with age, but its presence was not predictive of asthma symptoms at follow-up.

Heredity

Several studies have shown that a history of atopy or asthma in family members, particularly first-degree relatives, places an individual at higher risk for asthma persistence (21,63,68). Ryssing found that 67% of those with a "familial predisposition" were symptomatic at follow-up versus 58% without a family history (63). Blair found that 73% of those asthmatics having a first-degree relative with an atopic condition had chronic or recurrent asthma at follow-up (68). This compares with only 27% of those who were symptom-free at the end of the study.

Sex

Although the prevalence of asthma is higher in males, the rate of persistence into early adulthood appear to be higher in females. Kelly's follow-up data at age 28, however, suggest that this trend may not continue into later adulthood (72).

Respiratory Infection

Retrospective studies in adults generally show an association of chronic obstructive pulmonary disease (COPD) with a history of childhood respiratory disease (2,82). These studies have numerous methodological flaws, however, particularly for recall bias or lack of control populations.

The role of bronchiolitis in infancy as a risk factor for the development of persistent wheezing is discussed in depth later in this chapter. Several studies have noted an association between recurrent upper respiratory illnesses or croup in childhood and wheezing persistence or abnormal pulmonary functions studies later in childhood (2,4,83).

Age of Onset

Numerous studies show no correlation between age of onset of wheezing and the persistence of symptoms into later childhood and adulthood (4,65,67,68,75). Some studies have shown that children with the onset of symptoms later in childhood are at a higher risk for ongoing symptoms than are those with onset in the first 2 years of life (21,25), whereas others have found the opposite (69).

Asthma Therapy

Undertreatment of asthma also appears to be a risk factor for the continuation of reactive airway disease into adulthood (25,63). In addition, undertreatment has been suggested to lead to various degrees of fixed airway obstruction. The influx of inflammatory cells, particularly in the late-phase reaction of an asthma attack, has been hypothesized to result, over time, in some irreversible damage to the airways. Burrows found that patients with a chronic history of undertreated bronchospasm had a greater decline of 1-sec forced expiratory volume (FEV_1) with age than did asthmatics under good control (77).

Immunotherapy appeared to have little effect on asthma persistence in the few studies in which it has been addressed. Only Johnstone's study found that immunotherapy improved asthma outcome (84). He found that over a 4- to 14-year duration, 72% of those asthmatic children receiving allergen immunotherapy were symptom-free by age 16, as opposed to only 22% of placebo-treated controls. This study had a 40% dropout rate, however, suggesting that a high proportion of individuals were likely to have had an improvement in their symptoms and did not require further therapy or follow-up. The very low rate of improvement or remission in the placebo group is inconsistent with nearly all of the studies discussed earlier. The 72% improvement in the treated group, however, corresponds to the trends in the other studies in which immunotherapy was not considered.

Other epidemiological studies evaluating immunotherapy have found no effect on asthma outcome. In Rackemann and Edwards' landmark 20-year follow-up study of 449 childhood asthmatics, no difference was found in the 19 patients who received allergen immunotherapy (85). Kraepelien followed 100 asthmatic children receiving immunotherapy for 8–10 years (86). Only 12% were symptom-free and 55% were considerably improved, consistent with the outcome of other follow-up studies in which immunotherapy was not evaluated.

More recently, Jonsson's prospective study of previously hospitalized asthmatic children over two to three decades found no difference in outcome between those who had received immunotherapy and those who did not (69). In fact, 68% (38/56) of those not receiving immunotherapy were symptom-free at follow-up, as compared with 43% (26/61) of those who had been treated in this manner. This difference was not statistically different, but does indicate a trend toward treatment with immunotherapy in those asthmatics with more severe disease.

Johnstone suggested from his studies that specific immunotherapy for allergic rhinitis may prevent the ultimate development as asthma (75,84). This was based on the eventual development of asthma in 50% of children with allergic rhinitis who were in the placebo group in an immunotherapy study. There were only 22 subjects in this group, however. Furthermore, this observation has never been confirmed and is strongly tempered by many of the studies cited earlier, in which the onset of asthma occurs before or coincident with rhinitis (12,14,69,85). Hence, based on the availability of current data, there is no indication for initiating immunotherapy to prevent the onset of asthma or to alter its natural history.

Allergen Exposure

Ongoing exposure to inhalant allergens in sensitized individuals increases the likelihood of asthma persistence. This was shown most clearly in Sporik's prospective study of children to age 11, in whom levels of mite exposure correlated with not only the presence of asthma, but also its persistence (9). Long-term studies on environmental control avoidance measures are required to determine whether such measures affect asthma persistence. Although Johnstone found that the degree of dust-proofing appeared not to affect asthma outcome (75), more recent studies confirm the real benefit of dust mite avoidance on reducing bronchial hyperreactivity (87). Retrospective data also suggest that ongoing small-mammal exposure, and possibly pollen exposure, similarly increase the likelihood of persistent symptoms (34,36,69).

Smoking

Although parental or patient smoking is a risk factor for the prevalence of respiratory symptoms and diminished pulmonary function status, no definitive study has implicated smoking as a risk factor for the persistence of wheezing (4,21). In fact, some studies show no increased rate of wheezing in those patients who take up smoking in late adolescence (4,74). On the other hand, retrospective studies in adults with COPD (including asthma) have generally found a relation between smoking and asthma persistence or recurrence (2,77). As reviewed earlier, however, numerous studies have revealed a higher prevalence of respiratory illness as well as abnormal pulmonary function testing in children of smokers.

Breast-feeding

Studies conflict on the effect of breast-feeding on asthma persistence. While Geller-Bernstein (79) and Blair (68) found that breast-fed infants were statistically less likely to wheeze in late childhood and adolescence, other studies failed to show this association (4).

Miscellaneous Risk and Associated Factors

Children raised in northern England (an industrial area) were found to have a higher rate of asthma persistence than those in other locations. Those exposed to higher levels of air pollution were at higher risk for symptoms at age 15, but not at 20 or 25 (39). A history of pneumonia or whooping cough before age 7 was a risk factor for wheezing at age 16, but not at 23 (4). Similar to the possible risk of parental smoking, these findings show that the risk of early childhood exposure to irritants or infectious agents may initially result in symptomatic persistence, but that by early adulthood these symptoms resolve. Any subclinical effect on pulmonary status, or the ultimate effect on possible respiratory status in later adulthood, however, has not been evaluated. Young maternal age (15,17–18) and a history of recurrent abdominal symptoms were also found to be risk factors for ongoing symptoms (18).

A summary of the risk factors predictive of asthma persistence are listed in Table 6. In addition, factors that were and were not associated with (but not predictive of) persistent asthma are also listed. Britten found that the social class of an individual and the number of occupants of a child's bedroom were associated with ongoing symptoms, whereas Anderson did not (18,39).

Relation Between Bronchiolitis and Subsequent Wheezing or Asthma

Bronchiolitis is a viral infection of the lower respiratory tract occurring most commonly under 2 years of age. It is invariably associated with some degree of airway obstruction, although there is a wide spectrum of clinical severity. Numerous studies, both retrospective and prospective, have been performed evaluating the persistence of both clinical airway symptoms as well as the presence of functional airway abnormalities (Table 7) (79,81,89–95). However, difficulties are encountered in comparing these studies because of marked differences between them in (a) the time interval until follow-up evaluation, (b) the age of onset of the initial illness and its severity [varying from those severely affected and hospitalized in early infancy (89), to those younger than 2 years of age treated as outpatients for wheezing with respiratory infection (93)], and (c) the criteria established to determine persistent symptomatology. Nevertheless, consistent patterns occur, providing the practitioner with data to assess the risk and risk factors for the development of asthma after lower respiratory tract infection early in life.

Table 7 lists these studies in order of duration of follow-up. In general, the longer the duration of follow-up, the more likely it is that clinical symptoms of airway obstruction (wheeze, cough) will improve (91,94,95). Pullan retrospectively found that 38% of young infants with bronchiolitis experienced wheezing in the subsequent 4 years, but that by 10 years after the index illness, only 22% had recent wheezing (95).

Table 6 Factors Predictive of and Associated with Persistent Asthma

Definitely predictive[a]
Severity/frequency of symptoms
Concurrent allergic rhinitis
Family history of asthma in first-degree relative
Lower respiratory infection in infancy
Probably predictive[b]
Concurrent atopic dermatitis
Parental smoking
Overcrowded housing conditions in childhood
History of pneumonia with asthma
Possibly predictive[c]
Air pollution exposure as child
Undertreatment
Food allergy
Young maternal age
History of recurrent abdominal symptoms in early childhood
Erratically predictive[d]
Female sex
Smoking as adolescent/young adult
Lower social class
Absence of breast-feeding
Not predictive
Total IgE
Skin test reactivity
Eosinophilia
Onset age
Pneumonia without asthma before age 7
History of urticaria
No association with persistence
Birth weight/gestational age
Parental occupation
Birth order
History of measles
Presence of single parent

[a]Multiple studies show statistical significance.
[b]Multiple studies show statistical significance, occasional studies do not; *or* a limited number of studies show statistical significance.
[c]A majority of studies show statistical significance; *or* a single study shows statistical significance.
[d]Some studies show statistical significance, but many others do not.

Table 7 Bronchiolitis/Lower Respiratory Tract Infection Follow-up Studies

Author (Ref) Year	Study type	N	Onset age	F/U Time	Symptomatic at follow-up	Abnormal PFTs
Stokes et al. (88)	Retro No control	18	1½–5 mo	12–15 mo	67% (ongoing wheeze)	1. 40% increased thoracic gas volume 2. 75% abnormal airway resistance and/or conductance
Geller-Bernstein et al. (79)	Prosp No cont In + Outpt	80	6–24 mo(avg 13 mo)	4 yr (q6mo)	32% (ongoing wheeze in prior year)	
Welliver et al. (89)	Prosp No cont	38	Under 6 mo	4 yr	53% ever wheeze 32% over 3 episodes	
Sly and Hibbert (90)	Prosp No cont	48	½–10 mo (avg 3 mo)	5 yr (qlyr)	71% "asthmatic" 17% on daily meds 92% had further episodes	1. 3% FEV_1 <80% predicted 2. 30% FEV_1/EVC <80% 3. 60% + histamine challenge
Mok and Simpson (91)	Prosp Cont Outpt	200	Infancy	7 yr	60% symptomatic (47% wheeze, 36% cough)	1. If + sx, all flow studies within 80% predicted, but still significantly reduced v controls 2. If no sx, only FEV/FVC reduced vs controls 3. 38% + exercise challenge
McConnochie and Roghmann (92)	Retro Cont In + Outpt	77	Under 25 mo	7.7 yr	44% regularly wheeze in last 2 yr (13% control)	

					55% wheeze with colds (25% control) 18% on routine meds for asthma (4% cont) 22% wheeze with exercise (7% cont)	
Sims et al. (81)	Retro Cont	26	Under 12 mo	8 yr	56% (ongoing wheeze)	
Duiverman et al. (93)	Retro Cont	16	1–18 mo	2.5–12.8 yr (avg 8)	62% recurrent resp sx; 12% after age 6	1. If no sx, airway caliber (by force oscillometry) and histamine challenge normal 2. If + sx, 70% abnormal smooth-muscle tone and + histamine challenge
Pullan and Hey (94)	Retro Cont	130	Under 1 yr (avg 14 wk)	10 yr	42% ever wheeze (19% control) 38% in 1st 4 yr (15% control) 22% in last 2 yr (13% cont) 5% on beta-agonist No diff vs cont	1. 16% $FEV_1/FVC < 72\%$ (1.8% control) 2. 10% $FEV_1/FVC < 72\%$ with no further wheeze 3. 16% + exercise challenge (5% cont) 19% + histamine challenge (6% cont) 25% + exercise and/or histamine challenge (6% control) 4. All had normal nitrogen washout studies

F/U, follow-up interval; Retro, retrospective study; Inpt, inpatient study; sx, symptoms; Cont, controlled study or control group; PFT, pulmonary function studies; Prosp, prospective study; outpt, outpatient study; +, positive.

Duiverman retrospectively showed that 62% of infants had some degree of wheezing at follow-up, but only 12% remained symptomatic after age 6 (94).

Most prospective studies show higher rates of symptomatic persistence than do retrospective ones, probably indicating a recall bias, particularly when follow-up was by parental interview only. Milder symptoms of wheezing during infancy generally led to a lower incidence of persistence (32%) at follow-up (79). In contrast, when the index bronchiolitis episodes were more severe (requiring hospitalization), generally higher incidences of symptomatic persistence occurred, indicating that those with a specific diagnosis of bronchiolitis are more likely to having ongoing symptoms (81,89). Moreover, a study which included only infants with documented respiratory syncytial virus (RSV) disease demonstrated higher rates of persistence than any other study (91). In this latter study, 92% of infants had subsequent wheezing episodes and 71% had "symptoms suggestive" of asthma (by parental questionnaire) at 5 year follow-up, 42% of which had physician-diagnosed asthma (91).

Studies that include either general pediatric population control groups or control groups of pediatric asthmatic patients (92–95), have shown a significant increase in the likelihood of both clinical symptomatology and functional airway abnormalities in those children with bronchiolitis in infancy, when compared with age-matched controls. McConnochie et al. found that 44% of those infants who had bronchiolitis experienced wheezing in the 2 years before follow-up at 7.7 years, as opposed to 13.6% in a private practice pediatric population ($p < 0.0001$) (93). Of these, 18.6% had "current asthma" versus 4% of the control group ($p < 0.001$). Other patterns of recurrent lower respiratory symptoms, such as wheezing with exercise, also showed strong statistical significance in index cases versus controls (see Table 7). Although most studies found similar trends for lower airway symptomatology, Pullan found no difference at 10-year follow-up between index cases and controls for those children who required regular bronchodilator therapy (95).

A review of those studies evaluating pulmonary function show approximately a threefold risk of abnormal pulmonary function tests (PFTs) or increased bronchial reactivity following bronchiolitis. Abnormalities in airway resistance or specific conductance were found in 75% of infants 15 months after bronchiolitis (89), whereas 30% evidenced FEV_1/forced vital capacity (FVC) less than 80% 5 years post-bronchiolitis (91). Longer intervals of follow-up have found that pulmonary flow rates tend to eventually normalize to within normal limits (higher than 80% predicted) following bronchiolitis (92,94,95). Nevertheless, when compared with control groups, these values are still significantly reduced (96). Pullan found that 16% of the total index cases had FEV_1/FVC of less than 72% predicted, as opposed to only 1.9% of controls ($p < 0.005$) (95). Ten percent of infants with bronchiolitis but no subsequent wheezing for 12 years after the initial illness had FEV_1/FVC of less than 72%, as opposed to none of the 84 control patients without a history of wheezing.

Bronchial hyperreactivity occurred more often in ex-bronchiolitics than in controls. At 5 years follow-up, 60% had a positive bronchial histamine challenge (91), compared with 19% after 10 years (95); however, even this lower incidence was six times more frequent than in controls (95). Duiverman found 70% of those with symptoms at follow-up had abnormal smooth-muscle tone as measured by forced oscillometry (94), whereas those without symptoms were normal (94). All patients studied by Pullan had normal nitrogen washout studies, indicating the absence of persisting ventilatory abnormalities years after the bronchiolitis episode (95).

A summary of the associated risk factors for the persistence of wheezing following bronchiolitis is shown in Table 8. Those studies with younger index cases showed higher percentages of symptoms at follow-up (89,91,94). This finding is consistent with the persistent symptoms often seen after early lung damage from other types of lower respiratory tract infections of infancy, including pertussis and croup (97–99), as well as from other traumatic conditions such as respiratory distress syndrome (100), bronchopulmonary dysplasia (101), tracheoesophageal fistula (102), and foreign body aspiration (103). Even seemingly benign newborn respiratory conditions, such as transient tachypnea of the newborn, have been associated with persistent pulmonary abnormalities (104). These findings suggest that respiratory insults in infancy have the potential to significantly damage the lower airways, sometimes indefinitely.

Children with confirmed RSV bronchiolitis are at higher risk for persistent symptoms (91). Welliver et al. found that those infants demonstrating the highest RSV IgE titers in nasopharyngeal secretions were much more likely to have subsequent wheezing (70%) than those who did not develop an RSV IgE response (20%) (90).

Most studies show that the development of other atopic conditions (89,92,93), or a history of atopy in a first-degree relative (92,93,95,105), or both, are risk factors for persistent wheezing in infants with bronchiolitis. Other studies show that eosinophilia, an elevated serum IgE, and dust mite sensitivity during the initial illness are risk factors, al-

Table 8 Risk Factors for Persistence of Wheezing Following Bronchiolitis

Definite[a]	
Documented RSV infection	
Presence of RSV IgE titers	
Younger age at initial illness	
Probable[b]	
Associated atopy	
First-degree relative with atophy, particularly asthma	
Parental smoking	
Possible[c]	
Elevated IgE	
Poor socioeconomic background	
Bottle feeding	
Eosinophilia	
Specific IgE reactivity to dust mite	
Initial unresponsiveness to bronchodilators	
Doubtful	
Sex	
Other specific skin/RAST tests	
Other factors not associated with risk of persistence in single studies	
Race	Day-care
Family size	Force-air heat
Presence of dog/cat	Older sibling in preschool
General anesthesia	
Serum immunoglobulins	

[a]Multiple studies show statistical significance.
[b]Most studies show statistical significance, an occasional study does not.
[c]The majority of studies show statistical significance, but many do not; *or* a single study shows statistical significance; *or* studies show these to be risk factors for the development of bronchiolitis itself, but not necessarily for the persistence of wheezing after bronchiolitis.

though other specific allergic sensitivities (by skin test or RAST) are not (81,95). Even those studies that did not show these factors to be a risk for subsequent wheezing did show that they were still risk factors for the development of bronchiolitis itself (92,93).

Although Pullan found significantly more girls as index cases (95), other studies found boys to be at higher risk for symptomatic persistence (90,93). A single study found that infants of younger parents were at higher risk (92), but race, family size, and other socioeconomic variables have not been found to be significant risk factors (92,93,95). Likewise, many other environmental factors do not appear to be important. The primary exception is parental smoking, which in most studies has been shown to be a significant risk factor for both the acquisition of bronchiolitis and subsequent wheezing (79,81,91,93,95,106).

In studying the relative odds of future wheezing after bronchiolitis, McConnochie found that many of these factors have cumulative risk potential (Table 9) (93). The relative odds of wheezing at follow-up was 4 for those who had bronchiolitis without other atopy or without a smoking parent, 7 for those with bronchiolitis and a smoking parent, 15 for those with bronchiolitis and associated allergy, and 28 when all three factors were present. When these other risk variables were controlled, bronchiolitis was a more significant risk factor for future wheezing than the other two variables.

In summary, roughly two-thirds of infants experiencing bronchiolitis go on to have further recurrent wheezing episodes. Improvement does occur over time, particularly in terms of frequency of symptoms. Despite this symptomatic improvement, however, bronchial hyperreactivity persists. Even in those studies with the longest follow-up intervals, those index cases without wheezing have more frequent coughing and episodes of bronchitis. Although pulmonary function studies are usually within normal limits in these infants at follow-up, they are statistically below control values, and evidence of bronchial hyperreactivity persists. The long-term implications of these continuing abnormalities are unclear, but retrospective studies of adults do show a higher risk for increased symptoms and lower FEV_1 in those with a history of childhood respiratory illness, especially when younger than age 2 (2,107).

These findings indicate that there appears to be a propensity for those with familial atopic tendencies to be not only at risk for the persistence of wheezing after bronchiolitis, but for bronchiolitis itself. On the other hand, there is strong evidence that the infection itself may be a catalyst toward early manifestations of atopy and bronchial hyperreactivity (10). Hence, the ultimate chicken–egg dilemma has been only partially solved: Bronchiolitis does predispose to ongoing lower airway abnormality, but does a genetic propensity for airway hyperreactivity predispose an infant to bronchiolitis?

ATOPIC DERMATITIS

Well over a half of those with atopic dermatitis in childhood will evidence some persistent atopic dermatitis at follow-up at one to three decades (Table 10) (108–110). Rystedt et al. directly interviewed patients and performed physical examinations at frequent intervals for as long as 32 years in over 90% of patients (108). In 549 patients requiring hospital-

Table 9 Occurrence of Risk Factor Groups, Relative Odds of Wheezing, and Attributable Risk for Wheezing[a]

Upper respiratory tract allergy	Bronchiolitis	Passive smoking	Raw data	Occurrence	Relative odds	Population attributable risk
0	0	0	6/64	34.64	1.00	2.35
0	0	+	9/77	41.68	1.87	5.00
0	+	0	3/10	0.72	3.99	0.16
0	+	+	7/26	1.89	7.46	0.67
+	0	0	1/15	8.09	3.79	1.75
+	0	+	8/21	11.32	7.08	3.86
+	+	0	3/6	0.43	15.12	0.23
+	+	+	13/17	1.23	28.27	0.83
			50/236	100.00		14.85

[a]Symbols used: 0, absent; +, present.

Definitions are as follows: *Raw data* are presented as number of subjects wheezing/total number of subjects in each cell. *Occurrence* of risk factor groups in the pediatric practice population was based on the observed frequencies in the control and index groups and on the bronchiolitis attack rate of 4.27/100 children in the first 2 years of life. Figures represent frequency with which children were observed in each risk factor group per 100 children in the practice population. *Relative Odds* are those obtained from multivariate analysis. They range from 1.00, for children exposed to none of the risk factors in the model, to 28.27, for children who experience all three risk factors. *Population Attributable Risk* is presented as the number of children in each of the cells who report wheezing out of every 100 children in the practice population. Calculations are based on occurrence and on rate of wheezing in each risk factor group as predicted by logistic regression analysis. The total number of wheezing children per 100, 14.85, derived from predicted values, varies slightly from that derived from the observed values, 14.87.

Source: Ref. 93.

Table 10 Atopic Dermatitis: Follow-up Studies

Author (Ref)	N	Age of onset (yr)	Follow-up interval (yr)	Age at follow-up (yr)	Severity	Persistent (%)
Roth and Kierland (108)	271	Child	20	NS	Mild	60
	221				Severe	79
Musgrove and Morgan (109)	99	Under 5	15–17	NS	NS	57
Rystedt (107)	406	Under 14	24–32	24–44	Moderate	40
	549				Severe	62[a]

NS, not stated.

[a]Persistent hand eczema in 51% of severe, 35% of moderate cases. Severe disease persisted in 13% of severe onset cases, 3% overall.

izations for severe atopic dermatitis, 62% had continuing disease at a follow-up of 24–32 years (108). Forty percent of those with moderate atopic dermatitis who were evaluated as outpatients showed persistent disease at the same follow-up intervals (108). In a supportive 20-year follow-up study using retrospective questionnaires, patients with severe or moderate atopic dermatitis had a 79 and 60% persistence, respectively (109).

Despite the frequent chronicity of atopic dermatitis, the clinical severity generally diminishes. Only 13% of those initially presenting with severe eczema, and only 2–3% of the overall study population, continued to have severe disease at follow-up. The severity at initial presentation exists as the most significant risk factor for persistence of atopic dermatitis (108).

Other risk factors associated with disease continuation were (in decreasing order of significance): family history of atopic dermatitis, concurrent atopic disease, age of onset, and the female sex (107). These latter two factors were significant only in patients with severe symptoms. If all of these risk factors were present, there was an 80% chance of persistence at follow-up. If none of the factors were present, persistence declined to 15% (108).

About one-third of patients with chronic atopic dermatitis have a history of asthma, whereas one-half have a history of allergic rhinitis (108). A higher risk for the persistence of atopic dermatitis occurred in those with chronic asthma or allergic rhinitis or with the onset of symptoms before age 3 (108).

Although a family history of atopic dermatitis was a significant risk factor for persistence, a family history of other skin conditions or atopic disease was not. The presence of a positive family history for atopy or other skin conditions did increase the risk of acquiring atopic dermatitis, but did not increase the risk for persistence (108).

Similar to several studies with asthma, Rystedt found that 25% of the population initially studied had recurrences after prolonged symptom-free intervals (108). Most of the patients who had persistence or recurrence of atopic dermatitis experienced only hand involvement at follow-up. Fifty-one percent of those with severe symptoms at presentation, and 25% of those in the moderate group, had primarily hand eczema at follow-up. Approximately 10% of these cases were disabling (108).

Although those with severe and moderate atopic dermatitis exhibited a 45 and 26% incidence of elevated serum IgE, respectively, total IgE and total eosinophil counts did not correlate with persistence of atopic dermatitis. This is consistent with the findings in the asthma studies, which indicate the lack of prognostic value for IgE and eosinophilia. Positive patch testing also did not correlate with persistence (108). No relation was found between personality type, academic achievement, recreational activities, and financial success and the persistence of atopic dermatitis (110).

CHRONIC URTICARIA

Acute urticaria is generally self-limited, and its cause is usually identifiable. A certain proportion of these patients, however, will go on to develop chronic or recurrent urticaria. What time frame constitutes "chronic urticaria" is unclear. Nevertheless, several studies assessing the risk of urticaria persisting after existing for at least 6-weeks duration have found that one-half to two-thirds of these patients have continuing symptoms at 1–3 years follow-up (Table 11) (111–115). Longer follow-up has shown that approximately two-thirds remain symptom-free for prolonged periods (113,114). In one study of 86 patients of all ages with urticaria, the duration of the urticaria exhibited a mean of 4 years and a median of 1.5 years, indicating several cases had extremely long duration.

The prognosis of chronic urticaria with angioedema appears to be the same as chronic urticaria alone (111), although one study suggested a more prolonged course if both entities were present (116). Other generalizations can be made concerning the natural history of chronic urticaria. Age, sex, history of other atopic conditions, total serum IgE, eosinophil count, RAST analysis, and skin testing are of no value in predicting the natural course of urticaria. In general, those patients with an identifiable cause for their chronic urticaria have the same course of illness as those patients in whom no cause can be found, although exceptions exist (114).

The longer the urticaria persists, the worse the prognosis. Those patients with urticaria persisting for longer than 24 months had an 81% chance of symptomatic persistence 5–14 years after onset (113). As seen with other atopic conditions, disease severity in those with persistent symptoms generally tends to decrease over time.

Several other observations from these urticaria studies are worthy of note. Kauppinen found that 30% of those with acute urticaria (under 2-months duration) developed chronic urticaria (112). Harris found a mean duration of 16 months for urticaria in 52 children younger than age 16 (115). Most studies show that fewer than 25% and frequently fewer than 10% of patients have an identifiable cause for their chronic urticaria (111,112,114–116).

Table 11 Chronic Urticaria: Follow-up Studies

Author (Ref)	N	Age	Duration at onset	Follow-up interval	Asymptomatic at follow-up (%)	Symptomatic at follow-up (%)	Improved at follow-up (%)	Known etiology[a] (%)
Quaranta et al. (110)	86	33 yr (mean)	6 wk	3 yr	68	32	NS	10
Kauppinen et al. (111)	99	½–16 yr	2 mo	3.8 yr (mean)	47	53	36	25
Smith et al. (112)	100	NS	6–24 mo	6 mo–14 yr	52	48	NS	NS
	46		6 mo		67	33	22	
	38		6–24 mo		47	53	18	
	16		24 mo		19	81	NS	
Pecourd and Genton (113)	83	40 yr (mean)	6 mo	15–236 mo (mean 82)	65	35	6	26[b]
Harris et al. (114)	52	16 yr	6 wk	12 mo	58[c]	42	NS	21

NS, not stated.

[a]Those with food or food-additive triggered urticaria not included.

[b]13% of total group resolved with cessation of specific foods/additives/analgesics.

[c]37% had no symptoms for 12 months; 21% had no symptoms for 6 months.

FOOD ALLERGY AND INTOLERANCE

Reaction Types

Most adverse reactions to food begin in infancy. Approximately one-fourth of those with a positive family history of allergy in a first-degree relative will have a parentally reported adverse reaction to a food in the first 2 years of life (12,13). The immediacy of the adverse reaction, the severity, the type of offending food, the organ site involved, and whether the reaction is IgE-mediated, appear to affect the persistence of food allergy. In general, severe reactions that occur immediately and that are IgE-mediated persist for longer periods than do more vague, later onset, and non–IgE-mediated reactions. Immediate reactions occur within 4 hr of ingestion and usually involve milk, egg, legumes, fish, and nuts. These reactions often affect multiorgan systems, including the respiratory system. Delayed reactions more often involve grains, meats, and fruits and affect the gastrointestinal and dermatological systems exclusively. These delayed reactions almost never involve the respiratory system or cause anaphylaxis. Regardless of these categorizations, however, the ultimate prognosis for food allergies is good (discussed later).

Those children experiencing immediate-onset reactions to foods often have other evidence of atopic disease, a family history of atopy, and elevated serum IgE (117). These patients are more likely to have a correlation between double-blind, placebo-controlled food challenges (DBPCFC) and a positive skin test or RAST to the food involved (118,119). Dermatitis is the most common symptom experienced, followed by gastrointestinal upset, urticaria, and respiratory symptoms. Approximately 60% of childhood reactions to milk are of this immediate type, whereas 92% of reactions to eggs occur in this manner (118).

The delayed-onset reactivities to food usually occur in the first 3 years of life. Positive delayed-type DBPCFC results are rare after 3 years of age (119). Delayed reactions occur 3–4 hr after ingestion and are almost always confined to the gastrointestinal tract or skin (120). Bock found that no behavioral changes occurred in 1014 DBPCFC in 480 children referred for evaluation of food hypersensitivity. Similarly, no ear problems were found after challenge in children with a history of recurrent or persistent middle ear difficulties (119).

Prognosis

Double-blind, placebo-controlled food challenges are the gold standard for the diagnosis of true adverse reactivity to a food and are discussed in detail in Chapter 21.

As noted earlier (also see Chapter 21), most adverse reactions to food occurring in early childhood are mild and transient. Those with the delayed-type reactions are more likely to develop partial or complete tolerance to their food sensitivities (118,120). Reactions are more likely to persist if they are generalized, urticarial, or respiratory. Those with higher RAST or skin test reactivity also have an increased risk of persistent symptoms (117,118). After 1 year follow-up in all of the studies cited, no patient worsened in their sensitivity or reactivity (117–123).

Those patients with chronic symptoms generally continue to have positive RAST or skin test results to the offending food, although these reactions tend to diminish over time. Positive test results tend to lag behind clinical tolerance. Those with low positive testing values invariably develop tolerance. Dannaeus found that RAST titers to milk parallel the clinical course (118). Overall, these titers tend to increase between 12 and 18 months of age and decline thereafter. Conversely, Sampson found no correlation between the clinical course and skin reactivity to egg in children with atopic dermatitis (121). As has been observed with other types of atopic disease, total serum IgE is not predictive of outcome (117,123).

Bock followed 480 children from birth to age 3 referred for possible food intolerance (120). Twenty-eight percent of these children had some suspected reactivity to food, but these could be confirmed by challenge in only 8%. The average time until the food was back in the diet was 9 months. All but four patients were able to tolerate the offending food by age 3. He found an astonishingly high rate of reactivity to fruits and fruit juices. These reactions were generally dermatological or gastrointestinal, and they were not associated with any skin test reactivity. Orange was the primary offender, followed by tomato, apple, and grape.

In terms of severe reactions (anaphylactic, urticarial, asthmatic) Bock found that 80% occurred in the first year of life, with a mean age of onset at 6 months (122). Of nine children studied, all had milk reactions, one had soy reaction, and two had egg reactions. By age 3, three of nine were able to tolerate the offending foods in normal amounts, four were able to tolerate small quantities, and two remained reactive to even small quantities of the offending food.

Atopic dermatitis appears to be the most persistent of all food reactions (12,13,121). Sampson rechallenged 70 patients with challenge-proved food symptoms 1 year after presentation; two-thirds of these had persistent symptoms (122). Dannaeus followed 82 older children (mean age 4½ years) for 2–5 years: reactions in two-thirds of those with eczema persisted, while half of those with an asthmatic reaction persisted (117).

Specific Foods

One-third of those developing milk allergy do so after the first few exposures (117). Of those infants reacting, 60% have an immediate and more severe type of reactivity, whereas 40% have a delayed, less dramatic reaction. Dannaeus followed 47 infants 1–4 years after the development of milk sensitivity (117). At follow-up, 29% had developed complete tolerance, 32% were able to ingest small amounts without problem, 21% were improved, but had continued significant symptoms, and 18% were unchanged. In the delayed group, 3-4 developed complete tolerance and only 5% remained unchanged.

Reactivity to egg persists for longer periods. The reactions to egg occur in 90% of reactors by the first several exposures (123). Ford found the mean age of onset to be 17 months of age (123). He followed 25 patients with egg sensitivity for 2–2½ years; at follow-up 44% had developed complete tolerance.

Reactions to fish, nuts, and legumes have a higher tendency to persist, although the severity improves with time (117). In general, these reactions have a later onset than those to milk, egg, and fruit. There is a loose correlation between RAST reactivity to these foods and clinical course, although severe reactors are likely to have persistent symptoms.

CONCLUSION

Most allergic conditions are likely to persist, although they tend to improve over time. Even when these conditions appear to completely remit, they frequently recur, even after prolonged intervals. The clinical relevance of these observations are self-evident: clinicians may be cautiously optimistic about eventual outcome, but blind reassurance that an individual will outgrow allergies can be quite misleading. Furthermore, the foregoing review leaves little doubt that early environmental intervention must be studied in an attempt to minimize the persistence, the recurrence, and possibly the severity of respiratory allergies, particularly asthma, once they present. In addition, this information can be invaluable in advising parents about the prevention of atopic conditions in high-risk children.

Roughly 50–60% of children with asthma have symptoms at follow-up, even through three decades, the length of the longest follow-up studies. Most cases, however, become mild and episodic. Children tend to improve into their early teenage years, but approximately 25% of those who have seemingly "outgrown" their asthma have recurrence of symptoms in their late teens or 20s.

Those with the most severe allergic conditions or those with the presence of multiple concurrent atopic conditions are significantly more likely to have continuation of their symptoms. A strong family history of general atopy, an elevated total IgE, and positive specific allergy tests can identify an individual likely to develop allergies, but cannot predict if that individual will have prolonged symptomatic illness. Nevertheless, ongoing exposure to provocative factors, such as passive tobacco smoke and substantial house dust, appears to predispose to ongoing symptoms over the years. Empirically this should lead to aggressive environmental intervention, but this has not been specifically studied to ascertain if it affects ultimate outcome.

Any review of the natural history of an illness should attempt to answer two fundamental questions: (a) what are the ultimate implications of disease persistence? and (b) how does treatment or prevention alter disease outcome?

In nonasthmatic atopic conditions, the primary importance of persistence is in the realm of patient comfort. Ongoing problems with allergic rhinitis, atopic dermatitis, or urticaria may be disconcerting to a patient, but the inherent nature of these conditions and the myriad of safe treatment modalities available make prolonged or intractable morbidity unlikely. On the other hand, the implications of ongoing asthma on morbidity and mortality, although specifically unknown, are potentially quite severe. Adults with substantial pulmonary obstruction have repeatedly been shown to have accelerated declines in pulmonary flow studies (FEV_1) with age (124). In addition, FEV_1 appears to be the single most important predictor of morbidity and mortality in COPD (125). Retrospectively, adults with respiratory symptoms and diminished pulmonary function have stronger histories of childhood respiratory problems (2). On the other hand, adults with asthma and asthmatic bronchitis do not manifest an increased rate of FEV_1 decline with age, a phenomenon that appears restricted to only those with emphysema (77). We hope that continuation of many of the studies cited in this chapter will more definitely address the role of childhood asthma in the morbidity and mortality in COPD.

The influence of therapy on disease outcome, however, is unlikely to ever be adequately investigated, owing to the difficulties in studying large population groups, their medication regimens, and their environmental circumstances over many decades. Over short intervals, aggressive preventative measures and the extended use of anti-inflammatory inhaled medications, such as corticosteroids or cromolyn, are likely to prevent asthma morbidity in children. The major pathological role of inflammation in asthma has been recently stressed, as has the consequent recommendation of ongoing anti-inflammatory therapy, once again in an attempt to minimize disease morbidity (126). Unfortunately, how these interventions ultimately influence disease outcome, particularly into later adulthood when the complications of COPD arise, is unknown. To blindly recommend extensive environmental manipulation or expensive ongoing therapeutic interventions may be unnecessary. On the other hand, these interventions may improve the quality of daily life for an asthmatic with minimal risk. This, in conjunction with the general observation that any perpetual adverse stimulation of a body organ is likely to be harmful, appears to more than justify aggressive intervention in the childhood asthmatic.

REFERENCES

1. Smith JM. Epidemiology and natural history of asthma, allergic rhinitis, and atopic dermatitis (eczema). In: Middleton E, Reed CE, Ellis EF, et al., eds. Allergy: principles and practice, vol 2. St Louis: CV Mosby, 1988:891–929.
2. Burrows B, Knudson RJ, Lebowitz MD. The relationship of childhood respiratory illness to adult obstructive airway disease. Am Rev Respir Dis 1977; 115:751–760.
3. Cookson WOCM, Hopkin JM. Dominant inheritance of atopic immunoglobulin-E responsiveness. Lancet 1988; 1:86–88.
4. Anderson HR, Bland JM, Patel S, Peckham C. The natural history of asthma in childhood. J Epidemiol Community Health 1986; 40:121–129.
5. Peat JK, Britton WJ, Salome CM, Woolcock AJ. Bronchial hyperresponsiveness in two populations of Australian schoolchildren. II. Relative importance of associated factors. Clin Allergy 1987; 17:283–290.
6. Marsh DG. Immunogenetics of allergic disease. In: Middleton E, Reed CE, Ellis EF, et al, eds. Allergy: principles and practice, vol 1. St Louis: CV Mosby, 1988:94–105.
7. Andrae S, Axelson O, Bjorksten B, Fredrikkson M, Kjellman N-IM. Symptoms of bronchial hyperreactivity and asthma in relation to environmental factors. Arch Dis Child 1988; 63:473–478.
8. Gerritsen J, Koeter GH, de Monchy JGR, Knol K. Allergy in subjects with asthma from childhood to adulthood. J Allergy Clin Immunol 1990; 85:116–125.
9. Sporik R, Holgate ST, Platts-Mills TAE, Cogswell JJ. Exposure to house-dust mite allergen (Der p I) and the development of asthma in childhood. N Engl J Med 1990; 323:502–507.
10. Frick OL, German DL, Mills J. Development of allergy in children. Association with virus infections. J Allergy Clin Immunol 1979; 63:228–241.
11. Busse WW. Respiratory infections: their role in airway responsiveness and the pathogenesis of asthma. J Allergy Clin Immunol 1990; 85:671–683.

12. Van Asperen PP, Kemp AS. The natural history of IgE sensitisation and atopic disease in early childhood. Acta Paediatr Scand 1989; 78:239–245.
13. Cogswell JJ, Mitchell EB, Alexander J. Parental smoking, breast feeding, and respiratory infection in development of allergic diseases. Arch Dis Child 1987; 62:34–38.
14. Zeiger RS, Heller S, Mellon MH, et al. Effect of combined maternal and infant food allergen avoidance on development of atopy in early infancy: a randomized study. J Allergy Clin Immunol 1989; 84:72–89.
15. Rowntree S, Cogswell JJ, Platts-Mills TAE, Mitchell EB. Development of IgE and IgG antibodies to food and inhalant allergens in children at risk of allergic disease. Arch Dis Child 1985; 60:727–735.
16. Zeiger RS, Heller S, Mellon MH, Halsey JF, Hamburger RN, Sampson HA. Genetic and environmental factors affecting the development of atopy through age 4 in children of atopic parents: A prospective randomized study of food allergen avoidance. Pediatr Allergy Immunol (in press).
17. Van Asperen PP, Kemp AS, Mukhi A. Atopy in infancy predicts the severity of bronchial hyperresponsiveness in later childhood. J Allergy Clin Immunol 1990; 85:790–795.
18. Anderson HR, Bland JM, Peckham CS. Risk factors for asthma up to 16 years of age. Chest 1987; 91:127S–130S.
19. Kjellman B, Dalen G. Long-term changes in inhalant allergy in asthmatic children. Allergy 1986; 41:351–356.
20. Soothill JF, Stokes CR, Turner MV, Norma AP, Taylor B. Predisposing factors and the development of reaginic allergy in infants. Clin Allergy 1976; 6:305–319.
21. Foucard T, Sjoberg O. A prospective 12-year follow-up study of children with wheezy bronchitis. Acta Paediatr Scand 1984; 73:577–583.
22. Kaufman HS. Allergy in the newborn: skin test reactions confirmed by the Prausnitz–Kustner test at birth. Clin Allergy 1971; 1:363–367.
23. Martinez FD, Morgan WJ, Wright AL, Holberg CJ, Taussig LM. Diminished lung function as a predisposing factor for wheezing respiratory illness in infants. N Engl J Med 1988; 319:1112–1117.
24. Hopp RJ, Townley RG, Biven BE, Bewtra AK, Nair NM. The presence of airway reactivity before the development of asthma. Am Rev Respir Dis 1990; 141:2–6.
25. Lebowitz MD, Holberg CJ, Knudson RJ, Burrows B. Longitudinal study of pulmonary function development in childhood, adolescence, and early adulthood. Am Rev Respir Dis 1987; 136:69–75.
26. Burrows B, Halonen M, Lebowitz MD, Knudson RJ, Barbee RA. The relationship of serum immunoglobulin E, allergy skin tests, and smoking to respiratory disorders. J Allergy Clin Immunol 1982; 70:199–204.
27. Burrows B. The natural history of asthma. J Allergy Clin Immunol 1987; 80:373–377.
28. Charpin D, Kleisbauer JP, Lanteaume A, Razzouk H, Vervloet D, Toumi M, Fadel F, Charpin J. Asthma and allergy to house dust mites in populations living in high altitude. Chest 1988; 93:758–761.

29. Wen T. Mites and mite allergy in the Shanghai region of China. In: de Weck AL, Todt A, eds. Mite allergy. Brussels: UCB Institute, 1988:75–79.
30. Dowse GK, Turner KJ, Stewart GA, Alpers MP, Woolcock AJ. The association between *Dermatophagoides* mites and the increasing prevalence of asthma in village communities within the Papua New Guinea Highlands. J Allergy Clin Immunol 1985; 75:75–80.
31. Neuspiel DR, Rush D, Butler NR, Golding J, Bijur PE, Kurzon M. Parental smoking and post-infancy wheezing in children: a prospective cohort study. Am J Public Health 1989; 79:168–171.
32. Korsgaard J. Mite asthma and residency: a case–control study on the impact of exposure to house dust mites in dwellings. Am Rev Respir Dis 1983; 128:231–235.
33. Lau S, Falkenhorst G, Weber A, Werthmann I, Lind P, Buettner-Goetz P, Wahn U. High mite-allergen exposure increases the risk of sensitization in atopic children and young adults. J Allergy Clin Immunol 1989; 84:718–725.
34. Kjellman B, Petterson R. The problem of furred pets in childhood atopic disease. Allergy 1983; 38:65–73.
35. Suoniemi I, Bjorksten F, Haahtela T. Dependence of immediate hypersensitivity in the adolescent period on factors encountered in infancy. Allergy 1981; 36:263–268.
36. Bjorksten F, Suoniemi I, Koski V. Neonatal birch-pollen contact and subsequent allergy to birch pollen. Clin Allergy 1980; 10:585–591.
37. Peat JK, Britton WJ, Salome CM, Woolcock AJ. Bronchial hyperresponsiveness in two populations of Australian schoolchildren. III. Effect of exposure to environmental allergens. Clin Allergy 1987; 17:291–300.
38. Gelber L, Pollart SM, Chapman MD, Platts-Mills TAE. Serum IgE antibodies and allergen exposure as a risk factor for acute asthma [abstract]. J Allergy Clin Immunol 1990; 85:193.
39. Britten N, Davies JMC, Colley JRT. Early respiratory experience and subsequent cough and peak expiratory flow rate in 36 year old men and women. Br Med J 1987; 294:1317–1320.
40. Dodge R. The effects of indoor pollution on Arizona children. Arch Environ Health 1982; 37:151–215.
41. Ware JH, Ferris Jr. BG, Dockery DW, Spengler JD, Stram DO, Speizer FE. Effect of ambient sulfur oxides and suspended particles on respiratory health of preadolescent children. Am Rev Respir Dis 1986; 133:834–842.
42. Osebold JW, Gerschwin LJ, Zee YC. Studies on the enhancement of allergic lung sensitization by inhalation of ozone and sulfuric acid aerosol. J Environ Pathol Toxicol 1980; 3:221–234.
43. Riedel F, Kramer M, Scheibenboge C, Rieger CHL. Effects of SO_2 exposure on allergic sensitization in the guinea pig. J Allergy Clin Immunol 1988; 82:527–534.

44. Schilling RSF, Letai AD, Hui SL, Beck GJ, Schoenberg JB, Bouhuys AH. Lung function, respiratory disease, and smoking in families. Am J Epidemiol 1977; 106:274–283.
45. Ekwo EE, Weinberger MM, Lachenbruch PA, Huntley WH. Relationship of parental smoking and gas cooking to respiratory disease in children. Chest 1983; 84:62–668.
46. Colley JR, Holland WW, Corkhill RT. Influence of passive smoking and parental phlegm on pneumonia and bronchitis in early childhood. Lancet 1974; 1:529–532.
47. Lebowitz MD, Burrows B. Respiratory symptoms related to smoking habits of family adults. Chest 1976; 69:42–50.
48. Weiss ST, Tager JB, Speizer FE, Rosner B. Persistent wheeze: its relation to respiratory illness, cigarette smoking, and level of pulmonary function in a population sample of children. Am Rev Respir Dis 1980; 122:697–707.
49. Ware JH, Dockery DW, Spiro A, Speizer FE, Ferris BG. Passive smoking, gas cooking, and respiratory health of children living in six cities. Am Rev Respir Dis 1984; 129:366–374.
50. Burchfiel CM, Higgins MW, Keller JB, Howatt WF, Butler WJ, Higgins ITT. Passive smoking in childhood: respiratory conditions and pulmonary function in Tecumseh, Michigan. Am Rev Respir Dis 1986; 133:966–973.
51. Tager IB, Segal MR, Munoz A, Weiss ST, Speizer FE. The effect of maternal cigarette smoking on the pulmonary function of children and adolescents. Am Rev Respir Dis 1987; 136:1366–1370.
52. Hasselblad V, Humble OG, Graham MG, Anderson HS. Indoor environmental determinants of lung function in children. Am Rev Respir Dis 1981; 123:479–485.
53. Murray AB, Morrison BJ. The effect of cigarette smoke from the mother on bronchial responsiveness and severity of symptoms in children with asthma. J Allergy Clin Immunol 1986; 77:575–581.
54. Fergusson DM, Horwood LJ. Parental smoking and respiratory illness during early childhood: a 6 year longitudinal study. Pediatr Pulmonol 1985; 1:99–106.
55. Weitzman M, Gortmaker S, Walker DK, Sobol A. Maternal smoking and childhood asthma. Pediatrics 1990; 85:505–511.
56. Tashkin DP, Clark VA, Simmons M, Reems C, Coulson AH, Bourque LB, Sayre JW, Detels R, Rokaw S. The UCLA population studies of chronic obstructive respiratory disease: VII. Relationship between parental smoking and children's lung function. Am Rev Respir Dis 1984; 129:891–897.
57. Vedal S, Schenker MB, Samet JM, Speizer FE. Risk factors for childhood respiratory disease: analysis of pulmonary function. Am Rev Respir Dis 1984; 130:187–192.
58. O'Connor GT, Weiss ST, Tager IB, Speizer FE. The effect of passive smoking on pulmonary function and nonspecific bronchial responsive-

ness in a population based sample of children and young adults. Am Rev Respir Dis 1987; 135:800–804.
59. Collins MH, Moessinger AC, Kleinerman J, Bassi J, Rosso P, Collins AM, James LS, Blanc WA. Fetal lung hypoplasia associated with maternal smoking: a morphometric analysis. Pediatr Res 1985; 19:408–412.
60. Magnusson CGM. Maternal smoking influences cord serum IgE and IgD levels and increases the risk for subsequent infant allergy. J Allergy Clin Immunol 1986; 78:898–904.
61. Horwood LJ, Fergusson DM, Shannon FT. Social and familial factors in the development of early childhood asthma. Pediatrics 1985; 75:859–868.
62. Murray AB, Morrison BJ. It is children with atopic dermatitis who develop asthma more frequently if the mother smokes. J Allergy Clin Immunol 1990; 86:732–739.
63. Ryssing E, Flensborg EW. Prognosis after puberty for 442 asthmatic children examined and treated on specific allergologic principles. Acta Paediatr 1963; 52:97–105.
64. Buffum WP. The prognosis of asthma in infancy. Pediatrics 1963; 32:453–455.
65. Barr LW, Logan GB. Prognosis of children having asthma. Pediatrics 1964; 34:856–860.
66. Whatley JW, Guerrant JL. The prognosis of asthma in children. NC Med J 1965; 26:240–243.
67. Buffum WP, Settipane GA. Prognosis of asthma in childhood. Am J Dis Child 1966; 112:214–218.
68. Blair H. Natural history of childhood asthma: 20 year follow-up. Arch Dis Child 1977; 52:613–619.
69. Jonsson JA, Boe J, Berlin E. The long-term prognosis of childhood asthma in a predominantly rural Swedish county. Acta Paediatr Scand 1987; 76:950–954.
70. Friberg S, Bevegard S, Graff-Lonnevig V. Asthma from childhood to adult age. Acta Paediatr Scand 1988; 77:424–431.
71. Martin AJ, McLennan LA, Landau LI, Phelan PD. The natural history of childhood asthma to adult life. Br Med J 1980; 280:1397–1400.
72. Kelly WJW, Hudson I, Phelan PD, Pain MCF, Olinsky A. Childhood asthma in adult life: a further study at 28 years of age. Br Med J 1987; 294:1059–1062.
73. Strachan DP, Anderson HR, Bland JM, Peckham C. Asthma as a link between chest illness in childhood and chronic cough and phlegm in young adults. Br Med J 1988; 296:890–893.
74. Giles GG, Lickiss N, Gibson HB, Shaw K. Respiratory symptoms in Tasmanian adolescents: a follow up of the 1961 birth cohort. Aust NZ J Med 1983; 14:631–637.
75. Johnstone DE. A study of the natural history of bronchial asthma in children. Am J Dis Child 1968; 115:213–216.

76. Martin AJ, Landau LI, Phelan PD. Lung function in young adults who had asthma in childhood. Am Rev Respir Dis 1980; 122:609–616.
77. Burrows B, Bloom JW, Traver GA, Cline MG. The course and prognosis of different forms of chronic airways obstruction in a sample from the general population. N Engl J Med 1987; 317:1309–1314.
78. Blackhall M. Ventilating function in subjects with childhood asthma who have become symptom free. Arch Dis Child 1970; 45:363–366.
79. Geller-Bernstein G, Kenett R, Weisglass L, Tsur S, Lahav M, Levin S. Atopic babies with wheezy bronchitis. Allergy 1987; 42:85–91.
80. Kelly WJW, Hudson I, Phelan PD, Pain MCF, Olinsky A. Atopy in subjects with asthma followed to the age of 28 years. J Allergy Clin Immunol 1990; 85:548–557.
81. Sims DG, Gardner PS, Weightman D, Turner MW, Soothill JF. Atopy does not predispose to RSV bronchiolitis or postbronchiolitic wheezing. Br Med J 1981; 282:2086–2088.
82. Loren ML, Leung PK, Cooley R, Chai H, Bell TD, Buck VM. Irreversibility of obstructive changes in severe asthma in childhood. Chest 1978; 74:126–129.
83. Kuzemko JA. Natural history of childhood asthma. J Pediatr 1980; 97:886–894.
84. Johnstone DE, Dutton A. The value of hyposensitization therapy for bronchial asthma in children. A 14 year old study. Pediatrics 1968; 42:793–796.
85. Rackemann FM, Edwards MC. Asthma in children: a follow-up study of 688 patients after an interval of twenty years. N Engl J Med 1952; 246:815–823.
86. Kraepelien S. Prognosis of asthma in childhood with special reference to pulmonary function and the value of specific hyposensitization. Acta Paediatr Scand [Suppl] 1963; 140:92–96.
87. Platts-Mills TAE, Tovey ER, Mitchell EB et al. Reduction of bronchial hyperreactivity during prolonged allergen avoidance. Lancet 1982; 2:675–678.
88. Stokes GM, Milner AD, Hodges IGC, Groggins RC. Lung function abnormalities after acute bronchiolitis. J Pediatr 1981; 98:871–874.
89. Welliver RC, Sun M, Rinaldo D, Ogra PL. Predictive value of respiratory syncytial virus-specific IgE responses for recurrent wheezing following bronchiolitis. J Pediatr 1986; 109:776–780.
90. Sly PD, Hibbert ME. Childhood asthma following hospitalization with acute viral bronchiolitis in infancy. Pediatr Pulmonol 1989; 7:153–158.
91. Mok JYO, Simpson H. Symptoms, atopy, and bronchial reactivity after lower respiratory infection in infancy. Arch Dis Child 1984; 59:299–305.
92. McConnochie KM, Roghmann KL. Bronchiolitis as a possible cause of wheezing in childhood: new evidence. Pediatrics 1984; 74:1–10.

93. Duiverman EJ, Niejens HJ, van Strik R, Affourtit MJ, Kerrebijn KF. Lung function and bronchial responsiveness in children who had infantile bronchiolitis. Pediatr Pulmonol 1987; 3:38–44.
94. Pullan CR, Hey EN. Wheezing, asthma, and pulmonary dysfunction 10 years after infection with respiratory syncytial virus in infancy. Br Med J 1982; 284:1065–1069.
95. Kattan M, Keens TG, Lapierre JG, Levison H, Bryan AC. Pulmonary function abnormalities in symptom-free children after bronchiolitis. Pediatrics 1977; 59:683–688.
96. Johnston IDA, Anderson HR, Lambert HP, Patel S. Respiratory morbidity and lung function after whooping-cough. Lancet 1983; 2:104–1108.
97. Loughlin GM, Taussig LM. Pulmonary function in children with a history of laryngotracheobronchitis. J Pediatr 1979; 59:365–369.
98. Weiss ST, Tager IB, Munoz A, Speizer FE. The relationship of respiratory infections in early childhood to the occurrence of increased levels of bronchial responsiveness and atopy. Am Rev Respir Dis 1985; 131:573–578.
99. Coates AL, Bergsteinsson H, Desmond K, Outerbridge EW, Beaudry PH. Long-term pulmonary sequelae of premature birth with and without idiopathic respiratory distress syndrome. J Pediatr 1977; 90:611–616.
100. Smyth JA, Tabachrick E, Duncan WJ, Reilly BJ, Levison H. Pulmonary function and bronchial hyperreactivity in long-term survivors of bronchopulmonary dysplasia. Pediatrics 1981; 68:36–340.
101. Milligan DWA, Levison H. Lung function in children following repair of tracheo-oesophageal fistula. J Pediatr 1979; 95:24–27.
102. Givan D, Scott P, Jeglum E, Eigen H. Lung function and airway reactivity of children 3 to 10 years after foreign body aspiration. Am Rev Respir Dis 1981; 123(suppl):158S.
103. Shohat M, Levy G, Levy I, Schonfeld T, Merlob P. Transient tachypnoea of the newborn and asthma. Arch Dis Child 1988; 64:277–279.
104. Rooney JC, Williams HE. The relationship between proved viral bronchiolitis and subsequent wheezing. J Pediatr 1971; 78:397–406.
105. Fergusson DM, Horwood LJ, Shannon FT. Parental smoking and respiratory illness in infancy. Arch Dis Child 1980; 55:358–361.
106. Barker DJP, Osmond C. Childhood respiratory infection and adult chronic bronchitis in England and Wales. Br Med J 1986; 293:1271–1275.
107. Rystedt I. Prognostic factors in atopic dermatitis. Acta Derm Venereol 1985; 65:206–213.
108. Roth HL, Kierland RR. The natural history of atopic dermatitis. Arch Dermatol 1964; 89:209–214.
109. Musgrove K, Morgan JK. Infantile eczema: a long term follow-up study. Br J Dermatol 1976; 95:365–372.
110. Quarant JH, Rohr AS, Rachelefsky GS, Siegel SC, Katz RM, Spector SL, Mickey MR. The natural history and response to therapy of chronic urticaria and angioedema. Ann Allergy 1989; 62:421–428.

111. Kauppinen K, Juntunen K, Lanki H. Urticaria in children: retrospective evaluation and follow-up. Allergy 1984; 39:469–472.
112. Smith L, Wray BB, Stafford CT. Outcome of patients with chronic urticaria and angioedema. J Allergy Clin Immunol 1983;
113. Pecourd AR, Genton C. Outcome of 83 adults with chronic urticaria and angioedema. J Allergy Clin Immunol 1983; 71:128–133.
114. Harris A, Twarog FJ, Geha RS. Chronic urticaria in children: natural course and etiology. Ann Allergy 1983; 51:161–164.
115. Champion RH, Roberts SOB, Carpenter RG, Roger JH. Urticaria and angioedema: a review of 554 patients. Br J Dermatol 1969; 81:588–593.
116. Dannaeus A, Inganas M. A follow-up study of children with food allergy. Clinical course in relation to serum IgE- and IgG-antibody levels to milk, egg, and fish. Clin Allergy 1981; 11:533–539.
117. Dannaeus A, Johansson SGO. A follow-up study of infants with adverse reaction to cow's milk. Acta Paediatr Scand 1979; 68:37–382.
118. Bock SA, Atkins FM. Patterns of food hypersensitivity during sixteen years of double-blind, placebo-controlled food challenges. J Pediatr 1990; 117:561–567.
119. Bock SA. Prospective appraisal of complaints of adverse reactions to foods in children during the first 3 years of life. Pediatrics 1987; 79:683–688.
120. Sampson HA. Late-phase response to foods in atopic dermatitis. Hosp Pract 1987; 22:111–128.
121. Bock SA. Natural history of severe reactions to foods in young children. J Pediatr 1985; 107:676–680.
122. Ford RPK, Taylor B. Natural history of egg hypersensitivity. Arch Dis Child 1982; 57:649–652.
123. Burrows B, Earle RH. Course and prognosis of chronic obstructive lung disease. N Engl J Med 1969; 280:397–404.
124. Burrows B, Knudson RJ, Camilli AE, Lyle SK, Lebowitz MD. The "horse-racing effect" and predicting decline in forced expiratory volume in one second from screening spirometry. Am Rev Respir Dis 1987; 135:788–793.
125. McFadden ER Jr. Pathogenesis of asthma. J Allergy Clin Immunol 1984; 73:413–424.

21

Food Hypersensitivity in Infancy

S. Allan Bock

National Jewish Center for Immunology and Respiratory Medicine and University of Colorado Health Sciences Center, Denver, Colorado

Hugh A. Sampson

Johns Hopkins University School of Medicine, Baltimore, Maryland

DEFINITION OF TERMS

For eons the topic of food allergy has been the subject of mythology and misunderstanding. Practitioners, both medical and nonmedical, have had strongly held opinions about the effect of foods on people. The first adverse interaction between food and man is described in Genesis (1). Throughout the centuries, where records remain, adverse reactions to foods have been offered as an explanation for many of man's ills (2). This chapter will be devoted to examining the scientific basis of food hypersensitivity (allergy) and will endeavor to separate the information that currently exists based on properly controlled research from the opinions and impressions of practitioners whose claims often have a counterproductive effect on the laity.

The first problem encountered in discussions of food hypersensitivity is the definition of the word *allergy*. The term has been abused for so long that many authors in the field have chosen to substitute the term *hypersensitivity* when discussing adverse reactions to foods that can be proved to involve the immune system. When patients initially complain of symptoms associated with food ingestion, it would seem wise to counsel them to describe their symptoms as adverse reactions to the suspected food. One may then attempt to prove whether the specific suspected food is responsible for the reaction and then attempt to find the mechanism involved. A number of mechanisms are clearly associated with adverse symptoms following food ingestion, and greater precision of terminology must be established when trying to understand these reactions. This chapter examines those symptoms that have been proved to involve or are highly likely to involve immunological events, precipitated by food ingestion, that may properly be termed *food hypersensitivity* or *food allergy* (3,4).

Several additional terms have been applied to adverse reactions to foods. *Food intolerance* is often used (based on disaccharide enzyme deficiency) as a generic synonym for adverse reactions to food. However, the carbohydrate intolerances (e.g., lactose, sucrose, isomaltose intolerance), are illnesses for which specific biochemical, not immunological, mechanisms, are involved. Therefore, it would seem most appropriate to reserve the term *intolerance* for the diaccharidase deficiencies.

Toxic reactions may have two sources (5–7). There are natural toxins in our diet, including many natural carcinogens. There are endless examples, including toxins in "organically" grown food, such as the oxalates in rhubarb or the cyanides in the stones of apricots. Other intoxicants include contaminants such as aflotoxin, which is present only in low levels unless foods have been inappropriately stored and the mold producing aflotoxin has been allowed to produce copious amounts of the intoxicating substance. Accidental intoxication may occur when foods are contaminated in the manufacturing process. Attention has been given to the possible effects of pesticides, especially on young children. Some of these compounds may be passed to infants through breast milk (8–10).

The term *idiosyncratic* has been applied to many food reactions, but it does not have a clearly associated biochemical mechanism and, therefore, will not be used in this discussion. Strongly held beliefs about symptoms produced by certain foods under diverse circumstances may be classified as *psychological reactions*. Unfortunately, in our culture, this may now be the largest group of "adverse reactions to foods." Notions such as the production of behavioral aberrations by sugar ingestion are so rampant in the populous that even the medical profession has succumbed to perpetuation of these beliefs.

PREVALENCE

The exact frequency of occurrence of adverse reactions to foods, let alone determination of the frequency of true food hypersensitivity, has been an elusive figure. Methodological problems have complicated the acquisition of a definitive value for the incidence or prevalence of food hypersensitivity. A number of studies throughout the world have attempted, in various ways, to approach the determination of these figures, and the results of these studies have led to estimates from less than 1 up to 30% (11–20). (Of course, there are a group of enthusiasts who feel that food hypersensitivity affects 100% of children.)

Most of these studies suffer from one or more methodological deficiencies. Many of them investigate only one aspect of the problem (e.g., development of "allergy" to one or two foods). Although few foods cause adverse reactions during the first 2 years of life (primarily egg, milk, and soy), examination of all foods is needed to gain a true picture of the problem. A second major flaw in the cited studies (and others not listed) are definitions of symptoms. Persistent rhinitis in young children is often termed allergic, without any proof that the immune system is involved. Wheezing in infants has been attributed to foods by association, rather than by objective food challenge. Atopic dermatitis, an illness notorious for symptomatic fluctuation, has been blamed on foods because of improvement when the diet has been altered. This type of imprecision points to a major problem in most prevalence studies: lack of confirmation of the link between food and symptoms by properly controlled double-blind, placebo-controlled food challenge. Without this rigorous proof, it is hard to know if the true prevalence is closer to 1 or to 30%. Certainly, it is unacceptable to use such widely disparate figures to counsel families. One of the most useful pieces of numerical data concerning prevalence has been the finding by Burks that one-third of the children presenting to university dermatology and allergy clinics with atopic dermatitis will have food hypersensitivity (21).

Perhaps of assistance to physicians caring for infants is Bock's observation that 208/480 children had some symptom attributed to food during the first 3 years of life (19). Eighty percent of the initial complaints occurred during the first year of life. A second observation from the same study was the brief period of time during which the reactions persisted. For most children with previously confirmed reactions from food, the culprit was uneventfully reintroduced into the diet within a mean of 6 months. Few of these reactions could be shown to be "allergic," that is, could be shown to be associated with immune mechanisms. Thus, primary care practitioners caring for infants were frequently told about foods "causing symptoms" by the parents of their patients. These parents may be reassured that, if the problem is real, it should not persist for more than a few months, and careful systematic reintroduction of the food into the diet may promptly demonstrate the resolution of the problem. Symptoms caused by foods that appear to persist may require further evaluation, either by the primary care practitioner or by referral to an allergist familiar with food hypersensitivity in infants.

CLINICAL PRESENTATION OF FOOD HYPERSENSITIVITY

Symptoms and Signs

Gastrointestinal

Gastrointestinal symptoms (Table 1) are the first or second most common symptoms of an adverse reaction to food in children during the first 2 years of life (4,13,20). Gastrointestinal symptoms include acute vomiting and diarrhea as well as chronic, prolonged diarrhea. Abdominal pain and nausea, about which young children cannot complain, are often suspected by observation of their behavior, which often mimics the behavior of older children in whom these complaints can be verbalized. Acute vomiting and diarrhea are often easy to observe relative to food ingestion because there is a prompt onset of a rather impressive symptom and then often very prompt resolution. Vomiting and diarrhea caused by food hypersensitivity may be distinguished from intoxications and gastrointestinal infections by the prompt resolution of symptoms and prompt return of the young child's appetite after food avoidance. Some children with food allergy may often appear quite ill after food ingestion, with pallor and some lethargy developing; however, these symptoms usually resolve within minutes. When pallor persists, shock should be suspected, blood pressure measured, and epinephrine (Adrenalin) administered.

Table 1 Symptoms Confirmed During DBPCFC[a]

Gastrointestinal
Nausea, vomiting, abdominal pain (colic?), diarrhea, colitis
Cutaneous
Urticaria, atopic dermatitis, erythema
Respiratory
Rhinorrhea, sneezing, tearing, conjunctival swelling, laryngospasm, wheezing
Cardiovascular
Hypotension, collapse, shock
Nervous/behavioral
Migraine: controversial and not yet confirmed unequivocally in children
"Hyperactivity/irritability" rarely confirmed as only symptom

[a]DBPCFC, double blind, placebo-controlled food challenge.

Children with chronic diarrhea are more troublesome to evaluate because of the multiple pathogenic causes of chronic diarrhea. The differential diagnosis of chronic diarrhea in infancy comprises numerous conditions, especially infectious etiologies, which are beyond the scope of this review. However, food-associated chronic diarrheas are important considerations, once some of the more common etiologies have been eliminated by the initial evaluation. A variety of syndromes have been characterized in which diarrhea is often a major component.

Food Protein-Induced Enterocolitis. Enterocolitis induced by food protein is most frequently seen as adverse reaction to cow's milk or soy protein formulas in young infants (22–33). Symptoms consist primarily of vomiting or diarrhea, or their combination, and generally develop within the first 3 months of life. Not uncommonly, the infant will present dehydrated and quite ill. Diarrheal stools usually contain blood and increased numbers of eosinophils and polymorphonuclear neutrophils (PMNs). A jejunal biopsy characteristically reveals flattened villi, edema, and increased numbers of lymphocytes, eosinophils, and mast cells. Elimination of cow's milk or soy from the diet frequently results in resolution of symptoms within 72 hr. Vomiting or diarrhea generally occur within 1 to several hours after ingesting the offending food, but rarely may be delayed for as long as 20 hr (34). Serum antibody titers to the offending antigen may increase in response to the milk challenge (35), and there is an increase in the number of IgA- and IgM-containing cells in the jejunal mucosa (25,27,29,36). Secondary disaccharidase deficiency is not uncommon, presumably because of damage to the intestinal mucosa (33,37).

Food-Induced Colitis Syndrome. The syndrome of food-induced colitis is also most commonly due to adverse reactions to cow's milk or soy protein formulas, but involves primarily the colon, rather than upper small bowel (32,38–41). Similar to infants with the enterocolitis syndrome, these infants may present in the first 3 months of life with diarrhea, but generally do not appear ill. They are frequently detected because of the presence of gross or occult blood in the stool and, in many cases, these infants have no other evidence of bowel disease. Hematochezia usually clears within 72 hr of eliminating the offending food, but the length of time required for resolution of mucosal findings is highly variable and may take up to 1 month (32). Sigmoidoscopy will reveal mild patchy injection of the mucosa to severe friability with small aphthoid ulcerations. Colonic biopsy reveals infiltration of eosinophils within the lamina propria and into the surface and crypt epithelia (42). In severe cases with crypt destruction, PMNs were also prominent.

Food-Induced Malabsorption Syndrome (Excluding Celiac Disease). Malabsorption induced by food may present in the first several months of life with poor weight gain and diarrhea and, not infrequently, steatorrhea (24). Most infants will have some vomiting, and about 20% are reported to have atopic dermatitis and recurrent respiratory infections. Laboratory studies frequently reveal elevated serum IgA concentrations and elevated levels of IgG antibodies to cow's milk proteins. Endoscopy and intestinal biopsy reveal patchy villous atrophy, with a prominent mononuclear round cell infiltrate of the epithelium and lamina propria and some eosinophils, not unlike celiac disease, but generally less severe (43). Elimination of cow's milk (soy, egg, and wheat are also implicated) leads to resolution of clinical symptoms within days to several weeks and complete normalization of intestinal mucosa in 0.5–1.5 years.

Gluten-Sensitive Enteropathy. Also known as celiac disease, this enteropathy is the best-studied form of malabsorption syndrome. It is a mucosal disease of the small intestine, precipitated in susceptible individuals by gliadin, the alcohol-soluble portion of gluten found in wheat, oats, rye, and barley. Diarrhea, or frank steatorrhea, growth failure in children, abdominal distension or flatulence, malaise, and irritability are the most common forms of presentation. Mouth ulcers and a variety of extraintestinal manifestations, primarily secondary to malabsorption, are not infrequent. In some children, the diarrhea is not impressive, but they fail to thrive. Occasionally, the weakness and poor growth is reminiscent of neuromuscular disease. In patients with untreated celiac disease, intestinal biopsy reveals subtotal or total villous atrophy, with marked increase in intraepithelial lymphocytes. This disease itself has occupied volumes, and a complete review here is not possible, but the interested physician may profitably review several of the cited references on this subject (44–48).

Allergic Eosinophilic Gastroenteritis. A rare form of enteropathy, allergic eosinophilic gastroenteritis may present in the infant as abdominal pain, vomiting, diarrhea, and failure to thrive (49–53). In the mucosal form, patients often have atopic disease, elevated serum IgE, positive skin-prick tests to a variety of foods, and peripheral eosinophilia. Clinical symptoms correlate with the extent of eosinophil infiltration of the bowel wall. Infiltration of the mucosal layer corresponds to a syndrome of malabsorption, whereas infiltration of the muscular layer presents a clinical picture of obstruction. Rarely, infants with this syndrome may present with pyloric stenosis and outlet obstruction (54) or severe protein-losing enteropathy with generalized edema (55).

Food-Induced Pulmonary Hemosiderosis. Also called Heiner's syndrome, this is a rare disorder characterized by recurrent episodes of pneumonia associated with pulmonary infiltrates, hemosiderosis, anemia, and failure to thrive (56–58). These infants tend to have high precipitin titers to several cow's milk proteins. In other studies of patients with this syndrome, deposits of IgG, IgA, and C3 have been identified in lung biopsy material (59). Both antigen–antibody complexes and lymphocyte-mediated hypersensitivity responses to milk are postulated in the immunopathogenesis of this disorder. However, this is based primarily on the presence of elevated serum levels of milk-specific IgG antibodies and the in vitro proliferative response of patient lymphocytes to milk antigen.

Other Syndromes. Another more subtle condition appears in children with large volumes of milk intake, in whom protein and blood loss in the stool, anemia, and sometimes failure to thrive occur (60,61). The studies cited concerning this condition suffer from a lack of immunological data and do not explore the mechanism whereby the food produces the symptoms; thus, there is substantial data missing, the presence of which might enable more specific classifications of these "syndromes." There is one study that did examine biopsy specimens in children with the iron deficiency and protein loss syndromes. It did not find immunological changes like those found in protein enteropathy, suggesting that hypersensitivity is not involved in this syndrome (62).

A final and common, albeit unexplained, cause of chronic diarrhea, especially in the second year of life, is diarrhea associated with fruit juice ingestion. Along with the infectious diarrheas, this seems to be one of the most common causes of diarrhea in young children (19). Removal of fruit from the diet results in complete resolution of the symptoms. This adverse reaction usually does not persist, and small amounts of juice and fruit may often be immediately reintroduced into the diet. In the 1950s, oil in the peel of orange was felt to be toxic to the intestines of young children (63). More recently, Hyams and associates have proposed and demonstrated that malabsorption of natural carbohydrates may be the responsible mechanism (64,65).

Cutaneous

Cutaneous signs and symptoms are the other most common presentations of food hypersensitivity (see Table 1).

Urticaria Urticaria of abrupt onset and usually lasting only hours is common in young children with food hypersensitivity and may be rather dramatic. The urticaria may be accompanied by angioedema.

Recurring outbreaks of urticaria are uncommon, unless the offending food is eaten frequently. The urticaria may be triggered by ingestion, by contact, or by both. *Chronic* urticaria is rarely seen in children younger than 2 years of age and is rarely due to food hypersensitivity.

Atopic Dermatitis By contrast, atopic dermatitis is very common in children younger than 2 years of age, and 60% of individuals developing atopic dermatitis will do so in the first year of life. At times, it presents a severe management problem. Atopic dermatitis is usually characterized by extreme pruritus, but occasionally in very young children, it seems not to itch or otherwise disrupt their apparent well-being. The rash is usually an erythematous, papulovesicular eruption, often with crusting. It may progress to scaling and lichenification, but it is not unusual for infants, even with severe involvement, to experience complete resolution without detectable stigmata of the skin disease. In infancy, the rash is often distributed initially over the cheeks, neck, and extensor surfaces. With age, the flexor surfaces become more involved, with less eruption on the face. Much of the skin alteration seen by the physician is due to excoriation; in fact, atopic dermatitis has no primary skin lesion, but is identified by a constellation of symptoms (66,67). The incidence of atopic dermatitis (with or without food hypersensitivity) has apparently been increasing over the past 40 years, and it is now estimated to affect 10–12% of children (68).

The intensity of the evaluation of the young child with atopic dermatitis depends upon the severity and extent of involvement of the skin. In the mild situation in which few areas of the body are slightly involved, the history may be used as a guide to the initial plan recommended by the physician. If the mother or caretaker does not suspect any food to be causing an exacerbation of symptoms, then the youngster may be treated with topical medication; if the skin responds promptly to minimal medication, further evaluation may be unnecessary and not cost-effective.

At the opposite end of the spectrum is the youngster with severe and generalized skin involvement. A food hypersensitivity evaluation may be helpful, even in the absence of any history of foods suspected of causing a reaction. At least 30–35% of these severely affected children may be expected to have food hypersensitivity (21). Conversely a significant number will not have detectable food hypersensitivity; hence, the evaluation must be cost-effective in terms of expense and also the degree of dietary manipulation required of the family. Although firm rules cannot be proposed from the existing data, some suggestions may be helpful. When specific foods are suspected, skin testing for those foods may be undertaken. Given the results, the physician may suggest pursuit of an elimination diet or elect to postpone dietary manipulation and attempt topical measures to determine the response.

In circumstances in which no foods are suspected, skin tests could be undertaken for the food allergens known to be most likely to exacerbate atopic dermatitis (egg, milk, peanut, wheat, soy). Alternatively, the child may be placed on a strict elimination diet or an elemental diet for a few days. In our experience, when food hypersensitivity is a part of the problem, a very limited diet often makes the skin much easier to manage and less medication is required. When a child presents with very severe atopic dermatitis that may include infected skin, it is often necessary to make multiple changes concurrently and then determine the effective ones as the evaluation proceeds. For example, to control severely involved skin, it may be necessary to apply aggressive topical skin treatment (wet wraps over steroid cream), oral antibiotics, and an elimination diet. Then as the skin improves, the important components of the management may be identified. As discussed elsewhere in this chapter, we have found the elemental formulas to be very helpful in managing these youngsters.

The breast-feeding mother presents a particular challenge because it is often difficult to provide a nutritionally adequate diet to both mother and baby if many food groups are eliminated from the mother's diet. Occasionally, we have had to ask the mother to discontinue breast-feeding for a few days while the elemental formula is used. During this time the mother will need to use a breast pump to maintain her comfort and assure her milk supply so that breast-feeding can be reintroduced when appropriate. If the baby shows substantial skin improvement while on the elemental diet, then foods in the mother's diet may be suspected and eliminated if documented to cause repeat exacerbations; if not, then breast-feeding may be reintroduced and the mother does not have to worry about limiting her own diet.

Other Dermatoses. Less specific dermatoses have been noted in youngsters with food hypersensitivity, including erythema that does not have a pattern typical of either urticaria or atopic dermatitis and is not accompanied by a discrete eruption. The mechanism of these reactions is unclear; however, they are often closely associated with the presence of IgE, as detected by skin testing or radioallergosorbent test (RAST) (3).

Finally, it is extremely common for cutaneous and gastrointestinal manifestations to occur simultaneously, especially in infancy (19).

Respiratory

In infancy, respiratory tract symptoms (see Table 1), either as the sole manifestation of an adverse reaction to food or in concert with other manifestations, are much less common than cutaneous and gastrointestinal symptoms, yet respiratory symptoms are frequently attributed to foods (19). In the first 2 years of life, upper respiratory tract symptoms, particularly continuous rhinorrhea, or nasal airway congestion, are common childhood problems. However, the frequency with which these symptoms have been proved to be caused by foods is quite low. Several different studies have sought to attribute upper respiratory tract manifestations, including chronic rhinitis, rhinorrhea, and otitis media, to food hypersensitivity. Even in situations in which youngsters with these conditions are sensitized to foods identified by skin testing, elimination of foods from the diet and challenge to the foods have not regularly reproduced the incriminated respiratory symptoms (4,19). Examination of the data from the major centers studying food hypersensitivity in numerous children shows that the occurrence of upper respiratory tract symptoms caused by foods is much less common than either cutaneous or gastrointestinal symptoms (3,4,19–21,69–73). Moreover, respiratory tract symptoms typically are acute, rather than chronic, when triggered by foods (19–21,69–73).

Occasionally, when children have significant cutaneous and gastrointestinal manifestations of food hypersensitivity, they will also exhibit ocular signs and symptoms, including tearing and swelling of both the conjunctiva and the upper and lower eyelids. At times, these symptoms are accompanied by profuse rhinorrhea and sneezing. Contact reactions may also produce ocular symptoms. For example, youngsters who have milk hypersensitivity and in whom milk comes in contact with the eye exhibit very impressive ocular swelling, chemosis, and eyelid edema. This has also been noted with contact from eggs, various nuts, and peanuts.

As with upper respiratory tract symptoms, those of the lower respiratory tract, including cough, wheezing, breathlessness, "bronchitis," and bronchospasm, have been reported as manifestations of adverse food reactions. Perusal of the studies of several authors who have sought wheezing and asthma as manifestations of food hypersensitivity in young children have shown this to be an uncommon event (3,4,19,20,69–74). However, although wheezing in a child younger than 2 years of age usually occurs secondary to viral infections, acute wheezing may occasionally be due to food hypersensitivity. As a result, food hypersensitivity should be considered as a possible cause of intermittent acute and brief wheezing in infancy. Nevertheless, it is highly unlikely that wheezing will be the sole manifestation of food hypersensitivity. Furthermore, the connection between the food ingestion and the onset of wheezing is likely to be obvious, and the time between ingestion and onset of wheezing will almost always be brief.

Behavioral

It is often frustrating for parents and primary care practitioners to try to help fussy, unhappy, sleepless, "colicky" infants younger than 2 years of age who are unable to communicate their discomfort. It would certainly be attractive to find that most of these youngsters did have food hypersensitivity. Studies examining colic in young children have shown promising responses to food elimination in a few subjects (75–78). These studies have been faulted for methodological errors, but the weight of the evidence supports improvement in some children. One study of sleep disturbance in children, using double-blind, placebo-controlled food challenge, supports the contention that a few sleepless infants will experience improvement of their sleep disturbance if milk is removed from the diet (79). This study needs to be confirmed by other investigators. Removal of foods from the diet or feeding the infant an elimination diet for a few days should identify those youngsters in whom food is affecting sleep. It is not recommended that youngsters with these symptoms be placed on prolonged elimination or elemental diets. When more is learned about the biochemical mechanisms of food hypersensitivity, it may be possible to predict more precisely which of these infants with sleep disturbances would benefit from a food elimination diet.

Anaphylaxis

Fortunately, anaphylaxis in infancy caused by foods, or from any other cause, is extremely rare; however, when it occurs, it is potentially catastrophic. When an infant presents with cardiovascular collapse, it is often difficult to immediately identify food as a possible inciting factor. Most of these children will exhibit pallor and lethargy. Epinephrine administration under these circumstances is essential. Moreover, it is mandatory that the physician attempt to measure blood pressure; emergency rooms where infants are seen should have infant blood pressure-monitoring devices. If the youngster's blood pressure is below normal, then prompt administration of intravenous fluids may be crucial and lifesaving. Laryngospasm does occur in these youngsters, but the cardiovascular alterations pose the more prominent and probably more difficult problem to treat. Fortunately, fatalities in this aged group, even in situations when anaphylaxis has been precipitated, are exceedingly rare (80).

Timing

Prompt Onset

Currently, most research in food hypersensitivity in infancy suggests that most symptoms occur promptly after the ingestion of the food (Table 2). In fact, most youngsters will react within 2 hr and often within a few minutes, of ingestion of the food. All the aforementioned symptoms will usually be characterized by their prompt onset and fairly rapid disappearance.

Delayed Onset

Children younger than 2 years are also the group in whom delayed onset or late onset symptoms have been demonstrated by controlled challenge. In some of these infants, particularly those with atopic dermatitis, there is an immediate onset of symptoms, with prolongation of the eruption. Research in progress is demonstrating that this eruption has the characteristics of the late-phase reaction that has been well demonstrated in older patients with allergic rhinitis and asthma after challenges with inhalant allergens and occupational exposures. Young children may exhibit the delayed-onset chronic diarrhea patterns that have been well shown to be initiated by the gliadin fraction of wheat gluten, cow milk protein, and soy protein. It is characteristic of the protein enteropathies that it may take several days for the symptoms to begin and also several days for the diarrhea to resolve, once the food is removed from the diet. It is also important to know that soy protein and cow milk protein enteropathies are self-limited illnesses of young children; rarely, does one find these conditions in older children. In contrast, gluten-sensitive enteropathy is a lifelong disease, and there is data that the failure of patients to adhere to their gluten-free diet could result in chronic bowel problems and malignancy later in life.

Specific Foods

During the early years of life the list of foods demonstrated to elicit symptoms (Table 3) expands as the diversity of the diet widens. Ini-

Table 2 Onset of Reactions Observed During DBPCFC[a]

Many reactions within minutes
Most reactions within 2 hr
Rare IgE-mediated reactions over 2 hr
Non–IgE-mediated reactions (gastroenteritis) hours to days

[a]DBPCFC, double-blind, placebo-controlled food challenge.

Table 3 Foods Proved to Cause Food Hypersensitivity

Egg, peanut, milk, soy, wheat (80–85%)
Tree nuts, fish, shellfish (10%)
Pea, chicken, turkey, banana, other grains, other vegetables
Fruits and juice (especially in small children, non-IgE)
(Corn and chocolate *rarely* confirmed food villains)

tially, the incriminated foods are usually formulas composed of cow's milk and soy. Foods tend to be added to the diet of American children in a fairly predictable fashion, with grains and fruits added to the diet in the latter part of the first year. By the second birthday, most American children have a fairly diverse diet and, therefore, almost any food that might be ingested will have been included as a putative culprit. In one study for which foods were tabulated, the list of incriminated foods included milk, egg, soy, peanut, chocolate, corn, rice, wheat, and a multitude of fruit and fruit juices, with orange, tomato, and apple being the most frequently suspected (19).

In contrast with this list of incriminated foods, the list of foods shown by double-blind placebo-controlled food challenge to be responsible for the production of any of the symptoms discussed in the foregoing is much shorter. Examination of several studies using double-blind placebo-controlled food challenges to confirm histories in children younger than age two has shown that the offenders are milk, egg, peanut, soy, and wheat, in over 80% of children. Although other foods have produced reactions in this aged group, they are much less common, and two popular culprits, chocolate and corn, rarely cause food reactions (3,4,17,19–21,71–74,80).

Foods that pass through breast milk may assume importance in this age group. There is as yet no evidence that infants have ever reacted to proteins produced by the mother. By contrast, there are numerous reports of youngsters reacting to proteins *ingested* by their mothers (81–83). With the results of well-controlled studies as a basis for examination of this question, the major foods responsible for producing symptoms when passed through the breast milk are egg, milk, peanut, and soy. It has been most interesting to find that symptoms may be produced rapidly in the infant who nurses following maternal ingestion of the food protein. It would appear that as little as 15 minutes is sufficient to allow maternal absorption of peanut protein, passage into the breast milk, and then into the infant upon breast-feeding, which leads to a prompt onset of symptoms (Bock, SA, unpublished observation).

PATHOGENESIS AND IMMUNOLOGY

Differential Diagnosis

The differential diagnosis of food hypersensitivity includes several categories (Table 4). Probably the most common cause of adverse reactions to foods in North America, and a very common cause of adverse food reactions in young children, is carbohydrate intolerance. For most children younger than 2 years, the most important carbohydrate intolerance is lactase deficiency, leading to lactose intolerance. This usually occurs following a gastroenteritis, when there is damage to the brush border enzyme-producing apparatus, leading to a secondary deficiency of lactase. The problem is transient, but in some youngsters, does require the administration of a disaccharide-free formula for a time. Sucrase–isomaltase deficiency, which is much less common, also occurs in this aged group. In youngsters with chronic diarrhea, especially following gastroenteritis, the possibility of carbohydrate intolerance should be considered.

Toxic reactions from materials in infant foods have been reported. At the time this chapter was written there had recently been substantial public concern about the pesticide Alar contaminating children's apple juice. (This proved to be of little consequence.) Some of these intoxications are natural and others are due to contamination of food, as mentioned earlier in this chapter.

One of the most common causes of putative adverse food reactions are strongly held beliefs influencing feeding patterns. Observations associating the coincidental onset of symptoms with the administration of new foods is all too common in North America. Fads in feeding habits and the influence of "alternative practitioners" also have a significant influence in this area. Suffice to say that many primary care physicians will be confronted with dietary alterations that have been made because symptoms have been attributed to observations that have not been confirmed through objective challenge.

Table 4 Differential Diagnosis of Adverse Reaction To Foods

Deficiencies of intestinal enzymes (disaccharides)
Hypersensitivity/allergy (immunological)
Psychological (strongly held beliefs)
Noxious natural constituents (poisons)
Contaminants (microorganism, parasites, toxins, and chemicals)

Hypersensitivity or allergic mechanisms constitute the major mechanism and differential diagnostic category to which this chapter is devoted. In immunology over the past couple of decades, it has been common to consider hypersensitivity disorders in terms of the Gell and Coombs classification (types I, II, III, IV; 84). Although this classification system has been extremely useful for categorizing and investigating hypersensitivity reactions, it now seems likely that most hypersensitivity reactions involve more than one type of Gell and Coombs mechanism, since present knowledge suggests that most hypersensitivity reactions involve humoral and cellular components of the immune–inflammatory system.

Immunologic Mechanisms

Immunoglobulin E-Mediated Reactions

Immunoglobulin E-mediated hypersensitivity is the immune mechanism (Table 5) most strongly associated with adverse reactions to foods in young children. A reasonably pure example of an IgE-mediated reaction with mediators being released from tissue mast cells is the immediate hypersensitivity skin test. When a food protein (allergen) is placed into the skin, there is cross-linking between IgE molecules that are bound to cell membranes by high-affinity Fcε receptors. Ensuing

Table 5 Proposed Immune-Mediated Adverse Food Reactions in Infants

Type I: IgE-mediated	
Cutaneous	Urticaria/Angioedema, atopic dermatitis
Respiratory	Rhinoconjunctivitis, asthma
Gastrointestinal	GI anaphylaxis (nausea, colic, vomiting, diarrhea), infantile colic, allergic eosinophilic gastroenteritis, ? food-induced enterocolitis syndrome
Type III: Antigen–antibody complexes	
? Food-induced enterocolitis syndrome	
? Food-induced colitis syndrome	
? Food-induced malabsorption syndrome	
? Celiac disease	
? Food-induced pulmonary hemosiderosis	
Type IV: Cell-mediated hypersensitivity	
Celiac disease	
? Food-induced enterocolitis syndrome	
? Food-induced colitis syndrome	
? Food-induced malabsorption syndrome	
? Food-induced pulmonary hemosiderosis	

membrane and cellular interactions result in immediate release of histamine as well as other preformed mediators. The histamine is responsible for the wheal-and-flare reaction through vasodilatation and fluid leakage from blood vessels. The importance of other mediators, both preformed and those produced after cellular activation, are under intense investigation to determine their role in both the immediate and late-phase reaction. We should probably adopt the notion that IgE is necessary but not sufficient to produce these responses.

Immunoglobulin E-Mediated Cutaneous Late-Phase Reaction

It has now been repeatedly shown that the reaction just described is only the first part of the role IgE plays in a sequence of events that are termed the late-phase reaction. Within 2–4 hr after the immediate reaction, the late-phase changes begin, with an influx of neutrophils and eosinophils. The cellular influx is promoted by neutrophil and eosinophil chemotactic factors released from mast cells, endothelial cells, and probably other sources. The response is then protracted owing to the presence and ongoing production of all the recently described mediators of inflammation—platelet activating factor (PAF), prostaglandins, leukotrienes, major basic protein and eosinophilic cationic protein (both from eosinophils), oxygen free radical metabolites, and others. After 6–8 hr, the cellular infiltrate contains preponderantly mononuclear cells and eosinophils, with smaller numbers of neutrophils, basophils, and mast cells. Later biopsies, between 24–48 hr, detect a mononuclear cell infiltrate that appears identical with the classic type IV cell-mediated response (85–88).

The eosinophil has now been incriminated in the pathophysiology of atopic dermatitis owing to the detection of major basic protein, the major protein of eosinophilic granules, in active eczematous lesions. The major basic protein is able to damage skin epithelial cells and promote further mast cell degranulation (89).

Non–Immunoglobulin E-Mediated Reactions

There are some well-documented adverse reactions to foods which appear to involve the immune system and are either not IgE-mediated or IgE is only a limited component in the production of the symptoms. The protein enteropathies were mentioned earlier and include milk, soy, and gluten-sensitive enteropathies (celiac disease).

The histological characteristic of the protein enteropathies is a flattening of the intestinal mucosa. This appears to occur because of the rapid turnover of the upper layers of epithelial cells. The reproducing crypt cells are unable to replace the lost villous mucosal epithelial cells rapidly enough. There is still debate concerning the exact manner in which the immune system participates in the production of this lesion. The reason that this lesion is transient for milk and soy proteins, but is lifelong for gluten protein, is unknown (44–48).

The presence of increased IgG antibodies to cow's milk (or soy) compared with normal controls has led some to speculate that a type III hypersensitivity mechanism is responsible for this disorder. Others have suggested a type IV mechanism based upon the presence of increased lymphocyte proliferation in vitro in most patients with this disorder (26). Skin-prick test and RAST are generally negative in affected infants. However, in investigating two infants with this syndrome, Shiner et al. found increased mucosal IgE-containing plasma cells and degranulation of mast cells in response to milk challenge, along with deposition of IgG and C3 in intestinal connective tissue and basement membrane (90). More recently, Nolte demonstrated histamine release in response to milk antigen from dispersed intestinal mast cells of infants with this disorder (91). Taken together, these studies suggest a localized IgE-mediated mechanism may be, in part, responsible for this disorder.

In infants with the food-induced colitis syndrome, an oral challenge with the offending antigen will induce symptoms within hours to a few days. Sigmoidoscopy reveals an acute colitis. Histopathologically, glandular and epithelial architecture appear intact, with PMNs and eosinophils infiltrating the lamina propria. Both type III and type IV hypersensitivities are suggested as pathologic mechanisms because of increased serum antibodies, lymphocyte proliferative responses, and presence of activated T lymphocytes to food antigens (92).

Both type III and type IV hypersensitivity mechanisms are suggested in the etiology of the food-induced malabsorption syndrome, but no clear immunological mechanisms have been demonstrated. Morphological evidence and information generated in experimental animal models strongly implicates a type IV, cell-mediated mechanism in the pathogenesis of the intestinal lesion in celiac disease (92,93). However, experimental evidence in some patients and rodent models suggest that a cell-mediated response to gliadin alone is not sufficient for full expression of the enteropathy (94). Recent evidence suggests that a defect in mucosal digestion of gliadin in celiac patients may be responsible for the production of toxic peptides that contribute to the development of the intestinal lesion (95). Whether the elevated IgE and IgA antibodies to gliadin contribute to the pathogenesis of celiac disease is unclear. The increased levels of IgG-, IgA-, and IgM-containing immune complexes does not appear to correlate with disease activity in patients (96).

Studies of gluten-sensitive enteropathy have provided most of the available information about protein-induced malabsorption. The recommended procedure has involved placing the patient on a gluten-free diet, observing resolution of symptoms, performing a biopsy found to be normal, and performing a biopsy following a gluten challenge when the chronic diarrhea has returned. The α-gliaden fraction of gluten is clearly able to stimulate the immune system, as shown by the detection of antigliadin (or antireticulin) antibodies in patients who have the disease (97). Elegant organ culture studies undertaken by several investigators revealed that immunological interactions were significantly detectable at the time the abnormal histology was noted (44–46, 98, 99).

The role of IgE and atopy in general in the production of gluten-sensitive enteropathy has long been debated. A recent case-controlled study strongly suggests that there is no increased prevalence of atopy in subjects with gluten-sensitive enteropathy and their relatives compared with controls and their relatives. Despite some problems with precision in definition of terms, this is one of the best-controlled studies on this subject (100).

The immunopathogenetic mechanism(s) responsible for allergic eosinophilic gastroenteritis are unknown. A subset of patients have exacerbation of symptoms following the ingestion of food to which they have specific IgE antibodies, thus implicating a role for an IgE-mediated mechanism in some patients. Other evidence supporting this mechanism includes the presence of IgE-staining cells in jejunal tissue, elevated IgE in duodenal fluids, and the resolution of symptoms with removal of the implicated food from the diet (96). However, immune complex-mediated complement activation or lymphokine release from activated lymphocytes could also account for the massive influx of eosinophils into the bowel wall.

A rare and somewhat controversial syndrome is that of chronic lower respiratory tract disease associated with antibodies to cow's milk in the serum. This syndrome, known as Heiner's syndrome, has been reported with variable consistency. These infants exhibit pulmonary infiltrates and pulmonary hemosiderosis. They have been reported to present with anemia, failure to thrive, and chronic lung disease. Hemosiderin-laden macrophages have been found in gastric material aspirated from the stomach in the early morning and in lung biopsy specimens. The detection of precipitating antibodies to cow's milk led the original observers to remove cow's milk from the diet, after which they noticed a prompt improvement. Immunoglobulin E has not been shown to have any role in this condition. This illness would be better understood if a group of these youngsters were subjected to systematic and prolonged observation and study to determine the true role of the milk proteins. Case reports of this problem are so sporadic that it has been difficult to draw firm conclusions about the youngsters reported. The question also arises concerning the possibility that other food proteins might produce chronic pulmonary changes in youngsters with "idiopathic" lung diseases (56–59).

DIAGNOSIS

Laboratory

Skin Testing

Currently, the most useful laboratory test for identifying IgE-mediated food hypersensitivity in children of any age, including young children, is the prick/puncture skin test. Skin tests for foods have always had a bad reputation. This is primarily because of misinterpretation of skin testing and, therefore, a lack of understanding of the usefulness of the results. Skin tests merely detect antibody. This is true in any age, and it is true for any allergen. Skin test extracts must be verified—that is, they must be shown to detect antibody in those persons who have it, and they must be shown not to be nonspecifically irritating. This has been demonstrated to be true for foods often proved to cause symptoms. It has also frequently been said that skin testing in young children does not give useful information. On the contrary, several studies have shown that, beyond several months of age, skin tests have a high negative predictive accuracy. Skin testing for any food at any age has a lower positive predictive accuracy because of the ability of the skin test to detect the presence of antibody in patients in whom no symptoms occur when the food is ingested. This set of conditions—that is, the presence of IgE antibodies as detected by skin testing without concomitant symptoms during food ingestion—is properly termed *asymptomatic hypersensitivity*. These positive tests are not incorrect, nor are they "false-positive." Persons with IgE antibodies to foods detected by skin testing who have no symptoms upon ingestion of food may have marked symptoms that appear rapidly upon intravenous administration of the same food allergen. At present, the search continues for a test for food hypersensitivity with a higher positive predictive accuracy. Nevertheless, since there is such vast overdiagnosis of food "allergy" in our society, and since the negative skin test has a high negative predictive accuracy, it is a useful test for determining which patients are highly unlikely to have an IgE-mediated adverse reaction to food upon ingestion and, therefore, are unlikely to have food hypersensitivity (3,4,20,21,69–73,101–103).

Radioallergosorbent Testing

The radioallergosorbent test (RAST) is a most useful in vitro method for detection of IgE antibodies in the circulation. The major drawback to the RAST concerns its expense and the requirement for radioisotopes, especially in the use of the original test. A newer version of the RAST uses enzyme-linked immunosorbent assay (ELISA) technology for detection of the antibody. It is also important to note the vast laboratory differences in quality control of the in vitro specific IgE antibody tests, including the RAST. The RAST remains an excellent tool for research, but it cannot yet be recommended for regular clinical use. Both the RAST and skin testing are useful only for detecting IgE-mediated food hypersensitivity (103).

Mediator Levels

Measurement of circulating histamine levels has been undertaken following blinded food challenges. Elevated levels are demonstrable. Although useful for research purposes, measurement of blood histamine and other mediators released during food challenge cannot be recommended for routine clinical use (104).

Total Serum Immunoglobulin E

Measurement of serum immunoglobulins, particularly total IgE, has limited usefulness in this aged group. Unfortunately, total IgE measurements in any single person are not optimally predictive of the presence of symptomatic food or inhalant hypersensitivity. Because total IgE production is under strong genetic influence, it is quite common to find youngsters who have a high total IgE, with no detectable hypersensitivity. By the same token, it is not unusual to find youngsters with food or inhalant hypersensitivity who have normal total IgE measurements.

Intestinal Biopsy

Biopsy of the small bowel or colon for diagnosis of food protein-induced enteropathy or food protein-induced colitis is a test that should receive more attention. The true frequency of these illnesses is unknown, but it is probably underdiagnosed because of our reticence to undertake these biopsies in very young patients with chronic bowel symptoms. The chronic diarrheal syndromes, although transient, probably constitute the major source of non–IgE-mediated adverse reactions to foods that are likely to involve the immune system. Further study might illustrate the presence of IgE-mediated late-phase reactions in the intestines of such patients.

Food Challenge

The gold standard for identifying an adverse reaction to a food is the *double-blind, placebo-controlled food challenge* (DBPCFC). This procedure consists of administering the food to the infant or child in a blinded fashion so that all observers as well as the parent and patient are unaware of the contents of the challenge. Although this would seem an unnecessary step in children younger than 2 years of age, it must be remembered that parental observations in this aged group often lead to foods being eliminated from the diet because of a coincidental association between the ingestion of a food and the appearance of symptoms. For certain objective symptoms, such as vomiting, abrupt onset skin rashes, and some cases of diarrhea, the open administration of foods can be helpful in demonstrating the presence or absence of the adverse reaction. In particular, open challenges are useful for refuting histories of adverse reactions to foods. This is a particularly common finding in children younger than 2 years of age (19,105). The reason that blinded challenges are so important is that all of the studies cited that have used DBPCFC have found that 40–60% of the histories of adverse reaction cannot be confirmed. This makes history of adverse food reaction unacceptable as a tool for making an adequate diagnosis; thus, an unbiased test (DBPCFC) must be employed.

The DBPCFC is particularly easy to accomplish in youngsters younger than 2. Often the foods under suspicion are liquid (soy formula, cow's milk) that may easily be hidden in one of the available elemental formulas. The suspect food is given in incrementally increasing amounts until a reaction occurs or, if no symptoms are elicited, the food is returned to the diet in usual and customary portions. One should refer to a practical manual devised for the use of DBPCFC as an office procedure (105).

Food challenges utilized in non–IgE-mediated gastrointestinal food hypersensitivity are frequently modified, often eliminating the blinding and including a postchallenge bowel biopsy. In the cow's milk-induced enterocolitis syndrome, a challenge with milk (protein concentration up to 0.6 g/kg body weight) provokes adverse clinical manifestations, increased PMNs and eosinophils in the stool, peripheral leukocytosis 6–8 hr after milk ingestion, and villus atrophy of the duodenum and jejunum (33,106,107). Similar reactions may occur to soy protein (28,29,33,108,109), and up to 50% of patients sensitive to cow's milk will also react to soy protein, depending on the population under study (4,110).

Diagnosis of food-induced colitis similarly is dependent on an oral food challenge and postchallenge colonic biopsy to demonstrate the characteristic intestinal lesions, which may require 3–4 weeks to develop.

The diagnosis of the malabsorption syndrome is made by demonstrating biopsy evidence of small-intestinal mucosal injury, resolution with elimination of the responsible antigen from the diet, and recurrence of intestinal injury after challenge with the implicated antigen. Immunoglobulin A antibodies to gluten are present in over 80% of children with untreated celiac disease (111). In addition, patients with celiac disease frequently have high levels of IgG antibodies to a variety of foods, presumably reflecting their response to increased antigen absorption. Recently, measurement of intraepithelial lymphocytes within the rectal mucosa 6 hr after a rectal challenge with 2 g of a peptic–tryptic digest of gluten served as a simple, safe, and reliable test of gluten sensitivity. This test may obviate the need for oral gluten challenge, if confirmed by further studies (112).

TREATMENT

Avoidance

With young children in whom a definite diagnosis of food hypersensitivity has been made, two questions concerning treatment arise. First, is any treatment needed? Second, if treatment is needed what treatment should be applied? For some young children, the only adverse symptom they have to food is the repeated development of erythema or localized urticaria upon contact with that food. In these youngsters, no treatment need necessarily be prescribed as long as the rash that develops is merely an esthetic problem.

The major treatment for confirmed food hypersensitivity is manipulation of the diet so that the food culprit can be avoided, while still providing a nutritionally adequate diet. In infancy, food avoidance often means removal of one or more major foods, such as cow's milk or soy from the child's diet. In this situation, alternatives must be provided. When the youngster exhibits milk hypersensitivity, but can tolerate soy, then soy formula can be provided. On the other hand, when both foods have been incriminated, the child must be fed an elemental formula. Elemental formulas are nutritionally complete and, therefore, do not require additional dietary supplementation. Youngsters on a dairy product-free diet who are not receiving an alternative formula do need to have supplemental *calcium* in accordance with current dietary recommendations of elemental calcium (birth to 6 months = 360 mg; 6–12 months = 540 mg; 1–10 years = 800 mg). It is important to note that reactions to elemental diets are extremely rare, but have been reported, and should be suspected if the child appears not to tolerate the elemental diet (113–115).

In infants who are nursing, particularly during the first few months of life, maternal dietary manipulation may be required and must be done with care. Several dietary proteins rapidly cross into breast milk. If dairy products are removed from the mother's diet, it is crucial that her *calcium* intake be monitored; if it is insufficient, then supplementary calcium must be provided to a maximum of 1500 mg daily. Rarely, we have been confronted with a situation in which the maternal diet has been so limited that both the child and the mother are receiving inadequate nutrition. This is a circumstance that certainly must be avoided.

Medication

Several medications have been used to treat youngsters with adverse food reactions caused by food hypersensitivity. Studies of their efficacy have been either inadequately controlled or have shown the medications to be ineffective. Particularly in the infant-aged group, medication treatment is rarely required. Specifically, cromolyn sodium has not yet been shown to be effective in properly controlled studies for treatment of food hypersensitivity (116). Since an oral form of cromolyn is now available in the United States for treating mastocytosis, it may be tempting to try applying this treatment to youngsters who seem to have food hypersensitivity, especially if they seem to react to multiple foods. This temptation should be resisted, unless it can be shown that the drug is effective. In all cases, it must first be proved that the child has food hypersensitivity. The same comments and criticisms apply to the use of antihistamines in children with food hypersensitivity.

The immediate treatment of a patient experiencing an allergic reaction to a food is the same as the treatment for any other allergic reaction. During an acute allergic or anaphylactic reaction, the usual medical assessment measures include examination of airway patency, breathing effort, and circulatory status. The most immediate and important medication is epinephrine. In children younger than 2 years of age, a dose of 0.1–0.2 mL is appropriate. Some authors have recommended a per kilogram dose, but the dose is not really based upon controlled studies, and it is more important to quickly administer the medication and constantly monitor the child. Diphenhydramine given orally or intramuscularly may be given in addition to the epinephrine during the immediate reaction. Most often oral antihistamine is all that is required because the reaction is not life-threatening. For young children, a dosage of diphenhydramine of 5 mg/kg per day is recommended. This may be divided into four doses and continued until the reaction subsides. For the rare severe and prolonged reaction, the usual resuscitative measures should be employed, including intravenous support and ventilatory management if needed. In the rare patient with a reaction severe enough to require these tools, intravenous corticosteroids should be added to the program, realizing that they will require hours before they are of assistance.

There are rare diagnoses, such as secretory diarrheas and eosinophilic gastroenteritis, that may occur in infants and do require treatment with corticosteroids. In particular, severe eosinophilic gastroenteritis, which can be quite threatening to a youngster's health and nutrition, will respond dramatically to treatment with corticosteroids. The recommended starting dosage is 2 mg/kg per day and then, when the symptoms subside and eosinophilia has disappeared, the dose can be slowly tapered and discontinued. Usually the youngster's course can be monitored by following the peripheral eosinophil count.

Injection therapy for food hypersensitivity has never been shown in properly controlled trials to be effective in any-aged patient. Injections have been inflicted by a number of different techniques, but none have been shown to be efficacious. There is no justification whatever for giving allergy injections for foods to infants. Any use of allergy injection treatment should be viewed as experimental and should be administered only under properly supervised protocols.

NATURAL HISTORY AND PROGNOSIS

The natural history of food hypersensitivity (Tables 6–8) has two components: the development of the symptoms caused by food and the loss of the reactivity. The former subject is covered in Chapter 19 and the latter in Chapter 20. Several studies over the years have demonstrated that children with DBPCFC-proved food hypersensitivity do lose their

Table 6 Managing the Child Presenting With Adverse Food Reaction[a]

Eliminate food(s), use elimination diet to see if symptoms resolve.
Reintroduce foods in small amounts to see if tolerated or if reaction.
Rechallenge suspected foods at regular intervals.
Arrange for blinded food challenge if problem persists.

[a]**This approach is not for anaphylaxis or severe reactions.**

Table 7 Some Conclusions Based on Natural History Studies

Prolonged elimination of most foods is unnecessary, regular confirmation is important.
Cross-reactions between food families are rare—each food stands alone.
Food reactions may be lost at the rate of about 25% a year for foods listed.
Positive skin tests may persist for years, despite lack of symptoms during ingestion.
Life-threatening (anaphylactic) reactions in young children may be outgrown (egg, milk, soy); less likely in older children.

Table 8 Natural History of Food Allergy

Egg, milk, soy, and wheat likely to stop producing symptoms
Peanut and tree nuts unlikely to stop producing symptoms
Fish and shellfish probably unlikely to stop (little data in children)
Fruit and fruit juice: non–IgE-mediated reactions very likely to remit
Other grains and less common foods: little data available

reactivity with time (117–120). Particular predictable patterns of loss of symptoms are becoming clear from the studies. It is important to begin with children in whom DBPCFC have been used to prove that the problem exists so that the data upon which conclusions are drawn have validity. In studies for which this precaution is not followed, the results are often similar, but more difficult to interpret, because the initial status of the subjects is not known with certainty (121,122).

Loss of clinical reactivity appears to be more rapid in proximity to the initial diagnosis. Up to one-third of children will "lose" their clinical sensitivity over the first 1–3 years, and then a slower rate of resolution occurs thereafter. Hypersensitivity to milk, egg, soy, and wheat are more likely to disappear, whereas reactivity to peanut seems to persist indefinitely in many children. Problems with other nuts and fish are less troublesome in infants in whom these foods are usually withheld. Even in children in whom reactions are severe, loss of anaphylactic reactivity may be observed over time (80). These comments apply to children in whom DBPCFC has been found to be positive and in whom IgE has been implicated in the pathogenesis. In infants in whom adverse reactions can be documented, but in whom no mechanism has been found, the loss of clinical reactivity may occur even more quickly (19). However, all the studies in which IgE is detected show its presence remains detectable long after clinical reactivity may have disappeared. Thus, skin testing may not be used to determine whether or not clinical symptoms persist over time.

These observations have led to the development of recommendations for regular reintroduction of foods that produce reactions into the diet of food-allergic children (see Table 6). Although there is not universal agreement amongst investigators, the following guidelines may be helpful for the management of children who *do not* exhibit life-threatening food-allergic symptoms. In children between the age of 1 and 2 years in whom reactions to milk have occurred, reintroduction could be undertaken every 3–6 months. For soy and wheat the interval could be every 1–6 months, depending on the character and severity of the preceding reaction. If a reaction to peanut occurs during the first 2 years and the association between peanut and the symptoms makes peanut the likely culprit, then peanut should be avoided until after the third birthday. The same recommendation should be followed for egg, tree nuts (e.g., almonds, pecans, and walnuts), shellfish, and fish. For other foods little or no data exist and, consequently, useful recommendations are harder to evaluate. The recommended intervals may be altered by observations during accidental ingestion or particular concerns of parents, such as likely exposure to incriminated foods in day care settings (19,117–120).

VACCINE ADMINISTRATION IN EGG HYPERSENSITIVE CHILDREN

A significant problem for primary care practitioners caring for infants is the administration of measles, mumps, and rubella vaccine (MMR), and influenza vaccine in egg-allergic children. Both of these vaccines were grown in avian embryos and contained measurable amounts of egg protein (123), but MMR constituents are now grown on chicken embryo fibroblasts, and contain virtually no egg protein. Nevertheless, controversy remains about the safest manner in which to screen egg-allergic patients and how to administer the vaccine. The American Academy of Pediatrics makes specific recommendations for skin testing in a rather cumbersome 3-step procedure and then for administration of the vaccine if the skin test is positive (124). Several recent studies using MMR vaccine (125–128) and influenza vaccine (129) have tested variations of the "official" recommendations. Each of these studies has suffered from one main fault and a few minor ones. The major fault has been the absence of DBPCFC-proved egg hypersensitivity at the time of evaluation, with reliance instead upon history of egg-induced symptoms and egg skin tests. The reader of this chapter will, by now, realize the potential pitfalls of basing conclusions upon history and skin tests in the absence of DBPCFC. Since severe reactions to the small amount of egg in these vaccines is rare, even in egg-allergic children, studies of this nature require many patients to provide accurate conclusions. The study of Lavi (128) best supports the recommendations of the American Academy of Pediatrics.

The authors of this chapter each have experience with administration of MMR vaccine in children with DBPCFC-proved egg hypersensitivity. One of us has used prick or puncture skin testing with undiluted vaccine in proved egg-allergic children. In the absence of a positive skin test, the vaccine has been given in a single dose, and the patient observed for 1 hr. In the presence of a positive skin test, the vaccine is given in four doses of about 0.125 mL each. Thus far no systemic reactions have occurred in any of these children (Bock SA, unpublished observations). Unfortunately, the numbers are too small to rule out the possibility of an observation such as that described by Lavi et al. One of their three patients having a systemic reaction to MMR had only urticaria, by history, when ingesting egg, and the skin test was positive only by intradermal skin testing with diluted vaccine.

On the other hand, the other author (HAS) has a somewhat different approach to administering MMR to egg-allergic patients whose symptoms caused by egg ingestion were confirmed by DBPCFC. Three lines of evidence suggest that the MMR currently available is safe for use in children allergic to eggs. One hundred forty children with egg allergy, documented by DBPCFC, have been immunized with vaccine without difficulty. Of this group, 60 were prick skin tested with full-strength MMR and only 2 were considered positive (mean wheal diameter > 3 mm), and 5 demonstrated erythema only. Initially, intradermal skin testing was performed with 0.02–0.03 mL of MMR vaccine (1:100 dilution) before immunization. However, this practice was discontinued because it provoked sharp burning pain in most patients and controls and was found to yield many false-positive responses. Second, two patients were identified who had anaphylactic reactions to MMR. Neither patient had a history of egg hypersensitivity, prick skin test positivity to egg, nor evidence of egg-specific IgE antibodies. Finally, the MMR vaccine was analyzed with sensitive ELISAs capable of detecting picogram quantities of ovalbumin. This analysis indicated that less than 50 pg/dose of immunologically recognizable ovalbumin was present, a quantity unlikely to provoke any response. Given these observations, it seems unlikely that egg-allergic children are at any greater risk of anaphylaxis from MMR than the general population (130).

One must conclude that precautions must be taken when administering egg-containing vaccines to egg-allergic youngsters because there are rare children who may have systemic reactions to the vaccine. The administration of these vaccines should be undertaken only by personnel familiar with treatment of acute allergic reactions. However, the current recommendations are cumbersome and, if followed exactly, produce a great deal of discomfort in the child being inoculated. Thus, further research in this area is needed to derive a more efficient and less painful procedure.

UNPROVED DIAGNOSTIC AND THERAPEUTIC PRACTICES

Tests

Over the last several decades there has been an evolution of testing methods that have no proved efficacy. These procedures have involved methods such as the cytotoxic food test, including the "new" automated ALCAT, dilution neutralization skin testing, and sublingual testing. For the most part, these methods have not been applied to infants; however, the cytotoxic food test has been used in children of all ages. Since this test has generally become debunked, it has been replaced by ever more sophisticated, but equally unsubstantiated, methods. The latest testing methods involve measurements of circulating antibodies of the IgG4 subclass or measurement of "food immune complexes." Although these tests do measure the presence of antibody, and of immune complexes, they suffer from having never been correlated with double-blind, placebo-controlled food challenges. Therefore, almost all the claims made for the test are based merely on the detection of circulating antibodies and cannot be relied on to diagnose food hypersensitivity (131). These tests should be used only in experimental situations until their efficacy (or lack thereof) can be demonstrated. In the meantime, extravagant claims based upon their use should be countered by reference to the absence of application of the scientific method. Even in infants, observations may be subject to the placebo effect.

Diets

Over the years, several diets have been popularized for use in children with food hypersensitivity. Rarely, are these diets applied to children younger than 2 years of age. However, readers should be aware of their availability and, in certain areas of the country, enthusiasm for these diets does extend to young children. The most well-known of these is the so-called rotary or rotary-diversified diet. Since most young children with food hypersensitivity have a self-limited course, as pointed out in an earlier section, the application of any diet that tends to keep foods out of the diet, or maintains quantities at a minimum, is likely to appear efficacious. At this time, these diets should be considered experimental and should not be used for the treatment of true food hypersensitivity.

As discussed in Chapter 23, hypoallergenic formulas may be used in an attempt to prevent milk allergy and some atopic symptoms. In addition, formulas meeting the Food and Drug Administration (FDA) recommended definition of *hypoallergenic* may be used to treat almost all milk-allergic patients. To be approved as hypoallergenic, a manufacturer needs to demonstrate with 95% confidence that 90% of subjects with milk allergy documented by DBPCFC will not react to a given formula. From this definition it is clear that some caution must be exercised when giving a highly sensitive infant a hypoallergenic formula. *Hypoallergenic* does not mean *nonallergenic*, and there may be the rare infant who reacts to a hypoallergenic formula (115). There are now four formulas available in the United States that appear to meet the definition of hypoallergenic (although none have yet received FDA approval): Alimentum (Ross Laboratories); Nutramigen and Pregestemil (Mead Johnson), casein hydrolysates; and Neocate (Scientific Hospital Supplies), an elemental formula. Theoretically, Neocate should be the least allergenic, since it is formulated from amino acids, vitamins, and minerals to mimic the composition of human breast milk, whereas the hydrolysate formulas are generated from enzymatically degraded cow's milk casein. Tolerex (Vivonex) is a completely elemental formula that has been used as the sole source of nutrition in persons of all ages.

FUTURE CONSIDERATIONS

The critical reader of this chapter will be able to see several deficiencies in our current knowledge. The real prevalence of food-induced disease requires objective determination. The recent observation that cow's milk protein intolerance appears on the wane in Spain (possibly from the use of adapted formulas) is encouraging, but requires confirmation (132). More information about the pathogenesis of food hypersensitivity is certainly needed. There are several areas in which some preliminary data have been gathered, but further clarification is necessary, such as the importance of high spontaneous release of histamine and the role of histamine-releasing factors in food hypersensitivity (133,134). It is of great interest to investigators in this field to try to determine which biochemical mediators of inflammation are involved in food hypersensitivity, especially when compared with the biochemistry now unfolding from studies of allergic rhinitis and asthma. In particular, it would be most helpful if we could demonstrate the presence or absence of late-phase reactions in the pathogenesis of food hypersensitivity. Does atopic dermatitis have a late-phase component? Do protein enteropathies involve IgE and do they have a late-phase component? Does inflammation of the upper respiratory tract occur from food hypersensitivity with a greater frequency than has been identified?

Another area for which we need further understanding is that of non–IgE-mediated food hypersensitivity. Despite the great claims made about late and delayed food reactions and the involvement of foods in the production of arthritis, kidney disease, epilepsy, and migraine headache, there remains a great deal of anecdotal and testimonial information, with precious little confirmable science in this area. Understanding of the pathogenesis of "delayed" food reactions, if they exist, might improve our ability to diagnose and treat the conditions and to bring an end to some of the speculative diagnostic procedures and questionable treatments that are currently being prescribed, especially by alternative practitioners.

A major area in which important advances would be helpful is in the diagnosis of food hypersensitivity. The skin test is certainly a useful test, particularly for eliminating the probability of IgE-mediated food hypersensitivity. This is true in older children, and equally true in many infants. The RAST and ELISA remain useful as adjuncts in clinical diagnosis and as research procedures. The small-bowel biopsy, which has been mentioned in previous sections, can be extremely helpful, but in many centers there is resistance to undertaking small-bowel biopsies in young children for conditions that may be self-limited. Newer, noninvasive techniques and biochemical measurements that can be developed and obviate the use of the double-blind, placebo-controlled food challenge would certainly be welcome. In the meantime, more practitioners need to become skilled in the use of the double-blind food challenge, which is a technique that, after limited practice, becomes as routine as any other general office procedure. Certainly, we do not find this a cumbersome technique to apply for either routine clinical or for research purposes.

The area for which currently there is the least information is the relative merits of active pharmacologic prevention, as opposed to avoidance and reintroduction of foods into the diet. Certainly, for most children younger than 2 years of age, the latter is all that is needed because of the self-limited nature of this problem. However, there are youngsters in this aged group who do have true multiple food hypersensitivity and for whom some kind of treatment that would either hasten the natural history or block the biochemical reaction would be most helpful.

In conclusion, we hope that the reader of this chapter will have found that a useful approach can be developed to handle in an efficient and timely manner those children who present with a history of adverse reactions to foods. In the last two decades a great deal of information has been learned in this field and has allowed a systematic approach to be developed that aids the practitioner in coping with this most frequent of complaints.

REFERENCES

1. Genesis 3.
2. Cohen SG, Saaredra-Delgado AM. Through the centuries with food and drink, for better or worse. Allergy Proc 1989; 10:281–290.
3. Sampson HA. Role of immediate food hypersensitivity in the pathogenesis of atopic dermatitis. J Allergy Clin Immunol 1983; 71:473–480.
4. Bock SA, Atkins FM. Patterns of food hypersensitivity during sixteen years of double blind placebo controlled food challenges. J Pediatr 1990; 86:387–392.
5. Bryan F. Diseases transmitted by foods: a classification and summary. US Dept HHS, Public Health Service, Centers for Disease Control, HHS publ (CDC) 81–8237, 1981.
6. National Research Council, Committee on Food Protection. Toxicants naturally occurring in foods. National Academy of Sciences, Washington, DC, 1973.
7. Anderson JA, Sogn DD. Adverse reactions to foods. US Dept HHS, Public Health Services, NIH publ 84–2442, 1984.
8. Committee on Drugs, American Academy of Pediatrics. Transfer of drugs and other chemicals into human milk. Pediatrics 1989; 84:924–936.
9. Rogon WJ, Bagniewski W, Damstra T. Pollutants in human milk. N Engl J Med 1980; 302:1450–1453.
10. Bakken AF, Seip M. Insecticides in human milk. Acta Paediatr Scand, 1976; 65:535–539.
11. Halpern SR, Sellers WA, Johnson RB, et al. Development of childhood allergy in infants fed breast, soy or cow milk. J Allergy Clin Immunol 1973; 51:139–151.
12. Gerrard JW, MacKenzie JWA, Goluboff N. Cow's milk allergy: prevalence and manifestations in an unselected series of newborns. Acta Paediatr Scand [*Suppl*] 27:3–21.
13. Jakobsson I, Lindberg T. A prospective study of cow's milk protein intolerance in Swedish infants. Acta Paediatr Scand 1979; 68:853–859.
14. Stintzing G, Zetterstrom R. Cow's milk allergy, incidence and pathogenetic role of early exposure to cow's milk formula. Acta Paediatr Scand 1979; 68:383–387.

15. Heiner DC. Allergy to cow's milk. N Engl Soc Allergy Proc 1981; 2:198–203.
16. Kajosaari M. Food allergy in Finnish children aged 1 to 6 years. Acta Paediatr Scand 1982; 71:815–819.
17. Hattevig G, Kjellman B, Johansson SGO, Björkstén B. Clinical symptoms and IgE responses to common food proteins in atopic and healthy children. Clin Allergy 1984; 14:551–559.
18. Hattevig G, Kjellman B, Björkstén B. Clinical symptoms and IgE responses to common food proteins and inhalants in the first 7 years of life. Clin Allergy 1987; 17:571–578.
19. Bock SA. Prospective appraisal of complaints of adverse reactions to foods in children during the first 3 years of life. Pediatrics 1987; 79:683–688.
20. Zeiger RS, Heller S, Mellon MH, Forsythe AB, O'Connor RD, Hamburger RN, Schatz M. Effect of combined maternal and infant food-allergen avoidance on development of atopy in early infancy: a randomized study. J Allergy Clin Immunol 1989; 84:72–89.
21. Burks AW, Mallory SB, Williams LW, Shirrell MA. Allergic dermatitis: clinical relevance of food hypersensitivity reactions. J Pediatr 1988; 113:447–451.
22. Iyngkaran N, Robinson MJ, Prathap K, Sumithran E, Yadav M. Cow's milk protein-sensitive enteropathy. Arch Dis Child 1978; 53:20–26.
23. Iyngkaran N, Robinson MJ, Sumithran E, Lam SK, Puthucheary SD, Yadav M. Cow's milk protein-sensitive enteropathy. Arch Dis Child 1978; 53:150–153.
24. Kuitunen P, Visakorpi JK, Savilahti E, Pelkonen P. Malabsorption syndrome with cow's milk intolerance: clinical findings and course in fifty-four cases. Arch Dis Child 1975; 50:351–356.
25. Savilahti E. Immunochemical study of the malabsorption syndrome with cow's milk intolerance. Gut 1973; 14:491–501.
26. Fontaine JL, Navarro J. Small intestinal biopsy in cow's milk protein allergy in infancy. Arch Dis Child 1975; 50:357–362.
27. Bock SA, Remigio LK, Gordon B. Immunochemical localization of proteins in the intestinal mucosa of children with diarrhea. J Allergy Clin Immunol 1983; 72:262–268.
28. Ament ME, Rubin CE. Soy protein—another cause of the flat intestinal lesion. Gastroenterology 1972; 62:227–234.
29. Perkkiö M, Savilahti E, Kuitunen P. Morphometric and immunohistochemical study of jejunal biopsies from children with intestinal soy allergy. Eur J Pediatr 1981; 137:63–69.
30. Halpin TC, Byrne WJ, Ament ME. Colitis, persistent diarrhea, and soy protein intolerance. J Pediatr 1977; 91:404–407.
31. Vitoria JC, Camareno C, Sojo A, Ruiz A, and Rodriguez-Soriano J. Enteropathy related to fish, rice, and chicken. Arch Dis Child 1982; 57:44–48.

32. Gryloski JD. Gastrointestinal milk allergy in infants. Pediatrics 1967; 40:354–362.
33. Powell GK. Milk and soy induced enterocolitis of infancy. J Pediatr 1978; 93:553–560.
34. Hill DJ, Shelton MJ, Hosking CS. Manifestations of milk allergy in infancy: clinical and immunologic findings. J Pediatr 1986; 109:270–276.
35. McDonald PJ, Goldblum RM, Van Sickle GJ, Powell GK. Food protein-induced enterocolitis: altered antibody response to ingested antigen. Pediatr Res 1984; 18:751–755.
36. Pearson JR, Kingston D, Shiner M. Antibody production to milk proteins in the jejunal mucosa of children with cow's milk protein intolerance. Pediatr Res 1983; 17:406–412.
37. Iyngkaren N, Abdin Z, Davis K, et al. Acquired carbohydrate intolerance and cow milk protein-sensitive enteropathy in young infants. J Pediatr 1979; 95:373–378.
38. Lake AM, Whittington F, Hamilton SR. Dietary protein-induced colitis in breast fed infants. J Pediatr 1982; 101:906–910.
39. Berezin S, Schwarz SM, Glassman M, et al. Gastrointestinal milk intolerance of infancy. Am J Dis Child 1989; 143:361–362.
40. Ament ME, Rubin, CE. Soy protein—another cause of the flat intestinal lesion. Gastroenterology 1972; 62:227–234.
41. Jenkins HR, Pincott JR, Soothill JF, et al. Food allergy: the major cause of infantile colitis. Arch Dis Child 1984; 59:326–329.
42. Goldman H, Proujansky R. Allergic proctitis and gastroenteritis in children. Am J Surg Pathol 1986; 10:75–86.
43. Kosnai I, Kuitunen P, Savilahti E, Sipponen P. Mast cells and eosinophils in the jejunal mucosa of patients with intestinal cow's milk allergy and celiac disease of childhood. J Pediatr Gastroenterol Nutr 1984; 3:368–372.
44. Strober W, Falchuk ZM, Rogentine GN, et al. The pathogenesis of gluten-sensitive enteropathy. Ann Intern Med 1975; 83:242.
45. Falchuck ZM, Katz AJ, Shwachman H, et al. Gluten-sensitive enteropathy: genetic analysis and organ culture study in 35 families. Scand J Gastroenterol 1978; 13:839–843.
46. Jos J, Labbe F, Geny B, Griscelli C. Immunoelectron microscopic localization of immunoglobulin A and secretory component in jejunal mucosa from children with coeliac disease. Scand J Immunol 1979; 9:441–450.
47. Aurricchio S, Greco L, Troncone R. Gluten-sensitive enteropathy in childhood. Pediatr Clin North Am 1988; 35:157–187.
48. Kagnoff M. Immunopathogenesis of celiac disease. Immunol Invest 1989; 18:499–507.
49. Kettlehut BV, Metcalfe DD. Adverse reactions to foods. In: Middleton E Jr, Reed CE, Ellis EF, et al, eds. Allergy: principles and practice, vol. 2, 3rd ed. St Louis: CV Mosby 1988:1481–1502.

50. Katz AJ, Goldman H, Grand R. Gastric mucosal biopsy in eosinophilic (allergic) gastroenteritis. Gastroenterology 1977; 73:705–709.
51. Katz AJ, Twarog FJ, Zeiger RS, Falchuk M. Milk-sensitive and eosinophilic gastroenteropathy; similar clinical features with contrasting mechanisms and clinical course. J Allergy Clin Immunol 1984; 74:72–78.
52. Vandenplas Y, et al. Milk-sensitive eosinophilic gastroenteritis in a 10 day old boy. Eur J Pediatr 1990; 149:244–245.
53. Hill SM, Miller PJ. Colitis caused by food allergy in infants. Arch Dis Child 1990; 65:132–133.
54. Snyder JD, Rosenblum N, Wershil B, et al. Pyloric stenosis and eosinophilic gastroenteritis in infants. J Pediatr Gastroenterol Nutr 1987; 6:543–547.
55. Waldman TA, Wochner RD, Laster L, Gordon RS. Allergic gastroenteropathy. N Engl J Med 1967; 276:761–769.
56. Heiner DC, Sears JW, Kniker WT. Multiple precipitins to cow's milk in chronic respiratory disease. Am J Dis Child 1962; 103:634–654.
57. Holland NH, Hong R, Davis NC, West CD. Significance of precipitating antibodies to milk proteins in the serum of infants and children. J Pediatr 1962; 61:181–195.
58. Boat TF, Polmar SH, Whitman V, Kleinerman JI, Stern RC, Doershuk CF. Hyperreactivity to cow milk in young children with pulmonary hemosiderosis and cor pulmonale secondary to nasopharyngeal obstruction. J Pediatr 1975; 87:23–29.
59. Lee SK, Kniker WT, Cook CD, Heiner DC. Cow's milk-induced pulmonary disease in children. Adv Pediatr 1978; 25:39–57.
60. Wilson JF, Lahey NE, Heiner DC. Studies on iron metabolism V. Further observations on cow's milk induced gastrointestinal bleeding in infants with iron deficiency anemia. J Pediatr 1974; 84:335–343.
61. Woodruff CW, Clark JL. The role of fresh cow's milk in iron deficiency. I. Albumin turnover in infants with iron deficiency anemia. Am J Dis Child 1972; 124:18–23.
62. Lundstrom, U, Perkkio M, Savilahti E, Siimes M. Iron deficiency anemia with hyproteinemia. Arch Dis Child 1983; 58:438–441.
63. Ratner B, Untracht S, Malone J et al. Allergenicity of modified and processed food stuffs in oranges. Allergenicity of orange studied in man. J Pediatr 1953; 43:421–428.
64. Hyams JS, Leichter AM. Apple juice: an unappreciated cause of chronic diarrhea. Am J Dis Child 1985; 139:503–505.
65. Hyams JS, Etienne NL, Leichter AM, Thever TC. Carbohydrate malabsorption following fruit juice ingestion in young children. Pediatrics 1988; 88:64–68.
66. Blaylock WK. Atopic dermatitis: diagnosis and pathobiology. J Allergy Clin Immunol 1976; 57:62–79.
67. Hanifin JM, Rajka G. Diagnostic features of atopic dermatitis. Acta Derm Venerol [Suppl] 1980; 92:44–47.

68. Hanifin JM. Epidemiology of atopic dermatitis. Monogr Allergy 1987; 21:116–131.
69. May CD Objective clinical and laboratory studies of immediate hypersensitivity reactions to foods in children. J Allergy Clin Immunol 1976; 58:500–515.
70. Bock SA, Lee WY, Remigio LK, et al. Studies of hypersensitivity reactions to foods in infants and children. J Allergy Clin Immunol 1978; 62:327–334.
71. Sampson HA, McCaskill CM. Food hypersensitivity and atopic dermatitis: evaluation of 113 patients. J Pediatr 1985; 107:669–675.
72. Sampson HA. The role of food allergy and mediator release in atopic dermatitis. J Allergy Clin Immunol 1988; 81:635–645.
73. Burks AW. Antibody response to milk proteins in patients with milk protein intolerance documented by challenge. J Allergy Clin Immunol 1990; 85:921–927.
74. Onorato J, Merland N, Terral C, Michel FB. Placebo-controlled double-blind food challenge in asthma. J Allergy Clin Immunol 1986; 78:1139–1146.
75. Jakobsson I, Lindberg T. Cow's milk proteins cause infantile colic in breast-fed infants: a double-blind crossover study. Pediatrics 1983; 71:268–271.
76. Lothe L, Lindberg T. Cow's milk whey protein elicits symptoms of intractable colic in colicky formula-fed infants: a double-blind crossover study. Pediatrics 1989; 83:262–266.
77. Forsythe BWC. Colic and the effect of changing formulas: a double-blind multiple crossover study. J Pediatr 1989; 115:521–526.
78. Sampson HA. Infantile colic and food allergy: fact or fiction. J Pediatr 1989; 115:583–584.
79. Kuhn A, Mozin MJ, Rebuffat E, Sottiaux M, Muller MF. Milk intolerance in children with persistent sleeplessness: a double-blind crossover evaluation. Pediatrics 1989; 84:595–603.
80. Bock SA. Natural history of severe reactions to foods in young children. J Pediatr 1985; 107:676–680.
81. Jakobsson I, Lindberg T, Benediktsson B, et al. Dietary bovine β-lactoglobulin is transferred to human milk. Acta Paediatr Scand 1985; 74:342–345.
82. Machtinger S, Moss R. Cow's milk allergy in breast fed infants; the role of allergen and maternal secretory antibody. J Allergy Clin Immunol 1986; 77:541–547.
83. Host A, Husby S, Osterballe O. Prospective study of cow's milk allergy in exclusively breastfed infants. Acta Paediatr Scand 1988; 77:663–670.
84. Strobel S. Immunologically-mediated damage to the intestinal mucosa. Acta Paediatr Scand [*Suppl*] 1990; 365:46–57.

85. Dolovich J, Hargreave FE, Chalmers R, et al. Late cutaneous allergic responses in isolated IgE-dependent reactions. J Allergy Clin Immunol 1973; 52:38–46.
86. Solley GO, Gleich GJ, Jordan RE, Schroeter AL. Late phase of the immediate wheal and flare skin reaction: its dependence on IgE antibodies. J Clin Invest 1976; 58:408–420.
87. Sampson HA. Late phase response to food in atopic dermatitis. Hosp Pract 1987; 22:91–106.
88. Sampson HA. Pathogenesis of eczema. Clin Exp Allergy 1990; 20:459–467.
89. Leiferman KM, Ackerman SJ, Sampson HA, et al. Dermal deposition of eosinophil granule major basic protein in atopic dermatitis. Comparison with onchocerciasis. N Engl J Med 1985; 313:282–285.
90. Shiner M, Ballard J, Smith ME. The small intestinal mucosa in cow's milk allergy. Lancet 1975; 1:136–140.
91. Nolte H, Skov PS, Kruse A, Schiotz PO. Histamine release from dispersed human intestinal mast cells. Allergy 1989; 44:543–553.
92. McDonald TT. The role of activated T-lymphocytes in gastrointestinal disease. Clin Exp Allergy 1990; 20:247–252.
93. Ferguson A. Models of immunologically driven small intestinal damage. In: Marsh MN, ed. Immunopathology of the small intestine. Chichester: John Wiley & Co, 1987:225–252.
94. Troncone R, Ferguson A. Induction of intestinal cell-mediated immunity to gliadin in mice. In: Kumar P, Walker-Smith J, eds, Proceedings of the international symposium of coeliac disease. (in press)
95. Cornell HJ. Amino acid composition of peptides remaining after in vitro digestion of a gliadin sub-fraction with coeliac disease. Clin Chim Acta 1988; 176:279–290.
96. Saavedra-Delgado AM, Metcalfe DD. Interactions between food antigens and the immune system in the pathogenesis of gastrointestinal diseases. Ann Allergy 1985; 55:694–702.
97. Lycke N, et al. Production of antibodies to gliadin in intestinal mucosa of patients with celiac disease: a study at the single cell level. Gut 1989; 30:72–77.
98. Falchuk, ZM, Gebhard RL, Sessams C, et al. An in vitro model of gluten sensitivity enteropathy: effect of gliaden on intestinal epithelial cells of patients with gluten sensitive enteropathy in organ culture. J Clin Invest 1974; 53:487–500.
99. Fluge G, Andersen KJ, Aksnes L, Thunold K, et al. Brush border and lysomal marker enzyme profiles in duodenal mucosa of coeliac patients before and after organ culture. Scand J Gastroenterol 1982; 17:465–472.
100. Greco L, DeSeta L, D'Adamo G, et al. Atopy and celiac disease: bias or true relation? Acta Paediatr Scand 1990; 79:670–674.

101. Bock SA, Buckley J, Holst A, May CD. Proper use of skin tests with food extracts in diagnosis of hypersensitivity to food in children. Clin Allergy 1977; 7:375–383.
102. Bock SA, Lee WY, Remigio LK, et al. Appraisal of skin tests with food extracts for diagnosis of food hypersensitivity. Clin Allergy 1978; 8:559–564.
103. Sampson HA, Albergo R. Comparison of results of skin tests, RAST and double-blind, placebo-controlled food challenges in children with atopic dermatitis. J Allergy Clin Immunol 1984; 74:26–33.
104. Sampson HA, Jolie PL. Increased plasma histamine concentrations after food challenges in children with atopic dermatitis. N Engl J Med 1984; 31:372–376.
105. Bock SA, Sampson HA, Atkins FM, Zeiger RS, Lehrer S, Sachs M, Bush RK, Metcalfe DD. Double blind placebo controlled food challenge (DBPCFC) as an office procedure: a manual. J Allergy Clin Immunol 1988; 82:986–997.
106. Iyngkaran N, Robinson MJ, Prathap K, et al. Cow's milk protein sensitive enteropathy: combined clinical and histological approach to diagnosis. Arch Dis Child 1978; 53:20–26.
107. Wilson SJ, Walzer M. Absorption of undigested proteins in human begins. IV. Absorption of unaltered egg protein in infants. Am J Dis Child 1935; 50:49–54.
108. Butler HL, Byrne WJ, Marmer DJ, et al. Depressed neutrophil chemotaxis in infants with cow's milk and/or soy protein intolerance. Pediatrics 1981; 67:264–268.
109. Van Sickle GJ, Powell GK, McDonald PJ, Goldblum RM. Milk-and soy protein-induced enterocolitis: evidence for lymphocyte sensitization to specific food proteins. Gastroenterology 1985; 88:1915–1921.
110. Burks AW, Casteel HB, Fiedorek SC, et al. A prospective food challenge study of two different types of soy protein isolates in patients with possible milk or soy protein intolerance. (Presented at SPR, New Orleans, Jan 1991).
111. Scott H, Fausa V, Ek J, Brandtzaeg P. Immune response patterns in coeliac disease: serum antibodies to dietary antigens measured by an enzyme linked immunosorbent assay. Clin Exp Immunol 1984; 57:25–32.
112. Loft DE, Marsh MH, Crowe PT. Rectal gluten challenge and diagnosis of celiac disease. Lancet 1990; 335:1293–1295.
113. Bock SA. Probable allergic reaction to casein hydrolysate formula. J Allergy Clin Immunol 1989; 84:272.
114. Lipshitz CH, Hawkins HK, Guera, C, Byrd N. Anaphylactic shock due to cow's milk protein hypersensitivity in a breast fed infant. J Pediatr Gastroenterol Nutr 1988; 7:141–144.
115. Sampson HA, Bernhisel-Broadbent J, Yang E, Scanlon S. Safety of casein hydrolysate formula in children with cow milk allergy. J Pediatr 1991; 118:520–525.

116. Burks AW, Sampson HA. Double blind placebo controlled trial of oral cromolyn sodium in children with documented food hypersensitivity. J Allergy Clin Immunol 1988; 77:417–423.
117. Sampson HA, Scanlon S. Natural history of food hypersensitivity in children with atopic dermatitis. J Pediatr 1989; 115:23–27.
118. Bock SA, Atkins FM. The natural history of peanut allergy. J Allergy Clin Immunol 1989; 83:900–904.
119. Bock SA. The natural history of food hypersensitivity. J Allergy Clin Immunol 1982; 69:173–177.
120. Ford RPK, Taylor B. The natural history of egg hypersensitivity. Arch Dis Child 1982; 57:649–652.
121. Danaeus A, Inganäs M. A follow up study of children with food allergy, clinical course in relation to serum IgE and IgG antibody levels to milk, egg, and fish. Clin Allergy 1981; 11:537–539.
122. Bishop JM, Hill DJ, Hosking CS. Natural history of cow milk allergy: clinical outcome. J Pediatr 1990; 116:862–867.
123. O'Brien TC, Maloney CJ, Tauraso NM. Quantitation of residual host protein in chicken embryo derived vaccines by radial immunodiffusion. Appl Microbiol 1971; 21:780–782.
124. American Academy of Pediatrics. Report of the committee on infectious disease (red book). Elk Grove Village, IL: American Academy of Pediatrics Publication, 1988.
125. Herman JJ, Radin R, Schneiderman BS. Allergic reactions to measles (rubeola) vaccine in patients hypersensitive to egg protein. J Pediatr 1983; 102:196–199.
126. Greenberg MA, Birx DL. Safe administration of mumps–rubella vaccine in egg-allergic children. J Pediatr 1988; 113:504–506.
127. Kemp A, VanAsperen P, Mukhi A. Measles immunization in children with clinical reactions to egg protein. Am J Dis Child 1990; 144:33–35.
128. Lavi S, Zimmerman B, Koren G, Gold R. Administration of measles, mumps, and rubella virus vaccine (live) to egg-allergic children. JAMA 1990; 263:269–271.
129. Murphy KR, Strunk RC. Safe administration of influenza vaccine in asthmatic children hypersensitive to egg proteins. J Pediatr 1985; 106:931–933.
130. Fasano MB, Wood RA, Cooke SK, Sampson HA. Egg allergy and adverse reactions to measles, mumps, rubella vaccine. J Pediatr 1992; 120:878–881.
131. Sheffer AL, Lieberman PL, Aaronson PW, et al. Measurement of circulating IgG and IgE food immune complexes. J Allergy Clin Immunol 1988; 81:758–759.
132. Victoria JC, Sojo A, Rodriquez-Soriano J. Changing pattern of cow's milk protein intolerance. Acta Paediatr Scand 1990; 79:566–567.

133. May CD, Remigio L. Observation on high spontaneous release of histamine from leukocytes in vitro. Clin Allergy 1982; 12:229–241.
134. Sampson HA, Broadbent KR, Bernhisel-Braodbent J. Spontaneous release of histamine from basophils and histamine-releasing factor in patients with atopic dermatitis and food hypersensitivity. N Engl J Med 1989; 321:228–257.

22
The Wheezing Infant

Alan F. Isles

Royal Children's Hospital, Brisbane, Australia

Christopher J.L. Newth

Children's Hospital of Los Angeles, and University of Southern California School of Medicine, Los Angeles, California

Wheezing is one of the most frequently encountered respiratory symptoms of childhood. Although asthma is the most common cause of wheezing in older children, the differential diagnosis of wheezing in infancy is extensive, and it is inappropriate to label every wheeze as asthma, especially in the very young, without considering other possibilities. The diagnosis and management of wheezing in infancy has been made complicated by the use of imprecise and confusing diagnostic terms, such as wheezy bronchitis, recurrent bronchiolitis, and others. As well, there has been much controversy about the efficacy of bronchodilators in this age group.

PREDISPOSING ANATOMICAL AND PHYSIOLOGICAL FACTORS

A variety of anatomical and physiological factors combine to make the infant uniquely susceptible to respiratory illness (1). Peripheral airway resistance is greater in infants than in adults because the peripheral airways are disproportionately narrow (2). This explains, in part, why diseases such as bronchiolitis, which predominantly affect the small airways, have such an impact on infants. The relative lack of elastic recoil in the infant lung predisposes to early airway closure, even during tidal breathing (3). In disease states, this has the effect of predisposing to airway closure at a relatively high lung volume, resulting in ventilation–perfusion mismatching and a more profound disturbance of gas exchange than might be expected in older children. In addition, the pores of Kohn and the bronchoalveolar canals of Lambert (4) are either not present or are deficient in both number and size, which deprives infants of collateral ventilation and predisposes them to atelectasis during respiratory illness, further aggravating ventilation–perfusion mismatching and hypoxemia.

In infants, the angle of the ribs is almost horizontal. This is in contrast with the more oblique insertion in adults. The horizontal insertion decreases the efficiency of "bucket-handle" outward motion of the thoracic cage during inspiration. Subsequently, there is a greater tendency for the more compliant rib cage of the infant to distort, further decreasing the efficiency of diaphragmatic contraction during inspiration and increasing the work of breathing. In addition, the diaphragm of the infant has fewer type I (fatigue resistant) muscle fibers than the adult diaphragm, further predisposing the infant to respiratory failure in any condition that increases the respiratory load (5).

Even in normal infants, the number of mucous-secreting cells in the airway epithelium is proportionately greater in infants than in adults (6). Airway inflammation is, therefore, more likely to result in mucous plugging, atelectasis, and hypoxemia in infants. The latter is also likely to further aggravate the already increased pulmonary vascular resistance.

The developmental pharmacology of the respiratory system has been reviewed in detail by Isles and Newth (7). From a practical standpoint, the single most important issue relates to the bronchodilator responsiveness of infants compared with older children (8). There is a widely held view that infants lack bronchial smooth muscle (9) and, therefore, are unresponsive to bronchodilators. Although the literature in this area remains controversial, there is increasing evidence to suggest that this traditional view is incorrect. Recent studies on children with bronchopulmonary dysplasia have shown an airway response to bronchodilators as early as 25-weeks gestational age (10). Clinical studies of wheezy infants suggest a beneficial response to bronchodilator (11,12). Other studies, using more objective measures of lung function, have produced conflicting results. Hughes et al. found that albuterol (salbutamol) caused no improvement (13), whereas other studies have shown either deterioration (14) in respiratory mechanics or improvement in spirometry (15) in bronchiolitis. These differences may, in part, be methodological. The clinical studies generally assess response after several or multiple drug treatments, whereas the studies using objective measures of lung function are usually single-dose studies because of the inherent limitations of the measurement technique (15–17). The age of the infants studied and the cause of their wheezing is also likely to affect their response to medication. Many of the studies of bronchodilator responsiveness in infants have been performed during the recovery phase from acute bronchiolitis, a disease in which the airflow obstruction is predominantly due to edema and airway inflammation and not necessarily reflective of the pathology in infants with recurrent wheeze for other reasons. This lack of precise categorization has led to conflicting reports concerning responses to drugs—for example, O'Callaghan and others recently demonstrated that albuterol protected against bronchoconstriction induced by hypotonic airway challenge in infants younger than a year of age with recurrent wheezing (18). Previously, this same group published data showing wheezy infants younger than 18 months of age had no bronchodilator response to the same drug, but did respond to ipratropium (19).

AN APPROACH TO THE DIFFERENTIAL DIAGNOSIS OF WHEEZE IN INFANCY

Asthma is by far the most common cause of wheezing in older children and adults. In infants, however, the differential diagnosis is much broader and includes a wide range of congenital and acquired disorders (Table 1).

Age of Onset

Symptoms that begin in the first few weeks or months of life should arouse suspicion of an underlying congenital abnormality.

Nature of Symptoms

The nature of the symptoms often provides important clues to the likely underlying problem. A brassy-sounding cough, if present, is likely to be due to tracheal abnormality such as tracheomalacia. Wheezing that is both inspiratory and expiratory suggests fixed airway obstruction. Stridor in association with wheezing should always suggest an underlying congenital abnormality. Cyanotic spells can be due to recurrent aspiration or tracheomalacia.

Preceding History

Prematurity, especially if associated with intubation, mechanical ventilation, and repeated suctioning, may indicate an underlying airway

Table 1 Causes of Wheezing in Infants

- I. Congenital
  - A. Extramural
    1. Lobar emphysema
    2. Bronchogenic cyst
    3. Vascular ring
  - B. Intramural
    1. Primary tracheomalacia
    2. Tracheomalacia associated with tracheoesophageal fistula and vascular ring
    3. Tracheal stenosis
    4. Bronchial stenosis
  - C. Intraluminal
    1. Tracheal web
    2. Cystic fibrosis
- II. Acquired Causes
  - A. Extramural
    1. Cystic or mass lesions compressing trachea or bronchi
    2. Enlarged lymph nodes
  - B. Intramural
    1. Infections (e.g., bronchiolitis)
    2. Acquired tracheobronchial stenosis
    3. Tumors (e.g., carcinoid tumor)
    4. Asthma
    5. Bronchopulmonary dysplasia
  - C. Intraluminal
    1. Foreign body
    2. Mucous plugging secondary to infection or asthma
    3. Aspiration (gastroesophageal reflux)

problem such as tracheal or bronchial stenosis secondary to granulation tissue or scarring. Airway obstruction and recurrent or persistent wheeze are typical features of bronchopulmonary dysplasia. A history of gastroesophageal reflux should also be sought. Previous repair of a tracheoesophageal fistula introduces tracheomalacia, gastroesophageal reflux, and recurrent fistula into the differential diagnosis.

Chest Radiograph

Careful inspection of the chest radiograph can provide important clues to the underlying diagnosis. The lung fields should be inspected carefully for evidence of generalized or lobar hyperinflation. The vascularity of the two lungs and the individual lobes within should be examined carefully. The descending aorta should be identified. A right-sided aortic arch may indicate a vascular ring. Both the anteroposterior and lateral chest radiographs should be examined for evidence of tracheal displacement. The hilar region should be examined carefully in the lateral view, as this is the typical site for bronchogenic cysts and enlarged hilar lymph nodes. The tracheal outline should be inspected, especially in the lateral view, for evidence of narrowing that might suggest tracheomalacia or tracheal stenosis.

Investigation

The plain chest radiograph is the most useful initial investigation. Depending on the history and suggestive features outlined in the foregoing, a barium swallow and cinescreening of the airway may be indicated. More invasive investigation, such as bronchoscopy and conventional or ultrafast computed tomography (CT) examination, may be indicated, when intrinic airway abnormality is suspected (20).

SPECIFIC CONGENITAL CONDITIONS

Lobar Emphysema

Lobar emphysema is an important cause of respiratory distress in the first few months of life (21). Infants are usually symptomatic within the first few weeks of life, and almost all present within the first 3 months. Symptoms include tachypnea, lower rib retraction, and expiratory wheeze. Breath sounds may be diminished over the affected lobe, and the chest shape may be asymmetric. There may also be evidence of mediastinal displacement. Any lobe may be affected, but it is most commonly the left upper lobe. The chest radiograph typically shows marked hyperinflation and lucency of the affected lobe, with herniation across the anterior mediastinum. Radiographs in the newborn period may be confusing, as the affected lobe may be fluid-filled and, therefore, radiopaque. Treatment of congenital lobar emphysema is surgical excision to prevent progressive respiratory compromise or respiratory failure.

Bronchogenic Cysts

Bronchogenic cysts are usually found in close association with the trachea and major bronchi, the most common site being the region of the carina (21). Cough and wheeze are the usual symptoms. If tracheal or bronchial compression is severe, the infant may present with respiratory distress or failure. Typical radiographic findings are hyperinflation of one lung. The cyst itself is generally invisible, and compression or displacement of the esophagus is ordinarily evident on a barium swallow. The diagnosis is usually obvious on CT scan. Treatment is surgical removal of the cyst.

Vascular Ring

Tracheal compression from vascular anomalies can be divided into three main types (21). These are the following:

1. Double aortic arch
2. Rings in which the aorta and a combination of other vessels and rudimentary structures such as the ligamentum arteriosum cause the obstruction
3. A major artery of anomalous origin

The symptoms that result depend on the degree of tracheal narrowing and compression. There is commonly an inspiratory stridor or wheeze with expiratory wheezing. The cough is usually abnormal, and swallowing difficulties may also be a feature. The diagnosis can generally be made by barium swallow. Aortography may be necessary to define the vascular anatomy accurately before surgery. If an anomalous left pulmonary artery is present, bronchoscopy is indicated to exclude associated tracheal stenosis.

Tracheomalacia

Tracheomalacia may occur as a primary disorder or secondary to other conditions, such as tracheoesophageal fistula or vascular ring. The tracheomalacia may be localized to one segment of the trachea or be more generalized and may, on occasion, extend into the major bronchi as well. The symptoms that result obviously depend on the extent and severity of the tracheomalacia. Infants with localized tracheomalacia usually have an unusual harsh brassy-sounding cough, a moist chest with retained secretions, and a degree of expiratory wheeze. Wheezing may be minimal with quiet breathing, but commonly increases with activity or during intercurrent infection. When generalized tracheomalacia is present, the wheezing may be more prominent and, on occasion, may be associated with cyanotic spells. The tracheomalacia can be confirmed by cineradiography. Interpretation may not be easy, as a degree of dynamic collapse of the trachea during crying is normal. Bronchoscopy may be required to fully assess the extent of the tracheomalacia. Again, considerable experience is required, as anesthesia with neuromuscular blockade causing paralysis can obscure the diagnosis if the rigid ventilating bronchoscope is used. Flexible fiberoptic bronchoscopy in the spontaneously breathing, sedated infant can be more informative in this situation, if available. In most cases, no specific treatment is required, and improvement can be expected during the first 12–18 months of life. Children with repaired tracheoesophageal fistula retain an abnormal cough throughout childhood and frequently have detectable abnormalities on pulmonary function testing (22). On occasions, life-threatening cyanotic spells may require surgical intervention, such as aortopexy or external splinting of the trachea in the region of the tracheomalacia (23,24).

Tracheal Web, Tracheal Stenosis, and Bronchial Stenosis

Tracheal web and strictures are uncommon anomalies and usually present with both inspiratory and expiratory wheeze. As with tracheomalacia, symptoms are increased by activity and intercurrent infection. Tracheal stenosis is often associated with other abnormalities, such as pulmonary agenesis or aberrant left pulmonary artery or pulmonary sling (21). Tracheal stenosis may be a localized disorder or, more frequently, it is associated with complete or circumferential tracheal rings that narrow distally (the so-called rat-tailed trachea) (21). Endoscopy or bronchoscopy are required to define the nature and extent of the stenosis. Separate cardiac investigation, including angiography, may also be required. Bronchoscopy is usually indicated when the wheeze is both inspiratory and expiratory. Bronchial stenosis will cause inspiratory and expiratory wheeze and may be associated with focal hyperinflation or collapse on the chest radiograph.

Cystic Fibrosis

Cystic fibrosis is a common inherited condition affecting approximately 1:2000 white children, with a lower incidence in other population groups. In many areas, infants with cystic fibrosis are diagnosed shortly after birth in newborn-screening programs. If not diagnosed at birth, most will present in the first year of life with recurrent respiratory symptoms and failure to thrive. A small percentage of these children have recurrent or persistent wheezing owing to diffuse small-airway disease. Sometimes the wheezing may be a major management problem and, infrequently, even leads to respiratory failure. Mechanical ventilation in this situation is usually justified, since most infants can be weaned easily from the ventilator in 3–4 days after clearance of thick secretions. The wheezing often resolves in the first 1–2 years of life.

SPECIFIC ACQUIRED CONDITIONS

Bronchiolitis

Bronchiolitis is a disease of infants during the first year of life, being most common in those 6–12 months of age (21). It is characterized by inflammation and edema in bronchioles. Airflow obstruction results from accumulation of inflammatory mucus and cellular debris within the lumen of bronchioles, edema of the bronchiolar wall and, possibly, a degree of bronchiolar spasm (25). Partial airway obstruction causes gas trapping and hyperinflation, resulting in an increased work of breathing (25). Ventilation–perfusion mismatching causes hypoxia, the extent of which is dependent on the severity of the illness (25).

Respiratory syncytial virus (RSV) and parainfluenza virus are the most common etiologic agents, with RSV causing more than 90% of infections (26). Rarely, infection with adenovirus results in a more severe illness, characterized by obliterative bronchiolitis (21). Infection with RSV can occur at any time, but is most prevalent during the winter months, often occurring in epidemics. Parental smoking is a recognized risk factor for bronchiolitis (27).

Patients usually present with a history of an antecedent coryzal illness with a mild fever. This is followed by the onset of a harsh cough, tachypnea, chest retraction, and hyperinflation. Ausculatory findings include an expiratory wheeze and inspiratory crackles. The radiographic changes include hyperinflation and patchy consolidation and atelectasis. Hypoxia is usually present, with the severity being dependent on the severity of the illness. Apnea is a recognized complication during the initial phase of the illness (21).

The acute phase of bronchiolitis typically lasts 5–10 days, but it may be some weeks before symptoms fully resolve. On occasion, a more severe and protracted course is encountered (28). Mortality is rare in previously healthy children if appropriate intensive care facilities are readily available, but is a major risk in those with preexistent respiratory problems, such as bronchopulmonary dysplasia or congenital heart disease (18). The diagnosis is clinical and is dependent on a history of a prodromal illness with typical clinical and radiographic findings. Identification of a viral pathogen in respiratory secretions by immunofluorescence provides additional confirmatory evidence.

Treatment of the hospitalized infant includes monitoring of oxygenation and use of humidified oxygen to maintain a saturation in excess of 90%. Feeding problems are common and will often require the use of intravenous fluids. Nasogastric feeding tubes increase respiratory resistance and may aggravate incipient respiratory failure. Antibiotics are rarely necessary. The role of bronchodilator drugs in the treatment of bronchiolitis remains controversial. Most reports discourage their use because of a lack of proved efficacy. Sly et al, in a study of infants recovering from bronchiolitis, showed no improvement in lung mechanics from a single dose of albuterol (29). In contrast, Shuh et al. (12), in a recent placebo-controlled study of infants aged 6 weeks to 24 months with bronchiolitis, demonstrated an improvement in clinical score, oxygen saturation, and respiratory rate after two doses of nebulized albuterol. Corticosteroids are not beneficial.The role of ribavirin in the treatment of bronchiolitis remains controversial and was the subject of a recent symposium in which the safety and efficacy were extensively reviewed (30). The American Academy of Pediatrics has published recommendations for the use of ribavirin in patients with RSV infection. These include patients with congenital heart disease, bronchopulmonary dysplasia and other forms of chronic neonatal lung disease, prematurity, immunodeficiency, multiple congenital anomalies, and progressive respiratory failure (31). Groothuls et al. recently study showed that ribavirin administered early in the course of infection in high-risk patients significantly reduced the morbidity from RSV infection (32). Ribavirin is potentially teratogenic, so special care must be taken when using it to ensure the safety of caregivers.

A high percentage (50–90%) of infants who have an episode of bronchiolitis have recurrent episodes of wheezing (33). There are two possible reasons for this. First, the initial viral infection may trigger bronchial hyperreactivity. Second, there may be an inherited predisposition to bronchiolitis through inherited bronchial reactivity. Some studies have shown a higher prevalence of atopy in first-degree relatives of infants with bronchiolitis compared with controls (33). There is additional evidence that those who develop wheezing subsequent to bronchiolitis may have an immunological response different from other children. Welliver found RSV-specific IgE antibodies in nasopharyngeal secretions at the time of the initial episode (34).

Bronchiolitis may be associated with long-term sequelae other than asthma. Abnormalities in various measures of lung function have been described 8–10 years after bronchiolitis (27).

In general, the first episode of wheezing in an infant is called bronchiolitis, the second should be viewed suspiciously, and the third labeled as asthma, particularly when there is a supporting family history (35).

Gastroesophageal Reflux

Gastroesophageal reflux must always be considered in the differential diagnosis of wheezing and other respiratory symptoms in infants. Importantly, significant reflux can be present with little in the way of typical symptoms such as vomiting. Gastroesophageal reflux should be considered when there are prominent nocturnal symptoms.

The relation between reflux and respiratory symptoms has recently been reviewed by Orenstein and Orenstein (36). Reflux may be the primary cause of respiratory symptoms. Possible mechanisms include gross or microaspiration, reflex bronchoconstriction and increased bronchial hyperactivity, reflex bronchospasm, reflex central apnea, and reflex bradycardia (36). Reflex bronchoconstriction secondary to reflux is likely to occur only in the presence of esophagitis (37). In other patients, a primary respiratory condition (e.g., bronchopulmonary dysplasia) may be complicated by reflux. Coughing, greater negative intrathoracic and positive intra-abdominal pressures with increased respiratory effort, and hyperinflation with diaphragm flattening from the primary respiratory disease, predispose to reflux. Medications such as theophylline and, to a lesser extent, β-agonists when used in the treatment of the primary disorder may precipitate or aggravate gastric reflux by causing relaxation of the lower esophageal sphincter and increased gastric acid secretion.

As reflux is a common condition affecting about 20% of all infants, it can be difficult to establish an exact causal relation between reflux and respiratory symptoms in an individual patient (36). The presence of reflux can be defined by radiography, endoscopy, pH probe, or scintigraphy. No method is without its deficiencies, and the diagnosis of pathological gastroesophageal reflux is often a clinical decision, weighing the clinical features with the other supporting evidence. The presence of fat-laden alveolar macrophages in tracheobronchial secretions may be helpful, but there is a high false-positive rate (37).

Treatment of gastroesophageal reflux includes conservative measures with posturing, thickening of feeds, and altered feeding practices. The seated posture increases reflux and should be avoided (36). Prone positioning in bed with the head elevated is the preferred sleep posture. Pharmacologic treatment includes prokinetic agents, such as metoclopramide, and gastric acid suppressant therapy. Fundoplication must be considered in children with complex respiratory problems, such as bronchopulmonary dysplasia complicated by reflux that does not respond to medical management.

Smoking

A wide range of respiratory tract morbidity has been attributed to the exposure of infants and children to parental (especially maternal) smoking (38). Martinez et al., in a recent study (39), demonstrated a conclusive link between parental smoking and childhood asthma. Asthmatic children with smoking parents had increased airway responsiveness, when compared with asthmatic children with nonsmoking parents. Other studies have shown cord blood IgE concentrations to be increased in infants born to mothers who smoked during pregnancy (although conflicting studies exist), and infants born to mothers who smoked in pregnancy had a fourfold increased risk of developing a clinically manifest allergic state (40). In addition, Young et al. have shown recently that, although elevated airway responsiveness is present even at birth in normal healthy infants, elevated levels of airway responsiveness are related to parental smoking and a family history of asthma (41). Male children from smoking parents had increased skin test reactivity when compared with children from nonsmoking parents (39). On the basis of the foregoing data, it seems reasonable to postulate that early (even intrauterine) passive exposure to products of tobacco combustion may make an important contribution to the observed patterns of occurrence of bronchial hyperreactivity, atopy, and asthma (38). Passive smoking has demonstrable effects on IgE-mediated immune responses and may represent a pathway by which an environmental trigger could contribute to the pathogenesis of asthma and other respiratory disorders (38).

Asthma

Etiology

Asthma affects 10% or more of all young children. About 30% have the onset of their symptoms in the first year of life, and 50% by 2 years of age (42). Additionally, there is significant evidence that the frequency of asthma is increasing. Burr et al., in two identical surveys 15 years apart, showed that a history of current asthma symptoms increased from 5.2 to 12%, and a history of wheeze at any time increased from 17 to 22% (43). Hospital admission rates, especially for males have also increased during recent years (44).

In infancy, asthma is twice as common in boys as in girls (42). Schwartz et al. showed that for children 6 months to 11 years of age, the prevalence of asthma was 3% among white children and 7.2% among blacks. The prevalence of frequent wheeze was 6.2% among whites and 9.3% among blacks. They also identified other factors, such as young maternal age and central-city birth place, as being independent risk factors, suggesting that the intrauterine environment may play a priming role in the development of asthma (45).

Atopy or the genetic predisposition to asthma remains a major causative factor. Progress is being made in unraveling the underlying genetic defect, but this work is not yet complete (46). The relation between genetic predisposition and environmental factors remains poorly understood. In a 1985 study, Bertrand et al. showed that prematurely born children in whom respiratory disease did not develop during the neonatal period have evidence in later childhood of airflow limitation that is related to maternal hyperreactivity and not to their prematurity (47). In other words, uterine and airway smooth-muscle lability may be related. Other possible genetic links have been suggested. A retrospective study in Israel demonstrated that infants with transient tachypnea of the newborn had a much higher incidence of symptoms consistent with asthma and signs consistent with atopy (48). Furthermore, a prospective, controlled study from the United States has shown a much higher incidence (3.1 v 0.3%) of transient tachypnea of the newborn in infants of asthmatic mothers compared with (control) infants of nonasthmatic mothers (49).

Food allergies are common in infants. However, respiratory symptoms are the least common manifestation of allergic problems in this aged group and are rarely seen as the sole symptom of a positive food challenge (50). The widely held view that milk causes secretion of mucous has no scientific basis. Milk is the major source of calories, calcium, and other essential nutrients in infants, and dairy products should not be withdrawn from the diet without expert nutritional advice. In short, for the vast majority of infants with respiratory symptoms, dietary manipulation is totally unwarranted (50).

Viral respiratory infection is perhaps the single greatest risk factor for the development of asthma in infancy. Both clinical and epidemiological observations support the hypothesis that viral respiratory tract infection has a definite causal relationship in the development of airway reactivity and, particularly, in the causation of wheeze with subsequent viral infection. Microbiological studies of patients with acute asthma have shown no association between asthma and bacterial infection in childhood (51). Therefore, although antibiotics are frequently prescribed to wheezy infants, they are of no value unless there is an associated bacterial infection such as otitis media.

Viral respiratory infection accounts for 26–49% of asthma attacks in children, compared with 10% in adults (51). Atopy is apparently not an independent risk factor for the development of wheezing during a respiratory tract infection (51). Approximately 55–75% of symptomatic respiratory tract infections in asthmatic children result in exacerbation of asthma (52). Rhinovirus is an important precipitant of asthma in asthmatic individuals of all ages. In childhood, approximately 85% of rhinovirus infections trigger an episode of asthma (53). The importance of RSV as a cause of acute bronchiolitis and subsequent episodes of wheezing has already been discussed. Between 6 and 11 cases of virus-induced wheezing will be observed annually for each 100 children followed during the first 24 months of life (54). Other host factors, such as the number of siblings, socioeconomic status, and day-care attendance, alter the prevalence of viral infection in this age group (55).

A longitudinal study has demonstrated an increased frequency of viral respiratory tract infection in asthmatic children when compared with their nonasthmatic control siblings. Infection rates were 85.7% in the asthmatics compared with 56.3% in the controls (56,57). This increased susceptibility to infection was not found in nonasthmatic atopic subjects.

Pathology and Pathophysiology

Current concepts of the pathogenesis of bronchial hyperresponsiveness and asthma have been reviewed recently by Barnes (58) and by De Jongste et al. (59). The pathology and pathophysiology of asthma *in infancy* has been reviewed by Tabachnik and Levison (35). Airway inflammation, epithelial damage, mucosal edema, mucous secretion, and bronchial smooth-muscle spasm contribute to the causation of airflow obstruction. The relative contribution of each of these factors may vary from time to time. The role of smooth-muscle spasm in infants remains a controversial area. There is also a very strong association between asthma in infants and recurrent or persistent otitis media (60).

Clinical Presentation

In infancy, most episodes of wheezing are preceded by an upper respiratory tract infection. This may be followed by wheeze or cough or both. Depending on the severity of the airflow obstruction, there may be hyperinflation, tachypnea, subcostal, intercostal and suprasternal retraction. Occasionally, coughing, especially at night, may be the only asthmatic symptom. A small percentage of infants have rapidly progressive episodes that lead to respiratory failure. This group of asthmatic infants can be among the most difficult of all asthmatics to treat (Table 2).

Investigation

Investigations should be kept to an absolute minimum. A chest radiograph should always be obtained. If the child has atypical or recurrent symptoms, a sweat test may be indicated. Skin tests, IgE levels, and so on, are rarely helpful and should never be ordered routinely. α_1-Antitrypsin disease rarely causes symptoms in childhood and tests should not be requested routinely. Some measures of pulmonary function can

Table 2 Estimation of Severity of Exacerbations of Asthma in Infants

Sign/symptom	Mild	Moderate	Severe
Respiratory rate, resting or sleeping	Normal to 30% increase above the mean	30–50% increase above the mean	Increase over 50% above the mean
Alertness	Normal	Normal	May be decreased
Dyspnea[a]	Absent or mild; Normal suckling and feeding	Moderate; speaks in phrases or partial sentences; infant's cry softer and shorter, infant has difficulty suckling and feeding	Severe; speaks only in single words or short phrases; infant's cry softer and shorter, infant stops suckling and feeding
Accessory muscle use	No intercostal to mild retractions	Moderate intercostal retractions with tracheosternal retractions; use of sternocleidomastoid muscles; chest hyperinflation	Severe intercostal retractions, tracheosternal retractions with nasal flaring during inspration; chest hyperinflation
Color	Good	Pale	Possibly cyanotic
Auscultation	End expiratory wheeze only	Wheezing during entire expiration and inspiration	Breath sounds becoming inaudible
Oxygen saturation	>95%	90–95%	<90%
P_{CO_2}	<35	<40	>40

Note: Within each category, the presence of several parameters, but not necessarily all, indicate the general classification of the exacerbation
[a]Parent's or physician's impression of degree of child's breathlessness.

now be made routinely. Oximetry is widely available and provides a good measure of oxygenation. Actual measurement of lung function in infants is also possible in specialized facilities (61).

Treatment

Treatment must encompass both preventive measures and pharmacologic treatment.

Environmental Control. In the susceptible infant, every effort must be made to control the environment. Parents should cease smoking; dust and other inhaled irritants should be kept to a minimum.

Diet. Controversy exists over whether breast-feeding has a protective effect in the potentially atopic child. Some of the studies in this area were reviewed by Rachelefsky (42). Until a more definitive answer is available, it would seem reasonable to recommend breast-feeding until 6 months of age at least.

Immunotherapy. Immunotherapy has no role at all in the management of allergy and respiratory symptoms in infants (62).

Pharmacologic Treatment. Pharmacologic treatment remains the mainstay of treatment and should be individualized according to the frequency and severity of patients symptoms.

ANTIBIOTICS Although antibiotics are widely prescribed for intercurrent respiratory symptoms, there are no grounds at all for their routine use in asthma, even in infants. An associated otitis media or persisting mucopurulent nasal discharge for more than 4–5 days may be reasonable grounds for the introduction of antibiotics.

β-ADRENERGIC AGONISTS. Selective β-adrenergic agonists (albuterol and terbutaline) remain the agents of choice for the treatment of asthma in children. Their pharmacology has been reviewed by Weinberger (63). They should be regarded as effectively equipotent. Nonselective adrenergic agents, such as epinephrine have no role, except in the management of acute anaphylaxis and croup. β_2-adrenergic agonists may be administered orally, by wet nebulization, or by metered-dose aerosol or powder. Wet nebulization, and metered-dose aerosol or powder deliver the drug directly to the lung, providing rapid relief of symptoms with few side effects. Oral administration, although often easier in the infant, takes longer to work (typically 30–60 min) and is associated with a much higher frequency of side effects such as hyperactivity and sleep disturbance. The choice for the route of administration depends on the frequency and severity of the child's symptoms.

THEOPHYLLINE. Despite its continued widespread use in the United States, theophylline is receding in importance in other countries. Side effects, such as mood and behavior disturbance and sleep disturbance, are so common that they are frequently a major limiting factor in using the drug. Perhaps its strongest point is the availability of sustained-release formulations, which make it ideally suited for treatment of nocturnal asthma. It also has major practical benefits when a child has difficulty taking drugs in other forms, or when compliance needs to be monitored (serum drug concentrations). In the United States, theophylline is often used as a prophylactic or preventive drug. Few other countries appear to follow this practice (62). Weinberger has provided many extensive reviews of theophylline pharmacology, dosing guidelines, and interpretation of serum levels (63).

IPRATROPIUM BROMIDE. Ipratropium may be useful in the treatment of childhood asthma. The combination of albuterol and ipratropium is more effective than albuterol alone in the management of acute wheezing (64). It has few side effects and is also helpful in providing symptomatic relief for the coughing that can be so troublesome in asthma. Its peak effect is 30–60 min after administration; hence, it should always be administered in combination with a β-adrenergic agonist.

CROMOLYN. For children who require preventive treatment, cromolyn remains the drug of first choice (62,63). It has the major advantage of being free of major side effects and also reduces airway reactivity with long-term use. Newth et al. demonstrated its effectiveness in reducing asthma symptoms in a cohort of preschool children (65).

INHALED STEROIDS. Until recently, inhaled steroids were not available as a therapeutic option in this age group. The introduction of nebulized budesonide has been a major advance, as has the adaptation of face mask attachments for aerosol administration in this age group. The current indication for long-term inhaled steroid use is chronic asthma not adequately controlled with nonsteroidal agents. Budesonide and beclomethasone are effectively equipotent, but budesonide has the advantage of rapid clearance and a short half-life with fewer systemic side effects. Its topical/systemic ratio of activity is, therefore, superior to beclomethasone. Kerribijn has recently reviewed the use of topical corticosteroids in the treatment of childhood asthma (66). Bisgaard et al. reported a recent study on 77 children aged 11–36 months in whom budesonide by aerosol and mask resulted in significant clinical improvement, less oral steroid use, and fewer admissions to hospital (67). Freigang and Ashford assessed the effect of inhaled steroid [beclomethasone (400 μg/day)] administered by face mask to 17 children 12–26 months of age. All infants showed improvement in symptoms after 1 year, and all showed a decrease in the use of concomitant medication. Measures of adrenal function after 1 year showed no change (68). There remain concerns about the effect of inhaled steroids on growth, but the dysphonia and oral thrush frequently reported do not seem to be problems in infants and young children.

ORAL STEROIDS. Oral steroids are now used earlier and more aggressively in the treatment of acute exacerbations of asthma. Again

Weinberger has provided an extensive literature review focusing especially on safety aspects (63). Storr et al. in a important paper (69) demonstrated that a large dose of prednisone administered early in an acute attack was effective at aborting many episodes and preventing admission to hospital. Steroids are often used during symptomatic exacerbations, but fewer than 5% of patients would require long-term steroid therapy. The dose should be titrated to provide optimal symptom control with the fewest possible side effects. The dose should fluctuate according to the patients symptoms and, when possible, alternate-day steroid therapy should be the goal, if extended use becomes necessary.

Administration of Treatment. The age of the child, the severity of their symptoms, and their level of cooperation all influence decisions about the route of drug administration. Although the oral route is easiest, it is associated with the most side effects and is the least effective way of giving medication particularly if symptoms are severe. The nebulizer has traditionally been seen as the most effective way of giving medication to children and, at least during an acute symptomatic phase, this view is probably correct in this age group. There are now several reports of administering aerosols by spacer and face mask to young children (70,71). These novel devices are an alternative for the uncooperative child who refuses nebulizer therapy and, even for the cooperative patient, they can often replace the nebulizer for much of the daily medication during quiescent times, increasing parental freedom and mobility. Compliance with therapy is thereby encouraged. For example, with a child who is not responding to cromolyn the two options to be considered would be nebulized budesonide or an inhaled steroid by aerosol and mask. Parents are no longer dependent on the nebulizer and also have an effective way of giving β-adrenergic agonists if they are away from home and the child becomes symptomatic.

An Approach to Treatment of the Individual Patient. As previously stated, treatment must be individualized according to the frequency and severity of the patients symptoms. A systematic approach and specific guidelines can be found in the International Consensus statement (62) and in the review by Canny and Levison (72). A suggested approach to the management of infants with either episodic asthma (episodes of symptoms with no interval symptoms) and those with moderate to severe asthma (intermittent attacks with regular symptoms between) is contained in Table 3. Specific doses of asthma medication used during acute exacerbations of asthma in infants is listed in Table 4, modified from the National Asthma Education Program (73). Special

Table 3 Management of Infants With Episodic and Moderate to Severe Asthma

Episodic Asthma		Moderate to severe	
Mild:	β-Adrenergic agonist (orally or by inhalation)	Mild:	Regular cromolyn + β-agonist
Moderate:	Nebulized β-agonist ± nebulized ipratropium ± SR[a] theophylline	Moderate:	Inhaled steroid + β-agonist (either nebulized or by MDI + mask)
Severe:	Nebulized β-agonist with addition or oral ipratropium + SR theophylline + oral steroids	Severe:	As above for moderate, steroids during exacerbations or alternate days for chronic recalcitrant symptoms

[a]SR, sustained-release.

mention should be made of the group of infants often referred to as "fat happy wheezers." These infants have loud persistent wheezing, but little in the way of constitutional disturbance. The symptoms are usually of much greater concern to the child's parents and medical attendants. A trial of bronchodilator is indicated, but the response is usually disappointing and need not be continued. Careful parental counseling is important.

Acute Attacks. The management of acute asthma in this age group is little different from that in older children, except that medication doses are different and their overall response to treatment is often less dramatic. Oxygenation should be carefully monitored and supplemental oxygen given to maintain the oxygen saturation at greater than 94%. Inhaled β-adrenergic agonists remain the mainstay of treatment. There has been a trend in recent years to use these agents more and more aggressively as their safety has been better understood. With appropriate monitoring, nebulizer therapy every 30–60 min is now commonplace, and in the critically ill infant, continuous nebulized β-adrenergic agonists may be given safely (74). Intravenous β-adrenergic agonists may be administered if the infant is unresponsive to inhaled agents. Hypokalemia is a common side effect, and potassium supplementation and monitoring are crucial. The addition of ipratropium may

Table 4 Dosages of Drugs in Acute Exacerbations of Asthma in Infants

Drug	Available form	Dosage	Comment
Inhaled β-agonist			
Albuterol			
Nebulizer solution	0.5% (5 mg/mL)	0.1–0.15 mg/kg/dose up to 5 mg every 20 min for 1–2 hr (minimum dose 1.25 mg/dose)[a]	If improved, decrease to 1–2 hr; if not improved, use by continuous inhalation
		0.5 mg/kg/hr by continuous nebulization (maximum 15 mg/hr)	
Metaproterenol			
Nebulizer solution	5% (50 mg/mL)	0.1–0.3 mL (5–15 mg); do not exceed 15 mg	
	0.6% unit-dose vial of 2.5 mL (15 mg)	As above 5–15 mg; do not exceed 15 mg	
Corticosteroids			
Outpatients	Oral prednisone, prednisolone, or methylprednisolone	1–2 mg/kg/day in single or divided doses	Reassess at 3 days as only a short burst may be needed; no need to taper dose
Hospitalized patients	Methylprednisolone IV or PO	1–2 mg/kg/dose q6 hr for 24 hr, then 1–2 mg/kg/day in divided doses q 8–12 hr	Length depends on response; may only need a few days
Systemic β-agonist			
Epinephrine HCl	1:1000 (1 mg/ml)	0.01 mg/kg up to 0.3 mg subcutaneously every 20 min for 3 doses	Inhaled β_2-agonist preferred

Table 4 (Continued)

Drug	Available form	Dosage	Comment
Terbutaline	(0.1%) 1 mg/mL solution for injection in 0.9% NaCl	Subcutaneous: 0.01 mg/kg up to 0.3 mg every 2–6 hr as needed; intravenous: 10 μg/kg over 10 min loading dose; maintenance: 0.4 μg/kg/min: increase as necessary by 0.2 μg/kg/min and expect to use 3–6 μg/kg/min (74).	Inhaled β_2-agonist preferred
Methylxanthines			
Theophylline	Aminophylline (80% anhydrous theophylline)	Loading dose:[a] If theophylline concentration known: every 1 mg/kg theophylline will give 2 μg/mL increase in concentration. Loading dose:[a] If theophylline concentration is unknown:	

No previous theophylline: 6 mg/kg aminophylline	
Previous theophylline: 3 mg/kg aminophylline	
Constant infusion rates:[a] Infusion rates to obtain a mean steady-state concentration of 15 μg/mL:	
Age	
1–6 mo	0.5 mg/kg/hr aminophylline
6 mo–1 yr	1.0 mg/kg/hr aminophylline
1–9 yr	1.5 mg/kg/hr aminophylline
10–16 yr	1.2 mg/kg/hr aminophylline

[a]Check serum concentration at approximately 1, 12, and 24 hr after starting the infusion.

be useful (64), but, if used often, signs of atropinism may develop. Parenteral steroids should obviously be used, and the expected time course of action is about 3 hr. There is a limited role for the use of intravenous aminophylline in incipient respiratory failure, as it has a stimulant effect on the diaphragm (75) as well as the respiratory center. Theophylline does appear to have anti-inflammatory effects (76) in addition to its other properties, including bronchodilation. However, it is unclear whether these effects are additional to those of steroids. For the critically ill infant there can be no substitute for care in an appropriate pediatric intensive care facility with the capacity for routine respiratory monitoring and assisted ventilation when necessary. Figures 1–3 detail in algorithm form the home management (Figure 1), emergency department treatment (Figure 2), and hospital management (Figure 3) of acute exacerbations of asthma in infants, modified from the National Asthma Education Program (73).

Prognosis

The best data on the long-term prognosis come from the longitudinal study of asthma morbidity initiated by Williams et al. in the 1960s (77). A cohort of children have now been followed for close to 30 years. Briefly, the important observations are that there is a general trend for asthma to improve with age. For those with mild symptoms in childhood, there is about a 75% chance that they will "grow out" of their asthma (improve) as they grow older. For those with more severe childhood asthma, the prospect of growing out of their asthma is reduced to about 50%. Those with multiple admissions to hospital in the first 1–2 years, chest deformity, and severe eczema are more likely to carry their disease through to adult life.

Although Williams and McNicoll, in their prospective study, were unable to show that infants who wheezed only with infection had a different prognosis, other studies have suggested that there may be two distinct groups. Parkes et al., in a long-term follow-up study over 10 years, identified two groups (78). First, a large favorable prognosis group who have recurrent episodes of cough and wheeze with viral infection, who come from nonatopic families, and who have no other clinical or laboratory evidence of atopy. Such children can be expected to outgrow their asthma by school age or shortly after. The second group is smaller, and the children in this group have features considered unfavorable. These include coexistent eczema, allergic rhinitis and positive skin tests, asthma in one or both parents, and frequent severe wheeze in the first 2 years of life. It is possible that the two groups are not distinct, but part of the same continuum.

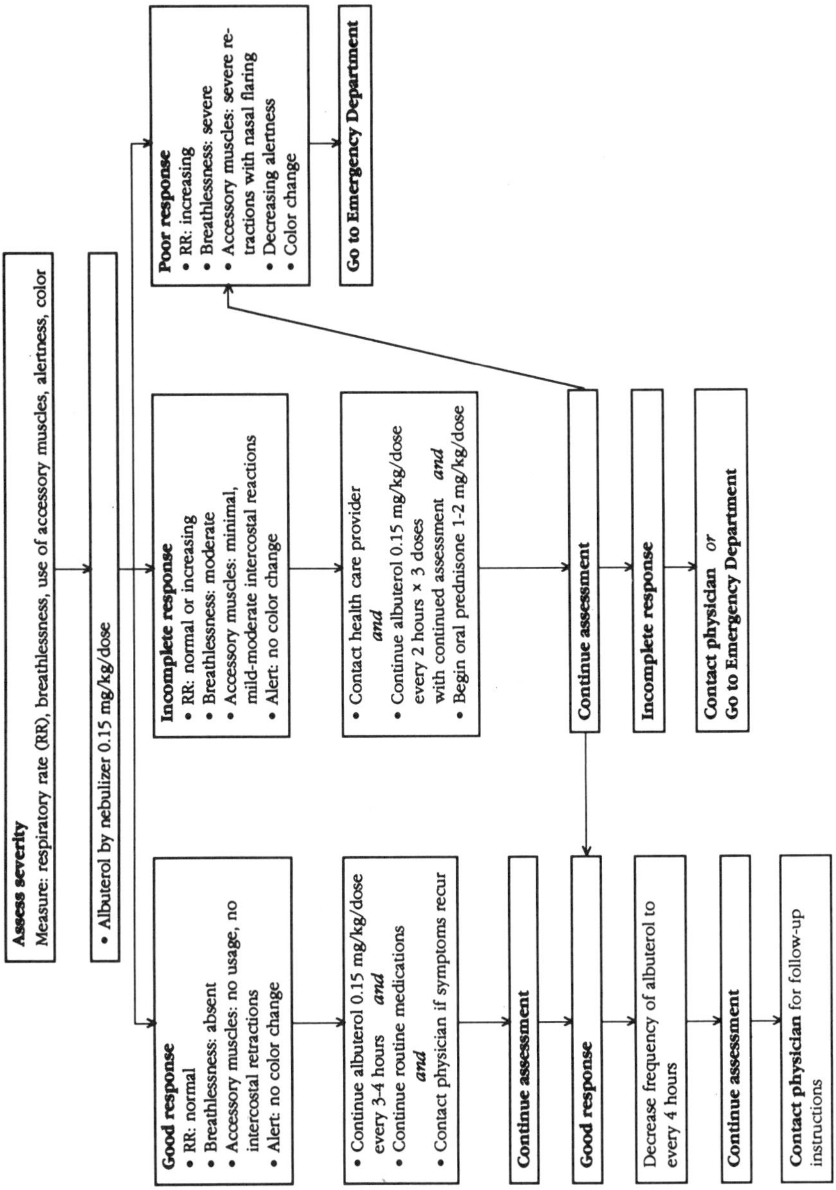

Figure 1 Acute exacerbations of asthma in infants: home management.

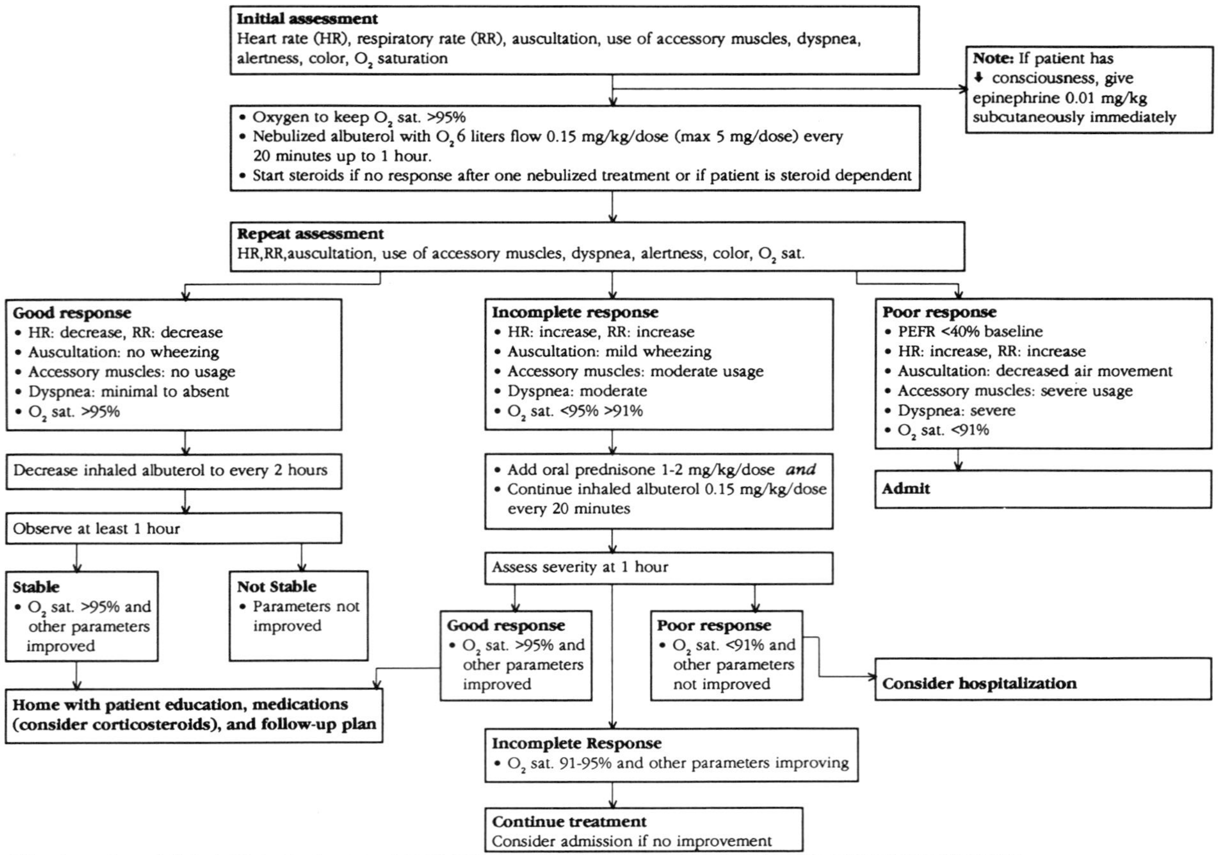

• Therapies are often available in physician's office. However, most acutely severe exacerbations of asthma require a complete course of therapy in an Emergency Department

Figure 2 Acute exacerbations of asthma in infants: emergency department management.

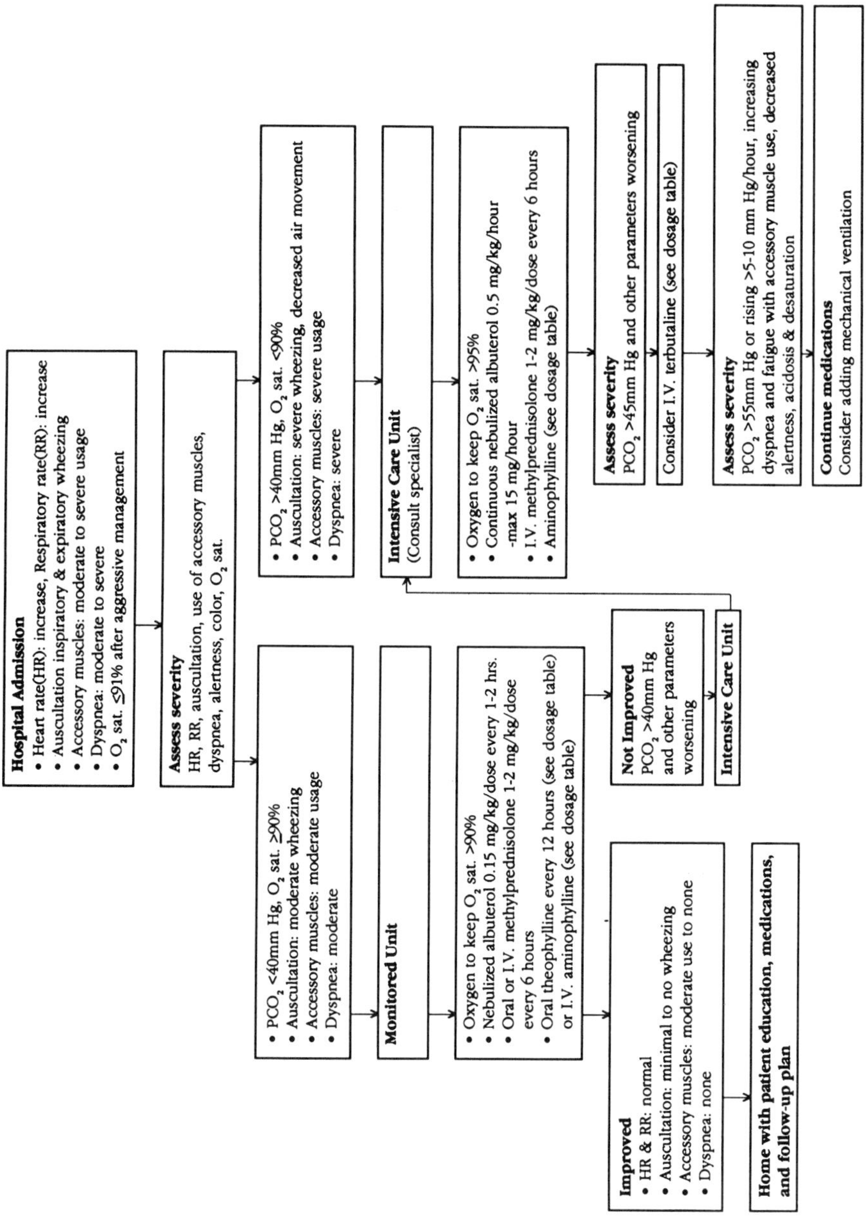

Figure 3 Acute exacerbations of asthma in infants: hospital management

Bronchopulmonary Dyplasia

With the increasing availability of neonatal intensive care and the aggressive treatment offered to very small premature infants, bronchopulmonary dysplasia (BPD) and other forms of chronic neonatal lung disease are an increasing part of pediatric pulmonary practice. A full review of BPD is beyond the scope of this chapter, but is reviewed elsewhere (79,80). In survivors of the acute phase of BPD, airway reactivity is very common (81), and overt asthma may be a major management problem in these infants. Airway reactivity appears to be a common component of the resolving airway injury in these infants. Gastroesophageal reflux is so common in infants with BPD that it must always enter into the differential diagnosis of continuing respiratory symptoms in this aged group.

Infants with severe BPD who are continuously oxygen-dependent and hospitalized are at special risk because of the high incidence of nosocomial viral infection in this situation. Many of these infants are so precariously poised physiologically that it takes little additional stress to precipitate acute respiratory failure. In this situation, respiratory failure is often a complex interaction between cardiac and respiratory factors.

Treatment of these exacerbations should ideally be carried out in a pediatric intensive care facility. Treatment involves adequate oxygenation, a trial of nebulized or intravenous β-adrenergic agonist and steroids.

In children with BPD who have a continuing asthma syndrome, a trial of nebulized cromolyn or, preferably, budesonide is certainly warranted. Some may require intermittent or continuous oral steroids. Treatment of other aggravating factors such as gastroesophageal reflux may also need to be vigorous.

Foreign Body

In young children, an inhaled foreign body must always enter into the differential diagnosis of acute or persistent wheezing. In the very young infant, an esophageal foreign body may present with respiratory symptoms from tracheal pressure. Questioning about the possibility of an inhaled foreign body should be a routine part of the initial evaluation of a wheezy infant. Regional differences in breath sounds or evidence of collapse or ball valve obstruction on the chest radiograph are suggestive features. When a foreign body is seriously suspected, bronchoscopy is indicated.

REFERENCES

1. Newth CJL. Recognition and management of respiratory failure. Pediatr Clin North Am 1979; 26:617–644.
2. Hogg JC, Williams J, Richardson JB, et al. Age as a factor in the distribution of lower airway conductance and in the pathologic anatomy of obstructive lung disease. N Engl J Med 1970; 282:1283–1287.
3. Bryan AC, Mansell AL, Levison H. Development of the mechanical properties of the respiratory system. In: Hodson W, ed. Development of the lung. New York: Marcel Decker, 1977.
4. Boyden EA. Notes on the development of the lung in infancy and early childhood. Am J Anat 1967; 121:749–762.
5. Keens T, Bryan AC, Levison H, et al. Development of fatigue resistant muscle fibers in the human diaphragm and intercostal muscles. Physiologist 1977; 20:50–54.
6. Matsuba K, Thurlbeck WM. Increased mucus glands in normal children compared to adults. Am Rev Respir Dis 1972; 105:708–710.
7. Isles AF, Newth CJL. Respiratory pharmacology. In: MacLeod S, Raddle IC, eds. Textbook of pediatric clinical pharmacology. Massachusetts: PSG Publishing, 1985: 188–208.
8. Lenny W, Milner AD. At what age do bronchodilators work? Arch Dis Child 1980; 58:279–283.
9. Polgar G, Weng TR. Functional development of the respiratory system. Am Rev Respir Dis 1979; 1120:625–695.
10. Rotschild A, Solimano A, Puterman M, Smyth J, Sharma A, Albersheim S. Increased compliance in response to salbutamol in premature infants with developing bronchopulmonary dysplasia. J Pediatr 1989; 115:984–991.
11. Mallol J, Barrueto L, Girardi G, et al. Use of nebulized bronchodilator in infants under 1 year of age: analysis of four forms of therapy. Pediatr Pulmonol 1987; 3:298–303.
12. Shuh S, Canny G, Reisman J, et al. Nebulized albuterol in acute bronchiolitis. J Pediatr 1990; 117:633–637.
13. Hughes DM, LeSouëf PN, Landau LI. Effect of salbutamol on respiratory mechanics in bronchiolitis. Pediatr Res 1987; 22:83–86.
14. Prendiville A, Green S, Silverman M. Paradoxical response to nebulized salbutamol in wheezy infants assessed by partial expiratory flow volume curves. Thorax 1987; 42:86–91.
15. Mallory GB Jr, Motoyama EK, Koumbourlis AC, Mutich RL, Nakiayama D. Bronchial reactivity in infants with respiratory failure with viral bronchiolitis. Pediatr Pulmonol 1989; 6:253–259.
16. Gupta SK, Wagener JS, Erenberg A. Pulmonary mechanics in healthy term neonates; variability in measurements obtained with a computerized system. J Pediatr 1990; 117:603–606.

17. Morgan WJ, Geller DE, Tepper R, Taussig LM. Partial expiratory flow volume curves in infants and young children. Pediatr Pulmonol 1988; 5:232–243.
18. O'Callaghan C, Milner AD, Swarbrick A. Nebulized salbutamol does have a protective effect on airways in children under 1 year of age. Arch Dis Child 1988; 63:479–483.
19. Lenny W, Milner AD. Alpha and beta adrenergic stimulants in bronchiolitis and wheezy bronchitis in children under 18 months of age. Arch Dis Child 1978; 53:707–709.
20. Newth CJL, Lipton MJ, Gould RG, Stretton M. Varying tracheal cross-sectional area during respiration in infants and children with suspected upper airway obstruction by computed cinetomography scanning. Pediatr Pulmonol 1990; 9:224–232.
21. Phelan PD, Landau LI, Olinsky A, eds. Respiratory illness in children, 3rd ed. Melbourne: Blackwell, 1990.
22. Smith GJ, Cooper DM. Laryngomalacia and inspiratory obstruction in later childhood. Arch Dis Child 1981; 56:345–349.
23. Filler RM, Rosselo PJ, Lebowitz RL. Life threatening anoxic spells caused by tracheal compression after repair of esophageal atresia; correction by surgery. J Pediatr Surg 1976; 11:739–748.
24. Filler RM, Buck JR, Bahoric A, Steward DJ. Treatment of segmental tracheomalacia and bronchomalacia by implantation of an airway splint. J Pediatr Surg 1982; 17:597–603.
25. Pagtakhan RD, Wohl ME, Chernick V. Bronchiolitis. Semin Respir Dis 1979; 1:123–130.
26. Henderson FW, Clyde WA, Collier AM, et al. The etiologic and epidemiologic spectrum of bronchiolitis in clinical practice. J Pediatr 1979; 95:183–190.
27. Pullan CR, Hey EN. Wheezing, asthma, and pulmonary dysfunction 10 years after infection with respiratory syncytial virus infection in infancy. Br Med J 1982; 284:1665–1669.
28. Hodges IG, Milner AD, Groggins RC, Stokes GM. Causes and management of bronchiolitis with chronic obstructive features. Arch Dis Child 1982; 57:495–499.
29. Sly PD, Lanteri CJ, Raven JM. Do wheezy infants respond to inhaled salbutamol? Pediatr Pulmonol 1991; 10:36–39.
30. Ribavirin therapy for respiratory syncytial virus infection [symposium]. Pediatr Infect Dis 1990; 9:9 (suppl).
31. American Academy of Pediatrics. Ribavirin therapy of respiratory syncytial virus. Pediatrics 1987; 79:475–478.
32. Groothius JR, Woodin KA, Katz R, et al. Early ribavirin treatment of respiratory syncytial viral infection in high-risk children. J Pediatr 1990; 117:792–798.
33. Phelan PD. Bronchiolitis: current concepts and controversies. Curr Ther (Aust) 1989:75–80.

34. Welliver RC, Sun M, Rinaldo D, Ogra PL. Protective value of respiratory syncytial virus-specific IgE responses for recurrent wheezing following bronchiolitis. J Pediatr 1986; 109:776–780.
35. Tabachnik E, Levison H. Infantile bronchial asthma. J Allergy Clin Immunol 1981; 67:339–347.
36. Orenstein SR, Orenstein DM. Gastroesophageal reflux and respiratory disease in childhood. J Pediatr 1988; 112:847–856.
37. Staugas R, Martin J. Binns G, Steven IM. The significance of fat-laden macrophages in the diagnosis of aspiration associated with gastro-esophageal reflux. Aust Paediatr J. 1985; 21:275–277.
38. Passive smoking—bronchial responsiveness and atopy [editorial]. Am Rev Respir Dis 1988; 138:507–509.
39. Martinez FD, Antognoni G, Macri F, Bonci E, Midulla F, DeCastro G, Ronchetti R. Parental smoking enhances bronchial responsiveness in 9 year old children. Am Rev Respir Dis 1988; 138:518–523.
40. Magnussen CG. Maternal smoking influences cord serum IgE and IgD levels and increases the subsequent risk for allergy. J Allergy Clin Immunol 1986; 78:898–904.
41. Young S, LeSouëf PN, Gellhoed GC, et al. The influence of a family history of asthma and parental smoking on airway hyper-responsiveness in early infancy. N Engl J Med 1991; 324:1168–1173.
42. Rachelefsky G, Siegel S. Asthma in infants and children. J Allergy Clin Immunol 1985; 3:3–17.
43. Burr ML, Butland B, King S, Vaughan-Williams E. Changes in asthma prevalence: two surveys 15 years apart. Arch Dis Child 1989; 64:1452–1456.
44. Anderson HR. Is the prevalence of asthma changing? Arch Dis Child 1989; 64:172–175.
45. Schwartz J, Gold D, Dockery DW, Weiss S, Speizer FE. Predictors of asthma and persistent wheeze in a national sample of children in USA. Am Rev Respir Dis 1990; 142:555–562.
46. Schneider L. Recent advances in pediatric allergy. Curr Opinion Pediatr 1990; 2:947–953.
47. Bertrand JM, Riley SP, Popkin J, Coates, AL. The long-term pulmonary sequelae of prematurity: the role of familial airway hyper-reactivity and the respiratory distress syndrome. N Engl J Med 1985; 312:742–745.
48. Shokat M, Levy G, Levy I, Schonfeld T, Merlob P. Transient tachypnoea of the newborn and asthma. Arch Dis Child 1989; 64:277–279.
49. Schatz M, Zeiger RS, Hoffman CP, Saunders BS, Harden KM, Forsythe AB. Increased transient tachypnea of the newborn in infants of asthmatic mothers. Am J Dis Child 1991; 145:156–158.
50. Bock SA. A critical evaluation of clinical trials in adverse reactions to food in children. J Allergy Clin Immunol 1986; 78:165–174.
51. Li TC, O'Connell E. Viral infection and asthma. Ann Allergy 1987; 59:321–331.

52. Minor TE, Dick EC, deMeo AN, et al. Viruses as precipitants of asthmatic attacks in children. J Am Assoc Med 1974; 227:292–298.
53. Minor TE, Dick EC, Baker JW, et al. Rhinovirus and influenza type A infection as precipitants of asthma. Am Rev Respir Dis 1976; 113:149–153.
54. Henderson AT, Clyde WA. The etiologic and epidemiologic spectrum of bronchiolitis in pediatric practice. J Pediatr 1978; 95:183–190.
55. Skoner D, Calliguri L. The wheezy infant. Pediatr Clin North Am 1988; 35:1011–1030.
56. Minor TE, Baker JW, Dick EC, et al. Greater frequency of viral respiratory infection in asthmatic children compared to non-asthmatic siblings. J Pediatr 1974; 85:472–477.
57. Cogswell JJ, Halliday DF, Alexander JR. Respiratory infections in the first year of life in children at risk of developing atopy. Br Med J 1982; 284:1011–1013.
58. Barnes P. New concepts in the pathogenesis of bronchial hyperresponsiveness and asthma. J Allergy Clin Immunol 1989; 83:1013–1025.
59. DeJongste JC, Kerrebijn KF. Asthma: mechanisms and management. Curr Opinion Pediatr 1990; 2:453–458.
60. Fireman P. Otitis media and its relationship to allergy. Pediatr Clin North Am 1988; 35:1075–1091.
61. Landau LI. New diagnostic approaches to lung disease. Curr Opinion Pediatr 1990; 2:487–494.
62. Warner JO, Götz M, Landau LI, et al. Management of asthma: a consensus statement. Arch Dis Child 1989; 64:1065–1079.
63. Weinberger M. Anti-asthmatic therapy in children. Pediatr Clin North Am 1989; 36:1251–1284.
64. Reisman J, Galdes-Sebalt M, Kazim F, Canny G, Levison H. Frequent administration by inhalation of salbutamol and ipratropium bromide in the management of acute severe asthma in children J Allergy Clin Immunol 1988; 81:16–20.
65. Newth CJL, Newth CV, Turner JAP. Comparison of nebulized sodium cromoglycate and oral theophylline in controlling symptoms of chronic asthma in preschool children. Aust NZ J Med 1982; 12:232–238.
66. Kerribijn KF. Use of topical corticosteroids in the treatment of childhood asthma. Am Rev Respir Dis 1990; 411:577–81.
67. Bisgaard G, Munch SL, Nielson JP, et al. Inhaled budesonide for the treatment of recurrent wheezing in early childhood. Lancet 1990; 336:649–651.
68. Freigang B, Ashford DR. Adrenal cortical function after long term aerosol steroid therapy in early childhood. Ann Allergy 1990; 64:342–344.
69. Storr J, Barry W, Barrell E, Lenney W. Effect of a single oral dose of prednisolone in acute childhood asthma. Lancet 1987; 8538:879–881.
70. Connor WT, Dolovich MB, Frame RA, Newhouse MT. Reliable salbutamol administration in 6–36 month old children by means of a metered dose inhaler and aerochamber with mask. Pediatr Pulmonol 1989; 6:263–267.

71. O'Callaghan C, Milner A, Swarbrick A. Spacer device with face mask attachment for giving bronchodilator to infants with asthma Br Med J 1989; 289:160–161.
72. Canny G, Levison H. Childhood asthma: a rational approach to treatment. Ann Allergy 1990; 64:406–416.
73. National Heart, Lung, and Blood Institute National Asthma Education Program Expert Panel Report. Guidelines for the diagnosis and management of asthma. Pediatr Asthma Allergy Immunol 1991; 5:57–188.
74. Portnoy L, Aggarwal J. Continuous terbutaline nebulization for the treatment of severe exacerbations of asthma in children. Ann Allergy 1988; 60:368–371.
75. Aubier M, DeTroyer A, Sampson M. Aminophylline improves diaphragmatic contractility. N Engl J Med 1981; 305:249–252.
76. Nielson CP, Crowley JJ, Morgan ME Vesta RE. Polymorphonuclear leukocyte inhibition by therapeutic concentration in theophyllin is medicated by cyclic-3′,5′-adenosine monophosphate. Am Rev Resp Dis 1988; 137:25–30.
77. Williams H, McNicol KN. Prevalence, natural history, and relationship of wheezy bronchitis and asthma in children: an epidemiological study. Br Med J 1969; 4:321–333.
78. Parkes ES, Golding J, Carswell F, et al. Pre-school wheezing and prognosis at 10 years of age. Arch Dis Child 1986; 61:642–646.
79. O'Brodovich H, Mellins RB. Bronchopulmonary dysplasia: unresolved neonatal acute lung injury. Am Rev Respir Dis 1985; 132:694–709.
80. Blanchard PW, Brown TM, Coates AL. Pharmacotherapy in bronchopulmonary dysplasia. Clin Perinatol 1987; 14:881–909.
81. Northway WH, Moss RB, Carlisle KB, et al. Late sequelae of bronchopulmonary dysplasia. N Engl J Med 1990; 323:1793–1799.

23

Prevention of Allergic Disease in Infancy

Robert S. Zeiger

Kaiser-Permanente Medical Center and University of California, San Diego, School of Medicine, San Diego, California

OVERVIEW OF PREVENTION

Although efforts to prevent allergic disease have been met with variable success over the past 60 years, a particular urgency exists today to develop efficacious preventive methods owing to the increase in atopic disease prevalence that is occurring throughout the world. Even though genetic and cellular manipulation of the atopic-prone subject may provide hope for prevention in the future, environmental engineering exists as the sole hope at the present time. Environmental engineering refers to active efforts directed at reducing the allergenic and adjuvant load to which an atopic-prone infant may be exposed. Chapters 18 and 19 emphasized the genetic and environmental risk factors critical to the development of atopy. The present chapter will (a) evaluate the successes and failures of investigative efforts directed at overcoming these risk obstacles, and (b) develop "practical" guidelines for the prevention of allergic disease.

One could direct efforts to prevent IgE-mediated disorders at any of the following stages of disease development (1):

1. Primary prevention: inhibition of IgE sensitization
2. Secondary prevention: deterrence of disease expression despite prior IgE sensitization

3. Tertiary prevention: suppression of symptoms after the occurrence of disease

Unfortunately, efforts to prevent allergic disease have met with considerable difficulty at all of these stages owing to limitations in scientific knowledge and societal compliance and resources to modulate the genetic, cellular, and environmental factors or forces, which together are responsible for the ultimate phenotypic expression of atopy.

Studies have suggested a critical time exists early in infancy in which the genetically programmed atopic-prone infant may be at an increased risk to become sensitized to allergens under certain environmental conditions. As such, prompt perinatal identification of such at-risk neonates would be important should preventive efforts prove efficacious, safe, and cost-effective. Research has uncovered several genetic and immunological factors and markers significantly associated with the subsequent development of allergic disease (Table 1); however,

Table 1 Risk Factors and Markers for Development of Atopy

Genetic and immunological		
	Atopic family history	
	Increased cord blood IgE	
	λ-MS.51 marker on chromosome 11q	
	Increased cord IgE-binding factors (soluble Fc RII)	
	Increased total serum IgE in infancy and childhood	
	Significant specific IgE antibody (skin or serum)	
	Decreased T cells (CD8+ subset) in infancy	
	Increased blood eosinophilia in infancy	
	Increased nasal eosinophilia or basophilia in infancy	
	Increased monocyte phosphodiesterase activity	
	Cord blood thrombocytopenia	
	Increased cord blood linoleic acid	
Specific environmental stimulation		
	Feeding practices	
		Brief breast-feeding
		Food allergens in breast milk
		Early solid foods
		Time of weaning
	Magnitude of allergen exposure	
	Early allergen exposure (food/inhalant, birth month)	
Nonspecific environmental stimulation		
	Pollutants including tobacco smoke	
	Infections (viral and bacterial)	

currently, none possess adequate sensitivity or specificity for practical screening of neonates to reveal those most at risk for atopy (see Chapter 5) (2,3). It is hoped that future research efforts may reveal better predictive markers. Such markers could include specific DNA polymorphisms when the genes for atopy are identified. Confirmation of the data suggesting that atopic risk may be associated with chromosome 11q (4) would certainly help in this effort.

PREVENTION OF FOOD ALLERGY

Although, over 50 years ago, Grulee and Sanford reported that breast-feeding compared with cow's milk feeding reduced the development of eczema sevenfold in a group of 10,000 infants (5), conflicting studies followed. The failure to appreciate and account for the many routes of food exposure may be responsible for some of these studies' disparate findings. Chicken's eggs, cow's milk, and peanut represent those foods in the United States most likely to induce food-specific IgE sensitization in infancy. The newborn potentially may become exposed to these and other food allergens through such routes as the placenta, breast milk, formula, solid food, and even, inadvertently, through airborne droplets or floor dusts. The relative importance of these routes in the development of food allergy and the successes or failures of preventive efforts to interfere with these exposures will be critically evaluated to develop useful prevention recommendations.

Avoidance of Allergenic Foods During Pregnancy

Although reportedly detected in early studies (6,7), specific IgE sensitization to foods in utero probably represents a rather rare event (possibly denoting false-positives assays), since such an occurrence has been detected in fewer than 0.3% of monitored pregnancies (8). Additional evidence against the existence of clinically meaningful specific IgE food sensitization in utero emanates from food allergen avoidance studies initiated during pregnancy. These studies have demonstrated a lack of effectiveness of such efforts during pregnancy to prevent the development of atopy in infancy (9,10). Specifically, two prenatally randomized studies reported that maternal diets void of milk, egg, and peanut (9), or with limited ingestion of milk or egg (10), compared with either normal (9) or high (10) exposure to these foods during the third trimester of pregnancy did not reduce the development of atopy in high–atopic-risk infants maintained on a hypoallergenic feeding regimen postnatally (breast-feeding or casein hydrolysate feeding until 3 months of age, solid foods after 4 months, and cow's milk after 6 months) (Table 2). No differences were found between these infants for (a) cord blood IgE levels, (b) incidence of food sensitization, or (c) development of atopic diseases at 6 to 18 months (9,10). Given the strong experimental evidence that intrauterine food sensitization occurs rarely, at best, and that restricted third-trimester maternal diets fail to affect atopic disease and IgE sensitization to egg, cow's milk, or peanut postnatally, it is inappropriate, futile, and potentially nutritionally harmful to mother and fetus (1,9,10) to implement such food avoidance regimens during pregnancy, with the intent of preventing food allergy.

Breast-feeding

Protective Effect of Breast Milk on Allergen Exposure and Absorption

By reducing both exposure to and intestinal absorption of food allergens, breast milk may decrease allergic sensitization. Specifically, breast milk functions to inhibit the increase in food antigen absorption that occurs early postnatally in newborn animals (11). Similarly, in humans, significantly higher antigen absorption occurs in preterm than in term neonates (12,13), which may place preterm or low-birth-weight infants at increased risk for developing IgE sensitization to foods, particularly cow's milk formula. In addition, a significant increase in peripheral blood histamine release to cow's milk was seen in preterm infants fed cow's milk, compared with banked breast milk, a response that correlated inversely with birth weight and gestational age (14). Consistent with these findings, a prospective randomized, and controlled study of 446 preterm neonates demonstrated that early exposure to cow's milk formula compared with banked breast milk increased the risk of developing allergic disease by 18 months (particularly eczema) (odds ratio 3.6 with 95% confidence interval 1.4–9.1) in the subgroup of neonates with an allergic family history (15). The specific factor(s) contained in breast milk responsible for these effects remain speculative, but include the protective capacity of human breast milk immunoglobulins, especially secretary IgA (sIgA), to inhibit intestinal absorption of food antigens (16), although conflicting data exist (17), and that of mucosal growth factor to facilitate early maturation of the gut (closure) (18).

As for the potential protective effect of breast milk sIgA, an uncontrolled study reported that total sIgA and milk-specific IgA antibodies to whole cow's milk and casein were significantly lower in breast milk from mothers of allergic compared with nonallergic infants (19).

In contrast with the foregoing study, a prospective controlled study of 123 high–atopic-risk neonates, followed from birth and breast-fed for at least 4 months, noted that maternal breast milk anti-cow's milk IgA levels were above the median significantly more frequently in those infants developing food allergy by 1 and 2 years (Zeiger RS, Machtingers, unpublished observations). The differing results of these two studies probably cannot arise solely from the study of atopic-prone neonates in the latter and unselected neonates in the former. Studies are needed to resolve these differences.

Effect of Breast Milk Compared with Cow's Milk Feeding on Allergic Sensitization and Allergic Disease.

Long-standing debate, raised over 50 years ago, still exists over whether breast-feeding prevents, reduces, delays, or increases the development of allergic disease. Even recent prospective natural history studies note conflicting results (20–26). Such disparate data may result from differences in study design, quality, size, and duration. Since several comprehensive reviews of this subject have been published recently (8,27,28), the subject will be discussed only briefly here. Discussion will concentrate on only those prospective studies that compared the effect of breast with cow's milk feeding on the development of atopy. For ease of discussion, they have been separated into those studies either reporting that breast-feeding was beneficial (Table 3) or not beneficial (Table 4) relative to the development of atopy. Although more published studies support the concept that breast-feeding reduces allergic disease development when compared with cow's milk formula-feeding, several more recent prolonged exclusive breast-feeding investigations of atopic-prone infants failed to demonstrate any allergy protective role of breast-feeding (see Table 4). The principal design weakness inherent in all these investigations (see Tables 3 and 4) was the failure to randomize the study groups, which may have led to biases in family recruitment and confounding variables. For example, breast-compared to formula-fed groups frequently reveal significantly less parental smoking, higher parental educational level, and greater home care, characteristics associated with health consciousness, which occurs more frequently in self-selected breast-feeding mothers (29). Such behaviors represent potential risk factors for the development of food and inhalant allergies, since they should be expected to delay solid food introduction, decrease exposure to viruses, and reduce second-hand smoke inhalation (3).

In addition to the failure to randomize groups, these breast and cow's milk comparison studies were individually flawed by such short-

Table 2 Prospective Randomized Controlled Studies of Hypoallergenic Dietary Regimens on the Development of Allergic Disease in Infants of Atopic Families

		Dietary regimens				Efficacy of dietary regimen	
Study (Ref)	Number	Maternal pregnancy	Maternal lactation	Infant	Follow-up (yrs)	Specific IgE sensitization	Atopic disease
Chandra et al.[82]	71	Entire (no egg, CM, peanut, fish, or beef)	Yes (same as pregnancy)	Exclusive breast for 5–6 mo	1.0	Not determined	Reduced eczema[a]
Falth-Magnusson et al.[9]	197	Third trimester (no egg, CM)	None	Breast +/or casein hydrolysate for 3 mo; solid foods > 4 mo; CM > 6 mo; egg/fish > 9 mo	1.5	Not significant	Not significant
Lilja et al.[10]	162	Third trimester (low egg, CM)	None	Breast +/or Soy for 6 mo; solids > 3 mo; CM > 6 mo (most); egg/fish > 9mo	1.5	Not significant	Not significant
Zeiger et al.[1]	288	Third trimester (no egg, CM, peanut)	Yes (same as pregnancy)	Breast +/or casein hydrolysate for 12 mo; Solids > 6 mo; CM, soy, corn > 12 mo; egg, peanut, fish > 24 mo	2.0	Reduced prevalence of CM IgE[b]	Reduced prevalence of food allergy[b]

Hattevig et al.[44]	115	None	Yes, (no egg, CM, fish, × 3 mo)	Breast +/or casein hydrolysate for 6 mo; CM and solids > 6 mo; egg/fish > 9 mo	1.5	Reduced number of tests for CM and/or egg IgE[b]	Reduced AD at 3[b] and 6 mo[a]
Chandra et al.[45]	97	None	Yes (no CM, egg, fish, peanuts, soy)	Exclusive breast for 6 mo; solids ~ 6 mo	1.5	Not determined	Reduced eczema[a]
Chandra et al.[45]	124	None	None (no breast feeding)	Exclusive casein hydrolysate, soy, or CM	1.5	Not determined	Reduced eczema with casein-hydrolysate[a]

CM, cow milk; AD, atopic dermatitis.
[a] $p < 0.05$
[b] $p < 0.01$
Source: Ref. 3.

Table 3 Prospective, Nonrandomized Studies of Effect of Breast Versus Cow Milk Feeding on Development of Allergy (Studies Reporting Benefit of Breast Feeding)

Investigator (Ref)	Year	B (n)/C (n)[a]	Interval (yr)	Eczema allergy outcome	Design weaknesses[b]
Grulee and Sanford[(5)]	1936	9749/1707	3/4	E: C = 7 × B	2, 3, 4, 5, 6
Matthew et al.[(136)]	1979	23/19	1	E: 13% B vs 47% C[c]	1, 2, 3, 5, 7, 8, 9
Saarinen et al.[(137)]	1979	25/19	3	E: at 3 yr ↓ B	2, 3, 5, 9
Ziering et al.[(138)]	1979	25/25	2	A: B = 34%; C = 65%	1, 2, 3, 5, 9
Chandra[(139)]	1979	37/37	3	E: 11% B vs 59% C[d]	2, 3, 5, 9, 10
Juto and Bjorksten[(140)]	1980	46/22	1	A: at 3 & 6 mo ↓ B[a]	1, 2, 3, 4, 5, 9
Gruskay[(53)]	1982	48/201	14	A: B ↓ 46% at 14 yr	2, 3, 5, 6
Businco et al.[(7)]	1983	34/41	2	A: B = 18%; C = 37%	1, 2, 3, 5, 9
Chandra et al.[(141)]	1985	72/48	2	E & AS: B = 17%; C = 52%	2, 3, 5, 9

[a]B, breast feeding; C, cow milk feeding; E, eczema; A, allergy; and AS, asthma.
[b]Design weaknesses: 1, late solids in B; 2, not randomized; 3, no blinding; 4, unselected sample; 5, compliance not documented; 6, lack of immunology; 7, environmental control in B; 8, dropout high; 9, small (n); and 10, B < 4 months.
[c]$p < .05$
[d]$p < 10^{-3}$
Source: Ref. 30.

comings as (a) nonblinded evaluations, (b) absence of immunological confirmation of diagnoses, (c) failure to document compliance to dietary regimen, (d) inadequate sample size, (f) brief duration of breast-feeding, and (g) differences in environmental control measures between groups. These limitations of study design preclude reaching definitive conclusions about the potential benefits of breast-feeding in reducing allergic disease. The detection of dietary allergens in breast milk (1) and the early sensitization of exclusively breast-fed infants to egg and milk (30–33) add complexity to this situation. These findings indicate that institution of maternal dietary restrictions during exclusive breast-feeding might be necessary to prevent food allergy.

Maternal Avoidance of Allergenic Food During Lactation

Food allergens in human breast milk have been implicated in causing food-specific IgE sensitization and food allergy in about 6% of infants of atopic parents, presumably exclusively breast-fed (32,33), with initial symptoms occurring at the time of the presumed initial direct food

Table 4 Prospective, Nonrandomized Studies of Effect of Breast Versus Cow Milk Feeding on Development of Allergy (Studies Nonsupportive of Benefit of Breast Feeding)

Investigator (Ref)	Year	B (*n*)/C (*n*)[a]	Interval (yr)	Outcome	Design weaknesses[b]
Kaufman[(142)]	1972	38/54	2	E > 50% B and C	1, 2, 3, 5, 8, 9
Halpern et al.[(143)]	1973	193/349	0.5–7	A = 16% B and C	1, 2, 3, 4, 5, 6, 9
Kaufman and Frick[(144)]	1976	38/56	2	E = 32% B; 23% C	1, 2, 3, 5, 8, 9
Hide and Guyer[(145)]	1981	204/62	1	A = 45% B; 53% C E = 10% B; 13% C	1, 2, 3, 5, 6, 7, 9
Gordon et al.[(146)]	1982	112/85	2	NS	1, 2, 3, 5, 9
Van Asperen et al.[(147)]	1984	54/25[c]	1.3	E = 52% B; 40% C	2, 3, 5, 8, 9
Van Asperen et al.[(147)]	1984	19/60[d]	1.3	E = 58% B; 45% C	2, 3, 5, 8

[a]B, breast feeding; C, cow milk feeding; E, eczema; and A, allergies.
[b]1, early solids; 2, nonrandomized; 3, no blinding; 4, unselected; 5, undocumented compliance; 6, lack of immunology; 7, dropout high; 8, (*n*) small; and 9, B < 3 mo.
[c]Breast feeding for only 2 mo.
[d]Breast feeding for only 4 mo.
Source: Ref. 30.

exposure (30,32). Moreover, milk-specific IgE has been reported commonly in, and even sometimes more often in, breast-fed than formula-fed infants (34,35). Nanogram concentrations of food allergens in breast milk may be responsible for this phenomenon. Thus far three bovine milk antigens [β-lactoglobulin (BLG), casein, and IgG; (19, 36–39)], chicken's egg ovalbumin (OVA; 40), and gliadin (41) have been detected in most samples of breast milk from mothers not avoiding these foods. These food allergens appear in breast milk within 2–6 hr and may persist for days after maternal ingestion of 4 oz (118 mL) of cow milk, one raw egg, or one slice of bread (19,37,38,40,41). As expected, food antigens are rarely detected in breast milk from mothers avoiding these food substances (19,37,42). Maternal handling of food antigens generally has been similar whether mother or infant are atopic or nonatopic (19,38,40), although other studies reported higher breast milk levels of cow's milk protein in infants who developed "atopic-like" symptoms (38) and colic (39). The wide overlap of values suggest that these findings may not be clinically relevant. Molecular sizing of the food antigens in breast milk suggest that these antigens may maintain their potential for infant sensitization (43). However, although the levels of food allergens in breast milk exist in sufficient quantity to trigger allergic reactions in sensitized infants, it is unknown whether such quantities can *prime* the infant's immune system to produce food-specific IgE.

Recognition of the existence of potentially allergenic food antigens in breast milk led to attempts to evaluate the effect of maternal diets during lactation on the development of atopy (44,45) (see Table 1). Avoidance of egg, cow's milk, and fish (n = 60) compared with an unrestricted diet (n = 50) during the first 3 months of lactation by atopic mothers, grouped according to attendance at one of two hospitals providing their health care in Sweden, in a prospective 18-month study, was reported to reduce eczema by 3 months (3 vs 22%, $p < 0.01$), 6 months (11 vs 28%, $p < 0.05$), but not 18 months in infants adhering to a similar hypoallergenic diet for 6 months (44). A lower prevalence of lactation-diet infants had detectable specific IgE to egg or milk at 3 months ($p = 0.06$), but not thereafter, possibly because of the introduction of milk and egg after 6 months. Infants in both the lactation- and normal-diet groups developed similar levels of total serum IgE and specific IgG antibodies to OVA and BLG from birth to 18 months (46). Restriction of milk and egg during lactation for only 3 months failed to suppress the IgG OVA or BLG responses after these foods were introduced to the infant after 6 months of life. The observation that serum levels of IgG antibodies to OVA increased in infants before introduction of eggs into the infants' diet implied that the nanogram per milliliter quantities of egg white antigen in breast milk might be sufficient to induce an IgG antibody response in the infants. Moreover, the association of an augmented IgG OVA response, with an increased specific IgE response to egg white, suggests that IgG OVA, rather than protecting against the development of an IgE response, merely represents the inherent immunological response of high-responder infants (46). The failure to randomize the groups, although shown demographically to be similar, weakens the study to some uncertain degree.

Confirmation of the foregoing findings was reported in a prospective, controlled study of 97 infants born to atopic parents (45). Mothers planning to breast-feed exclusively for 6 months received random allocation to either a lactation diet, avoiding milk products, eggs, fish, peanuts, and soy, or a diet with *no* restrictions. The specific dietary regimen of the infants after 6 months was unfortunately omitted. The lactation-restricted diet appeared to halve the cumulative incidence of eczema by 18 months [11/49 (22%) vs 21/48 (48%), $p < 0.05$] (45). Since the relation of the eczema to food sensitization was not investigated immunologically or by food challenge, the results of this study must be considered with reservations.

It is essential to confirm the foregoing findings by more definitive randomized studies that correlate disease occurrence with food sensitization before maternal lactation avoidance diets are universally recommended to prevent food allergy and atopic dermatitis in infancy.

Effect of Soy Feeding on Development of Atopy (Table 5)

Initial retrospective studies (50–52) extolled the value of soy formula feeding in reducing atopy. A subsequent prospective randomized study by the same group (47) reported that soy feeding reduced asthma and perennial rhinitis by 3 years without affecting the development of atopic dermatitis in infancy or hay fever during childhood. The failure of soy feeding to affect atopic dermatitis (the atopic condition most associated with food allergy) cast doubt on the findings and led to subsequent investigations (45,48,49,54,148). These randomized prospective studies of infants, generally from atopic families, uniformly failed to demonstrate any reduction in the development of atopy in infancy and childhood derived from soy compared with cow's milk feeding (45,48, 49,54,148). These findings are consistent with studies that verified the immunogenic and allergenic capacity of soybean protein (55–58). These results suggest that intact soybean protein formulas should not be considered hypoallergenic nor used in attempts to prevent food allergy in infancy.

Table 5 Prospective Randomized Studies of Soy (S) Versus Cow's Milk (CM) Feedings on Development of Allergy in Infancy

Study (Ref)	S (*n*)/CM (*n*)	Allergy outcome
Johnstone and Dutton[47]	115/120	Asthma $<$ 3 yr ($p < .05$) Chronic rhinitis $<$ 6 yr ($p < .01$) No difference in eczema/hay fever by 10 yr
Brown et al.[48]	85/196	No difference in allergies by 1.5 yr
Kjellman and Johansson[49]	23/25	No difference in allergies by 3 yr (soy = 74%; cow's milk = 60%)
Miskelly et al.[148]	228/233	No difference in allergies by 1 yr
Chandra et al.[45]	40/41	No difference in eczema by 1.5 yr

Source: Ref. 8.

Effect of Hypoallergenic Protein Hydrolysate Formula Feeding on Development of Allergic Disease

Allergenicity and Immunogenicity

In the 1940s, protein hydrolysate formulas, prepared by extensively hydrolyzing casein to peptides below 1500 Da, were developed to treat infants with gastrointestinal food intolerances, food allergies, and malabsorption. Such molecular-sized peptides generally contain from six to nine amino acids that, subsequently, have been shown to behave nonimmunologically upon injection into animals (59). The extensive hydrolysis attempted to reduce or eliminate allergenicity and immunogenicity, but retain nutritional adequacy and palatability at reasonable cost. Preclinical screening of these hydrolysates revealed (a) absence of animal passive cutaneous anaphylaxis (PCA) [suggesting a relative molecular mass (M_r) < 3400 Da], (b) absence of any intact proteins, (c) over 99% of the peptides with an M_r of less than 1500 Da, and (d) less than 1 millionth of the protein determinant equivalence of the original protein (60). Recently, these hydrolysates (Nutramigen), as well as the more recently developed casein hydrolysate (Alimentum), were shown by double-blind, placebo-controlled food challenges (DBPCFC) (the gold standard in food testing) and then in open consumption to be tolerated in 23 consecutive and documented milk-allergic infants (determined by positive DBPCFC to cow's milk) (61).

Commercially available protein hydrolysates in the United States reveal different characteristics (Table 6). The two casein hydrolysates,

Table 6 Protein Hydrolysate Formulas: Composition, Cost, Allergenicity, and Immunogenicity

Brand	Nutramigen	Alimentum	Good Start
Year introduced	1942	1989	1989
Hydrolysate	Casein	Casein	Whey
Oil	Corn	Safflower	Coconut/palm
Carbohydrate	Corn syrup solids	Sucrose tapioca	Lactose-14%
Cost/32 oz	\$3.02	\$2.60	\$1.43
% > 1.5kd	None	< 1%	> 20%
Antigen (μg/g)[a]	0.4	1.3	752
USP guinea pig assay	Negative	Negative	Negative
Reactions in milk-allergic	Rare	Rare	May be frequent

[a]Sampson HA, et al., J Pediatr 1991; 118:520–525.
Source: Ref. 8.

Nutramigen and Alimentum, represent extensively hydrolyzed formulations (60,61). On the other hand, the whey hydrolysate, Good Start, has been only partially hydrolyzed and, therefore, contains large quantities of peptides larger than 4000 Da, determined by sodium dodecylsulfate–polyacrylamide gel electrophoresis, (SDS–PAGE), and more than 2–3 log higher levels of immunologically identifiable cow's milk proteins, determined by enzyme-linked immunosorbent assay (ELISA), than either of the casein hydrolysates (60). The hypoallergenicity of the casein hydrolysates (Nutramigen and Alimentum) was documented recently by Sampson et al. (60) with 95% confidence that at least 90% of milk-allergic children should be able to consume either without reactions (60) (a level of confidence designated as *hypoallergenic* by the American Academy of Pediatrics). In contrast, the partially hydrolyzed whey hydrolysate (variously named in the world as Good Start, LH, or Alfare) in quantities from 1 to 5 mL led to allergic reactions in five consecutive milk-allergic infants (63). Although the casein hydrolysates have received hypoallergenic labeling and the safety, and hypoallergenicity of Nutramigen has been documented by 50 years of safe commercial use in milk-sensitive infants and children (1,64–68), they are not completely nonallergenic, since in rare instances, they have been implicated in allergic reactions (69,70) or intolerance (71,72) in cow's milk-sensitive subjects. It remains prudent, therefore, for cow's milk-allergic patients to ingest these casein hydrolysates for the first time in the presence of physicians experienced and equipped to treat anaphylaxis (8,61). These findings should dissuade clinicians from using partially-hydrolyzed milk protein formulas in cow's milk-allergic patients (1,60,63,71).

Prevention of Atopy

For prevention of atopic disease, ideally one should use the least immunogenic and allergenic formula. In experiments employing animal-sensitizing models, Nutramigen exhibited no sensitizing capacity, whereas formulas, such as evaporated milk, purified intact lactose-free casein, chicken, and soy led to sensitization in 100, 90, 70, and 55% of animals, respectively (72). These data prompted (73) the use of protein hydrolysates such as Nutramigen for infant feeding or supplementation in studies evaluating the capacity of various dietary regimens to prevent the development of allergic disease in infants at high risk for atopy. Zeiger et al. (1) noted that Nutramigen (as part of a hypoallergenic dietary regimen), compared with cow's milk feeding, from birth in non–breast-fed infants or as a supplement to breast-feeding was associated with a lower prevalence of formula allergy and milk-specific IgE by 1 year in infants at risk for atopy

[0% (n = 89) in the Nutramigen group compared with 4.3% (n = 161) in the cow's milk group, (p = 0.053, two-tail)]. In addition, the hypoimmunogenicity of Nutramigen was documented by its capacity, compared with cow's milk formula, to inhibit the IgG BLG response before and after cow's milk introduction (Figure 1). Such findings confirm the preliminary study of Eastham et al. (74) who reported that five infants fed a casein hydrolysate (Nutramigen), compared with five given cow's milk formula for three months, developed significantly lower whey hemagglutinins before and after cow's milk intake. In addition, Zeiger et al. reported that casein hydrolysate-fed infants demonstrated a decreased BLG IgG response similar to that observed in infants solely breast-fed until 1 year, whether or not a maternal lactation diet free of cow's milk was adopted (see Figure 1) (1). These findings extend those of Kletter et al. (75), who noted that infants solely breast-fed for 3 months (n = 44) had reduced cow's milk IgG responses and suppression of the peak response after addition of cow's milk, compared with a group fed cow's milk from birth (n = 165). These findings reveal reduced immunogenicity of casein hydrolysate formula (Nutramigen) and exclusive breast-feeding in unselected infants (74,75) and also in at-risk atopic infants (1), those most expected to mount strong immunological responses.

Confirming the foregoing beneficial effect of protein hydrolysate formulas, Chandra et al. (45,54) noted, in two prospective, randomized controlled studies in non–breast-fed atopic-prone infants, that casein (45) or whey (54) hydrolysate, compared with cow milk or soy feeding, was associated with a lower cumulative incidence of eczema by 6 months (54) and 18 months (45) (see Table 2). Unfortunately, immunological and food challenge confirmation was omitted from one (45) and incomplete in the other study (54).

These studies require confirmation before protein hydrolysate formulas are proclaimed effective and safe for the prevention of atopy in high–atopic-risk infants when breast-feeding is not a choice or when formula supplementation is desired. The casein hydrolysates may be preferable (8,60) to the partial whey hydrolysates for purposes of allergy prevention. Casein hydrolysates are hypoallergenic (60) and hypoimmunogenic (8) (see Figure 1), whereas the partial whey hydrolysates may induce milk-specific IgE (54) and are more likely to cause anaphylaxis in an infant who has become sensitized to cow's milk from other sources (8).

Delayed Introduction of Solid Foods

The effect of solid food ingestion on the development of eczema by ages 2 and 10 years and asthma by age 4 years was analyzed in an unselected, uncontrolled, prospective birth cohort study of 1265 New

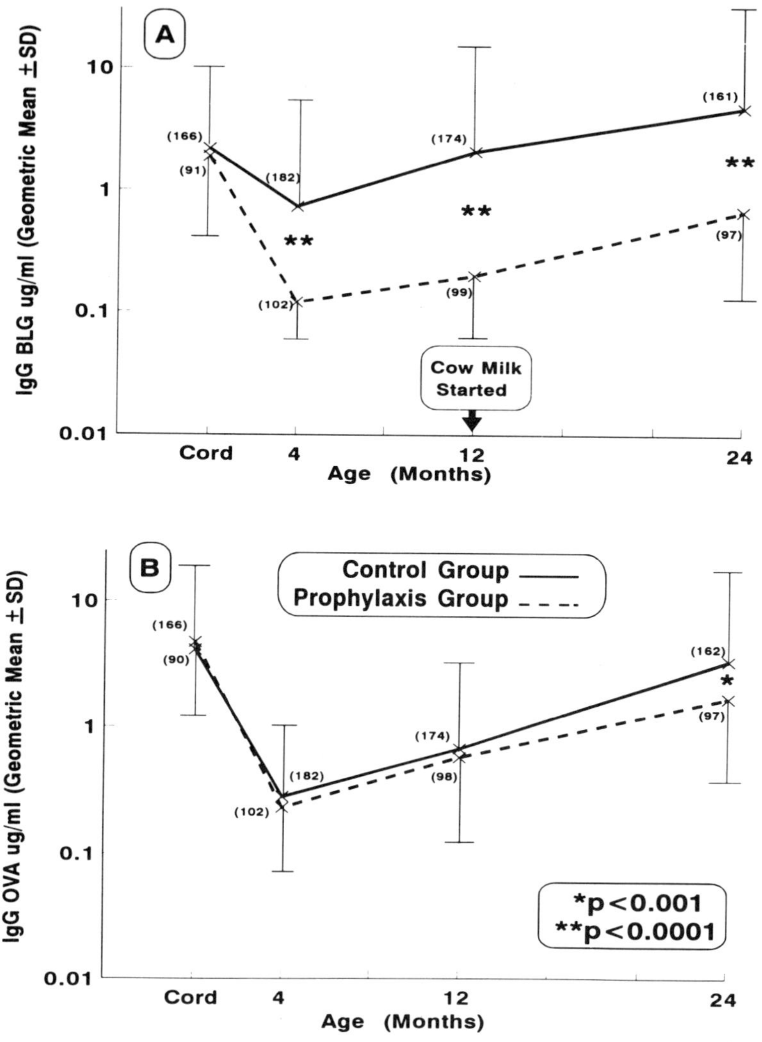

Figure 1 IgG Beta-lactoglobulin (BLG) (A) and IgG Ovalbumen/Ovomucoid (OVA) (B) response from birth to 2 years in prophylactic-treated and control groups. (Reprinted from Zeiger RS, Heller S, Mellon MH, et al.). Genetic and environmental factors effecting the development of atopy through age 4 in children of atopic parents: A prospective randomized study of food allergen avoidance. Pediatr Allergy Immunol (in press).

Zealand neonates in which 1067 or 84% were evaluated at 10 years (76–79). The prevalence of eczema related significantly to parental atopy and solid-feeding patterns. A 2.5-fold greater incidence of eczema by 2 years occurred in infants of atopic parents. On the other hand, the development of asthma was not related to solid food feeding (79). A statistically significant linear relation existed between the number of solid foods introduced during the first 4 months of life and the ensuing incidence of one episode of eczema by 2 years (76) and 3 years (77) and recurrent or chronic eczema by 10 years (78). Moreover, there was an almost threefold increase in the risk of recurrent or current eczema by 10 years in infants ingesting four or more solid foods, compared with infants not receiving solid foods by 4 months (78). Limitations of this series of reports include chart review, rather than objective determination of disease etiology either immunologically or by food challenge.

A prospective nonrandomized study of 115 infants from atopic families evaluated the effect of delaying solid food introduction on the development of eczema and food allergy (80). Eczema developed by 1 year in only 14% of infants exclusively breast-fed for 6 months, compared with 35% ($p < 0.01$) in a group of breast-fed infants in whom solid foods were introduced at 3 months of age (80). The failure to randomize the groups weakens the impact of the study's findings.

Taken together, such findings suggest that early exposure to multiple foodstuffs may predispose infants, particularly those at risk for atopy, to recurrent or chronic eczema. In contrast, it has been reported that the benefit of delaying the introduction of solid foods may merely postpone the development of food allergy (81). Nevertheless, the weight of evidence suggests that the neonate, with his or her immature gastrointestinal system, poorly excludes multiple allergens or large quantities of allergens that may prime the IgE-sensitizing system in atopic-prone infants. Delaying solid food feeding until after 6 months has many advocates; additional confirmatory studies would solidify such pronouncements.

Maternal and Infant Avoidance of Allergenic Foods

The existence of multiple potential sources of food exposure in infants led to the suggestion that it probably would be necessary to institute dietary restriction in both infant and mother to optimally minimize food allergen exposure (73). Two studies have examined the effect of such combined maternal and infant dietary avoidance regimens (see Table 2) (1,82). In a prospective, randomized controlled study of atopic-prone infants exclusively breast-fed for 6 months. Chandra et al. (82) reported a reduced incidence of eczema by 1 year in the group whose mothers excluded milk, egg, peanut, fish, and beef throughout *pregnancy and lactation*, compared with a group whose mothers maintained an unrestricted diet. Casein, BLG, or OA was rarely detected in the breast milk of mothers practicing dietary restriction compared with control mothers ($p < 0.01$), demonstrating relative compliance in the diet-restricted group. Study weaknesses included (a) a partial self-selection to the respective groups, (b) absence of immunological or food challenge confirmation of a food basis for the eczema, and (c) lack of blinding (82).

In a prenatally randomized, physician-blinded, parallel controlled trial Zeiger et al (1) compared the effect of combined maternal and infant food allergen avoidance (prophylaxis group) with currently recommended maternal- and infant-feeding practices, on the development of allergic disease by 2 years in infants born to documented allergic parents. The diet regimen of the prophylaxis group ($n = 103$) included *(a) maternal avoidance of milk, egg, and peanut during both the third trimester of pregnancy and lactation, and (b) infant breast or Nutramigen feedings and avoidance of solid foods for 6 months; milk, corn, soy, citrus, and wheat for 1 year; and egg, peanut, and fish for 2 years.* The control group ($n = 185$) followed standard pregnancy diets and American Academy of Pediatrics-recommended infant-feeding practices. The prevalences of atopic disorders were reduced at 1 year owing to lower prevalences of food allergy in the prophylaxis group (Figure 2). Specific IgE sensitization to foods, determined by skin-prick tests, were reduced significantly in infants in the prophylaxis group at 1 year owing to a lower prevalence of milk-specific IgE [1% in the prophylaxis compared with 9% in the control group, ($p = 0.01$)]. Serum IgE was marginally lower only at 4 months in the prophylaxis compared with the control group ($p = 0.07$). The prevalences of allergic rhinitis, asthma, and inhalant IgE were similar in both groups (1).

The effectiveness of the prolonged combined maternal and infant dietary avoidance regimen practiced in the foregoing study (1), contrasts with that of Lilja et al. (83), who did not observe a reduction in food atopy when maternal and infant food avoidance were practiced for less than 6 months postnatally. Lilja et al. (83) reported that both the restricted and nonrestricted diet groups developed similar IgG responses to BLG and OVA from birth to 18 months of age. In contrast, Zeiger et al. (1) documented significantly suppressed IgG BLG responses from 4 to 24 months (8) (see Figure 1) and IgG OVA by 24 months (Figure 1) in the prophylactic diet compared with control group. Such findings

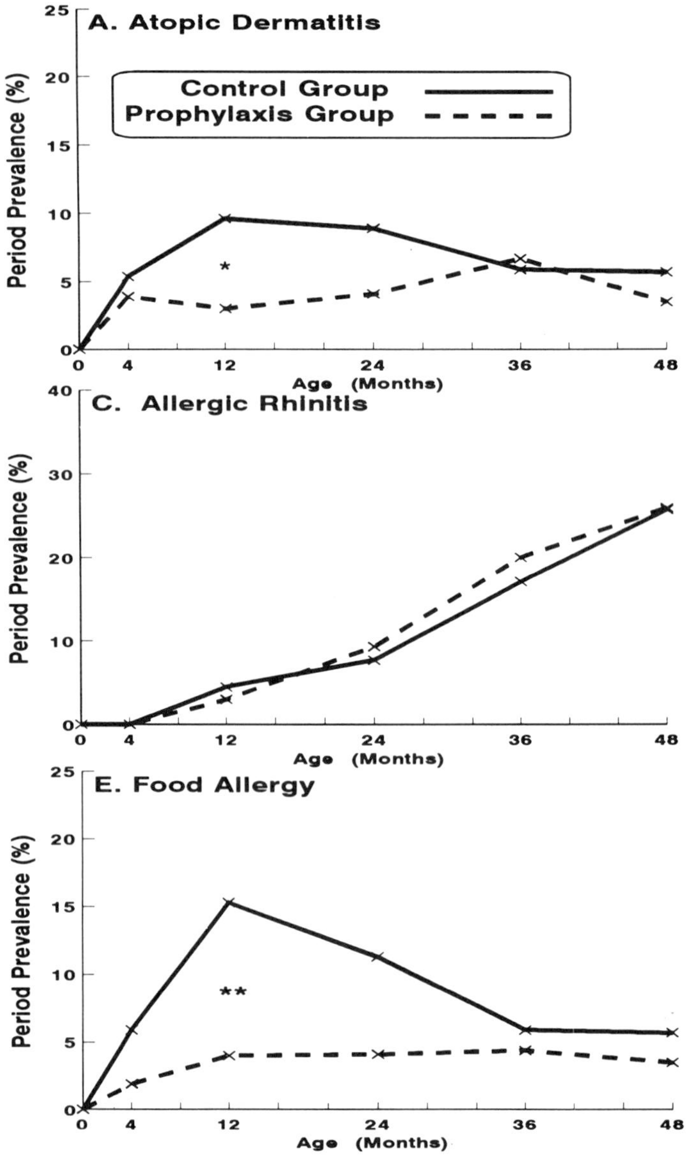

Figure 2 Period prevalences of atopic disorders from birth to 4 years in prophylactic-treated and control groups. (Reprinted from Zeiger RS, Heller S, Mellon MH, et al.). Pediatr Allergy Immunol (in press).

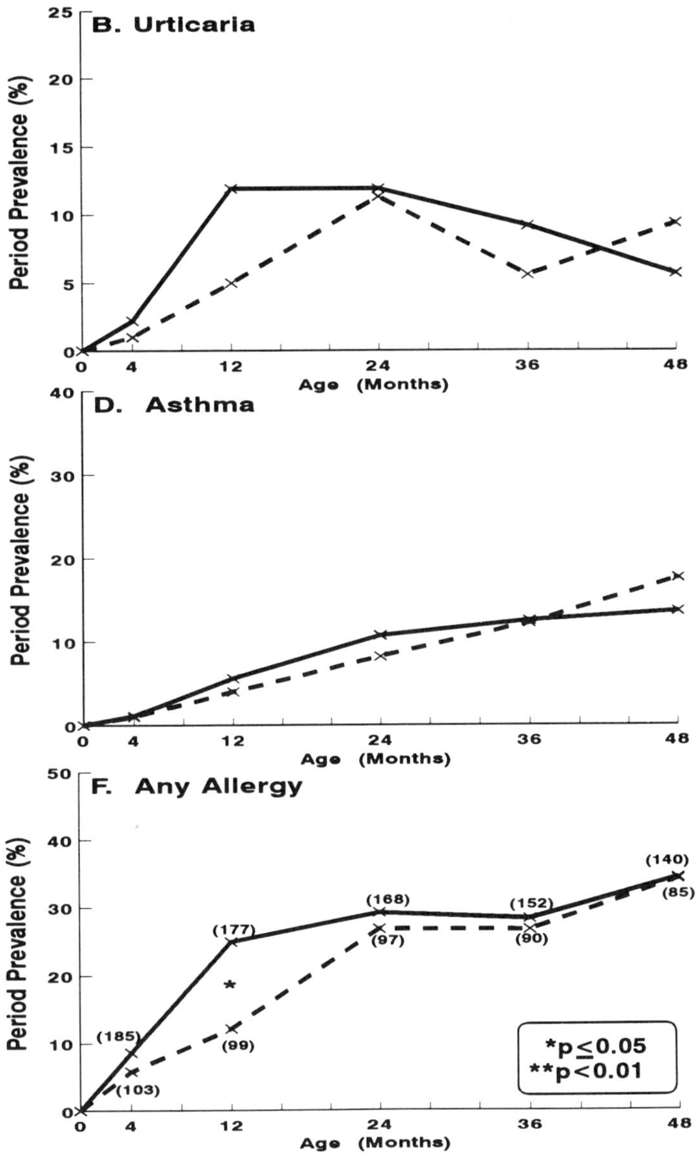

Figure 2 (Continued)

suggest that a prolonged avoidance of allergenic foods may be necessary to optimally prevent or reduce the development of food allergy. The optimal duration of dietary avoidance remains speculative, but between 6 and 12 months is suggested by previous studies (1,80).

On the other hand, it has been postulated that small quantities of, or delay in introduction of, food allergens such as cow's milk potentially could increase, rather than decrease allergic sensitization in humans, analogous to such a phenomenon documented in animal studies (84). Recent data does not support a similar phenomenon in humans (1,8,85). A prospective, randomized study reported that delayed cow's milk ingestion during the first year of life in infants of allergic parents significantly decreased the cumulative prevalence of cow's milk allergy, reduced the cumulative prevalence of specific IgE sensitization to cow's milk, and suppressed the IgG BLG response before and after cow's milk introduction, compared with a control group supplemented or maintained on cow's milk formula from birth (see Figure 1) (1,8). Host et al. (85) also noted a significantly lower incidence of cow's milk allergy in exclusively breast-fed infants (0.5 %), compared with formula-supplemented infants (2.2%), in a longitudinal study of 1749 Danish neonates. Inadvertent exposure to up to 4 oz (118 mL) of cow's milk formula in the nursery was possibly responsible for sensitization of the exclusive breast-fed group. The quantity of cow's milk protein present in 4 oz of cow's milk formula approaches 1 g of BLG. It would require approximately 10^5- to 10^6-fold more breast than cow's milk to provide the infant with similar quantities of BLG (85). Such an analysis places the immunizing capacity of breast milk in more appropriate perspective. These observations suggest that, at least for cow's milk, delay in its introduction is not associated with increased sensitization in either high–atopic-risk (1) or unselected neonates (85).

In summary, strict, prolonged food avoidance by mother and infant for more than 6 months appears to reduce the development of food allergy, but not allergic respiratory disorders during early infancy. The benefit may be brief and limited to the first year of life owing to the frequent remissions in food allergy by 2 years and the elimination of the responsible foods from the diets of the food-allergic infants. The benefits attained by the combined maternal and infant avoidance regimens cannot be attributed to the pregnancy diet, since, as discussed earlier, prenatal sensitization to foods is rare (8), and prenatal maternal dietary restrictions when examined separately in prospective randomized studies failed to prevent food allergy in infancy (9,10). *As such, allergenic food prevention diets should be discouraged during preg-*

nancy, since such practices do not prevent atopy, but have the potential to inflict nutritional harm to mother and fetus by suppressing normal third-trimester weight gain (1,9).

PREVENTION OF INHALANT ALLERGY

Inhalant Allergen Sensitization in Infancy

Experimental studies in both human and animal models have identified an increased risk for primary sensitization to inhalant allergens during early postnatal life. Holt et al. (86), in a recent review, emphasized that the initial T-cell response to an initial encounter with an inhalant allergen may set the immunological stage for allergic sensitization and development of allergic rhinitis and asthma in later years. As noted earlier, the immature mucosal immune response during infancy, when exposed to critical concentrations of allergens and environmental pollutants or adjuvants, may be responsible for the increased risk of IgE sensitization noted during infancy and early childhood (87). The stage of maturity at the time of initial allergen exposure assumes critical importance in both humans and animals. In contrast with IgE isotype-specific tolerance developing in adult high-IgE–responder rats with initial exposure to inhaled allergens, similar newborn rates cannot be tolerized to identical allergen exposure until after weaning (87), a phenomenon similar to that discussed previously for food sensitization and tolerance in animals (88).

The consequence of inhalant exposure early postnatally on the development of allergic sensitization and respiratory disease has been studied and reviewed recently (3). Exposure to elevated levels of the *Dermatophagoides* antigen Der p I in amounts in excess of 2 μg/g of household dust in carpets and bedding measured during infancy was related to both an increased prevalence of positive skin tests and increased concentrations of specific IgE to dust mite by age 5 in infants with atopic parents (89). Additionally, Der p I levels in household dust in excess of 10 μg/g of dust measured during infancy was associated with a fivefold increased risk of developing atopic asthma at age 11 in a cohort of 67 subjects prospectively followed from birth (90). Moreover, the age of the first wheezing episode was inversely related to the level of Der p I exposure at 1 year in all subjects, which was particularly prominent in the atopic children (90). In a similar series of experiments, Warner et al. (91) explored the influence of household exposure to mite, cat, pollen, and fungal allergens on primary sensitization in 68 atopic asthmatic children studied at ages 2–14. Air samples of each child's postnatal bedroom, taken at the corresponding month of the child's birth, were analyzed for inhalant allergens in an attempt to extrapolate exposure during infancy to later sensitization. This group noted (a) a significant association of Der p I and cat allergenic Fel d I in the air and the presence of mite- and cat-specific IgE in the children, respectively; (b) a higher risk for the development of cat allergy in homes with cats present at birth; (c) Fel d I in homes without cats ever in residence, suggesting introduction of Fel allergen indirectly by clothing, shoes, or other sources; and (d) tree, but not grass pollen or mold, indoor exposure correlating with children's skin test sensitivity (91). Further support for the importance of early inhalant exposure comes from a retrospective questionnaire study that noted that exposure to pollen and cat allergens during the first 6 postnatal months appeared to increase the risk for IgE sensitization and allergic disease in teenagers (92). Moreover, mite exposure at the time of disease manifestations appears etiologically related to atopic dermatitis in a case–control study of children and young adults. In this study, no data were available for mite exposure in infancy and the subsequent development of chronic atopic dermatitis (93).

Despite the relation of inhalant allergen exposure during infancy to the development of specific inhalant sensitization and allergic disease (90,91), specific inhalant sensitization generally is not detected before 2 years of age (1,89,94,95). Such observations suggest that early allergen exposure primes the T-cell system to form allergen-specific T-memory cells, but must await some future critical event(s) (i.e., maturation of the respiratory mucosal immune system, or greater and more continuous allergen exposure) to induce specific IgE antibody (3,86).

As noted in Chapter 19, even the month of one's birth appears related to cord blood IgE levels and the development of specific inhalant sensitization and respiratory disease (3). Specifically, springtime births are associated with higher cord blood IgE levels (96–98) and with grass and tree pollen sensitization and allergy (99–101), whereas the early fall months are associated with lower cord blood IgE levels (55) and with mite (101–103) and ragweed (104) sensitization. Although some investigators recommend family planning based on these associations of birth month and sensitization and disease, more definitive data are required before such recommendations appear appropriate. Nevertheless, such data support the premise that there is an early postnatal period of increased risk for allergic sensitization.

Role of Adjuvants and Pollutants

Pollutants, including smoke, ozone, oxides, and diesel fumes, present significant health hazards related to allergic disease as discussed in Chapter 19 and reviewed recently (3). These pollutants have the capacity to serve as adjuvants, which increase allergen sensitization in animal models (105–107) and in humans (108–110). The allergy consequences of passive smoke inhalation on children are considerable and include increased persistent wheezing (111–115), reduced level and rate of increase of pulmonary function (116,117), abnormal fetal lung changes (118), increased bronchial hyperreactivity (119–121), an earlier onset of asthma or allergic rhinitis (92), and increased serum IgE levels (122,123). One unconfirmed study reported that exposure to maternal smoke during pregnancy significantly increased the risk of allergic disease by 18 months (124). The capacity of components in cigarette smoke to augment IgE sensitization and respiratory disease in animals (125,126) and humans (127–129) demonstrates the capacity of cigarette smoke to modulate the allergic response. The immunomodulatory-enhancing properties of cigarette smoke and other pollutants on atopy and allergic inflammatory responses in predisposed subjects, especially those with atopic predispositions, may be responsible, in part, for the increasing prevalence of allergic disorders reported throughout the world. Methods to prevent such exposures should be evaluated for their effectiveness to prevent or reduce allergic disease.

Other Nonspecific Environmental Adjuvants

Microbial infections and their products, particularly viral, may act as adjuvants or cofactors in the induction of IgE sensitization, as noted in animals and humans (3,130,131) and discussed in Chapter 19. Mechanisms for this effect have been reviewed recently (132). With the increase in day-care attendance and concomitant increase in viral respiratory infections, efforts to reduce viral exposure in infancy will face major obstacles.

Pharmacologic agents may also modulate several limbs of the allergy sensitization process. Progesterone administration during pregnancy appears to increase cord blood IgE levels (6), corticosteroid administration in humans reduces Fc RII on monocytes and lymphocytes (133), and cytotoxic agents and low-dose radiation switch animals from IgE low- to high-responders (134). Unnecessary exposure of the developing fetus and newborn to these and other similar modulating agents should be prevented.

IMPLICATIONS AND RECOMMENDATIONS FOR THE PREVENTION OF ATOPY

From the foregoing discussion, it is clear that more definitive data must be obtained before universal prevention recommendations are pronounced. Randomized, prospective controlled studies, preferably double-blind, should be directed toward determining the relative efficacy, practicality, and cost of implementing preventive measures such as protein hydrolysate feeding, maternal lactation diet, and delay in introduction of allergenic foods in the attempt to reduce food allergy. In addition, well-designed studies should determine whether elimination of environmental pollutants (parental smoking pre- and postpartum) and aeroallergens, such as dust mite and danders (postnatally), will affect such atopic disorders as asthma, allergic rhinitis, and atopic dermatitis. Dust-mite avoidance (anti-mite measures) when added to a maternal and infant food allergen avoidance diet in infancy was recently reported to significantly reduce asthma in addition to reducing eczema by age one year.[149] Parental compliance, motivation, and resources will present major obstacles to the success of these preventive efforts. Specifically, the well-controlled studies discussed earlier emphasized that parental compliance was far from optimal, despite apparent motivation and resources provided by the studies (1,9,135). One can anticipate less success when preventive efforts are implemented in uncontrolled, unstructured settings such as seen in clinical practice. With this in mind, both primary and secondary allergy prevention may generate less success, practicality, and appeal than first envisioned. Given the multiple obstacles encountered during environmental engineering, dietary and inhalant avoidance efforts can, at best, serve only as stopgap measures until more effective and universally acceptable genetic or cellular engineering methods are developed. Future scientific breakthroughs will identify and isolate the essential allergic gene(s), which then could be altered or switched-off by directed genetic engineering. In addition, immune and inflammatory cells, cytokines instrumental in IgE synthesis, mediator release, and target-organ sensitivity are realistic areas for modulation and preventive efforts within this decade. However, currently, clinicians interested in preventing allergic disorders, must direct their efforts to manipulating the environmental factors responsible for sensitization and disease expression.

Therefore, only preliminary dietary and environmental recommendations are available for the prevention of allergic disease. These recommendations are based on and modified from the more stringent measures found beneficial in the aforementioned studies. As more compelling evidence emerges, these recommendations will be revised. However, they must not be promulgated or proselytized universally but, if indicated, given to highly motivated parents of infants at high risk for developing allergic disease (Table 7 and Appendix).

Table 7 Practical Recommendations for the Prevention of Allergic Disease in High-Risk Offspring

Strategy	Method or measure
1. Identify at-risk infant prenatally or early postnatally	a. Document highly atopic families biparental, parent and sibling) or b. Document elevated cord blood igE
2. Avoid infant exposure to	
a. Food allergens	
In breast milk	a. Maternal lactation diet without egg, milk, or peanut b. Supplement maternal diet daily with 1500 mg elemental calcium
In infant diet	a. Breast-feed for 4–6 mo b. Supplement or wean with suitable protein hydrosylate formula c. Delay solid foods until 6 mo, then add least allergenic first d. After 1 yr, add biweekly or monthly, if tolerated: milk, wheat, soy, corn, citrus, egg, peanut, fish, delay egg, peanut, and fish longer in food-atopic infants
b. Inhalant allergens	a. Home mite, mold, pet avoidance b. Air-conditioners, air purifiers
3. Avoid nonspecific environmental enhancers	a. No smoking prenatally or postnatally b. Reduce pollution c. Minimize infections (avoid early day-care, encourage breast feeding)

Source: Ref. 8.

APPENDIX I: SOUTHERN CALIFORNIA PERMANENTE MEDICAL GROUP ALLERGY DEPARTMENT

Introduction of Foods to Infants at High Risk for Food Allergy

Introduction

Allergists have desired to prevent, reduce, or delay the onset of allergic illnesses caused by foods and other allergens for decades. Although no foolproof method exists, recent studies suggest that delaying the introduction of allergenic foods to infants at risk for allergies may reduce food allergy within the first year of life. Unfortunately, food avoidance appears to have *no* effect on the development of asthma or inhalant allergies.

One problem with strict diets is the potential development of nutritional deficiencies if adequate food substitutions are not eaten. Therefore, such diets *must* be undertaken only with professional supervision. The benefits and risks of such a food avoidance program must be determined for each individual family, depending on specific considerations such as the degree of risk of developing allergies and overall parental compliance.

Description

The diet of infants with a high risk of developing allergy should avoid highly allergenic foods, such as milk, egg, peanut, nuts, soy, corn, and fish, during the first 1–2 years. Breast-feeding is encouraged, but nursing mothers are to avoid milk, egg, and peanut consumption. If formula is preferred, hydrolyzed infant formulas such as Nutramigen and Alimentum are recommended; soybean and cow's milk formulas are avoided.

Indication

Studies have shown that this avoidance diet may reduce food allergies in infants of documented allergic parents. This diet does not appear to reduce chronic asthma, chronic rhinitis, or inhalant allergies.

Adequacy

This diet is nutritionally adequate for infants if breast milk or recommended formula and a variety of allowed foods are provided in adequate amounts. Fluoride is suggested after 3 months of age when local water levels of fluoride are low. Nursing women on milk restriction require calcium supplementation of 1500 mg calcium daily.

Nursing Mother

1. Avoid milk, egg, and peanuts during lactation.
2. 1500 mg supplement calcium daily.

Infant

1. Prolong breast-feeding for at least 4–6 months.
2. Hydrolyzed milk formula is recommended if infant is supplemented or not breast-fed.
3. Add solids as follows
   Birth to 6 months: breast milk or hydrolyzed formula (Nutramigen or Alimentum).
   6–12 months; vegetables, rice, meat, fruit.
   12–18 months: add the following food groups if tolerated every 2–4 weeks: milk, wheat, corn, citrus, soy.
   After the above foods have been tolerated, and depending on your physician's recommendations, then egg, peanut, and fish may be added.
4. Avoid any foods suspected of causing food allergy. Notify physician of these foods so that he or she may evaluate the situation relative to further consumption.

Food group	Foods allowed	Foods to avoid
6–12 mo		
Baked goods	Plain rice cakes	All others
Cereal	Beech-Nut rice cereal	All others
Dessert	None	All
Fats	Safflower oil	Mayonnaise, peanut oil, soy oil, all others
Fruit	Strained, fresh, canned, or frozen without added citrus	All citrus fruits and berries
Fruit juice	Any without added citrus orange juice	Orange or citrus juices
Meat	Strained, junior or fresh liver, chicken, ham, pork, turkey, veal; fresh-cooked beef, lamb	[a]Strained and junior beef, lamb; any mixed or high meat dinners, breaded meats; chicken or meat sticks; fish; shellfish
Meat substitutes	None	Tomato or tomato products; corn; eggs, peanut butter; tofu; cheese; legumes; soy
Vegetables	[a]Most single-ingredient strained and junior vegetables; fresh vegetables; [a]most canned or frozen vegetables	Creamed corn, creamed spinach, creamed green beans, creamed peas,[a] some mixed vegetables, legumes, soy, tofu

Food group	Foods allowed	Foods to avoid
12–18 mo		
Baked goods	Arrowroot cookies, Toddler biscuits, animal cookies, baby pretzels, Zwieback; [a]commercial or homemade baked goods without eggs or peanut products	Any containing egg or peanut products; Be aware of type of vegetable oil used
Beverages	Cow's milk or soy-based formulas; whole cow's milk, Gatorade, fruit drinks	[a]Powdered fruit beverages containing egg; Orange Julius
Bread	Homemade or commercial egg-free breads, pita bread, rice cakes	Breads with egg as an ingredient; challah; egg bagels
Cereal and breakfast foods	Dry or jarred cereals, toasted oat rings	Prepared mixes for pancakes, waffles, biscuits, muffins
Dessert	[a]Most strained and junior desserts; popsicles; gelatin; [a]commercial or homemade desserts without egg or peanut products	Junior puddings; any containing egg or peanut products
Fats	[a]Most margarines, butter, corn or safflower oil, sour cream, cream cheese, nondairy creamer, avocado	Peanut oil; [a]margarine containing peanut oil; mayonnaise
Fruit juice	All	None
Juice	All	None
Meat	Strained, junior, or fresh meat; poultry; high meat dinners	Strained and junior dinners (avoid eggs, egg noodles); fish, shellfish
Meat substitute	Tofu; cheese	Eggs; peanut butter
Vegetables	Strained, junior, fresh, frozen, canned	Any prepared with an egg batter or cream sauce made with egg; fried in peanut oil

After 18 Months

Egg and egg products may be added to the diet if infant does not demonstrate allergies to these products. Fish and peanut products may be added to the diet at your physician's recommendations if infant does not demonstrate allergies to these products. Avoid whole peanuts because of possibility of choking.

[a]These foods may not be allowed on this diet depending on the ingredients. Read the label or contact the manufacturer for product information.

Source: Special thanks given to Barbara Gordon, R.D., Children's Hospital & Medical Center, San Diego, California, from whose diet form the above was modified.

APPENDIX II: Representative Potentially Allergenic Foods: Identification and Avoidance

Foodstuff	Hidden ingredients listed on label	Foods to avoid	Substitutes
Milk	Casein Caseinate Whey Lactalbumin Sodium caseinate Lactose Nonfat milk solids Cream Calcium Caseinate	Cheese Cottage cheese Ice cream, yogurt Creamed soups and sauces Butter and many margarines Baked goods made with milk Some "nondairy" products Candy (creams and milk chocolate) Custards and puddings	Mocha Mix Coffee Rich Nutramigen Soy formulas (Isomil, Prosobes) Tofu Milk-free baked goods (often french bread) Pareve foods Supplement for calcium and vitamin D
Egg	Albumin Egg whites Egg yolks	Many baked goods Egg noodles Custards, pudding Mayonnaise, some salad dressings Hollandaise sauce Meringues Many egg substitutes (Egg-beaters) Some batter-fried foods	Egg-free baked goods[a] Spaghetti Rice Some egg substitutes[a] (read label)

Foodstuff	Hidden ingredients listed on label	Foods to avoid	Substitutes
Wheat	(Enriched) flour Wheat germ Wheat bran Wheat starch Gluten Food starch Vegetable starch Vegetable gum Rye Oatmeal Barley Buckwheat	Baked goods made with wheat flour Crackers Macaroni Spaghetti Noodles Gravies, thickened sauces Fried food coating Baking mixes Soy sauce Hot dogs with wheat filler Batter-fried foods Some sausages	Wheat-free breads,[a] crackers (rice cakes, special breads) Certain cold cereals (corn, rice flour, tapioca) Flours: rice, potato
Soy	Soy flour Soybean oil Vegetable oil Soy protein Soy protein isolate Textured vegetable protein (TVP) Vegetable starch Vegetable gum	Soy sauce Teriyaki sauce Worcestershire sauce Tuna packed in-vegetable oil Tofu Baked goods or cereals that include soy	Nutramigen
Corn	Cornmeal Corn starch Corn oil Corn syrup (solids) Corn sweetner Corn alcohol Vegetable oil Vegetable starch Vegetable gum Food starch	Some baked goods Corn tortillas (chips, tacos) Popcorn Some cold cereals Corn syrup Pancake syrup Many candies Most baking powders	Wheat flour tortillas Thickeners: wheat, potato or rice flour Beet or cane sugar Maple syrup or honey Baking soda and cream of tartar (for leavening agent)
Chocolate	Cocoa Cocoa butter	Candy Baked goods Colas	Carob products

Foodstuff	Hidden ingredients listed on label	Foods to avoid	Substitutes
Beef	Animal shortening Animal lard Animal gelatin	Soups Bouillon Beef gravies and sauces Hot dogs Cold cuts	Pure vegetable shortening
Pork	Animal shortening Animal lard	Bacon Sausage Hot dogs Baked beans and soups with pork	All beef hot dogs and cold cuts Vegetarian baked beans Pure vegetable shortening

Source: Adapted from Ref. 150.

[a]Products available from Ener-G Foods, P.O. Box 84487, Seattle, WA 98124-5787 (1-800-331-5222).

REFERENCES

1. Zeiger RS, Heller S, Mellon MH, et al. Effect of combined maternal and infant food-allergen avoidance on development of atopy in early infancy: a randomized study. J Allergy Clin Immunol 1989; 84:72–89.
2. Croner S, Kjellman NIH. Development of atopic disease in relation to family history and cord blood IgE levels. Eleven-year follow up in 1654 children. Pediatr Allergy Immunol 1990; 1:14–20.
3. Zeiger RS. Development and prevention of allergic disease in childhood In: Middleton E Jr, Reed CE, Ellis EE, et al., eds. Allergy: principles and practice, 3rd ed. St Louis: CV Mosby, 1992 (in press).
4. Cookson WOCM, Faux J, Sharp PA, Hopkin JM. Linkage between immunoglobulin E responses underlying asthma and rhinitis and chromosome 11q. Lancet 1989; 1:1292–1294.
5. Grulee CG, Sanford HN. The influence of breast and artificial feeding on infantile eczema. J Pediatr 1936; 9:223–225.
6. Michel FB, Bousquet J, Greillier P, et al. Comparison of cord blood immunoglobulin E and maternal allergy for the prediction of atopic disease infancy. J Allergy Clin Immunol 1980; 65:422–430.
7. Businco L, Marchetti F, Pelligrini G, Berlini R. Predictive value of cord blood IgE levels in "at-risk" newborn babies and influence of type of feeding. *Clin. Allergy* 1983; 13:503–508.
8. Zeiger RS. Prevention of food allergy in infancy. *Ann Allergy* 1990; 65:430–441.

9. Falth-Magnusson K, Kjellman NIM. Development of atopic disease in babies whose mothers were receiving exclusion diet during pregnancy—a randomized study. J Allergy Clin Immunol 1987; 80:868–875.
10. Lilja G, Dannaeus A, Foucard T, et al. Effects of maternal diet during late pregnancy and lactation on the development of atopic diseases in infants up to 18 months of age—in-vivo results. Clin Exp Allergy 1989; 19:473–479.
11. Udall JN, Colony P, Fritze L, et al. Development of gastrointestinal mucosal barrier. II. The effect of natural versus artificial feeding on intestinal permeability to macromolecules. Pediatr Res 1981; 15:245–249.
12. Axelsson I, Jakobsson I, Lindberg T. Macromolecular absorption in preterm and term infants. Acta Paediatr Scand 1989; 78:532–537.
13. Moller G, Bernsau I, Muller W. Cow milk protein antigens and antibodies in serum of premature infants during the first 10 days of life. J Pediatr 1986; 109:869–873.
14. Lucas A, McLaughlan P, Coombs RRA. Latent anaphylactic sensitization of infants of low birth weight to cows' milk protein. Br Med J 1984; 289:1254–1256.
15. Lucas A, Brooke OG, Morley R, et al. Early diet of preterm infants and development of allergic or atopic disease: randomized prospective study. Br Med J 1990; 300:837–840.
16. Walker WA, Hanson D. The mechanisms of allergic reactions and local antibody production in infancy. Clin Disord Pediatr Nurtr 1985; 4:75–95.
17. Savilahti E, Jarvenpaa AL, Raiha N. Serum immunoglobulin in preterm infants. Comparison of human milk and formula feeding. Pediatrics 1983; 72:312–316.
18. Kleinman RE, Walker WA. Antigen processing and uptake from the intestinal track. Clin Rev Allergy 1984; 2:25–37.
19. Machtinger S, Moss R. Cow's milk allergy in breast-fed infants: the role of allergen and maternal secretory IgA antibody. J Allergy Clin Immunol 1986; 77:341–347.
20. Aberg N, Engstrom I, Lindberg U. Allergic diseases in Swedish school children. Acta Paediatr Scand 1989; 78:246–252.
21. Cogswell JJ, Mitchell EB, Alexander J. Parental smoking, breast feeding, and respiratory infection in development of allergic diseases. Arch Dis Child 1987; 62:338–344.
22. Kramer M, Moroz B. Do breast-feeding and delayed introduction of solid foods protect against subsequent atopic eczema? J Pediatr 1981; 98:546–550.
23. Taylor B, Wadsworth J, Golding J, Butler N. Breast feeding, eczema, asthma, and hayfever. J Epidemiol Community Health 1983; 37:95–99.
24. Savilahti E., Tainio VM, Salmenpera L, et al. Prolonged exclusive breast feeding and heredity as determinants in infantile atopy. Arch Dis Child 1987; 62:269–273.

25. Poysa L, Remes K, Korppi M, Juntunen-Backman K. Atopy in children with and without a family history of atopy. 1. Clinical manifestations, with special reference to diet in infancy. Acta Paediatr Scand 1989; 78:896–901.
26. Poysa L, Korppi M, Remes K, Juntunen-Backman K. Atopy in childhood and diet in infancy. A nine-year follow-up study I. Clinical manifestations. Allergy Proc. 1991; 12:107–111.
27. Burr ML. Does infant feeding affect the risk of allergy? Arch Dis Child 1983; 58:561–565.
28. Kramer MS. Does breast feeding help protect against atopic disease? Biology, methodology, and a golden jubilee of controversy. J Pediatr 1988; 112:181–190.
29. Myers MG, Fomon SJ, Koontz FP, et al. Respiratory and gastrointestinal illnesses in breast and formula fed infants. Am J Dis Child 1984; 138:629–632.
30. Zeiger, RS, Heller S, Mellon M, et al. Effectiveness of dietary manipulation in the prevention of food allergy in infants. J Allergy Clin Immunol 1986; 78: (part 2):224–238.
31. Warner JO. Food allergy in fully breast-fed infants. Clin Allergy 1980; 10:133–136.
32. Van Asperen PP, Kemp SS, Mellis CM. Immediate food hypersensitivity reactions on the first known exposure to the food. Arch Dis Child 1983; 58:253–256.
33. Gerrard JW. Allergy in breast-fed babies to ingredients in breast milk. Ann Allergy 1979; 42:69–72.
34. Hattevig G, Kjellman B, Johansson SGO, and Bjorksten B. Clinical symptoms and IgE responses to common food problems in atopic and healthy children. Clin Allergy 1984; 14:551–559.
35. Kaplan MS, Solli NJ. Immunoglobulin E to cow's milk protein in breast fed atopic children. J Allergy Clin Immunol 1979; 64:122–126.
36. Stuart CA, Twiselton R, Nicholas MF, Hide DW. Passage of cow's milk protein in breast milk. Clin Allergy 1984; 14:533–535.
37. Jakobsson I, Lindberg R, Benediktsson B, Hansson BG. Dietary bovine β-lactoglobulin is transferred to human milk. Acta Paediatr Scand 1985; 74:342–345.
38. Axelsson I, Jakobsson I, Lindberg T, Benediktsson B. Bovine β-lactoglobulin in the human milk. A longitudinal study during the whole lactation period. Acta Paediatr Scand 1986; 75:702–707.
39. Clyne PS, Kulczycki A. Human breast milk contains bovine IgG. Relationship to infant colic? Pediatrics 1991; 87:439–444.
40. Cant A, Narsden RA, Kilshaw PJ. Egg and cow's milk hypersensitivity in exclusively breast-fed infants with eczema, and detection of egg protein in breast milk. Br Med J 1985; 291:932–935.
41. Troncone R, Scarcella A, Donatiello A, et al. Passage of gliadin into human breast milk. Acta Paediatr Scand 1987; 76:453–456.

42. Cavagni G, Paganelli R, Caffarelli C, et al. Passage of food antigens into circulation of breast-fed infants with atopic dermatitis. Ann Allergy 1988; 61:361–365.
43. Kilshaw PJ, Cant AJ. The passage of maternal dietary proteins in human breast milk. Int Arch Allergy Appl Immunol 1984; 75:8–15.
44. Hattevig G, Kjellman B, Siqurs N, et al. Effect of maternal avoidance of eggs, cow's milk, and fish during lactation upon allergic manifestations in infants. Clin Exp Allergy 1989; 19:27–32.
45. Chandra RK, Shakuntla P, Hamed A. Influence of maternal diet during lactation and use of formula feeds on development of atopic eczema in high risk infants. Br Med J 1989; 299:228–230.
46. Hattevig G, Kjellman B, Sigurs H, et al. The effect of maternal avoidance of eggs, cow's milk and fish during lactation on the development of IgE, IgG, and IgA antibodies in infants. J Allergy Clin Immunol 1990; 85:108–115.
47. Johnstone DE, Dutton AM. Dietary prophylaxis of allergic diseases in children. N Engl J Med 1966; 274:715–719.
48. Brown EB, Josephson BM, Levine HS, Rosen MA. A prospective study of allergy in a pediatric population. Am J Dis Child 1969; 63:388–393.
49. Kjellman NIM, Johansson SGO. Soy versus cow's milk in infants with a biparental history of atopic disease: development of atopic disease and immunoglobulins from birth to 4 years of age. Clin Allergy 1979; 9:347–358.
50. Glaser J, Johnstone DE. Soybean milk as a substitute for mammalian milk in early infancy: with special reference to prevention of allergy to cow's milk. Ann Allergy 1952; 10:433–439.
51. Glaser J, Johnstone DE. Prophylaxis of allergic disease in the newborn. JAMA 1953; 153:620–622.
52. Johnstone DE, Glaser J. Use of soybean milk as an aid in prophylaxis of allergic disease in children. J Allergy 1953; 24:434–436.
53. Gruskay FL. Comparison of breast, cow, and soy feedings in the prevention of onset of allergic disease. A 15-year prospective study. Clin Pediatr 1982; 21:486–491.
54. Chandra RK, Singh G, Shridhara B. Effect of feeding whey hydrolysate, soy and conventional cow milk formulas on incidence of atopic disease in high risk infants. Ann Allergy 1989; 63:102–106.
55. Mortimer ER. Anaphylaxis following ingestion of soybean. J Pediatr 1961; 58:90–92.
56. Bush RK, Cohen M. Immediate and late onset asthma from occupational exposure to soybean dust. Clin Allergy 1977; 7:369–373.
57. Peters GA. Bronchial asthma due to soybean allergy. Ann Allergy 1965; 23:270–272.
58. Dannaeus A, Johansson SGO, Foucard T, Ohman S. Clinical and immunological aspects of food allergy in childhood. I. Estimation of IgG, IgA, and IgE antibodies to food antigens in children with food allergy and atopic dermatitis. Acta Paediatr Scand 1977; 66:31–37.

59. Singh B, Lee K-C, Fraga E, et al. Minimum peptide sequences necessary for priming and triggering of humoral and cell-mediated immune responses in mice: use of synthetic peptide antigens of defined structure. J Immunol 1980; 124:1336–1343.
60. Knights RJ. Processing and evaluation of the antigenicity of protein hydrolysates. Clin Dis Pediatr Nutr 1985; 4:105–115.
61. Sampson HA, Bernhisel-Broadbent J, Yang E, Scanlon SM. Safety of casein hydrolysate formula in children with cow milk allergy. J Pediatr 1991; 118:520–525.
62. Pahud JJ, Monti JC, Jost R. Allergenicity of whey protein: its modifciation by tryptic in vitro hydrolysis of the protein. J Pediatr Gastroenterol Nutr 1985; 4:408–413.
63. Businco L, Cantani A, Longhi AL, Giampietro PG. Anaphylactic reactions to a cow's milk whey protein hydrolysate (Alfa-Re, Nestle) in infants with cow's milk allergy. Ann Allergy 1989; 62:333–335.
64. Kuitunen P, Visakorpi JK, Savilahti E, Pelkonen P. Malabsorption syndrome with cow's milk intolerance. Clinical findings and course in 54 cases. Arch Dis Child 1975; 50:351–356.
65. Whitington PF, Gibson R. Soy protein intolerance: four patients with concomitant cow's milk intolerance. Pediatrics 1977; 59:730–732.
66. Freier S, Kletter B, Gery I, et al. Intolerance to milk protein. J Pediatr 1969; 75:623–631.
67. Whitfield MF, Barr DGD. Cow's milk allergy in the syndrome of thrombocytopenia with absent radius. Arch Dis Child 1976; 51:337–343.
68. Jakobsson I, Lindberg T. A prospective study of cow's milk protein intolerance in Swedish infants. Acta Paediatr Scand 1979; 68:853–859.
69. Lifschitz CH, Hawkins HK, Guerra C, Byrd N. Anaphylactic shock due to cow's milk protein hypersensitivity in a breast-fed infant. J Pediatr Gastroenterol Nutr 1988; 7:141–144.
70. Bock SA. Probable allergic reaction to casein hydrolysate formula [correspondence]. J Allergy Clin Immunol 1989; 84:272.
71. Ellis MH, Short JA, Heiner DC. Anaphylaxis after ingestion of a recently introduced hydrolyzed whey protein formula. J Pediatr 1991; 118:74–77.
72. McLaughlan P, Anderson KJ, Coombs RRA. An oral screening procedure to determine the sensitizing capacity of infant feeding formulae. Clin Allergy 1981; 11:311–318.
73. Schatz M, Zeiger RA, Mellon M, Porreco R. The course and management of asthma and allergic disease during pregnancy. In: Middleton E, Reed CE, Ellis EF, eds. Allergy:principles and practice. St Louis: CV Mosby, 1983; 935–986.
74. Eastham EJ, Lichauco T, Grady MI. Antigenicity of infant formulas: role of immature intestine on protein permeability. J Pediatr 1978; 93:561–564.

75. Kletter B, Gery I, Freier S, Davies AM. Immune response of normal infants to cow milk. II. Decreased immune reactions in initially breast fed infants. Int Arch Allergy 1971; 40:667–671.
76. Fergusson DM, Horwood LJ, Beautrais AL, et al. Eczema and infant diet. Clin Allergy 1981; 11:325–331.
77. Fergusson DM, Horwood LJ, Shannon FT. Risk factors in childhood eczema. J Epidemiol Community Health 1982; 36:118–122.
78. Fergusson DM, Horwood LJ, Shannon FT. Early solid feeding and recurrent childhood eczema: a 10-year longitudinal study. Pediatrics 1990; 86:541–546.
79. Fergusson DM, Horwood LJ, Shannon FT. Asthma and infant diet. Arch Dis Child. 1983; 58:48–51.
80. Kajosaari M, Saarinen UM. Prophylaxis of atopic disease by six months; total solid food elimination. Arch Paediatr Scand 1983; 72:411–414.
81. Saarinen UM, Kajosaari M. Does dietary elimination in infancy prevent or only postpone a food allergy? A study of fish and citrus allergy in 375 children. Lancet 1980; 1:166–167.
82. Chandra RK, Puri S, Suraiya C, Cheema PS. Influence of maternal food antigen avoidance during pregnancy and lactation and on the incidence of atopic eczema in infants. Clin Allergy 1986; 16:563–571.
83. Lilja G, Dannaeus A, Foucard T, et al. Effects of maternal diet during late pregnancy and lactation on the development of IgE and egg- and milk-specific IgE and IgG antibodies in infants. Clin Exp Allergy 1991; 21:195–202.
84. Jarrett EEE. Perinatal influences on IgE responses. Lancet 1985; 2:797–799.
85. Host A, Husby S, Osterballe O. A prospective study of cow's milk allergy in exclusively breast-fed infants. Acta Paediatr Scand 1988; 77:663–670.
86. Holt PG, McMenamin C, Nelson D. Primary sensitization to inhalant allergens during infancy. Pediatr Allergy Immunol 1990; 1:3–13.
87. Holt PG, Vines J, Britten D. Suppression of IgE responses by antigen inhalation: failure of tolerance mechanisms in newborn rats. Immunology 1988; 63:591–593.
88. Strobel D, Ferguson A. Immune responses to fed protein agents in mice. 3. Systemic tolerance or priming is related to age at which antigen is first encountered. Pediatr Res 1984; 18:588–594.
89. Rowntree S, Cogswell JJ, Platts-Mills TAE, Mitchell EB. Development of IgE and IgG antibodies to food and inhalant allergens in children at risk of allergic disease. Arch Dis Child 1985; 60:727–735.
90. Sporik R, Holgate ST, Platts-Mills TAE, Cogswell JJ. Exposure to house-dust mite allergen (Der p I) and the development of asthma in childhood. A prospective study. N Engl J Med 1990; 323:502–507.
91. Warner JA, Little SA, Pollock I, et al. The influence of exposure to house dust mite, cat, pollen and fungal allergens in the home on primary sensitization in asthma. Pediatr Allergy Immunol 1990; 1:79–86.

92. Suoniemi I, Bjorksten F, Haahtela T. Dependence of immediate hypersensitivity in the adolescent period on factors encountered in infancy. Allergy 1981; 36:263–268.
93. Harving H, Korsgaard J, Dahl R, et al. House dust mites and atopic dermatitis. A case–control study on the significance of house dust mites as etiologic allergens in atopic dermatitis. Ann Allergy 1990; 65:25–31.
94. Hattevig G, Kjellman B, Bjorksten B. Clinical symptoms and IgE responses to common food proteins and inhalants in the first 7 years of life. Clin Allergy 1987; 17:571–578.
95. Van Asperen PP, Kemp AS, Mellis CM. Skin test reactivity and clinical allergen sensitivity in infancy. J Allergy Clin Immunol 1984; 73:381–386.
96. Croner S, Kjellman NIM. Predictors of atopic disease: cord blood IgE and month of birth. Allergy 1986; 41:68–70.
97. Kimpen J, Callaert H, Embrechts P, Bosmans E. Cord blood IgE and month of birth. Arch Dis Child 1987; 62:478–482.
98. Halonen M, Stern D, Lyle S, et al. Relationship of total serum IgE levels in cord and 9-month sera of infants. Clin Exp Allergy 1991; 21:235–241.
99. Bjorksten F, Suoniemi I, Koski V. Neonatal birch pollen contact and subsequent allergy to birch pollen. Clin Allergy 1980; 10:585–591.
100. Bjorksten F, Suoniemi I. Time and intensity of first pollen contacts and risk of subsequent pollen allergies. Acta Med Scand 1981; 209:299–303.
101. Businco L, Cantani A, Farinella F, Businco E. Month of birth and grass pollen or mite sensitization in children with respiratory allergy: a significant relationship. Clin Allergy 1988; 18:269–274.
102. Korsgaard J, Dahl R. Sensitivity to house dust, mite, and grass pollen in adults. Clin Allergy 1983; 13:529–536.
103. Beck HI, Hagdrup HK. Atopic dermatitis, house dust mite allergy and month of birth. Acta Derm Venereol (Stockh) 1987; 67:448–451.
104. Settipane RJ, Hagy GW. Effect of atmospheric pollen on the newborn. RI Med J 1979; 62:477–482.
105. Matsumara Y. The effects of ozone, nitrogen dioxide, and sulfur dioxide on the experimentally induced allergic respiratory disorder in guinea pigs. Am Rev Respir Dis 1978; 102:430–447.
106. Osebold JW, Gershwin LJ, Zee YC. Studies on the enhancement of allergic lung sensitization by inhalation of ozone and sulfuric acid aerosol. J Environ Pathol Toxicol Oncol 1980; 3:221–234.
107. Riedel F, Kramer M, Scheibenbogen C, Rieger CHL. Effects of SO_2 exposure on allergic sensitization in the guinea pig. J Allergy Clin Immunol 1988; 82:527–534.
108. Ishizaki T, Koisumi K, Ikemore R, et al. Studies of prevalence of Japanese cedar pollinosis among the residents in a densely cultivated area. Ann Allergy 1987; 58:265–270.

109. Andrae S, Axelson O, Bjorksten B, et al. Symptoms of bronchial hyperreactivity and asthma in relation to environmental factors. Arch Dis Child 1988; 63:473–478.
110. Aberg N. Asthma and allergic rhinitis in Swedish conscripts. Clin Allergy 1989; 19:59–63.
111. Fergusson DM, Horwood LJ. Parental smoking and respiratory illness during early childhood. Pediatr Pulmonol 1985; 1:99–106.
112. Schenker MB, Samet JM, Speizer FE. Risk factors for childhood respiratory disease. The effect of host factors and home environmental exposures. Am Rev Respir Dis 1983; 128:1038–1043.
113. Burchfiel CM, Higgins MW, Keller JB, et al. Passive smoking in childhood. Respiratory conditions and pulmonary function in Tecumsch, Michigan. Am Rev Respir Dis 1986; 133:966–973.
114. Neuspiel DR, Rush D, Butler NR, et al. Parental smoking and post-infancy wheezing in children: a prospective cohort study. Am J Public Health 1989; 79:168–171.
115. Burr ML, Miskelly FG, Butland BK, et al. Environmental factors and symptoms in infants at high risk of allergy. J Epidemiol Community Health 1989; 43:125–132.
116. Tager IB, Weiss ST, Munoz A, et al. Longitudinal study of the effects of maternal smoking on pulmonary function in children. N Engl J Med 1983; 309:699–703.
117. Vedal S, Schenker MB, Samet JM, Speizer FE. Risk factors for childhood respiratory disease. Analysis of pulmonary function. Am Rev Respir Dis 1984; 130:187–192.
118. Chen MF, Kimizuka G, Wang NS. Human fetal lung changes associated with maternal smoking during pregnancy. Pediatr Pulmonol 1987; 3:51–58.
119. Murray AB, Morrison BJ. The effect of cigarette smoke from the mother on bronchial responsiveness and severity of symptoms in children with asthma. J Allergy Clin Immunol 1986; 77:575–581.
120. Andrae S, Axelson O, Bjorksten B, et al. Symptoms of bronchial hyperreactivity and asthma in relation to environmental factors. Arch Dis Child 1988; 63:473–478.
121. Martinez FD, Antognoni G, Macri F, et al. Parental smoking enhances bronchial responsiveness in nine-year-old children. Am Rev Respir Dis 1988; 138:518–523.
122. Kjellman NIM. Effect of parental smoking on IgE levels in children. Lancet 1981; 1:993–994.
123. Ronchetti R, Macri F, Ciofetta G, et al. Increased serum IgE and increased prevalence of eosinophilia in 9-year-old children of smoking parents. J Allergy Clin Immunol 1990; 86:400–407.
124. Magnusson CGM. Maternal smoking influences cord serum IgE and IgD levels and increases the risk for subsequent infant allergy. J Allergy Clin Immunol 1986; 78:898–904.

125. Zetterstrom O, Nordvall SL, Bjorksten B, et al. Increased IgE antibody response in rats exposed to tobacco smoke. J Allergy Clin Immunol 1985; 75:594–598.
126. Nublein RR, Ruschoff J, Rieger CHL. Tobacco smoke enhances allergic bronchial sensitization in the guinea pig. Pediatr Allergy Immunol 1990; 1:26–33.
127. Venables KM, Dally MB, Nunn AJ, et al. Smoking and occupational allergy in workers in a platinum refinery. Br Med J 1989; 299:939–942.
128. Zetterstrom O, Osterman K, Machado L, Johansson SGO. Another smoking hazard: raised serum IgE concentration and increased risk of occupational allergy. Br Med J 1981; 283:1215–1217.
129. Venables KM, Topping MD, Howe W, et al. Interaction of smoking and atopy in producing specific IgE antibody against a hapten protein conjugate. Br Med J 1985; 290:201–204.
130. Frick OL, German DF, Mills J. Development of allergy in children. I. Association with virus infection. J Allergy Clin Immunol 1979; 63:228–241.
131. Welliver RC, Wong DT, Sun M, et al. The development of respiratory syncytial virus-specific IgE and the release of histamine in nasopharyngeal secretions after infection. N Engl J Med 1981; 305:841–846.
132. Busse WW. The relationship between viral infections and onset of allergic diseases and asthma. Clin Exp Allergy 1989; 19:1–9.
133. Melewicz FM, Zeiger RS, Mellon MH, et al. Increased IgE-dependent cytotoxicity by blood mononuclear cells of allergic patients. Clin Exp Immunol 1981; 43:526–533.
134. Katz DH. Recent studies on the regulation of IgE antibody synthesis in experimenal animals and man. Immunology 1980; 41:1–24.
135. Poysa L, Remes K, Korppi M, Launiala K. Compliance with a dietary manipulation programme in families wtih infants prone to atopy. Acta Paediatr Scand 1988; 77:563–568.
136. Matthew DJ, Norman AP, Taylor B, Turner MW. Prevention of eczema. Lancet 1977; 1:321–324.
137. Saarinen UM, Backman A, Kajosaari M, Siimes MA. Prolonged breastfeeding as prophylaxis for atopic disease. Lancet 1979; 1:163–166.
138. Ziering RW, O'Connor R, Mellon M, et al. University of California in San Diego prophylaxis of allergy in infancy study: an interim report. J Allergy Clin Immunol 1979; 63:199.
139. Chandra RK. Prospective studies of the effect of breast feeding on incidence of infection and allergy. Acta Paediatr Scand 1979; 68:691–694.
140. Juto P, Bjorksten B. Serum IgE in infants and influence of type of feeding. Clin Allergy 1980; 10:593–600.
141. Chandra RK, Puri S, Cheema PS. Predictive value of cord blood IgE in the development of atopic disease and role of breast feeding in its prevention. Clin Allergy 1985; 15:517–522.

142. Kaufman HS. Diet and heredity in infantile atopic dermatitis. Arch Dermatol 1972; 105:400–404.
143. Halpern SR, Sellars WA, Johnson RB, et al. Development of childhood allergy in infants fed breast, soy, or cow milk. J Allergy Clin Immunol 1973; 51:139–151.
144. Kaufman HS, Frick OL. The development of allergy in infants of allergic parents: a prospective study concerning the role of heredity. Ann Allergy 1976; 37:410–415.
145. Hide DW, Guyer BM. Clinical manifestations of allergy related to breast and cow's milk feeding. Arch Dis Child 1981; 56:172–175.
146. Gordon RR, Ward AM, Noble DA, Allen R. Immunoglobulin E and the eczema–asthma syndrome in early childhood. Lancet 1982; 1:72–74.
147. Van Asperen PP, Kemp AS, Mellis CM. Relationship of diet in the development of atopy in infancy. Clin Allergy 1984; 14:525–532.
148. Miskelly FG, Burr ML, Vaughan-Williams E, et al. Infant feeding and allergy. Arch Dis Child. 1988; 63:388–393.
149. Arshad SH, Matthews S, Gant C, Hide DW. Effect of allergen avoidance on development of allergic disorders in infancy. Lancet 1992; 339:1493–97.
150. Adams EJ, Mahan LK. Nutritional care in food and allergy intolerance. In: Krause KMW, Mahan LK, eds. Food, nutrition, and diet therapy. Philadelphia: WB Saunders, 1984.

APPENDIX

National Asthma Education Program Report: Four Components of the Management of Asthma During Pregnancy and Lactation

INTRODUCTION

Effective management of asthma for pregnant women relies on four integral components:

1. Objective measures for assessing and monitoring maternal lung function and fetal well-being to make appropriate therapeutic recommendations
2. Measures to avoid or control asthma triggers in the patient's environment
3. Pharmacologic therapy
4. Patient eduction

Goals of Therapy for Pregnant Women

Goals for the management of asthma in pregnant women—as for all asthma patients—are:

1. Control of symptoms, including nocturnal symptoms
2. Maintenance of normal activity levels, including exercise

Chapter 5 from the National Asthma Education Program Report of the Working Group on Asthma and Pregnancy; modified from Ref. 1.

3. Maintenance of pulmonary function as close to normal levels as possible
4. Prevention of acute exacerbations of asthma
5. Avoidance of adverse effects from asthma medications

An important additional goal for the management of asthma in pregnant women is the birth of a healthy baby.

Principles of Therapy for Pregnant Women

Asthma is a chronic condition with acute exacerbations. Continuing attention is required to control symptoms, prevent exacerbations, and reduce chronic airway inflammation. Prevention of exacerbations is particularly important. This includes avoidance of triggers, and for allergic patients, the avoidance of allergens, especially in the indoor environment. It also includes regular (daily) and aggressive use of anti-inflammatory medication for many patients.

Anticipatory or early intervention in treating acute exacerbations of asthma reduces the likelihood of the episode progressing to severe airway obstruction and impaired maternal or fetal oxygenation. Both nonpharmacologic and pharmacologic therapies should be considered. Optimal use of nonpharmacologic measures is important because it may reduce the requirement for medication. Therefore, patients, if allergic, should avoid exposure to house-dust mites, animal dander, pollen, and mold spores. Patients should avoid irritant triggers, especially active and passive exposure to tobacco smoke.

Although it is generally desirable to use as few medications as possible, it is essential to strive for normal lung function and blood oxygenation to ensure normal oxygen supply to the fetus. Inhaled medications are preferred; however, systemic drugs should be employed when inhaled medications are not sufficient to control symptoms and normalize pulmonary function.

Although some not yet fully defined risk may be associated with asthma medication during pregnancy, it is to be emphasized that the greater risk to the fetus is uncontrolled asthma. The Working Group on Asthma and Pregnancy strongly recommends that asthma should be aggressively treated in pregnant women just as it should be in nonpregnant patients. Studies to date have identified few risks to the fetus from drugs employed in treating asthma. The known risk of uncontrolled asthma, causing morbidity in the mother and hypoxemia in the fetus, is far greater than any known risks to the mother or fetus from asthma medications.

COMPONENT 1: OBJECTIVE MEASURES FOR ASSESSMENT AND MONITORING

Maternal Lung Function

Pulmonary function tests are essential for assessing the severity of asthma in order to make appropriate therapeutic recommendations. Asthma is characterized by variable airflow obstruction that is often at its worst at night or on arising. Measurements of pulmonary function performed during the day in the physician's office may offer incomplete insight into the course of the asthma throughout the 24-hr day. Home measurement of pulmonary function is important for assessing circadian variation in pulmonary function and for documentation that asthma is the cause of nocturnal awakening. Patients' and physicians' perceptions of the severity of asthma are often insensitive, making a quantitative assessment of airflow obstruction highly desirable. Furthermore, it can be extremely difficult for the patient and her physician to differentiate breathlessness associated with pregnancy, anxiety, or asthma without objective measures of lung function.

Pulmonary function has traditionally been assessed by spirometry. The volume of air expired in 1 sec from maximum inspiration (FEV_1) is the single best measure of pulmonary function for assessing severity. Therefore, it is recommended that office spirometry be conducted in the initial assessment of all pregnant patients being evaluated for asthma, and periodically thereafter, as appropriate.

The peak expiratory flow rate (PEFR) is the greatest flow velocity that can be obtained during a forced expiration, starting with fully inflated lungs, and it correlates well with FEV_1. The PEFR can be measured reliably with inexpensive, portable peak flowmeters. However, because PEFR measures only large-airway function, the PEFR is not the most sensitive measurement of airflow obstruction. Thus, PEFR measurements are insufficient to make a diagnosis or to fully evaluate the physiological impairment associated with asthma. Nevertheless, monitoring PEFR is extremely useful in following both the course of asthma and a patient's response to therapy. Peak flow rates can also help differentiate asthma from other causes of dyspnea during pregnancy.

Use PEFR to assess symptoms and predict exacerbations of asthma. It is recommended that PEFR be used as the objective parameter to follow in assessing symptoms and making therapeutic recommendations when such recommendations depend on the severity of airflow obstruction. PEFR monitoring is especially valuable for detecting deterioration of asthma, predicting acute exacerbations, and assessing response to therapy. Availability of PEFR measurements not only allows formulation of a management plan with criteria for both intensification of therapy and recourse to medical assistance but also facilitates telephone communication with health care providers. Maintenance of as near-normal pulmonary function as possible is desirable during pregnancy; those patients in whom there is any concern in this regard should be supplied with a home peak flow meter device. In general this includes all women with moderate to severe asthma. These patients should record PEFR upon arising in the morning, and approximately twelve hours later. Patients should bring PEFR records to each prenatal visit.

Use PEFR to adjust asthma therapy. Predicted values of PEFR are in the range of 380 to 550 liters per minute for women and do not change during the course of pregnancy. Rather than employing the predicted value, it is often better to establish a personal best PEFR for each patient at a time when asthma is well controlled. Recommendations for changes in asthma therapy may then be based on deviations from this personal best level. For more complete discussion, see the National Asthma Education Program *Expert Panel Report: Guidelines for the Diagnosis and Management of Asthma.*

Fetal Monitoring

The goal of managing the pregnancy of a woman with asthma is to optimize maternal pulmonary function and to identify those fetuses at risk for intrauterine growth retardation and adverse outcome. In the absence of maternal or fetal decompensation, an additional goal should be to provide a normal family-centered birthing experience. Prevention of adverse fetal outcome is complicated. Ill-informed concern for fetal health early in pregnancy may defer appropriate drug therapy. Moreover, in the third trimester, fetal evaluation is sometimes overlooked during an asthma exacerbation. Finally, there are multiple methods available for fetal evaluation; more research is needed to determine which method correlates best with good fetal outcome.

Therefore, principles for management of the fetus during a pregnancy complicated by asthma should include the following:

There is little additional risk from mild or well-controlled asthma.

Other coexistent conditions such as hypertension or diabetes increase risk.

Patients with severe or uncontrolled asthma deserve increased surveillance.

Consultation with a perinatologist is recommended when serious fetal problems are suspected.

The most common errors leading to adverse outcome are underestimation of asthma severity and undertreatment of exacerbations.

Fetal evaluation during the pregnancy of a woman with asthma is longitudinal and uses different techniques, according to gestational age and risk factors. Because accurate determination of gestational age is crucial in making obstetrical decisions, early (12–20 weeks) sonography should be performed for most patients, especially when accurate clinical dating is not possible or if asthma is moderate or severe. Early obstetrical sonography will provide a benchmark against which fetal growth can be measured. Monitoring of pregnant patients with asthma starts with an evaluation of progressive fetal growth. Growth during the second and third trimesters is determined by careful serial measurements of fundal height. Confirmation with sequential sonographic evaluations of fetal growth is indicated if asthma is uncontrolled or if growth retardation is suspected. In the third trimester, electronic fetal heart rate monitoring (nonstress test or contraction stress test) and ultrasonic determinations of fetal behavior (biophysical assessment) should be used, if needed, to assure fetal well-being. Indications for electronic fetal monitoring include growth retardation, moderate to severe asthma, asthma exacerbation, and decreased fetal movements. The type of monitoring chosen and its frequency depend on many factors: for many patients, weekly testing is sufficient; if fetal problems are suspected the frequency increases. Daily maternal recording of fetal activity, or "kick counts," should be encouraged. Several methods are used and appear to improve perinatal outcome in both low- and high-risk pregnancies.

If there is serious maternal decompensation, as in an acute exacerbation of asthma with an incomplete or poor response or with significant maternal hypoxemia, previous fetal monitoring is irrelevant, and intensive fetal monitoring should begin and continue until maternal status is stable. One reasonable approach to antepartum fetal assessment is continuous electronic fetal heart rate monitoring. It is rarely necessary to deliver a fetus by emergency cesarean section for acute asthma complicated by respiratory failure. In most cases, fetal distress can be successfully treated by aggressive ventilation and medical management.

Careful fetal monitoring is essential when women with asthma are admitted in labor. In low risk patients, continuous electronic fetal monitoring may not be necessary. Fetal assessment can be accomplished by 20 minutes of electronic monitoring—the so called admission test. Subsequently, for patients with mild or moderate asthma that is well controlled and with a reassuring admission test, intermittent auscultation, peak expiratory flow rate measurements, or electronic fetal heart rate monitoring may be sufficient. Intensive fetal monitoring is recommended for those patients who enter labor with uncontrolled or severe asthma and have a nonreassuring admission test or other risk factors. This may be performed by either continuous electronic fetal heart rate monitoring or intermittent auscultation (every fifteen minutes in the first stage of labor; every five minutes in the second stage of labor). During the course of labor, intensive fetal monitoring may be considered to guide appropriate obstetrical and asthma management decisions (See Charts 7 and 8).

COMPONENT 2: MEASURES TO AVOID OR CONTROL ASTHMA TRIGGERS

Environmental Control

Eliminating adverse environmental exposures is critically important in controlling asthma during pregnancy. Irritants and allergens that provoke acute symptoms may also increase airway hyperresponsiveness, which, in turn, may increase vulnerability to further irritant or allergen exposure. Nonspecific irritants include tobacco smoke, dusts, strong odors, and environmental air pollutants. Certainly, if the patient herself is smoking, she should be strongly encouraged to quit and referred to an appropriate smoking cessation program.

If allergy plays a role in an individual patient's asthma, environmental control measures to avoid these specific allergens are paramount. All warm-blooded pets, including small rodents and birds, produce dander, urine, and saliva that can cause allergic reactions. To eliminate exposure to animal dander, the animal should be removed from the house. Removal of the pet may not afford immediate relief, even when followed by vigorous cleaning, because dander remains in the home for many months. Recent studies indicate that the residual allergen can be rendered nonallergenic by application of a 3% tannic acid spray, which is commercially available. If the pet cannot be removed from the house, it should, at the very least, be kept out of the pregnant women's bedroom at all times. If there is forced-air heating in a home where a pet resides, the air ducts into the bedroom should be sealed. An electric baseboard heater can be used if necessary. Weekly washing of the pet may reduce exposure somewhat by decreasing the amount of dander and dried saliva deposited on carpets and furnishings.

House dust mites appear to play a major role in the causation of allergic asthma. Because they are dependent for survival on moisture from the atmosphere, they occur in environments where the relative humidity is usually greater than 50%. Mite allergen is found throughout the home: in mattresses, pillows, carpets, upholstered furniture, bed covers, clothes, and soft toys. Mite antigen is easily demonstrated in the air during housecleaning activities, but it is present in only very small amounts in undisturbed air. Mite antigen control includes encasing mattresses in airtight, plastic covers, either encasing pillows or washing them weekly, and washing the bedding weekly in water of 130°F (54.4°C). If allergic to house dust mites, the pregnant woman should not vacuum and should remain away from home for about 1 hr after house cleaning activity. If this is not possible, wearing a mask while vacuuming may be helpful. Additional measures that may be indicated include use of an acaracide (mite killer) on the carpets and avoidance of lying on upholstered furniture. In areas of very high humidity, consideration should be given to a dehumidifier or air-conditioner. The use of humidifiers is discouraged because they provide moisture that may encourage mite growth. Home humidity levels should be maintained at less than 50%.

Indoor exposure to mold and cockroach allergens may be important in homes with specific problems with dampness (molds) or infestation (cockroaches). Outdoor allergen exposure can be reduced by avoiding outdoor activities during the warmer months from midmorning until dusk, the period of highest prevalence for pollens and some mold spores. The use of an air-conditioner during these same months will allow the doors and windows to remain closed, effectively preventing outdoor pollen and mold spores from entering the home.

Immunotherapy

The principal concern with the use of allergy immunotherapy during pregnancy has been the occurrence of systemic reactions (anaphylaxis). Induction of uterine contractions following anaphylaxis and resultant abortion have been reported, although rarely. Patients at increased risk for anaphylaxis include those who are receiving increasing doses of antigen, who have extreme sensitivity, or who are exposed to high levels of ambient allergens. Accordingly, the general recommendation is that immunotherapy should not be started during pregnancy, but that ongoing immunotherapy may be continued at the current dose. Exceptions would be if immunotherapy has been started only recently or if the patient is experiencing frequent reactions that have prevented achieving an effective dose. Furthermore, patients who have demonstrated a tendency to have systemic reactions should have their treatment discontinued. Extra caution is required during the patient's pollen season when she may be at greater risk of experiencing a systemic reaction; therefore, a reduction in dose during this period should be considered.

Vaccines

It is generally recommended that influenza vaccine be given each year to patients with moderate and severe asthma. Influenza is a killed vaccine, and there is no evidence suggesting that it is associated with any maternal or fetal risk, although it has been recommended that it should be given after the first trimester as an extra precaution.

COMPONENT 3: PHARMACOLOGIC THERAPY

Discussion of this component opens with a statement of the general principles of pharmacologic management and a listing of preferred medications and selection criteria for pregnant women with asthma. Following are the protocols for management of asthma during pregnancy, the protocols for management of exacerbations of asthma during pregnancy, and the protocols for management of asthma during labor and delivery. There are no randomized prospective human studies of asthma pharmacotherapy during pregnancy. The following recommendations are based on the published safety and efficacy data and the experience of the working group members.

General Principles of Pharmacologic Management

INTEGRATE ASTHMA CARE WITH OBSTETRICAL CARE. The obstetrical care provider must be involved in asthma care. Consultation with an asthma specialist is appropriate, as indicated, for evaluation of the role of allergy and irritants, complete pulmonary function studies, or evaluation of the medication plan if there are complications in achieving goals of therapy. A team approach is required if there is more than one clinician managing the asthma and the pregnancy.

OBTAIN INFORMATION ON ASTHMA STATUS DURING PRENATAL VISITS Collect the following information:

1. Day and nighttime symptoms
2. Peak flow measures or spirometry reading
3. Medication use

USE STEP-CARE PHARMACOLOGIC THERAPY. An aim of therapy is to use the minimum medication needed to maintain control with the least risk for adverse effects. The step-care approach, in which the number of medications and frequency of administration are increased as necessary to establish control (step-up) and reduced when possible to maintain control (step-down), is used to achieve this aim.

In general, every asthma patient must have an inhaled β_2-agonist available for rescue treatment of acute symptoms. This rescue treatment also has a step-care pattern: medications are added as necessary to control symptoms. The increase is often temporary and depends on the severity and duration of the asthma exacerbation as well as the patient's response. (Note, however, that increasing use of rescue treatment by the patient is an indication to review the medication plan and possibly to increase preventive therapy.)

Maintenance therapy, or chronic management of asthma, also uses a step-care approach and is based on severity of disease: mild, moderate, or severe.

MONITOR CONTINUALLY. Continual monitoring, which includes objective measures of lung function, is necessary to assure that therapeutic goals are met.

While the patient is achieving control of asthma, PEFR variability greater than 10–20% and continued presence of chronic symptoms indicate a need to reevaluate the patient's technique in using medication, any environmental aggravators and the patient's efforts to control them, the presence of concomitant upper respiratory disease and, finally, the possibility that medications need to be increased.

Once asthma control is established, regular follow-up visits in conjunction with prenatal visits, continue to be essential. Clinicians need to monitor and review the treatment plans, the medications, and the patient's management techniques (i.e., for using medicines and peak flowmeters, for controlling the environment).

Preferred Medications and Selection Criteria for Pregnant Women With Asthma

The choice of a specific medication plan during pregnancy is based on the following considerations:

1. Available animal and human gestational data
2. Efficacy
3. Preference for drugs administered by inhalation
4. Preference for older medications with greater experience during pregnancy and documented clinical investigation.

Given these considerations, the specific drugs listed in Table 1 are currently preferred by the Working Group on Asthma in Pregnancy

Table 1 Preferred Drugs and Dosages for Asthma and Associated Conditions[a]

Drug class	Specific drug	Dosage
Bronchodilator	Inhaled β_2-agonist[b]	2 puffs every 4 hr as needed
	Systemic terbutaline	0.25 mg subcutaneous 2.5–5.0 mg by mouth tid
	Theophylline	Oral: Dose to reach serum concentration level of 8–12 μg/mL Intravenous: See Table 3
Anti-inflammatory	Cromolyn sodium	2 puffs qid (inhalation) 2 sprays in each nostril bid–qid (intranasal for nasal symptoms)
	Beclomethasone	2–5 puffs bid–qid (inhalation) 2 sprays in each nostril bid (intranasal for allergic rhinitis)
	Prednisone	See Table 3
	Methylprednisolone	See Table 3
	Hydrocortisone	See Table 3
Antihistamine	Chlorpheniramine	4 mg by mouth up to qid 8–12 mg sustained-release bid
	Tripelennamine	25–50 mg by mouth up to qid 100 mg sustained-release bid
Decongestant	Pseudoephedrine	60 mg by mouth up to qid 120 mg sustained-release bid
	Oxymetazoline	Intranasal spray or drops up to 5 days
Cough	Guaifenesin Dextromethorphan	2 tsp by mouth qid
Antibiotic	Amoxicillin	3 weeks therapy for sinusitis

[a]Given the considerations and data described in the text, these specific drugs are preferred by the working group for use during pregnancy.
[b]The available information does not permit determination of a preferred inhaled β_2-agonist.

for the management of asthma and associated conditions during pregnancy. However, it should be noted that lack of inclusion of a specific medication on this list does not necessarily imply that it is inappropriate for use during pregnancy. Table 2 lists drugs for asthma and associated conditions that generally should be avoided during pregnancy.

Step-Care Pharmacologic Management of Asthma During Pregnancy

Treatment plans for asthma during pregnancy are based on the goals of therapy, the general principles for managing asthma, and information on the use of medications during pregnancy. This section and its accompanying charts present application of these principles to development of treatment protocols based on the severity of disease. The step care approach recommends increasing the number and frequency of medications with increasing asthma severity. Once control of asthma is established and sustained for several weeks, a reduction in therapy, or step-down, is carefully considered in order to identify the minimum therapy required to maintain control.

Chronic Mild Asthma (Chart 1)

Inhaled β_2-agonists by themselves are usually sufficient therapy for mild, intermittent asthma. If symptoms disappear and pulmonary function normalizes with inhaled β_2-agonists, they can be used indefinitely on an as-needed basis. However, their daily use, or even more often than three times a week, usually indicates a need for anti-inflammatory therapy (see following section: Chronic Moderate Asthma).

Oral theophylline does not usually give prompt bronchodilation and, therefore, is not recommended for episodic asthma.

Chronic Moderate Asthma (Chart 2)

The category of moderate asthma includes those patients who have symptoms that are uncontrolled or that are poorly regulated by episodic

Table 2 Drugs for Asthma and Associated Conditions That Generally Should Be Avoided During Pregnancy

Alpha-adrenergic compounds (other than pseudoephedrine)
Epinephrine
Iodides
Sulfonamides (in late pregnancy)
Tetracyclines
Quinalones

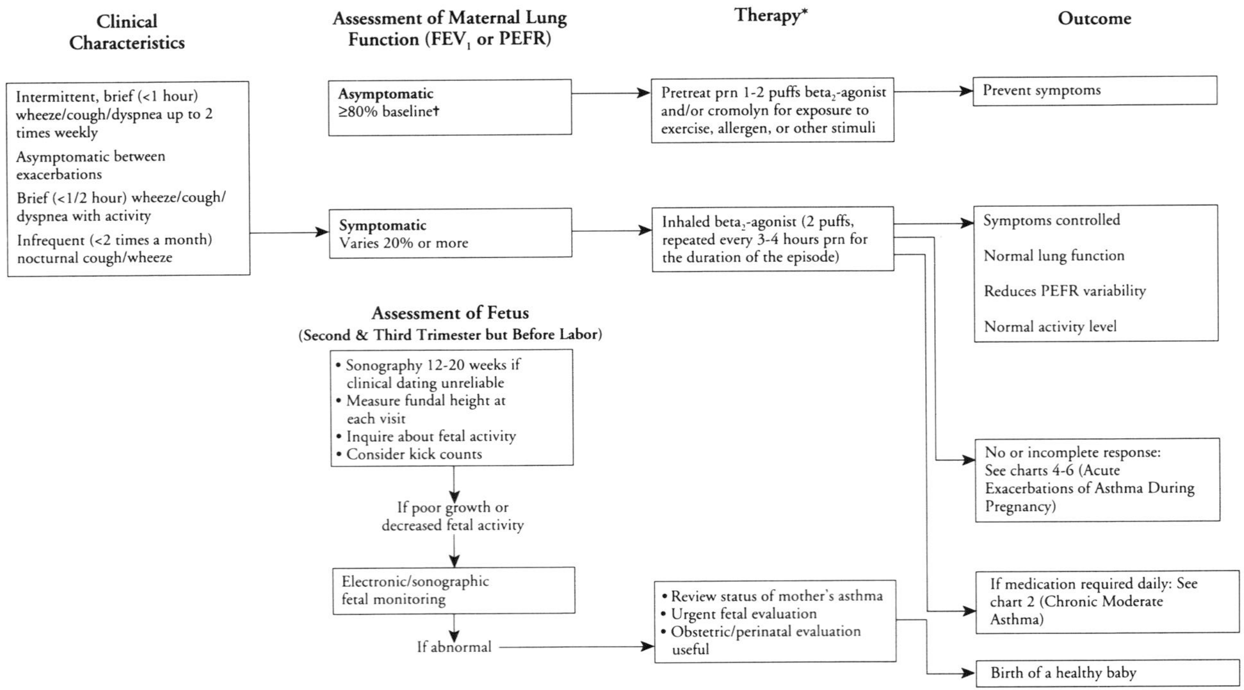

†PEFR percent baseline refers to the norm for the individual, established by the clinician. This may be percent predicted based on standardized norms or percent of patient's personal best.

***All therapy must include patient education about prevention (including environmental control where appropriate) as well as control of symptoms.**

Chart 1 Management of Asthma During Pregnancy: Chronic Mild Asthma

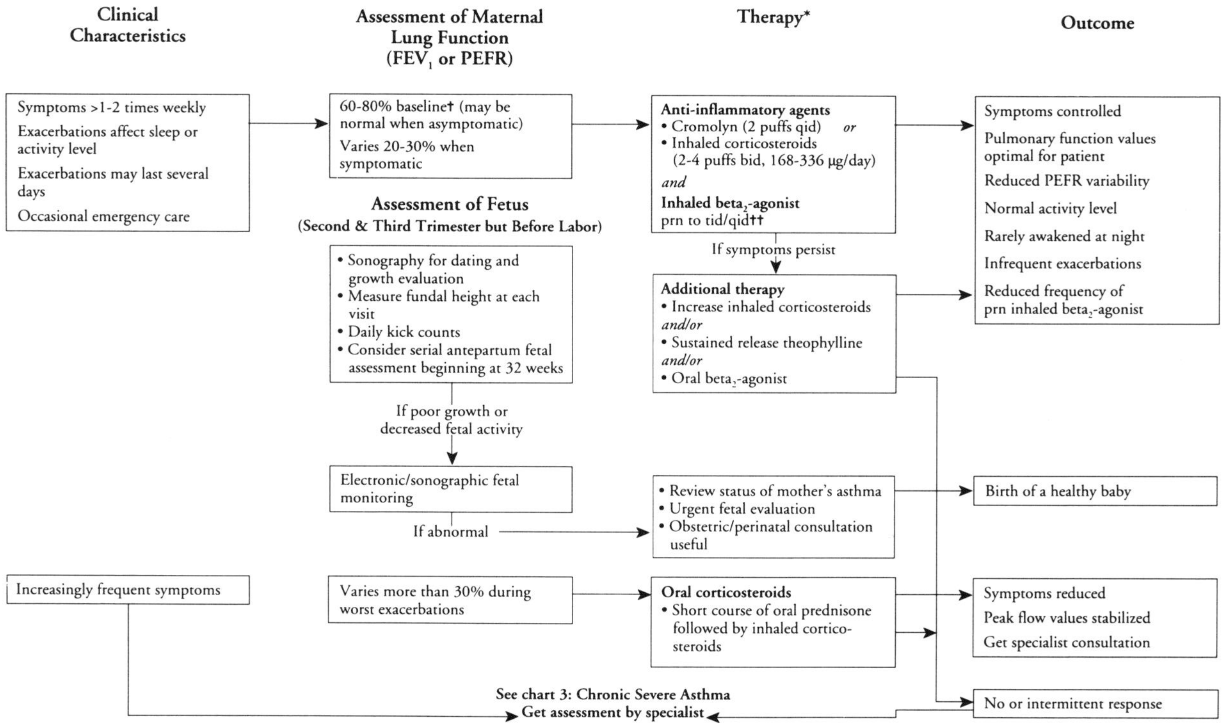

†PEFR percent baseline refers to the norm for the individual, established by the clinician. This may be percent predicted based on standardized norms or percent of patient's personal best.
††If exceed 3-4 doses a day, consider additional therapy other than inhaled beta$_2$-agonist.

***All therapy must include patient education about prevention (including environmental control where appropriate) as well as control of symptoms.**

Chart 2 Management of Asthma During Pregnancy: Chronic Moderate Asthma

administration of a β_2-agonist. Some patients have frequent (more than twice-a-week) symptomatic exacerbations of asthma. Other patients do not have acute exacerbations and can regulate symptoms by modulation in life-styles, but their pulmonary functions (FEV_1 or PEFR 60–80% of predicted range) indicate potential compromises in airway function or maternal–fetal oxygenation. These patients have very "fragile" control of asthma. Many asthma specialists think that all patients with moderate asthma should receive inhaled anti-inflammatory medication to diminish airway inflammation and airway hyperresponsiveness.

Anti-inflammatory Agents. Anti-inflammatory agents are the primary therapy in moderate asthma.

Cromolyn sodium is virtually devoid of side effects and is the most effective nonsteroidal anti-inflammatory drug for asthma currently available. Its efficacy is less predictable than that of inhaled corticosteroids and a 4- to 6-week trial may be necessary to determine benefit in individual patients.

Inhaled corticosteroids provide effective asthma control with minimal side effects at recommended doses. Immediate benefit may not be evident, however, because suppression of symptoms and PEFR improvement are often not maximal until 2–4 weeks of treatment. A spacer should be considered not only to reduce oropharyngeal candidiasis but also to improve respiratory tract penetration and to reduce the possibility of systemic effects.

A burst, or short tapering course, of oral corticosteroids is indicated when asthma is uncontrolled by any combination of bronchodilators, cromolyn sodium, or inhaled corticosteroids, even at increased doses. Such deterioration of asthma is characterized by gradual reductions in PEFR (approximately 20%) that fail to have a sustained response to inhaled bronchodilators, by greater intolerance of activities or exercise, and by the development of nocturnal symptoms. For example, a short course of 40 mg/day prednisone (single or divided) for up to 1 week, followed by up to 7–14 days of tapering doses, may be effective. At the end of this therapeutic deescalation, oral corticosteroids can be stopped; if asthma symptoms do not occur and pulmonary functions remain normal, no additional oral steroid therapy is necessary. However, if the burst of prednisone does not control symptoms, is effective for fewer than 10–24 days, or is repeated frequently, the patient has severe asthma and obviously needs additional therapy.

Nedocromil sodium has properties similar to cromolyn, but because it is a newer drug, there is less documented clinical experience with it during pregnancy.

Bronchodilators. The physician has several choices:

As-needed (PRN) *inhaled* β_2*-agonist* must be available for treatment of acute exacerbations.

Regular administration of inhaled β_2*-agonists* may be effective. However, as noted earlier, some studies have raised questions about the effectiveness and safety of regularly scheduled use of inhaled β_2-agonist. It is recommended that regularly scheduled inhaled β_2-agonist treatment should be kept to a minimum. Because well-controlled asthma requires minimal use of inhaled β_2-agonists, an increased use—or even a daily use—generally indicates the need to institute or intensify regular anti-inflammatory therapy.

Sustained-release theophylline or long-acting oral β_2*-agonist* once a day in the evening may be helpful for the patient with primarily nocturnal symptoms because the currently available inhaled β_2-agonists have a limited duration of action—4–6 h. However, when patients who use sustained-release theophylline (or oral β_2-agonist) to control nocturnal symptoms also take anti-inflammatory medication, they may be able to discontinue the bronchodilator use after 4–6 weeks.

If theophylline is the primary bronchodilator, β_2-agonist therapy can be administered episodically on an as-needed basis.

Chronic Severe Asthma (Chart 3)

Patients with severe asthma should be evaluated by an asthma specialist.

Patients whose asthma is uncontrolled on maximal doses of bronchodilators and inhaled anti-inflammatory agents may need systemic corticosteroids on a routine basis. In such cases, the physician will use long-term oral corticosteroids.

Anti-inflammatory medication. Daily anti-inflammatory medication is recommended to suppress and prevent airway inflammation and airway responsiveness.

Inhaled corticosteroids in higher doses (336–840 μg a day or more), are recommended as the primary inhaled anti-inflammatory therapy. Use of a spacer device will reduce oropharyngeal candidasis, improve delivery of the medication, and reduce the possibility of systemic effects.

Cromolyn sodium (2 puffs four times a day) may be given in addition to inhaled corticosteroids.

Oral coriticosteroids on a long-term basis are often required.

1. In this case, the lowest possible dose (alternate-day or single daily dose) should be used and administered under the supervision of an asthma specialist.
2. Patients must be monitored closely for corticosteroid adverse side effects. Prolonged use of oral corticosteroids may be associated with

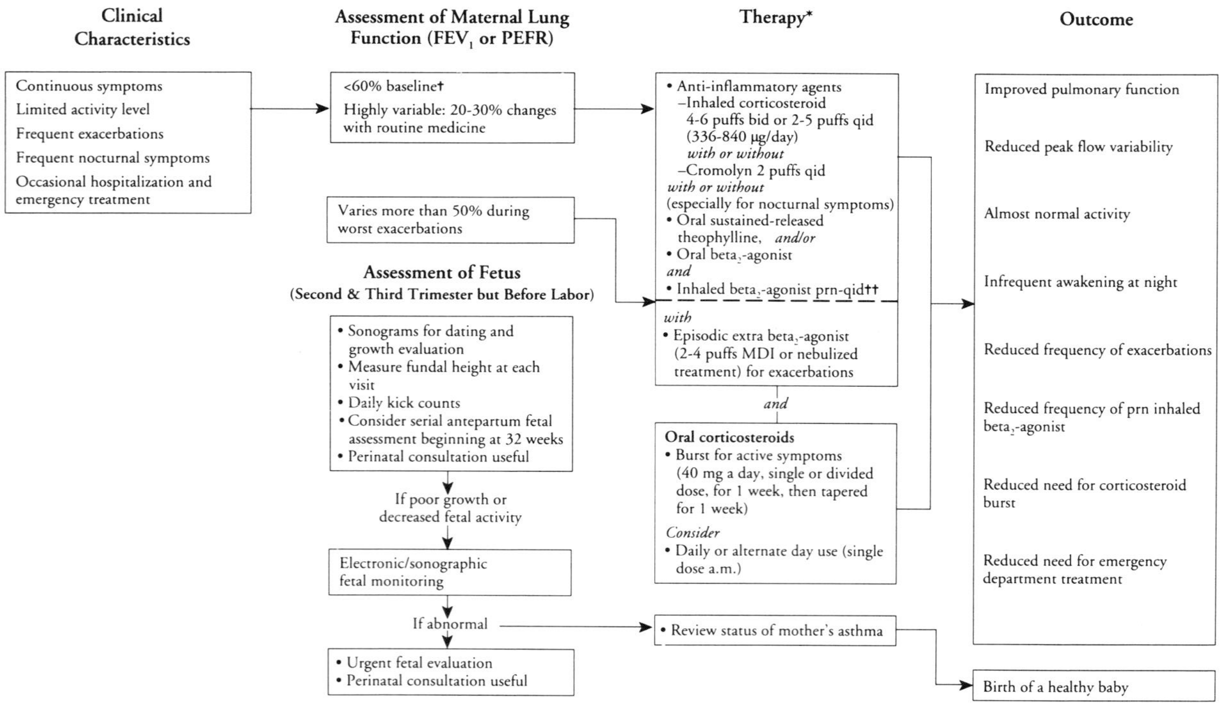

Note: Individuals with severe asthma should be evaluated by an asthma specialist.

†PEFR percent baseline refers to the norm for the individual, established by the clinician. This may be percent predicted based on standardized norms or percent of patient's personal best.

††If exceed 3-4 doses a day, consider additional therapy other than inhaled $beta_2$-agonist.

***All therapy must include patient education about prevention (including environmental control where appropriate) as well as control of symptoms.**

Chart 3 Management of Asthma During Pregnancy: Chronic Severe Asthma

increased risk of gestational diabetes, preeclampsia, and intrauterine growth retardation. The evaluation of these possibilities may be most appropriately managed in consultation with an obstetrician specializing in high-risk pregnancy care.

3. Attempts should be made to reduce oral corticosteroids with persistent administration of high doses of inhaled corticosteroids (e.g., 800 μg/day or more). Monitoring for clinical signs of adrenal insufficiency is important when a patient is being transferred from oral to inhaled corticosteroids.

Bronchodilator medication.

Inhaled β_2-agonists must be available as needed for treatment of asthma symptoms and acute exacerbations.

Sustained release theophylline and/or a long acting oral β_2-agonist may be given, especially to control nocturnal symptoms.

Regular administration of inhaled beta2 agonists may be effective, although it is recommended that their use be kept to a minimum.

Management of Exercise-Induced Asthma

Exercise-induced asthma (EIA)—which untreated can limit and disrupt normal lives—is the term for airway narrowing that occurs minutes after the onset of vigorous activity. Exercise-induced asthma should be anticipated in all asthma patients; most have the airway hyperirritability that leads to this condition.

Diagnosis of Exercise-Induced Asthma

A good history is the most important diagnostic tool. Symptoms of asthma should not interfere with the pregnant patient's usual activities or exercise. If indicated, an exercise challenge can be used to establish the diagnosis. It can be conducted in a formal laboratory setting. It can also consist of measurements of PEFR or FEV_1 before and after the patient undertakes whatever task caused the symptoms. A 15% decrease in PEFR or FEV_1 at 5–10 min after exercise is compatible with EIA.

Exercise-induced asthma is caused mainly by smooth-muscle constriction. It generally reaches its peak 5–10 min after stopping the vigorous activity and usually resolves in another 20–30 min.

Management Strategies for Exercise-Induced Asthma

The goal of management is to enable patients to participate in any activity they choose without experiencing asthma symptoms. Patients who are taking regularly scheduled anti-inflammatory therapy may have sufficient control of asthma such that it is not provoked by exercise.

Exercise-induced asthma can be prevented with inhalation of beta$_2$-agonist 5 to 60 minutes before exercise; the pretreatment is helpful for up to several hours. Cromolyn is also acceptable. If the patient still experiences symptoms with exercise, two puffs of inhaled beta$_2$-agonist should relieve the symptoms, and the dose should be increased for future exercise pretreatment. Combined beta$_2$ agonists and cromolyn pretreatment may be effective when neither one suffices on its own.

Management of Exacerbations of Asthma During Pregnancy

Exacerbations of asthma are acute or subacute episodes of progressively worsening shortness of breath, cough, wheezing, or chest tightness, or a combination of these symptoms. Respiratory distress is common. Exacerbations are characterized by decreases in expiratory airflow that can be documented and quantified by measurement of lung function (PEFR or spirometry).

This section looks first at general considerations and treatment goals for exacerbations of asthma during pregnancy and then presents, in general terms and with accompanying charts, methods for managing asthma exacerbations in home, emergency department, and hospital settings.

General Considerations

Prevention and early treatment to reverse symptoms are the best strategies for management of asthma exacerbations. Important elements of this early treatment to prevent deterioration and abort the exacerbation include:

1. Written action plans to help the patient to manage asthma exacerbations at home according to a plan prearranged with the physician
2. Recognition of early indicators of an exacerbation, including worsening PEFR or FEV_1
3. Prompt communication between patient and health care provider about any serious deterioration and its treatment
4. Appropriate intensification of antiasthma medications, including in many cases a short course of systemic corticosteroids
5. Removal of or withdrawal from any allergic or irritant trigger in the environment because treatment is less effective if there is continued exposure.

Pregnant patients with potentially fatal asthma include those patients with a history of the following:

Prior intubation for asthma

Two or more hospitalizations for asthma in the past year
Three or more emergency care visits for asthma in the past year
Hospitalization or an emergency care visit for asthma within the past month
Current use of systemic corticosteroids or recent withdrawal from systemic corticosteroids
Past history of syncope or hypoxic seizure caused by asthma
Prior admission for asthma to a hospital-based intensive care unit
Serious psychiatric disease or psychosocial problems.

Individuals with one or more of these risk factors require particularly intensive patient education, close monitoring, and prompt care. They should be counseled to seek medical care early during an exacerbation and instructed about the availability and appropriate use of ambulance services.

Treatment Goals

The principal goals of treatment in exacerbations of asthma are as follows:

1. Rapid reversal of airflow obstruction, thereby relieving respiratory distress. Repetitive administration of inhaled β_2-agonists best achieves this rapid reversal of airflow obstruction (2,3). Early addition of systemic corticosteroids speeds the rate of improvement among patients who fail to respond incompletely to inhaled β_2-agonists (4).
2. Prevention of potential fetal hypoxemia by administering supplemental oxygen to maintain maternal arterial oxygen saturation greater than or equal to 95%. In rare instances, severe alveolar hypoventilation requires mechanically assisted ventilation. Be alert to reverse of expected hypocarbia (P_{CO_2} increased to 35 mmHg indicates serious hypoventilation during pregnancy). Fetal monitoring is essential because significant fetal hypoxemia may occur in the absence of maternal hypoxemia.
3. Reduction of the rate of recurrent severe asthma symptoms by intensifying the patient's antiasthma medication regimen upon discharge from the emergency department. Often a short course of oral corticosteroids is useful.

Crucial to successful achievement of these treatment goals is close monitoring of the patient's condition and response to treatment with serial measurements of lung function. These measurements provide quantification of the severity of the asthma exacerbation and of the extent of improvement with treatment. The ranges of PEFR and FEV_1

in the protocols are general guidelines, not precise criteria. The PEFR and FEV_1 results should be seen as aids in a monitoring and decision-making process that also takes into account such other factors as the patient's history, current symptoms, and physical findings.

Home Management of Acute Exacerbations of Asthma During Pregnancy (Chart 4)

Successful management of exacerbations of asthma requires early initiation of antiasthma therapy. When pregnant patients are able to initiate treatment at home, they not only avoid delays in treatment, but also add to their sense of control over their asthma and their lives. The degree of care provided in the home depends on the physician's and the patient's experience and the availability of emergency care. (For example, patients who live in rural settings may, by necessity, have to manage asthma exacerbations at home.) Many patients who have moderately severe to severe asthma will have the equipment and medications at home necessary for treating and monitoring an asthma exacerbation.

For an individual patient, the optimal management strategy evolves out of patient and physician experience with what "works" and what does not in treating acute exacerbations. General guidelines applicable to most patients are presented in Chart 4.

1. Home PEFR determinations are an integral part of home management strategies. They make it possible for the patient to obtain information, which can then be shared with the clinician, concerning the severity of the exacerbation and the response to treatment.
2. Patients are encouraged to use inhaled β_2-agonist medications with increased frequency during an exacerbation and, under certain circumstances, begin or increase the dose of systemic corticosteroids.
3. Patients should not delay in seeking medical help if the asthma exacerbation is severe, if therapy does not give rapid improvement, if sustained improvement is not achieved, if there is further deterioration, or if the fetal kick count decreases. Furthermore, severe exacerbations in the third trimester of pregnancy are best managed with concurrent fetal monitoring.
4. Recovery from an acute exacerbation is often gradual. Medications for acute therapy may need to be continued for several days to sustain relief of symptoms and improvement in PEFR. However, patients should seek medical care rather than rely on bronchodilator therapy in excessive doses or for prolonged periods of time.

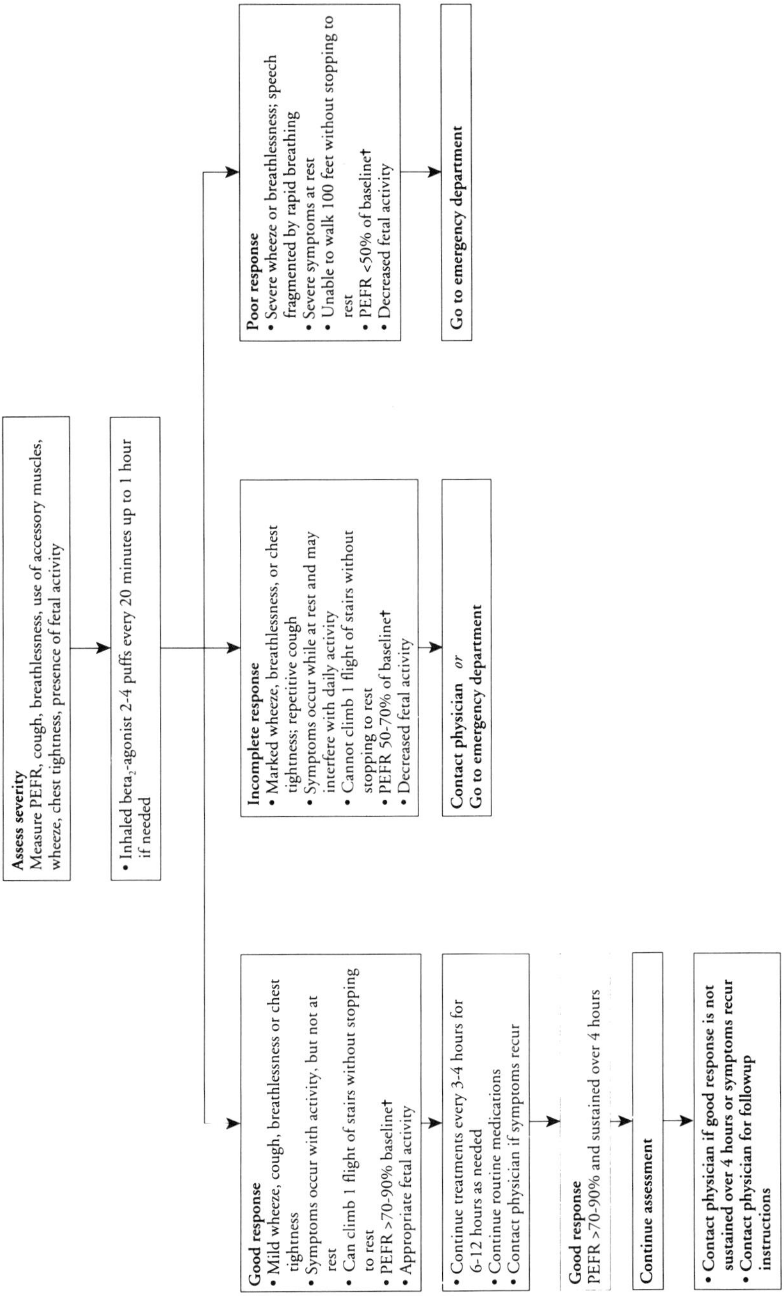

†PEFR percent baseline refers to the norm for the individual, established by the clinician. This may be percent predicted based on standardized norms or percent of patient's personal best.

Chart 4 Acute Exacerbations of Asthma During Pregnancy: Home Management

5. Pursed-lips breathing and other forms of controlled breathing may help to maintain calm during a period of respiratory distress, but they do not bring about any improvement in lung function.
6. *Not* recommended are the following home management techniques:
   Drinking large volumes of liquids or breathing warm, moist air (e.g., the mist from a hot shower)
   Rebreathing into a bag held tightly at the nose and mouth
   Using over-the-counter antihistamines, asthma, and cold remedies.

Hospital-Based Emergency Department Management and Hospital Management of Acute Exacerbations of Asthma During Pregnancy (Charts 5 and 6)

Severe exacerbations of asthma are potentially life-threatening. Care must be expeditious. Emergency care for pregnant patients may occur in labor and delivery units based on individual hospital policies. However, in this report for simplicity, emergency care will be said to occur in the emergency department.

Effective therapies may be available in a physician's office. However, serious maternal exacerbations require close observation, frequent treatment, and repetitive measurements of maternal lung function and fetal monitoring in the third trimester. Most moderate and severe exacerbations of asthma during pregnancy require prompt transfer to and a complete course of therapy in an emergency department or hospital (5).

Assessment. In the emergency department, a brief history and physical examination pertinent to the exacerbation are appropriate before treatment. A more detailed history and complete physical examination should be performed once therapy has been started.

BRIEF HISTORY. Important questions to ask in obtaining a brief history concern the following:

Time of onset and cause of present exacerbation of asthma
Severity of symptoms, including exercise limitation and sleep disturbance
All current medications
Prior hospitalizations and emergency department visits for asthma, particularly with the past year
Prior episodes of respiratory insufficiency due to asthma (loss of consciousness or intubation and mechanical ventilation)
Significant prior cardiopulmonary disease
Expected date of delivery for the infant
Obstetrical problems or risk factors.
Presence or absence of fetal activity.

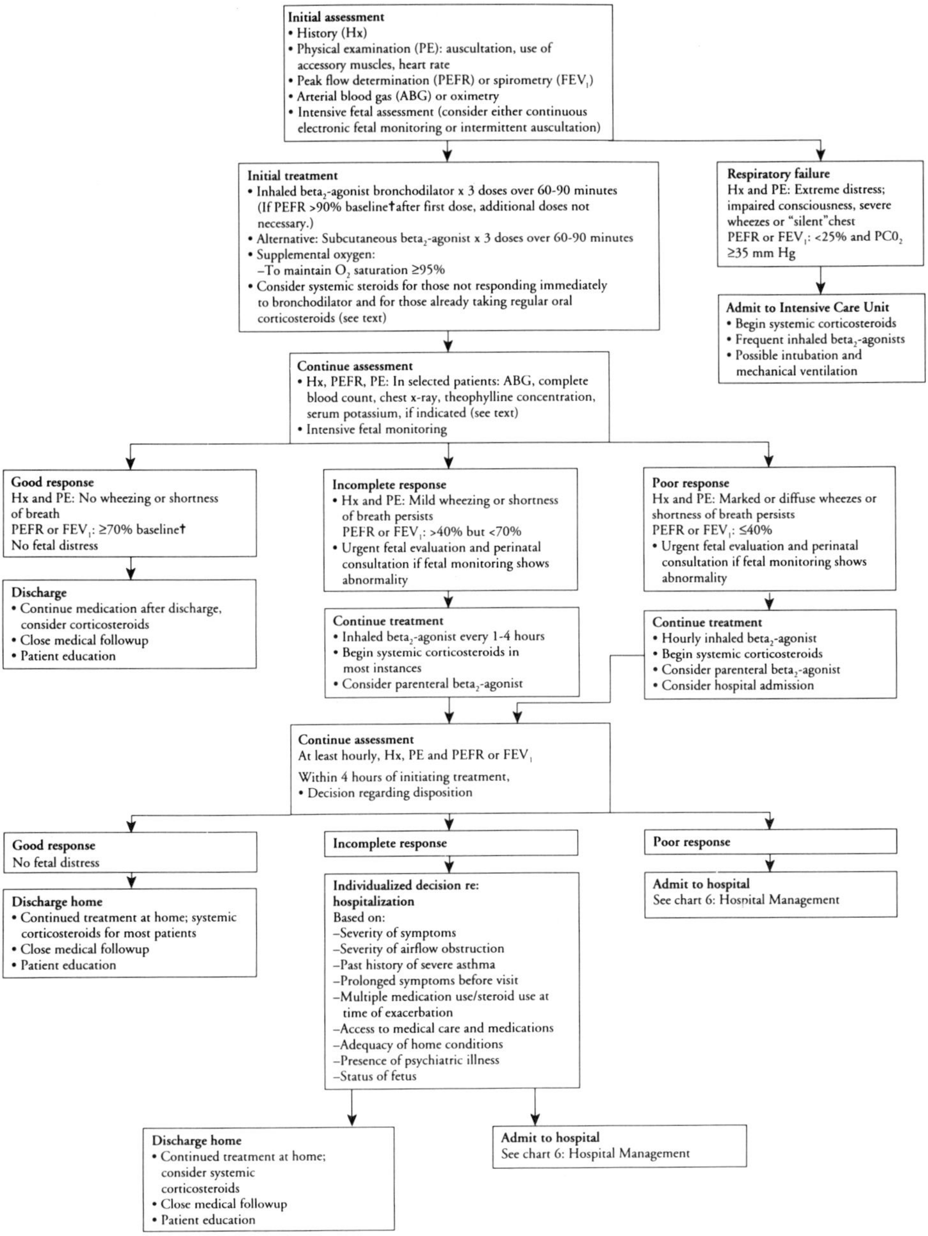

*Therapies are often available in a physician's office. However, most acute severe exacerbations of asthma require a complete course of therapy in an emergency department.
†PEFR percent baseline refers to the norm for the individual, established by the clinician. This may be percent predicted based on standardized norms or percent of patient's personal best.

Chart 5 Acute Exacerbations of Asthma During Pregnancy: Emergency Department Management

Initial assessment
- Detailed medical history (Hx)
- Complete physical examination (PE)
- Expiratory flow measurement: PEFR or FEV_1
- Chest radiograph
- Arterial blood gas/oximetry (see text)
- Intensive fetal assessment (consider either continuous electronic fetal monitoring or intermittent auscultation)

Special attention for:
- –past history of respiratory failure
- –suspicion of intrauterine growth retardation
- –uterine irritability
- –complicating medical conditions
- –history of steroid-induced complications (e.g., psychosis)

Treatment
- Inhaled $beta_2$-agonists up to every 1-2 hours
- Systemic corticosteroids; e.g., IV methylprednisolone 60-80 mg every 6-8 hours
- Supplemental oxygen to maintain 0_2 saturation ≥95%
- Consider IV aminophylline or oral theophylline

Continued assessments
- Hx, PE, PEFR or FEV_1 (measured at least twice daily; before and after bronchodilator desirable)
- Intensive fetal monitoring until patient stabilized

Improved
Suggested goals prior to discharge:
- Hx and PE: Minimal or no wheezing; ≤1 awakening at night with mild symptoms; good activity tolerance
- PEFR or FEV: ≥70% of baseline†
- No fetal distress

Preparation for discharge
- Inhaled $beta_2$-agonist no more than every 3-4 hours
- Oral corticosteroids; role of inhaled corticosteroids discussed in text
- Oral theophylline if indicated
- Adequate oxygen saturation breathing room air
- Provide patient education, especially
  - –medication use, including inhaler technique
  - –PEFR measurement at home
  - –need for followup and chronic care (contact with physician within 7-10 days of discharge recommended)

Home with patient education, medications, and followup plan

Intensive Care Unit
- PCO_2 ≥35 mm Hg with PEFR or FEV_1 <25%
- Deterioration despite maximal therapy

ICU treatment
- Nebulized $beta_2$-agonists every 30-60 minutes; may supplement with parenteral $beta_2$-agonist
- IV corticosteroids
- IV aminophylline
- Oxygen supplementation
- Intubation and mechanical ventilation for hypercapnic respiratory failure

Transfer ICU

Not improved
Deterioration despite maximal therapy
Fetal monitoring indicates abnormality; seek urgent fetal evaluation and perinatal consultation

†PEFR percent baseline refers to the norm for the individual, established by the clinician. This may be percent predicted based on standardized norms or percent of patient's personal best.

Chart 6 Acute Exacerbations of Asthma During Pregnancy: Hospital Management

PHYSICAL EXAMINATION. Objectives of the physical examination include:

Assessment of the severity of the exacerbation. Predictors of severe airflow obstruction include pulsus paradoxus (greater than or equal to 12 mmHg fall in systolic blood pressure during inspiration), use of accessory muscles of respiration, diaphoresis, and inability to recline with head elevated less than 30 degrees.

Identification of complications (e.g., pneumonia, atelectasis, pneumothorax, or pneumomediastinum).

Assessment of overall patient status, including level of alertness, fluid status, and presence of cyanosis, respiratory distress, and wheezing. [Wheezing can be an unreliable indicator of obstruction; in rare cases, extremely severe obstruction may be accompanied by a "silent chest" (6)]

Assessment of fetus.

FUNCTIONAL ASSESSMENTS. Such assessments are as follows:

In the emergency department assessment of PEFR or FEV_1 at least hourly. *In the hospital*, measurements should optimally be made before and after bronchodilator therapy at least twice daily.

In both the emergency department and hospital measurements should be made of arterial oxygen saturation by pulse oximetry (where available).

In both the emergency department and hospital intensive fetal monitoring should be instituted and continued until the exacerbation is controlled (see p. 579).

LABORATORY STUDIES. *In the emergency department* such laboratory studies as complete blood count (CBC), chest roentgenogram (with appropriate shielding), and serum theophylline concentration are rarely needed for initial assessment, and their performance should not be permitted to delay initiation of treatment.

After initial treatment in the emergency department (a) a CBC is appropriate in patients with fever or purulent sputum. (b) Chest roentgenogram should be obtained in patients suspected of a complicating cardiopulmonary process. Appropriate shielding should be used. (c) Serum theophylline concentration should be measured in patients taking theophylline before presentation.

Arterial blood gas (ABG) measurements should be performed to evaluate arterial carbon dioxide tension (P_{CO_2}) in patients with obvious hypoventilation, cyanosis, or severe distress after initial treatment, especially if PEFR is less than 200 L/min or FEV_1 is less than or equal to 40% of predicted. Patients with arterial P_{CO_2} greater than or equal to

30 mmHG will require repeated ABG measurements to monitor their response to treatment.

Oximetry can be used to follow oxygen saturation. Measures of arterial blood gases are required if oxygen saturation remains below 95% when patient is receiving supplemental oxygen.

CHARACTERISTICS IDENTIFYING PATIENTS AT PARTICULAR RISK FOR LIFE-THREATENING DETERIORATION. Patients are at particular risk for life-threatening deterioration under the following conditions:

Less than 10% improvement in PEFR or FEV_1 in the emergency department
Prior history of life-threatening exacerbations
A PEFR of less than 100 l/min or FEV_1 less than 25% of predicted
The P_{CO_2} greater than or equal to 35 mmHg

Treatment. In the emergency department and hospital, the primary therapies are repeated administration of inhaled β_2-agonist bronchodilators and systemic corticosteroids. Supplemental oxygen should be given to patients with significant hypoxemia and to all patients when arterial oxygen monitoring is not available and if fetal heart rate abnormalities are detected. Other treatment may include methylxanthines and antibiotics.

β_2-AGONISTS. Recommended doses are given in Table 3

Reversal of airflow obstruction is most effectively achieved by the repetitive administration of inhaled β_2-agonist bronchodilators.
Inhalation of a β_2-agonist solution aerosolized by nebulizer is favored, although some studies raise the possibility that supervised delivery by metered-dose inhaler (MDI) with a spacer device may be equally effective.
Onset of action for inhaled β_2-agonist is less than 5 min; repetitive administration produces incremental bronchodilation.
Duration of action in severe asthma is not precisely known.
Three doses spaced every 20–30 min can safely be given as initial therapy to patients without comorbid cardiovascular disease. Thereafter, the frequency of administration varies according to severity of patients' symptoms and occurrence of adverse side effects. In patients without underlying cardiovascular disease, administration as frequently as every 1–2 h is safe for periods of severe airflow obstruction.

SYSTEMIC CORTICOSTEROIDS. Recommended doses are given in Table 3.

Table 3 Doses of Drugs in Acute Exacerbations of Asthma During Pregnancy

β-Agonists
- Inhaled
  - Albuterol 2.5 mg (0.5 mL of a 0.5% solution, diluted with 2–3 mL of normal saline) *or*
  - Metaproterenol 15 mg (0.3 mL of a 5% solution, diluted with 2–3 mL of normal saline); *or*
- Subcutaneous
  - Terbutaline 0.25 mg

Methylxanthines
- Intravenous loading dose: Aminophylline 6 mg/kg, theophylline 5 mg/kg
- Intravenous maintenance dose: Aminophylline 0.5 mg/kg/hr, theophylline 0.4 mg/kg/hr adjusted to keep theophylline level between 8–12 μg/mL

Corticosteroids
- Intravenous
  - Methylprednisolone 1 mg/kg IV bolus every 6–8 hr *or*
  - Hydrocortisone 2.0 mg/kg IV bolus every 4 hr *or*
  - Hydrocortisone 2.0 mg/kg IV bolus, then 0.5 mg/kg/hr continuous intravenous infusion
- Oral
  - A typical oral regimen that may be used as a substitute for intravenous corticosteroids might be prednisone or methylprednisolone 60 mg given immediately, then 60–120 mg/day in divided doses, tapered over several days at the discretion of the physician.
  - With improvement in the patient's condition (e.g., stabilized PEFR), corticosteroids are usually tapered to a single daily dose of oral prednisone or methylprednisolone (e.g., 60 mg/day), or divided doses (e.g., 20 mg three times a day), then gradually further reduced over 7–14 days.
  - If the patient requires a prolonged course of oral corticosteroids, side effects may be minimized by a single morning dose given on alternate days.

In the emergency department: Immediate administration of systemic corticosteroids are warranted in patients with severe exacerbations of asthma in whom no improvement is observed after the initial dose of β_2-agonist, or in those patients who developed an exacerbation despite the regular use of oral corticosteroids (3,7–9). Patients with severe airflow obstruction (PEFR less than 200 L/min or FEV_1 less than or equal to 40% of predicted) after the initial hour of treatment should be given systemic corticosteroids.

In the hospital: Systemic corticosteroids speed the resolution of severe asthma exacerbations refractory to bronchodilator therapy and should be given to all patients admitted to the hospital for severe asthma.

OXYGEN. Supplemental oxygen should be administered to the pregnant patient to achieve an arterial oxygen saturation of greater than or equal to 95%.

In the absence of available continuous oxygen saturation monitoring, supplemental oxygen should be administered to all patients.

METHYLXANTHINES. See Table 3 for recommended doses.

In the emergency department: Intravenous aminophylline is not recommended. It has been demonstrated that in the first 4 hr of treatment aminophylline provides no additional benefit to optimal inhaled β_2-agonist therapy (10–12). When used in combination with repetitively administered β_2-agonist bronchodilators, intravenous aminophylline causes increased adverse side effects without effecting additive bronchodilation (12–14).

In patients currently taking a theophylline-containing preparation, serum theophylline concentration should be determined: maintenance theophylline may be considered if the patient is hospitalized. Monitoring theophylline levels is imperative. In the last trimester of pregnancy, theophylline clearance is reduced, and doses need to be decreased accordingly. The theophylline level should be maintained between 8 and 12 μg/mL to reduce adverse effects that may result from changes in drug disposition in the pregnant patient.

ANTIBIOTICS. The use of antibiotics is generally reserved for those patients with purulent sputum (discolored because of polymorphonuclear leukocytes, not eosinophils), especially when combined with fever. The presence of bacterial sinusitis should be treated with antibiotics if suspected.

Some treatments—anticholinergics, hydration, and chest physical therapy–are generally not beneficial; others—mucolytics and sedation—should be avoided.

ANTICHOLINERGICS. Ipratropium bromide in metered-dose inhaler form does not appear to benefit patients receiving intensive bronchodilator therapy with β_2-agonists. In contrast, ipratropium bromide nebulizer solution may be of some benefit for patients with severe exacerbations, but it is not currently available in the United States.

HYDRATION. Among adults intravenous or oral administration of large volumes of fluids does *not* play a role in the management of severe asthma. However, pregnant patients may become dehydrated as a result of increased respiratory rate and decreased oral intake. Dehydration may cause urine contractions. Assessment of fluid status should be made (urine output, urine specific gravity, mucous membrane moisture, electrolytes), and appropriate corrections provided.

CHEST PHYSICAL THERAPY. In general, among patients with normal respiratory muscle strength and effective cough, chest physical therapy is not beneficial and may be unnecessarily stressful for the severely breathless patient. However, in selected patients who manifest severe hypersecretion of mucus or atelectasis as part of their asthma exacerbation, postural drainage, chest vibration and percussion, and other techniques of chest physical therapy may be beneficial.

MUCOLYTICS. Administration of mucolytic agents (e.g., acetylcysteine, potassium iodide) in severe exacerbations of asthma may worsen cough or airflow obstruction and should be *avoided*.

SEDATION. Because of their respiratory depressant effect, anxiolytic, hypnotic, and narcotic drugs should be *strictly avoided* in severely ill asthma patients.

With intensive therapy, unpleasant side effects (e.g., palpitations, tremulousness, sense of inner raciness, headache) may occur, but injurious adverse reactions (e.g., significant cardiac arrhythmias or myocardial ischemia) are rare.

Treatment of impending respiratory failure (pregnant patients with severe asthma and an arterial $P\text{CO}_2$ greater than or equal to 35 mmHg after intensive therapy) should be in an intensive care unit. In general, if there is steady deterioration in clinical signs and symptoms despite intensive therapy for asthma, the pregnant patient should be intubated and mechanically ventilated when the $P\text{CO}_2$ is greater than or equal to 45 mmHg and rising.

An arterial line should be placed for continuous blood pressure, heart rate, and blood gas monitoring. Mechanical ventilation of an asthma patient is difficult and always requires the assistance of a qualified specialist.

All pregnant patients admitted to intensive care units should have consultation with an asthma specialist. Consultation should also be considered for patients with multiple hospital admissions.

Patient Discharge

FROM THE EMERGENCY DEPARTMENT

1. Release of the pregnant patient from the emergency department depends on the patient's response to treatment.
2. In general, consider pregnant patients for hospitalization if their PEFR is less than 200 L/min, or FEV_1 remains less than or equal to

40% of predicted, or if the PEFR is between 200 and 300, or FEV_1 is greater than 40%, but less than 70% when the following factors pertain: persistent symptoms; evidence of pneumonia; past history of severe asthma; prolonged increase in asthma symptoms before the emergency department visit; use of multiple antiasthma medications, especially of systemic corticosteroids, at the time of the exacerbation; nonreassuring fetal assessment; uterine irritability; inadequate access to medications and medical care; poor home situation; comorbid psychiatric illness.

3. Avoid prolonged (more than 2–4 hr) detention of pregnant asthma patients in the emergency department awaiting a good response to treatment. Extended treatment in a holding area or overnight unit with sufficient monitoring and nursing care may be appropriate.
4. For patients with a rapid response, require a 30- to 60-min period of observation after the last dose of bronchodilator to ensure stability of response before discharge to home.

At emergency department discharge:

1. Prescribe at least 3–5 days of treatment to be continued after discharge. Most regimens should include a course of oral corticosteroids to reduce the rate of recurrent severe asthma symptoms and to treat the underlying pathology of the exacerbation.
2. Emphasize the need for continuous, regular care in an outpatient setting. A follow-up medical appointment is necessary within 7 days to ensure complete resolution of the exacerbation and to review the long-term medication plan.
3. Consider issuing a peak flowmeter and providing patient education on how to make and record daily PEFR measurements.
4. Review discharge medications and inhaler technique. Where appropriate, provide patient education on avoidance of asthma triggers.
5. Notify the physicians managing the patient's asthma and pregnancy, by telephone if possible.

FROM THE HOSPITAL

1. Before discharge, the pregnant patient's medication must be adjusted to an oral or inhaled regimen. The optimal timing of this transition is not precisely established, but the general approach is to wait until the patient is minimally symptomatic, with no or minimal wheezing corresponding to a PEFR or FEV_1 value between 60 and 70% of predicted.

2. During the first 24 hr after this medication adjustment, closely observe patients for possible deterioration. Because changing from intravenous to oral corticosteroids usually involves a significant dose reduction, relapse may occur.
3. Discharge most patients with a β_2-agonist bronchodilator by metered-dose inhaler, dry powder inhaler, or compressor-driven nebulizer, to be used no more than every 3 or 4 hr.
4. Confirm the patient's ability to maintain good lung function with near normal PEFR.
5. Before discharge, confirm the adequacy of arterial oxygen saturation while breathing room air for patients who received supplemental oxygen during their hospitalization. The preferred method of measurement is pulse oximetry.
6. Initiate inhaled corticosteroids at the first follow-up visit during the prednisone taper. Alternatively, begin inhaled corticosteroids along with the oral corticosteroid therapy before discharge from the hospital; this approach may enhance patient adherence.
7. If theophylline is used, base the oral dose of theophylline on the dose required to achieve serum concentration levels between 8 and 12 μg/mL and initiate careful monitoring to keep the theophylline level between 8 and 12 μg/mL.
8. Set a follow-up appointment for 3–7 days after discharge.
9. Provide patient education:
   Educate patients about their discharge medications and the importance of a followup medical visit in an outpatient regular-care setting.
   Educate patients in the use of peak flow meters to monitor their lung function at home.
   Review inhaler technique.
   Recommend fetal "kick count" recording during exacerbations in the third trimester

Management of Asthma During Labor and Delivery (charts 7, 8)

General Considerations

To manage the patient with asthma during labor and delivery, it is recommended that the patient's regularly scheduled asthma medications (inhaled cromolyn, beclomethasone, and/or oral theophylline) be continued during labor and delivery. The patient's PEFR should be measured upon admission to labor or delivery, and subsequently every

Assessment at Admission
- Medical history
- Physical examination
- Expiratory flow measurement (PEFR or FEV_1)
- Careful fetal monitoring (consider electronic fetal monitoring for at least 20 minutes–admission test)

Well controlled asthma
(PEFR/FEV_1 ≥80% baseline, no/minimal symptoms)
- Continue routine asthma medications
- Administer hydrocortisone every 8 hours until postpartum if systemic steroids were taken within 4 weeks
- If labor is induced, avoid 15-methyl prostaglandin F_2 alpha
- Analgesia
  - Avoid morphine and meperidine
  - Consider fentanyl
  - Consider lumbar epidural

Continue assessment
- PEFR/FEV_1 every 12 hours
  or
  if symptoms develop
- Continued intermittent fetal monitoring
  - Intensive fetal monitoring recommended if admission test indicates abnormality or other risk factors present
  - If abnormal, urgent fetal evaluation with perinatal consultation

Continue treatment for asthma and for labor

Exacerbation of asthma
(PEFR/FEV_1 ≤80% baseline
Symptoms: wheeze, cough, breathlessness or chest tightness)
- Anesthesia consultation useful

Treatment
- Inhaled $beta_2$-agonist
- IV corticosteroids
- Hydrocortisone (100 mg every 8 hours) if systemic steroids taken within 4 weeks
- Oxygen to maintain O_2 saturation ≥95%
- Analgesia
  - Avoid narcotic analgesics
  - Consider epidural analgesia

Continue assessment
- PEFR/FEV_1
- Oxygen saturation
- Intensive fetal monitoring (consider either continuous electronic fetal monitoring or intermittent auscultation)
  - If abnormal, urgent fetal evaluation with perinatal consultation

- Continue treatment for asthma
- Continue efforts for vaginal delivery

Chart 7 Management of Asthma During Labor

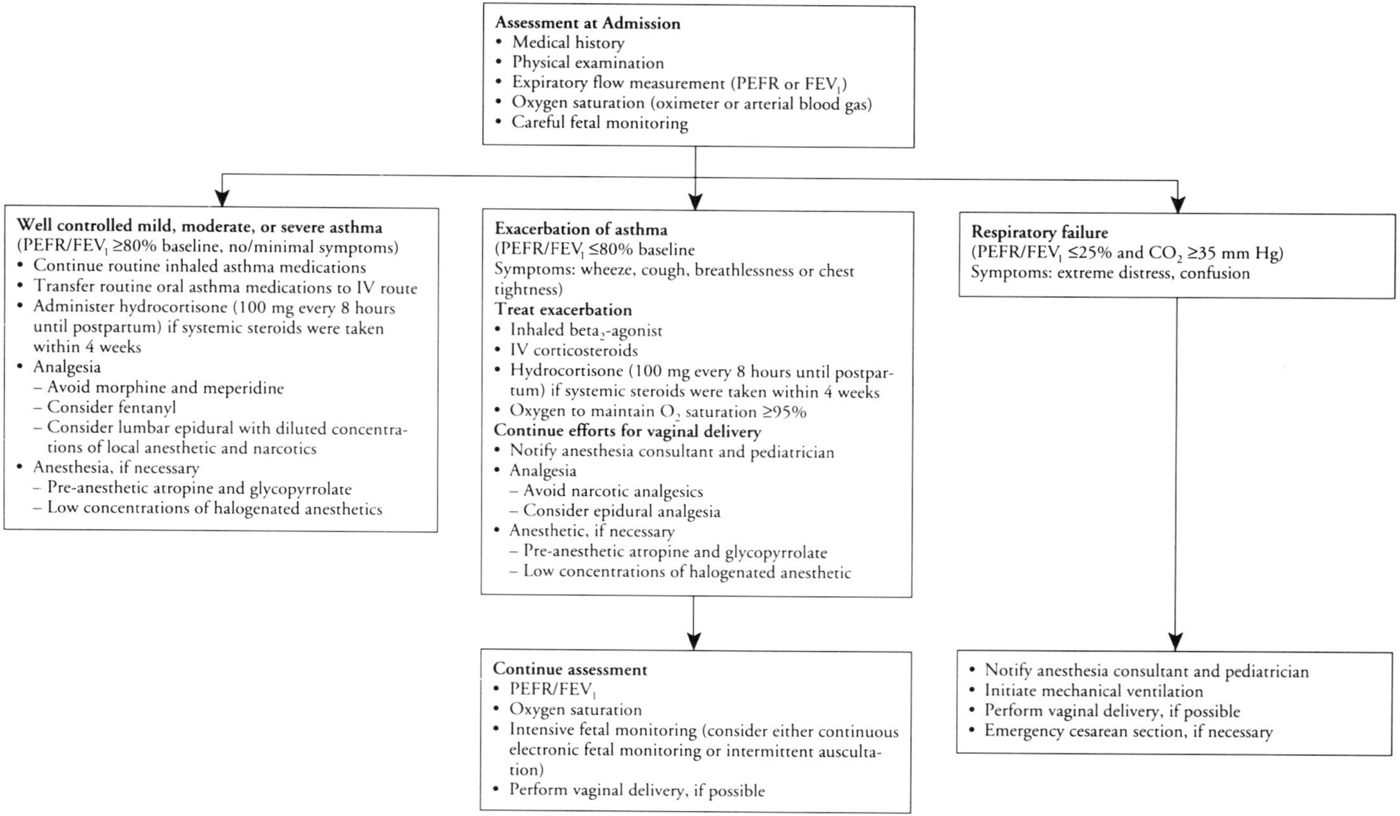

Chart 8 Management of Asthma During Delivery

12 hours. If asthma symptoms develop, PEFR should be measured after asthma treatments (see Managing Exacerbations). The patient should be kept well hydrated and be provided adequate analgesia to limit the risk of bronchospasm. Patients who have required chronic systemic corticosteroids or several short courses of systemic corticosteroids during pregnancy should be given 100 mg hydrocortisone every 8 hours until 24 hours postpartum to treat for possible adrenal suppression. Fetal monitoring during labor and delivery is described on page 579.

For labor induction, the use of 15-methyl prostaglandin $F_{2\alpha}$ should be avoided because it is a synthetic analogue of prostaglandin $F_{2\alpha}$ that has been reported to cause bronchospasm in patients with asthma (15). Use of prostaglandin E_2 has been reported to cause bronchospasm (16); however, a recent report has shown that it can safely be used in the patient with asthma for therapeutic abortion or labor induction with a dead fetus (17). Use of intravaginal or intracervical prostaglandin E_2 gel for cervical ripening before labor induction has not been reported to cause bronchospasm (18,19).

Analgesic and Anesthetic Considerations

When choosing a narcotic analgesic to use in the patient with asthma, consideration must be given to the propensity of that agent to cause histamine release that may precipitate bronchospasm. Morphine and meperidine, therefore, should be avoided, and a preferred agent may be fentanyl. Narcotic analgesics do cause respiratory depression and should be not used if there is an acute asthma exacerbation.

Lumbar epidural analgesia reduces oxygen consumption and minute ventilation during first- and second-stage labor, which offers patients with asthma considerable benefit (20). Dilute concentrations of local anesthetics and narcotics administered by continuous epidural infusion technique offer consistent analgesia and minimize motor blockade for labor and delivery (21). In the patient with an asthma exacerbation, epidural analgesia has been reported to enhance the response to bronchodilator therapy (22). However, bronchospasm has been reported in approximately 2% of patients with asthma receiving regional anesthesia (23).

If a general anesthetic is necessary, preanesthetic use of atropine and glycopyrrolate may provide a bronchodilatory effect (24). For induction, ketamine is the agent of choice because it decreases airway resistance (25) and can prevent bronchospasm (26). Low concentrations of halogenated anesthetics can provide the patient with asthma with bronchodilatation (27), allowing high inspired concentrations of oxygen and avoiding maternal awareness of the surgery, and does not appear to contribute to postpartum hemorrhage (28).

Postpartum Hemorrhage

The pharmacologic treatment of postpartum hemorrhage in a patient with asthma is different because many of the commonly used oxytocic drugs for treatment of uterine atony may worsen bronchospasm. Oxytocin is the drug of choice for postpartum hemorrhage. However, if additional agents are required, methylergonovine, as well as ergonovine, should be avoided because they may cause bronchospasm (29). If their use is unavoidable, pretreatment with methylprednisolone is recommended. The use of 15-methyl prostaglandin $F_{2\alpha}$ should also be avoided because it is a synthetic analogue of prostaglandin $F_{2\alpha}$ that is a bronchoconstrictor and may worsen asthma (15). If prostaglandin treatment is necessary, the safest analogue is E_2, which is less likely to cause bronchospasm. If there is severe uterine hemorrhage, a 20-mg prostaglandin E_2 suppository can be administered rectally, thereby avoiding the "washout" effect caused by continued vaginal bleeding.

Preterm Labor

The treatment of preterm labor in a patient already receiving asthma medication creates the risk of dangerous drug interactions. During an asthma exacerbation, uterine contractions are common and usually do not progress to preterm labor. Typically, with successful treatment of the acute asthma exacerbation, uterine contractions usually abate without therapy. However, if progressive cervical change occurs before term, tocolytic therapy should be instituted. The use of multiple different beta$_2$-agonists should be avoided. If a patient is already taking a systemic beta$_2$-agonist for her asthma, the alternative tocolytic agent, magnesium sulfate, is recommended for uterine contractions. Magnesium sulfate may be safer than the beta$_2$-agonists as tocolytic therapy, and it may provide some bronchodilation. There are no theoretical contraindications to the use of calcium channel blockers, such as nifedipine. However, there are no reports of concurrent use to treat women with asthma with preterm labor. The use of indomethacin is relatively contraindicated in the patient with asthma. However, because aspirin intolerance occurs in only a few patients with asthma, for those patients who have previously demonstrated ability to tolerate aspirin and other nonsteroidal anti-inflammatory agents, indomethacin can be considered. Consultation with an asthma specialist may be helpful for those asthma patients who also have rhino-sinusitis, given the association between aspirin sensitivity and nasal polyps.

COMPONENT 4: PATIENT EDUCATION

Patient education is a powerful tool for helping patients gain the motivation, skill, and confidence to control their asthma (30,31). Patient education should begin at the time of diagnosis and be integrated with continuing care. All members of the health care term should participate in the process.

Building a Partnership

Much of the day-to-day responsibility for managing asthma falls on the patient and her family. Active participation by the clinician, the patient, and the family in a partnership can improve adherence to the treatment plan and stimulate improvements in asthma management (32,33). This partnership concept includes open communication, joint development of a treatment plan by the clinician and patient, and encouragement of the family's efforts to improve prevention and treatment of the patient's symptoms. An important step in building the partnership is to ask questions early at each visit to identify the patient's main concerns about and expectations for treatment. Patients can focus fully on the clinician's recommendations only after these have been addressed (34).

The medicolegal implications of pharmacologic management of asthma during pregnancy warrant specific consideration. It is recommended that, through patient education, the clinician should

1. Acknowledge that, although relatively few medications have been proved harmful during pregnancy, no medication for asthma, allergy—or any condition—can be considered absolutely safe
2. Discuss the potential direct and indirect consequences for the mother and for the baby of inadequately controlled asthma, emphasizing that the recommended medications are safe enough to be preferable to the uncontrolled asthma that would result if the medications are not used
3. Discuss the medication choices available and the rationale for the selection of a particular treatment plan
4. Document the discussion in the patient's record and that informed consent for the treatment plan was obtained

The Content of Teaching

Patient education involves helping patients understand asthma, helping patients learn and practice the skills necessary to manage asthma, and supporting patients for adopting appropriate asthma management behaviors and adhering to the treatment plan. Providing information contributes, but is not enough by itself, to accomplish these objectives. Developing the patient's asthma management skills and confidence that she can control asthma is also required.

Areas and topics to be considered in patient education for asthma include the following:

Definition of asthma (with an emphasis on the chronic nature of asthma and goals of therapy)
Key points about signs and symptoms of asthma (the main symptoms of acute asthma episodes, the variability of symptoms among patients, the need to recognize and treat even mild symptoms, the importance of PEFR measurements in detecting early symptoms)
Characteristic changes in the airways of asthma patients and the role of medications (inflammation, bronchospasm, and excessive thick mucus; inhaled steroids, cromolyn, and bronchodilators)
Asthma triggers and how to avoid or control them (allergens and irritants, viral respiratory tract infections, and exercise)
Treatment (the need for individualized continuing care, adverse effects and how to reduce them, the need for preventive treatment, the importance of early treatment of acute episodes)
Patient fears concerning medication (responses to common fears include the following: inhaled steroids are safe and efficacious; toxicity effects can be minimized by reducing the dosage; asthma medications are not addictive; continuous use does not reduce effectiveness.)
Use of written guidelines (including medication plans for maintenance therapy and managing exacerbations as well as criteria for detecting onset of symptoms, initiating treatment for acute episodes, seeking emergency care, and recognizing when long-term treatment is less than optimal)
Use of written diaries (to record asthma triggers, symptoms, actions taken, and PEFR to see patterns and report to the clinician)
Correct use of inhalers
Criteria for premedicating to prevent onset of symptoms (before exercise, before exposure to allergens, cold air, or irritants)
Optimal use of home peak expiratory flow rate monitoring (to help decide when to initiate or terminate treatment, when to seek emergency care, or when to consider additional chronic treatment because of, for example, high variability in PEFR readings or evening dips below morning PEFR levels)
Evaluation of results of treatment plan (review whether the goals of therapy are being achieved; identify any adherence problems to

overcome barriers or to negotiate changes in the treatment plan. Adherence to the treatment plan is enhanced when the plan is simplified as much as possible and when the plan considers both the patient's ability to afford the medications and the payment method.)

Fears and misconceptions (asthma is not caused by psychological factors; most deaths are related to undertreatment and are rare in children; people with asthma should live full and active lives; with proper treatment asthma does not lead to permanent lung disability.)

Family understanding and support (need for family education about asthma, need for help in managing an acute exacerbation)

Feelings about asthma (need for acknowledging negative feelings and their validity; possible need for obtaining referrals to self-management programs, counseling, and social services).

Psychological Support

Pregnancy is a time of psychological stress because of changes in body image, the physical symptoms accompanying pregnancy, and fears concerning the pregnancy, labor, delivery, and the developing fetus. Many pregnant women experience emotional lability and ambivalence about the pregnancy. In the patient who has asthma, there are additional concerns. The stress associated with normal pregnancy may aggravate asthma in some predisposed women. Furthermore, the morbidity of asthma may compound the stresses of pregnancy. There may also be additional fears about the effect of the asthma or the medications taken for the asthma on the developing infant.

Suggestions for psychological management for the patient with asthma during pregnancy include the following:

DISCUSSION. Allow the patient ample opportunity to express her fears and concerns.

EDUCATION. Factual information should be given to the patient concerning

The lack of adverse effects of properly managed asthma on pregnancy

The possible effects of pregnancy on the course of asthma

What is known about the effects of the medication taken for asthma on the developing infant

The anticipated course of labor and delivery

The patterns of inheritance of asthma and allergic diseases

Possible strategies to reduce the risk for the infant.

SUPPORT. Support and reassurance can be provided by the physician through frequent scheduled appointments and easy accessibility at other times.

SAMPLE PATIENT EDUCATION HANDOUT: "GOOD NEWS AND GREAT TIPS FOR PREGNANT WOMEN WITH ASTHMA"

Asthma Can Be Controlled During Pregnancy

You are breathing for two now, and you need to keep your asthma under close control. By taking the steps listed in this handout, you can both control your asthma and protect your baby.

If you do not take these steps, you could lose control of your asthma. Your wheezing, coughing, and shortness of breath could deprive your baby of oxygen and slow your baby's growth inside you. Your baby could be less healthy and smaller when born. Your baby could even come too early. Your baby's chances of dying could be greater. But these things do not need to happen!

Here are the steps for you to take to control your asthma and protect your baby:

1. **Work with your doctor.**
   Keep your appointments.
   Ask your doctor all the questions you have. (Writing them down before each visit is a good idea. It helps you remember them all.)
   Tell your doctor about any symptoms you have.
   Tell your doctor of any concerns you have about your medicines or the other parts of your treatment plan.
   Make sure you know what your doctor wants you to do before you leave the office.
2. **Take your medicines.**
   Follow directions exactly about how much and when to take your asthma medicines.
   Do not stop taking your asthma medicines unless your doctor directs you to.
   Before you take *any* new medicines or over-the-counter drugs get your doctor's OK.

Remember: Using asthma medications during pregnancy is much safer than letting your asthma get out of control. Such asthma medicines as inhaled β-agonist, cromolyn, and inhaled steroids are safe for pregnant woman. The babies of women who control their asthma are just as healthy as those of women without asthma. So: Take your medicines and control your asthma!

3. **Watch your asthma and treat symptoms fast.**
   Pregnancy is a time of change. Your asthma can change too and can get worse, better, or stay the same. If this is your first pregnancy, there is no way to predict what will happen with your asthma. If you have been pregnant before, your asthma is most likely to change—or not change—as it did before. It is very important for you to follow your asthma closely.
   Use a peak flowmeter each day so you can find any changes in your asthma and act early.
   Know your warning signs when your asthma is getting worse.
   Make a plan with your doctor for dealing with any sign that your asthma is getting worse. Use it.
4. **Stay away from asthma triggers.**
   Stay away from your asthma triggers—things that you know start your asthma. Dusty or damp places, animals, tobacco smoke, very cold air, and food with sulfite or MSG in them are some examples of triggers.

When you follow these four steps you can be sure you are doing the best for yourself and your baby.

Answers to Some Common Questions

Most asthma medicines are safe for pregnant women. It is very important for your baby's health that you keep your asthma under good control!

You can exercise if you exercised before you became pregnant. Exercise is important and you should be able to be physically active without having asthma symptoms. Talk to your doctor about this.

You can get allergy shots. Allergy shots can be continued if you were getting them before you were pregnant. But allergy shots should not be started for the first time while you are pregnant.

You can get flu shots. These are made from dead viruses that will not harm you or your baby.

Problems with asthma rarely occur during labor. If symptoms do occur, you will receive prompt treatment.

You can safely breast-feed. Very little asthma medicine will get to your baby through your breast milk. This small amount will not affect your baby.

We cannot predict whether your child will have asthma. Your child is more likely to have asthma if both you and the baby's father have asthma or allergies.

REFERENCES

1. National Heart, Lung, and Blood Institute, National Asthma Education Program. Executive summary expert panel report: guidelines for the diagnosis and management of asthma. Washington, DC: US Government Printing Office, 1991.
2. Brenner BE. Bronchial asthma in adults: presentation to the emergency department. Part 1: pathogenesis, clinical manifestations, diagnostic evaluation, and differential diagnosis. Am J Emerg Med 1983; 1:50–70.
3. McFadden ER Jr. Therapy of acute asthma. J Allergy Clin Immunol 1989; 84:151–158.
4. Fanta CH, Rossing TH, McFadden ER Jr. Glucocorticoids in acute asthma: a critical controlled trial. Am J Med 1983; 74:845–851.
5. Brenner BE. Bronchial asthma in adults: presentation to the emergency department. Part 2: sympathomimetics, respiratory failure, recommendations for initial treatment, indications for admission, and summary. Am J Emerg Med 1983; 1:306–333.
6. Shim CS, Williams MH Jr. Evaluation of the severity of asthma: patients versus physicians. Am J Med 1980; 68:11–3.
7. Harris JB, Weinberger MM, Nassif E, Smith G, Milavetz G, Stillerman A. Early intervention with short courses of prednisone to prevent progression of asthma in ambulatory patients incompletely responsive to bronchodilators. J Pediatr 1987; 110:627–633.
8. Harrison BD, Stokes TC, Hart GJ, Vaughn DA, Ali NJ, Robinson AA. Need for intravenous hydrocortisone in addition to oral prednisolone in patients admitted to hospital with severe asthma without ventilatory failure. Lancet 1986; 1:181–184.
9. Littenberg B, Gluck EH. A controlled trial of methylprednisolone in the emergency treatment of asthma. N Engl J Med 1986; 314:150–2.
10. Fanta CH, Rossing TH, McFadden ER Jr. Treatment of acute asthma. Is combination therapy with sympathomimetics and methylxanthines indicated? Am J Med 1986; 80:5–10.
11. Rossing TH, Fanta CH, Goldstein DH, Snapper, JR, McFadden ER Jr. Emergency therapy of asthma: comparison of the acute effects of parenteral and inhaled sympathomimetics and infused aminophylline. Am Rev Respir Dis 1980; 122:365–371.
12. Siegel D, Sheppard D, Gelb A, Weinberg PF. Aminophylline increases the toxicity but not the efficacy of an inhaled beta-adrenergic agonist in the treatment of acute exacerbations of asthma. Am Rev Respir Dis 1985; 132:283–286.

13. Fanta CH, Rossing TH, McFadden ER Jr. Emergency room treatment of asthma: relationships among therapeutic combinations, severity of obstruction, and time course of response. Am J Med 1982; 72:416–422.
14. Josephson GW, MacKenzie EJ, Lietman PS, Gibson G. Emergency treatment of asthma. A comparison of two treatment regimens. JAMA 1979; 242:639–643.
15. Fishburne JI Jr, Brenner WE, Braaksma JT, Hendricks CH. Bronchospasm complicating intravenous prostaglandin $F_{2\alpha}$ for therapeutic abortion. Obstet Gynecol 1972; 39:892–896.
16. Fraser IS, Brash JH. Comparison of extra- and intra-amniotic prostaglandins for therapeutic abortion. Obstet Gynecol 1974; 43:97–103.
17. Towers CV, Rojas JA, Lewis DF, Asrat T, Nageotte MP, Briggs GG. Usage of prostaglandin E_2 (PGE_2) in patients with asthma. Am J Obstet Gynecol 1991; 164:(part 2):295.
18. Lao TT, Huengsburg M. Labour and delivery in mothers with asthma. Eur J Obstet Gynecol Reprod Biol 1990; 35:183–190.
19. Rayburn WF. Prostaglandin E_2 gel for cervical ripening and induction of labor: a critical analysis. Am J Obstet Gynecol 1989; 160:529–534.
20. Hagerdal M, Morgan CW, Sumner AE, Gutsche BB. Minute ventilation and oxygen consumption during labor with epidural analgesia. Anesthesiology 1983; 59:425–427.
21. Chestnut DH, Pollack KL, Laszewski LJ, Bates JN, Choi WW. Continuous epidural infusion of bupivacaine–fentanyl during the second stage of labor. Anesthesiology 1989; 71:A841.
22. Younker D, Clark R, Tessem J, Joyce TH III, Kubicek M. Bupivacaine–fentanyl epidural analgesia for a parturient in status asthmaticus. Can J Anesth 1987; 34:609–612.
23. Fung DL. Emergency anesthesia for asthma patients. Clin Rev Allergy 1985; 3:127–141.
24. Gal TJ, Suratt PM. Atropine and glycopyrrolate effects on lung mechanics in normal man. Anesth Analg 1981; 60:85–90.
25. Corssen G, Gutierrez J, Reves JG, Huber FC Jr. Ketamine in the anesthetic management of asthmatic patients. Anesth Analg 1972; 51:588–596.
26. Hirshman CA, Downes H, Farbood A, Bergman NA. Ketamine block of bronchospasm in experimental canine asthma. Br J Anaesth 1979; 51:713–718.
27. Kingston HG, Hirshman CA. Perioperative management of the patient with asthma. Anesth Analg 1984; 63:844–855.
28. Marx GF, Kim YI, Lin CC, Halevy S, Schulman H. Postpartum uterine pressures under halothane or enflurance anesthesia. Obstet Gynecol 1978; 51:695–698.
29. Crawford JS. Bronchospasm following ergometrine [letter]. Anesth 1980; 35:397–398.
30. Feldman CH, Clark NM, Evans D. The role of health education in medical management of asthma. Clin Rev Allergy 1987; 5:195–205.

31. Mellins RB. Patient education is key to successful management of asthma. J Respir Dis 1989; 10 (suppl):S47–S52.
32. Schulman BA. Active patient orientation and outcomes in hypertensive treatment. Med Care 1979; 17:267–280.
33. Clark NC. Asthma self-management education: research and implications for clinical practice. Chest 1989; 95:1110–1113.
34. Korsch BM, Gozzi EK, Francis V. Gaps in doctor–patient communication. I. Doctor–patient interaction and patient satisfaction. Pediatrics 1968; 42:855–871.

Index

About the Editors

MICHAEL SCHATZ is Staff Allergist, Department of Allergy, Kaiser-Permanente Medical Center, San Diego, California, and Associate Clinical Professor, Department of Medicine, the University of California, San Diego,School of Medicine.The author or coauthor of over 80 journal articles and book chapters and coeditor of one book, he is a Fellow of the American College of Physicians, the American Academy of Allergy and Immunology, the American College of Allergy and Immunology, and the American College of Chest Physicians. Dr. Schatz received the B.S. degree (1968) in medicine and the M.D. degree (1970) from Northwestern University, Evanston, Illinois.

ROBERT S. ZEIGER is Chief, Department of Allergy, Kaiser-Permanente Medical Center, San Diego, California, and Clinical Professor, Department of Pediatrics, the University of California, San Diego. The author or coauthor of over 80 journal articles and book chapters and coeditor of one book, he is a Fellow of the American Academy of Allergy and Immunology and the American Academy of Pediatrics. Dr. Zeiger received the B.A. degree (1963) in political science from Tulane University, New Orleans, Louisiana, and the M.D. degree (1969) and the Ph.D. degree (1969) in anatomy from the State University of New York Downstate Medical Center, Brooklyn, New York.